Optic Neuropathies: Current and Future Strategies for Optic Nerve Protection and Repair

Optic Neuropathies: Current and Future Strategies for Optic Nerve Protection and Repair

Editors

Rongkung Tsai
Neil R. Miller

MDPI • Basel • Beijing • Wuhan • Barcelona • Belgrade • Manchester • Tokyo • Cluj • Tianjin

Editors
Rongkung Tsai
Institute of Medical Sciences
Tzu Chi University
Hualien 970
Taiwan

Neil R. Miller
Wilmer Eye Institute
Johns Hopkins University
Baltimore
United States

Editorial Office
MDPI
St. Alban-Anlage 66
4052 Basel, Switzerland

This is a reprint of articles from the Special Issue published online in the open access journal *International Journal of Molecular Sciences* (ISSN 1422-0067) (available at: www.mdpi.com/journal/ijms/special_issues/Strategies_Optic_Neuropathies).

For citation purposes, cite each article independently as indicated on the article page online and as indicated below:

LastName, A.A.; LastName, B.B.; LastName, C.C. Article Title. *Journal Name* **Year**, *Volume Number*, Page Range.

ISBN 978-3-0365-7505-6 (Hbk)
ISBN 978-3-0365-7504-9 (PDF)

Contents

Preface to "Optic Neuropathies: Current and Future Strategies for Optic Nerve Protection and Repair" vii

Neil R. Miller and Rong-Kung Tsai
Optic Neuropathies: Current and Future Strategies for Optic Nerve Protection and Repair
Reprinted from: *Int. J. Mol. Sci.* **2023**, *24*, 6977, doi:10.3390/ijms24086977 1

Samuel J. Spiegel and Alfredo A. Sadun
Solutions to a Radical Problem: Overview of Current and Future Treatment Strategies in Leber's Hereditary Neuropathy
Reprinted from: *Int. J. Mol. Sci.* **2022**, *23*, 13205, doi:10.3390/ijms232113205 7

Kimberly A. Wong and Larry I. Benowitz
Retinal Ganglion Cell Survival and Axon Regeneration after Optic Nerve Injury: Role of Inflammation and Other Factors
Reprinted from: *Int. J. Mol. Sci.* **2022**, *23*, 10179, doi:10.3390/ijms231710179 23

Ajay Ashok, Sarita Pooranawattanakul, Wai Lydia Tai, Kin-Sang Cho, Tor P. Utheim and Dean M. Cestari et al.
Epigenetic Regulation of Optic Nerve Development, Protection, and Repair
Reprinted from: *Int. J. Mol. Sci.* **2022**, *23*, 8927, doi:10.3390/ijms23168927 39

George Saitakis and Bart K. Chwalisz
Treatment and Relapse Prevention of Typical and Atypical Optic Neuritis
Reprinted from: *Int. J. Mol. Sci.* **2022**, *23*, 9769, doi:10.3390/ijms23179769 55

Ryan G. Strickland, Mary Anne Garner, Alecia K. Gross and Christopher A. Girkin
Remodeling of the Lamina Cribrosa: Mechanisms and Potential Therapeutic Approaches for Glaucoma
Reprinted from: *Int. J. Mol. Sci.* **2022**, *23*, 8068, doi:10.3390/ijms23158068 95

Aoife Smyth, Breedge Callaghan, Colin E. Willoughby and Colm O'Brien
The Role of miR-29 Family in TGF- Driven Fibrosis in Glaucomatous Optic Neuropathy
Reprinted from: *Int. J. Mol. Sci.* **2022**, *23*, 10216, doi:10.3390/ijms231810216 115

Tzu-Lun Huang, Jia-Kang Wang, Pei-Yao Chang, Yung-Ray Hsu, Cheng-Hung Lin and Kung-Hung Lin et al.
Neuromyelitis Optica Spectrum Disorder: From Basic Research to Clinical Perspectives
Reprinted from: *Int. J. Mol. Sci.* **2022**, *23*, 7908, doi:10.3390/ijms23147908 129

Yi-Fen Lai, Ting-Yi Lin, Pin-Kuan Ho, Yi-Hao Chen, Yu-Chuan Huang and Da-Wen Lu
Erythropoietin in Optic Neuropathies: Current Future Strategies for Optic Nerve Protection and Repair
Reprinted from: *Int. J. Mol. Sci.* **2022**, *23*, 7143, doi:10.3390/ijms23137143 147

Steven L. Bernstein, Yan Guo, Zara Mehrabian and Neil R. Miller
Neuroprotection and Neuroregeneration Strategies Using the rNAION Model: Theory, Histology, Problems, Results and Analytical Approaches
Reprinted from: *Int. J. Mol. Sci.* **2022**, *23*, 15604, doi:10.3390/ijms232415604 167

Lillian M. Toomey, Melissa G. Papini, Thomas O. Clarke, Alexander J. Wright, Eleanor Denham and Andrew Warnock et al.
Secondary Degeneration of Oligodendrocyte Precursor Cells Occurs as Early as 24 h after Optic Nerve Injury in Rats
Reprinted from: *Int. J. Mol. Sci.* **2023**, *24*, 3463, doi:10.3390/ijms24043463 . . . . **187**

Omri Zveik, Ariel Rechtman, Nitzan Haham, Irit Adini, Tamar Canello and Iris Lavon et al.
Sera of Neuromyelitis Optica Patients Increase BID-Mediated Apoptosis in Astrocytes
Reprinted from: *Int. J. Mol. Sci.* **2022**, *23*, 7117, doi:10.3390/ijms23137117 . . . . **203**

Hui-Chen Cheng, Sheng-Chu Chi, Chiao-Ying Liang, Jenn-Yah Yu and An-Guor Wang
Candidate Modifier Genes for the Penetrance of Leber's Hereditary Optic Neuropathy
Reprinted from: *Int. J. Mol. Sci.* **2022**, *23*, 11891, doi:10.3390/ijms231911891 . . . . **221**

Ofira Zloto, Alon Zahavi, Stephen Richard, Moran Friedman-Gohas, Shirel Weiss and Nitza Goldenberg-Cohen
Neuroprotective Effect of Azithromycin Following Induction of Optic Nerve Crush in Wild Type and Immunodeficient Mice
Reprinted from: *Int. J. Mol. Sci.* **2022**, *23*, 11872, doi:10.3390/ijms231911872 . . . . **235**

Kayo Sugitani, Takumi Mokuya, Shuichi Homma, Minami Maeda, Ayano Konno and Kazuhiro Ogai
Specific Activation of Yamanaka Factors via HSF1 Signaling in the Early Stage of Zebrafish Optic Nerve Regeneration
Reprinted from: *Int. J. Mol. Sci.* **2023**, *24*, 3253, doi:10.3390/ijms24043253 . . . . **247**

Heung-Sun Kwon, Karl Kevala, Haohua Qian, Mones Abu-Asab, Samarjit Patnaik and Juan Marugan et al.
Ligand-Induced Activation of GPR110 (ADGRF1) to Improve Visual Function Impaired by Optic Nerve Injury
Reprinted from: *Int. J. Mol. Sci.* **2023**, *24*, 5340, doi:10.3390/ijms24065340 . . . . **259**

Ming-Hui Sun, Kuan-Jen Chen, Chi-Chin Sun and Rong-Kung Tsai
Protective Effect of Pioglitazone on Retinal Ganglion Cells in an Experimental Mouse Model of Ischemic Optic Neuropathy
Reprinted from: *Int. J. Mol. Sci.* **2022**, *24*, 411, doi:10.3390/ijms24010411 . . . . **273**

Rong-Kung Tsai, Keh-Liang Lin, Chin-Te Huang and Yao-Tseng Wen
Transcriptomic Analysis Reveals That Granulocyte Colony-Stimulating Factor Trigger a Novel Signaling Pathway (TAF9-P53-TRIAP1-CASP3) to Protect Retinal Ganglion Cells after Ischemic Optic Neuropathy
Reprinted from: *Int. J. Mol. Sci.* **2022**, *23*, 8359, doi:10.3390/ijms23158359 . . . . **285**

Vittorio Porciatti and Tsung-Han Chou
Using Noninvasive Electrophysiology to Determine Time Windows of Neuroprotection in Optic Neuropathies
Reprinted from: *Int. J. Mol. Sci.* **2022**, *23*, 5751, doi:10.3390/ijms23105751 . . . . **301**

Preface to "Optic Neuropathies: Current and Future Strategies for Optic Nerve Protection and Repair"

Optic neuropathies are conditions in which there is damage to the optic nerve (ON) caused by a variety of causes, including glaucoma, inflammation, gene abnormalities, ischemia, trauma, and toxicity. ON damage triggers a process of axon degeneration, inflammatory cytokine upregulation, breakdown of the blood–optic nerve barrier, and, eventually, the induction of apoptosis of retinal ganglion cells (RGCs), resulting in optic atrophy. To date, there is no effective treatment for most optic neuropathies; however, because the damage initially is axogenic, there may exist a window of therapeutic opportunity before the death of RGCs. Thus, the search for effective treatments for various optic neuropathies before there is permanent damage to prevent or limit visual dysfunction and the development of methods to stimulate axon and/or RGC regeneration to restore vision after damage has occurred is pivotal.

This reprint collected 19 articles published in this Special Issue of *IJMS* which covers the molecular mechanisms to protect RGCs and/or axonal damage, translational research, gene therapy, regenerative medicine, and neuroprotection for glaucoma. We are grateful to all of the authors who contributed to this special issue.

Rongkung Tsai and Neil R. Miller
Editors

International Journal of
Molecular Sciences

MDPI

Editorial

Optic Neuropathies: Current and Future Strategies for Optic Nerve Protection and Repair

Neil R. Miller [1] and Rong-Kung Tsai [2,3,*]

1 Wilmer Eye Institute, Johns Hopkins University School of Medicine, 600 N. Wolfe St., Baltimore, MD 21205, USA; nrmiller@jhmi.edu
2 Institute of Eye Research, Hualien Tzu Chi Hospital, Buddhist Tzu Chi Medical Foundation, Hualien 970, Taiwan
3 Institute of Medical Sciences, Tzu Chi University, Hualien 970, Taiwan
* Correspondence: rktsai@tzuchi.com.tw

Citation: Miller, N.R.; Tsai, R.-K. Optic Neuropathies: Current and Future Strategies for Optic Nerve Protection and Repair. *Int. J. Mol. Sci.* **2023**, *24*, 6977. https://doi.org/10.3390/ijms24086977

Received: 21 March 2023
Accepted: 6 April 2023
Published: 10 April 2023

Processes that damage the optic nerve, including elevated intraocular pressure, trauma, ischemia, and compression, often cause visual loss for which there is no current treatment. It has long been believed that patients who experience damage to the optic nerve will never regain useful vision because the nerve cannot regenerate or repair itself. This belief is based on three assumptions: (1) a mammalian retinal ganglion cell (RGC) cannot be prevented from dying once its cell body or its axon has been injured; (2) an injured mammalian RGC whose axon has degenerated cannot be induced to extend a new axon; and (3) even if an injured mammalian RGC could be induced to regenerate, the regenerating axon cannot be directed toward its correct target in the central nervous system (CNS) [1]. In fact, accumulating evidence from experimental studies in mammals, including nonhuman primates, shows that, under certain conditions, RGCs can be prevented from dying despite injury to the cell bodies or their axons, injured RGCs whose axons have degenerated can be induced to extend new axons, and regenerating axons can reach their correct targets in the CNS. Several steps are necessary for the successful treatment of optic nerve injuries. First, the death of RGCs that have been (or have the potential to be) damaged must be prevented. Second, living RGCs whose axons have degenerated must be induced to extend new axons toward their targets in the CNS. Finally, a process of synaptic connection and refinement must occur so that appropriate RGCs are connected to the appropriate target in a retinotopic distribution. Prevention of the death of RGCs usually is referred to as neuroprotection, whereas restoration of the optic nerve function after injury is called neurorepair. In this issue, 18 well-respected scientists and their colleagues review or report the results of their original research in the fields of optic nerve protection, repair, or both.

1. Reviews

The optic nerve, similar to most pathways in the mature central nervous system, cannot regenerate if injured, and within days, RGCs begin to die. Research over the past two decades has identified several strategies to enable RGCs to regenerate axons the entire length of the optic nerve, in some cases leading to modest reinnervation of di- and mesencephalic visual relay centers. A review by Wong and Benowitz [2] primarily focuses on the role of the innate immune system in improving RGC survival and axon regeneration, and its synergy with manipulations of signal transduction pathways, transcription factors, and cell-extrinsic suppressors of axon growth. Research in this field hopefully will identify clinically effective strategies to improve vision in patients with currently untreatable losses within 5–10 years.

Epigenetic factors are known to influence tissue development, functionality, and their response to pathophysiology. In their review, Ashok et al. [3] focus on different types of epigenetic regulators and their associated molecular apparatus that affect the optic nerve. They emphasize that a comprehensive understanding of epigenetic regulation in optic nerve development and homeostasis should help unravel novel molecular pathways and pave the way to design blueprints for effective therapeutics to address optic nerve protection, repair, and regeneration.

The goal of neuroprotection in optic neuropathies is to prevent loss of RGCs and to preserve their function. The ideal time window for initiating neuroprotective treatments should be the preclinical period at which RGCs start losing their functional integrity before dying. In their review, Porciatti et al. [4] discuss the noninvasive electrophysiological test known as the pattern electroretinogram (PERG) and emphasize that it can assess the ability of RGCs to generate electrical signals under a protracted degenerative process in both clinical conditions and experimental models, which may have both diagnostic and prognostic value and provide the rationale for early treatment. They emphasize that a PERG also can be used to longitudinally monitor the acute and chronic effects of neuroprotective treatments. Finally, they point out that user-friendly versions of the PERG technology are commercially available for both clinical and experimental use.

One of the most interesting therapies for a variety of acute optic neuropathies is erythropoietin (EPO), which has been shown to have neuroprotective properties in extra-hematopoietic tissues, especially the retina. It is postulated that EPO may interact with its heterodimer receptor (EPOR/βcR) to exert its anti-apoptosis, anti-inflammatory, and anti-oxidation effects in preventing RGC death through different intracellular signaling pathways. In their review, Lai et al. [5] summarize the current pre-clinical studies on EPO in treating glaucomatous optic neuropathy, optic neuritis, NAION, and traumatic optic neuropathy. In addition, they explore future strategies of EPO for optic nerve protection and repair, including advances in EPO derivates and EPO deliveries. These strategies hopefully will lead to a new chapter in the treatment of these and other optic neuropathies.

Primary open angle glaucoma (POAG), a chronic optic neuropathy, remains the leading cause of irreversible blindness worldwide. It is driven in part by the pro-fibrotic cytokine transforming growth factor beta (TGF-β) and leads to extracellular matrix remodeling at the lamina cribrosa of the optic nerve head. Despite an array of medical and surgical treatments targeting the only known modifiable risk factor, raised intraocular pressure, many patients still progress and develop significant visual field loss and eventual blindness. The search for alternative treatment strategies targeting the underlying fibrotic transformation in the optic nerve head and trabecular meshwork in glaucoma is ongoing. MicroRNAs are small non-coding RNAs known to regulate post-transcriptional gene expression. Extensive research has been undertaken to uncover the complex role of miRNAs in gene expression and miRNA dysregulation in fibrotic diseases. MiR-29 is a family of miRNAs which are strongly anti-fibrotic in their effects on the TGF-β signaling pathway and the regulation of extracellular matrix production and deposition. In their review, Smyth et al. [6] discuss the anti-fibrotic effects of miR-29 and the role of miR-29 in ocular pathology and in the development of glaucomatous optic neuropathy. A better understanding of the role of miR-29 in POAG may aid in developing diagnostic and therapeutic strategies for patients with this common optic neuropathy.

A reduction in intraocular pressure remains the only proven treatment for POAG, but it does not prevent further neurodegeneration. In their review, Strickland et al. [7] discuss the three major classes of cells in the human optic nerve head (ONH) that provide support for the lamina cribrosa, lamina cribrosa (LC) cells, glial cells, and scleral fibroblasts, all of which are essential in maintaining healthy RGC axons and demonstrate responses to glaucomatous conditions through extracellular matrix remodeling. The authors discuss these responses and emphasize that understanding the major remodeling pathways in the ONH may be key to developing targeted therapies that reduce deleterious remodeling.

Optic neuritis is an inflammatory condition involving the optic nerve and is the most common acute optic neuropathy in young adults. Optic neuritis can be idiopathic or represent an early manifestation of demyelinating diseases, mostly multiple sclerosis (MS), at least in the Western hemisphere. Other causes include antibody-driven optic neuritis associated with neuromyelitis optica spectrum disorder (NMOSD), myelin oligodendrocyte glycoprotein antibody disease (MOGAD), chronic/relapsing inflammatory optic neuropathy (CRION, often a form of MOGAD), sarcoidosis, and a variety of infectious causes such as Lyme disease, Cat Scratch disease, syphilis, and tuberculosis. Appropriate and timely diagnosis is essential to rapidly decide on the appropriate treatment, maximize visual recovery, and minimize recurrences. Saitakis and Chwalisz [8] review the currently available state-of-the-art treatment strategies for many of these forms of optic neuritis, both in the acute phase and in the long term. The authors also discuss emerging therapeutic approaches and novel steps in the direction of achieving remyelination.

As noted in the review by Saitakis and Chwalisz [8], one of the causes of acute optic neuritis, particularly that associated with simultaneous or sequential transverse myelitis, is the aquaporin 4 (AQP4) antibody-driven condition called neuromyelitis optica. Over the past decade, there have been significant advances in the biologic knowledge on NMOSD, which have resulted in the identification of variable disease phenotypes, biomarkers, and complex inflammatory cascades involved in the disease pathogenesis. Ongoing clinical trials are looking at new treatments targeting NMOSD relapses. The review by Huang et al. [9] is intended to provide an update on recent studies regarding issues related to NMOSD, including the pathophysiology of the disease, the potential use of serum and cerebrospinal fluid cytokines as disease biomarkers, the clinical utilization of ocular coherence tomography, and the comparison of different animal models of NMOSD.

Non-arteritic anterior ischemic optic neuropathy (NAION) is the most common cause of sudden optic nerve (ON)-related vision loss in humans. Fortunately, there are several animal models of the condition. In particular, the rodent NAION model (rNAION) closely resembles clinical NAION in its pathophysiological changes and physiological responses and enables analyses of the specific responses to sudden ischemic axonopathy and of the effectiveness of potential treatments. However, there are anatomic and genetic differences between human and rodent optic nerves, and the inducing factors for the human disease and the model are different. These variables can result in marked differences in lesion development between the two species, as well as differences in the possible responses to various treatments. Bernstein et al. [10] discuss these issues as well as some of the species-associated differences that may be related to ischemic lesion severity and responses. These differences may be important when assessing the potential of any treatment that appears beneficial in rNAION to have a similar effect in human NAION.

Leber hereditary optic neuropathy (LHON) is the most common primary mitochondrial DNA disorder. It is characterized by bilateral severe central subacute vision loss due to specific loss of RGCs and their axons. Historically, treatment options have been quite limited, but ongoing clinical trials show promise, with significant advances being made in the testing of free radical scavengers and gene therapy. Spiegel and Sadun [11] summarize the management strategies and rationale of treatments based on current insights from molecular research. Their review includes preventative recommendations for unaffected genetic carriers, current medical and supportive treatments for those affected, and emerging evidence for future potential therapeutics.

2. Original Research

The activation of G-protein-coupled receptor 110 (GPR110) has been shown to stimulate neurite extension in developing neurons and after axon injury in adult mice. In the first paper in this issue, Kwon et al. [12] report that intravitreal injection of GPR110 in adult mice after optic nerve crush significantly reduced axon degeneration and improved axon integrity, RGC preservation, and visual function in wild-type but not in gpr110 knockout mice. They suggest that targeting GPR110 may be a viable strategy for functional recovery after optic nerve injury.

Toomey et al. [13] remind us that secondary optic nerve degeneration occurs after primary optic nerve injury. This spread of damage is thought to relate to mechanisms such as oxidative stress, apoptosis, and blood–brain barrier (BBB) dysfunction that, in turn, damage oligodendrocyte precursor cells (OPCs). However, there may be a time period for therapeutic intervention before permanent damage to the BBB and oligodendrocytes render any treatment useless. To address this issue, these investigators performed a partial optic nerve transection in adult rats and assessed BBB dysfunction, oxidative stress, and proliferation in OPCs. They found that even at 1 day post-injury, there was considerable BBB breach and oxidative DNA damage in OPCs, resulting in apoptosis. The investigators thus emphasize the need to consider early oxidative damage to OPCs in therapeutic efforts to limit secondary degeneration following primary optic nerve injury.

Some animal species have the potential for partial or complete regeneration of neural tissue. Sugitani et al. [14] point out that the fish optic nerve can spontaneously regenerate, with visual function being fully restored within 3–4 months after optic nerve injury. However, the regenerative mechanism behind this remains unknown. These investigators focus on the expression of three Yamanaka factors (Oct4, Sox2, and Klf4: OSK), all well-known inducers of induced pluripotent stem (iPS) cells in the zebrafish retina after optic nerve injury. They found that after optic nerve injury, mRNA expression of OSK was rapidly induced in RGCs, that heat shock factor 1 (HSF1) mRNA was most rapidly induced in the RGCs within 30 min, and that activation of OSK mRNA was completely suppressed by the intraocular injection of HSF1 morpholino prior to optic nerve injury. Their results suggest that the sequential activation of HSF1 and OSK might provide an avenue for RGC regeneration with return of the optic nerve function.

Pioglitazone (PGZ) is a drug that selectively stimulates the nuclear receptor peroxisome proliferator-activated receptor gamma (PPAR-γ) and to a lesser extent PPAR-α. It modulates the transcription of the genes involved in the control of glucose and lipid metabolism in various tissues. Sun et al. [15] assessed the protective effect of PGZ on RGCs when given for 4 weeks before photochemically induced NAION (see the paper in this issue by Bernstein et al. [10]) in diabetic and non-diabetic mice. They found that when given for 4 weeks before NAION induction, PGZ confers significant preservation of RGCs in both diabetic and non-diabetic mice assessed 2 weeks after completion of the 4-week treatment. These results suggest that if one could identify a population at high risk for ION (e.g., patients who already had NAION in one eye and who thus have a 15–20% risk of NAION in the fellow eye or patients who experienced post-cataract surgery ION in one eye and who require cataract surgery in the fellow eye), pre-treatment with a drug such as PGZ might reduce RGC damage and thus prevent severe visual loss in the fellow eye if NAION were to occur.

The most common mutation causing LHON is at site 11778 and is transmitted (similar to all mtDNA) to all maternal lineages. However, not everyone harboring the 11778 mutation develops LHON and men are much more often affected than woman. Nuclear modifier genes have been presumed to affect the penetrance of LHON, but conventional genetic methods have failed to clarify these issues. Cheng et al. [16] performed both whole exome sequencing (WES), a technique used to capture all genetic variations, and genome-wide association studies (GWAS), that generally involve targeted genotyping of specific and pre-selected variants using microarrays, to assess seventeen members of five families, all of whom had the 11778 mutation. Seven of these members had LHON, whereas ten were asymptomatic carriers. Using these techniques, the investigators found several mitochondrial genes with a high percentage of variants as well as several candidate nuclear modifier genes. They conclude that both WES and GWAS can provide highly efficient candidate gene screening functions for patients with a molecular genetic component.

Azithromycin is an antibiotic that also has been shown to be neuroprotective in some studies. Zloto et al. [17] assess the neuroprotective potential of intraperitoneal azithromycin after optic nerve crush injury in wild-type mice and in severely immunodeficient NOD scid gamma (NSG) mice. They found reduced apoptosis and improved RGC preservation in both WT and NSG mice, but much more in the WT than in the NSG. Their results suggest that azithromycin acts by immunomodulation. These findings have implications for the development of drugs to preserve RGCs after acute optic neuropathies.

Another drug that has been shown to exhibit RGC protection is granulocyte colony-stimulating factor (GCSF); however, the mechanisms by which this occurs are unclear. To investigate the mechanisms involved in RGC protection by GCSF, Tsai et al. [18] examined the transcriptome profiles of GCSF-treated adult rat retinas using microarray technology after induction of NAION (rNAION, see the paper by Bernstein et al. [10] in this issue) and demonstrated that GCSF modulates a new pathway, TAF9-P53-TRIAP1-CASP3, to control RGC death and survival after optic nerve infarct.

The AQP4 autoantibodies found in most patients with NMOSD are believed to cross the blood–brain barrier, target astrocytes, activate complement, and eventually lead to astrocyte destruction, demyelination, and axonal damage. However, it is still not clear what the primary pathological event is. Zveik et al. [19] hypothesize that the interaction of AQP4-IgG and astrocytes leads to DNA damage and apoptosis. These investigators studied the effects of sera from seropositive NMO patients and healthy controls (HCs) on astrocyte immune gene expression and viability. They found that sera from seropositive NMO patients led to higher expression of apoptosis-related genes and triggered more apoptosis in astrocytes and a higher expression of immunological genes, including BH3-interacting domain death agonist (BID), compared with sera from HCs. Furthermore, NMO sera increased DNA damage and led to a higher expression of immunological genes that interact with BID (TLR4 and NOD-1). Their findings suggest that sera of seropositive NMO patients may cause astrocytic DNA damage and apoptosis and that this may be one of the mechanisms implicated in the primary pathological event in NMO, thus providing new avenues for therapeutic interventions.

Finally, we are grateful to all the invited researchers who contributed to this Special Issue dealing with optic nerve regeneration and repair. Hopefully, these contributions will have both new and lasting impacts on our quest to restore vision to those who suffer from both acute and chronic optic nerve damage.

Author Contributions: Conceptualization, N.R.M. and R.-K.T.; methodology, N.R.M. and R.-K.T.; validation, N.R.M. and R.-K.T.; data curation, N.R.M. and R.-K.T.; writing-original draft preparation, N.R.M.; writing-review and editing, N.R.M. and R.-K.T. All authors have read and agreed to the published version of the manuscript.

Conflicts of Interest: The authors declare no conflict of interest.

References

1. Miller, N.R. Optic Nerve Protection, Regeneration, and Repair in the 21st Century: LVIII Edward Jackson Memorial Lecture. *Am. J. Ophthalmol.* **2001**, *132*, 811–818. [CrossRef] [PubMed]
2. Wong, K.A.; Benowitz, L.I. Retinal Ganglion Cell Survival and Axon Regeneration after Optic Nerve Injury: Roles of Inflammation and Other Factors. *Int. J. Mol. Sci.* **2022**, *23*, 10179. [CrossRef] [PubMed]
3. Ashok, A.; Pooranawattanakul, S.; Tai, W.L.; Cho, K.-S.; Utheim, T.P.; Cestari, D.M.; Cheng, D.F. Epigenetic Regulation of Optic Nerve Development, Protection, and Repair. *Int. J. Mol. Sci.* **2022**, *23*, 8927. [CrossRef] [PubMed]
4. Porciatti, V.; Chou, T.-H. Using Noninvasive Electrophysiology to Determine Time Windows of Neuroprotection in Optic Neuropathies. *Int. J. Mol. Sci.* **2022**, *23*, 5751. [CrossRef] [PubMed]
5. Lai, Y.-F.; Lin, T.-Y.; Ho, P.-K.; Chen, Y.-H.; Huang, Y.-C.; Lu, D.-W. Erythropoietin in Optic Neuropathies: Current Future Strategies for Optic Nerve Protection and Repair. *Int. J. Mol. Sci.* **2022**, *23*, 7143. [CrossRef] [PubMed]
6. Smyth, A.; Callaghan, B.; Willoughby, C.E.; O'Brien, C. The Role of miR-29 Family in TGF-ß Driven Fibrosis in Glaucomatous Optic Neuropathy. *Int. J. Mol. Sci.* **2022**, *23*, 10216. [CrossRef] [PubMed]
7. Strickland, R.G.; Garner, M.A.; Gross, A.K.; Girkin, C.A. Remodeling of the Lamina Cribrosa: Mechanisms and Potential Therapeutic Approaches for Glaucoma. *Int. J. Mol. Sci.* **2022**, *23*, 8068. [CrossRef] [PubMed]
8. Saitakis, G.; Chwalisz, B.K. Treatment and Relapse Prevention of Typical and Atypical Optic Neuritis. *Int. J. Mol. Sci.* **2022**, *23*, 9769. [CrossRef] [PubMed]
9. Huang, T.-L.; Wang, J.-K.; Chang, P.-Y.; Hsu, Y.-R.; Lin, C.-H.; Lin, K.-H.; Tsai, R.-K. Neuromyelitis Optica Spectrum Disorder: From Basic Research to Clinical Perspectives. *Int. J. Mol. Sci.* **2022**, *23*, 7908. [CrossRef] [PubMed]
10. Bernstein, S.L.; Guo, Y.; Mehrabian, Z.; Miller, N.R. Neuroprotection and Neuroregeneration Strategies Using the rNAION Model: Theory, Histology, Problems, Results, and Analytical Approaches. *Int. J. Mol. Sci.* **2022**, *23*, 15604. [CrossRef] [PubMed]
11. Spiegel, S.J.; Sadun, A.A. Solutions to a Radical Problem: Overview of Current and Future Treatment Strategies in Leber's Hereditary Optic Neuropathy. *Int. J. Mol. Sci.* **2022**, *23*, 13205. [CrossRef]

12. Kwon, H.-S.; Kevala, K.; Qian, H.; Abu-Asab, M.; Patnaik, S.; Marugan, J.; Kim, H.-Y. Ligand-Induced Activation of GPR110 (ADGRF1) to Improve Visual Function Impaired by Optic Nerve Injury. *Int. J. Mol. Sci.* **2023**, *24*, 5340. [CrossRef]
13. Toomey, L.M.; Papini, M.G.; Clarke, T.O.; Wright, A.J.; Denham, E.; Warnock, A.; McGonigle, T.; Bartlett, C.A.; Fitzgerald, M.; Anyaegbu, C.C. Secondary Degeneration of Oligodendrocyte Precursor Cells Occurs as Early as 24 h after Optic Nerve Injury in Rats. *Int. J. Mol. Sci.* **2023**, *24*, 3463. [CrossRef] [PubMed]
14. Sugitani, K.; Mokuya, T.; Homma, S.; Maeda, M.; Konomo, A.; Ogai, K. Specific Activation of Yamanaka Factors via HSF1 Signaling in the Early Stage of Zebrafish Optic Nerve Regeneration. *Int. J. Mol. Sci.* **2023**, *24*, 3253. [CrossRef] [PubMed]
15. Sun, M.-H.; Chen, K.-J.; Sun, C.-C.; Tsai, R.-K. Protective Effect of Pioglitazone on Retinal Ganglion Cells in an Experimental Mouse Model of Ischemic Optic Neuropathy. *Int. J. Mol. Sci.* **2023**, *24*, 411. [CrossRef] [PubMed]
16. Cheng, H.-C.; Chi, S.-C.; Liang, C.-Y.; Yu, J.-Y.; Wang, A.-G. Candidate Modifier Genes for the Penetrance of Leber's Hereditary Optic Neuropathy. *Int. J. Mol. Sci.* **2022**, *23*, 11891. [CrossRef] [PubMed]
17. Zloto, O.; Zahavi, A.; Richard, S.; Friedman-Gohas, M.; Weiss, S.; Goldenberg-Cohen, N. Neuroprotective Effect of Azithromycin Following Induction of Optic Nerve Crush in Wild Type and Immunodeficient Mice. *Int. J. Mol. Sci.* **2022**, *23*, 11872. [CrossRef] [PubMed]
18. Tsai, R.-K.; Lin, K.-L.; Huang, C.-T.; Wen, Y.-T. Transcriptomic Analysis Reveals That Granulocyte Colony-Stimulating Factor Triggers a Novel Signaling Pathway (TAF9-P53-TRIAP1-CASP3) to Protect Retinal Ganglion Cells after Ischemic Optic Neuropathy. *Int. J. Mol. Sci.* **2022**, *23*, 8359. [CrossRef] [PubMed]
19. Zveik, O.; Rechtman, A.; Haham, N.; Adini, I.; Canello, T.; Lavon, I.; Brill, L.; Vaknin-Dembinsky, A. Sera of Neuromyelitis Optica Patients Increase BID-Mediated Apoptosis in Astrocytes. *Int. J. Mol. Sci.* **2022**, *23*, 7117. [CrossRef] [PubMed]

International Journal of
Molecular Sciences

MDPI

Review

Solutions to a Radical Problem: Overview of Current and Future Treatment Strategies in Leber's Hereditary Opic Neuropathy

Samuel J. Spiegel [1,*] and Alfredo A. Sadun [2]

[1] Gavin Herbert Eye Institute, University of California, Irvine, CA 92617, USA
[2] Jules Stein and Doheny Eye Institute, University of California, Los Angeles, CA 90095, USA
* Correspondence: sjspiege@hs.uci.edu

Abstract: Leber's Hereditary Optic Neuropathy (LHON) is the most common primary mitochondrial DNA disorder. It is characterized by bilateral severe central subacute vision loss due to specific loss of Retinal Ganglion Cells and their axons. Historically, treatment options have been quite limited, but ongoing clinical trials show promise, with significant advances being made in the testing of free radical scavengers and gene therapy. In this review, we summarize management strategies and rational of treatment based on current insights from molecular research. This includes preventative recommendations for unaffected genetic carriers, current medical and supportive treatments for those affected, and emerging evidence for future potential therapeutics.

Keywords: leber's hereditary optic neuropathy; optic neuropathy; mitochondrial disorder; mitochondrial optic neuropathy; hereditary optic neuropathy; neuro-ophthalmology; idebenone

Citation: Spiegel, S.J.; Sadun, A.A. Solutions to a Radical Problem: Overview of Current and Future Treatment Strategies in Leber's Hereditary Opic Neuropathy. *Int. J. Mol. Sci.* **2022**, *23*, 13205. https://doi.org/10.3390/ijms232113205

Academic Editors: Neil R. Miller and Rongkung Tsai

Received: 27 September 2022
Accepted: 26 October 2022
Published: 30 October 2022

1. Introduction

Leber's Hereditary optic neuropathy (LHON) is one of the inherited hereditary mitochondrial optic neuropathies. Inherited optic neuropathies have been estimated to affect 1 in 10,000 individuals and are an important cause of visual impairment [1]. LHON has been reported to be the most common primary mitochondrial DNA disorder with epidemiological estimates ranging from 1 in 27,000 to 40,000 [2]. Clinically, it primarily presents in individuals in the second or third decade of life. Typically, these young adults experience unilateral, painless, subacute central or cecocentral scotomas, impaired color vision, and visual acuity loss with involvement of the contralateral eye in the following weeks to month. It is a clinical diagnosis which is subsequently confirmed by blood testing for mitochondrial DNA (mtDNA) analysis. The 3 most common mtDNA mutations (*m.3460G>A*, *m.11778G>A*, and *m.14484T*>C mutations) account for 90–95% of cases [3–5]. Genetics (mitochondrial and likely nuclear) and environmental factors may lend to respiratory chain dysfunction leading to retinal ganglion cell (RCG) dysfunction, cell death and vision loss. Currently most persons affected will have irreversible severe visual impairment.

To date, treatments have been limited and there is no curative therapy. The European union has authorized the use of Idebenone in patients with LHON and current consensus guidelines recommend its use in affected individuals [2]. Although efficacious treatment options are limited for those affected by LHON, recent years have seen an upsurge of scientific advancements in the understanding of the disease process and search for potential therapeutics.

LHON is uniquely placed for scientific study as most cases occur from identifiable point mutations, it affects a unique and measurable cellular line, and is one of the more commonly inherited mitochondrial disorders. Clinicians and scientists have been working on further defining the clinical disease course of LHON in combination with the molecular impact of genetic and environmental factors. This review will discuss the natural disease course and molecular mechanisms in the development of LHON to allow for an in-depth review of the current and future treatment strategies in LHON. It is this multifaceted understanding of specific pathways of damage and their influence on LHON and visual outcomes which have provided insights to allow for the creation of novel therapeutic strategies. Additionally, as LHON has become a model for mitochondrial disorders, the advancements in this field serve to inform research of other related disorders.

2. Natural Disease Course

LHON has been subcategorized into disease states to help further define and approach clinical interventions (Table 1). It is important to understand these key time markers within the disease process for the clinical and therapeutic implications. Broadly individuals with LHON mtDNA mutations can be classified into carriers and affected symptomatic patients.

Table 1. Disease Classification.

Disease Classification
Asymptomatic (mutation carriers)
Preclinical
Subacute (<6 months)
Dynamic (6–12 months)
Chronic (>12 months)

Currently, the asymptomatic phase is defined as any individual who is a carrier of one of the known causative mutations but is not experiencing visual loss. Due to highly variable, incomplete penetrance, LHON individuals may never develop vision loss. Carriers and pre-symptomatic patients may demonstrate clinical findings in the absence of subjective vision changes. Inferotemporal retinal nerve fiber layer (RNFL) swelling can be seen on fundoscopic exam or Optical Coherence Tomography (OCT) and is not indicative of progression to vision loss [6,7]. Pre-symptomatic patients additionally may have subtle clinical findings such as mild dyschromatopsia, reduced contrast sensitivity, and ultimately will show fundus changes such as telangiectatic vessels. More recent studies have also demonstrated subnormal electroretinogram and visual evoked potentials in these patients [6]. OCT angiography studies have shown that microvascular changes occur in the temporal sector and may precede RNFL changes and mirror the ganglion cell layer changes [8–10]. The optic disc microangiopathy, seen as telangiectatic vessels, may occur in both asymptomatic and acute stages of the disease. Its role in the pathogenesis of LHON is currently not well understood [8]. Pre-clinical or pre-symptomatic individuals may eventually go on to develop vision loss. Some may define conversion to the affected stage when loss of macular RGCs occur while visual acuity is still normal; however, most define conversion when the onset of vision loss occurs.

Those who convert from asymptomatic to symptomatic states typically do so in their second or third decade of life [11]. Disease onset is characterized by subacute, central vision loss occurring sequentially in the contralateral eye within weeks to months of the first eye in >97% of individuals [12,13]. Visual function will decline in the following months with significant impairments in visual acuity and color vision. Visual fields demonstrate dense central or cecocentral scotomas and OCT will show loss of macular retinal ganglion cells (RGCs). The evolution and progression of disease occurs during the acute/subacute phase. Most individuals will continue to lose visual acuity during the first six months, at which point central vision loss may stabilize, but quantitative clinical metrics may continue to decline (for example visual field loss and OCT measurements). Why vision loss is catastrophic and not more gradual is still not well understood. Evidence is limited given the lack of longitudinal studies in pre-clinical patients. Currently mechanical and metabolic mechanisms are hypothesized in the development of conversion to symptomatically affected patient.

Metabolic changes within nerve fibers lead to increased mitochondrial and axonal stasis, eventually producing axonal swelling. Mechanically, the laminar portion of the optic nerve is anatomically unable to accommodate swelling, thereby leading to vascular insufficiency and triggering catastrophic retinal ganglion cell loss [8,14–16]. It is the papillomacular bundle (PMB) which is selectively lost early in the disease course and this pathologic process affects the smallest fibers first [17]. Further understanding of changes seen from carrier to pre-symptomatic to symptomatic is needed to better understand disease conversion.

After about 1 year stability occurs, and it is at this time patients are considered to have transitioned to the chronic phase of the disease [18,19]. Some individuals will show improvement between 18–24 months after onset of disease. There may be reduction of the central scotoma or in many cases a fenestration of the central scotoma may lead to an opening of a central visual island allowing improved central acuity. Recovery is currently most dependent on mutation subtype and age at onset. The best potential for recovery is seen in those younger than age 12 at onset and those with the m.14484T>A variant [20]. Additionally subacute presentation and large optic discs predispose to better recovery. Adults with the *m.11778G>A* mutation have been found to have the worst visual outcomes [13,21]. Most patient remain severely affected and rarely are visual acuities better than 20/200.

It should be noted that the disease state categories above are applied to help define disease process for clinical and scientific trials; however, it is becoming further elucidated that the LHON phenotype is fairly heterogenous. There is variability between each mutation in regard to timing, severity and outcomes. Additionally, within specific subgroups of genetic mutations there is variability given environmental and genetic heterogeneity within the population, for example mtDNA haplogroup polymorphisms [22].

There appears to be two important subcategories of clinical manifestation that has been termed LHON Type I and Type II. Type I is likely to be a mtDNA mutation in the context of nDNA which is susceptible. This gene-gene process may be inevitable. Type II may be Type I cases in which environmental factors are key and lead to conversion. This might explain several distinctions in presentation. Type I is abrupt (sub-acute), and Type II is more insidious. Type I occurs about age 20 and Type II often after age 40. Type II is almost always associated with a major exposure to smoke or smoking. Type II is more likely to recover if the patients risk factor is removed. Most importantly, in Type I there is profound loss of both structure (OCT-RNFL) and function (VFs), but in Type II there is often a structure-function mismatch (RNFL is partly preserved) [12].

3. Molecular Background and Pathophysiology

Mitochondrial respiration is driven by redox reactions, organized through mitochondrial electron transport chain complexes. The complex I (a NADH:Ubiquinone oxidoreductase) proton pump is the first step in the respiratory chain and couples electron transfer with proton translocation across the mitochondrial membrane. This complex contains 45 subunits, 7 of which are mtDNA encoded [23]. The 3 most common mtDNA mutations affect mitochondrial Complex I at the ND1 (*m.3460G>A*), ND4 (*m.11778G>A*), and ND6 (*m.14484T>C*) subunits. Complex I then uses two co-factors: coenzyme Q (ubiquinone, CoQ) and Cytochrome c (cyt c) to transfer electrons to the succeeding respiratory complexes (Figure 1). LHON mutation *m.3460G>A* has been demonstrated to alter the catalytic activity of Complex I with subsequent impairment in mitochondrial respiration and all three mutations impair mitochondrial respiration and reduce complex I-drive ATP synthesis. Of particular importance, the electrons produce reactive oxygen species (ROS). There is also, to a lesser extent, a reduction in ATP synthesis. Figure 2 shows why the retinal ganglion cell (RGC), with a long non-myelinated retinal nerve fiber layer (RNFL) is particularly vulnerable to this process. The generation of ROS occur when electrons spill from the transfer between Complex I and CoEnzymeQ10 and react with molecular oxygen, triggering a cascade of deleterious downstream reactions and eventual apoptosis [24]. Most of the energy required by neurons is to re-establish the membrane potential after an action potential. Fortunately, this only has to happen at the

Nodes of Ranvier as myelin covers the remaining membrane. However, RGCs being unmyelinated in the eye, have anatomical and biochemical elements that predispose them for failure. Since RCGs contain the bioenergetically demanding unmyelinated RNFL, they have a high concentration of mitochondria most concentrated in the prelaminar and intralaminar portions (Figure 2). This predisposes them to mitochondrial dysfunction [24,25]. Specifically, due to the adverse surface to volume characteristics, the thin axons of the papillomacular bundle and their corresponding RGCs are most vulnerable and are selectively lost early in LHON (Figure 3). It is this selective loss that has allowed researchers to further delve into pathophysiologic biomolecular mechanisms by which mitochondrial impairment creates the devastating cascade of apoptosis. From this research various therapeutic models have been attempted and are being further investigated.

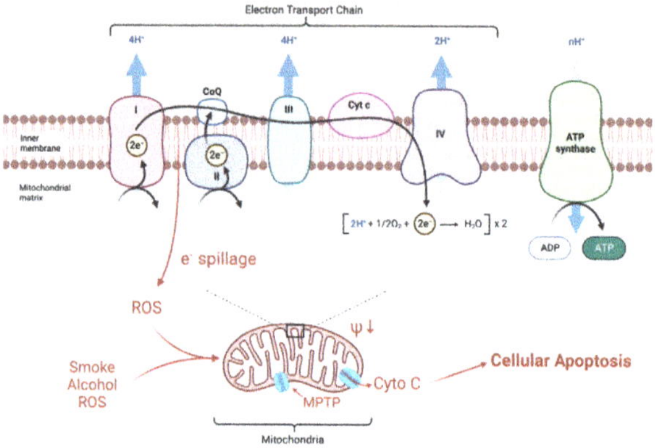

Figure 1. Electrons are transferred along the chain of complexes for oxidative phosphorylation. The energy is largely stored as a proton gradient that is later exploited for the production of ATP. Mutations of Complex I, as seen in LHON, produce a minor impairment of ATP production (about 20%), but also a greater production of ROS (10X) by spillage of electrons at the attempted transfer to Co Enzyme Q10. These ROS change the electrical potential across the mitochondrial membrane which, in crossing a critical threshold, can open the mitochondrial permeability transition pore (MPTP) releasing cytochrome C (Cyto C) and initiating apoptosis of the RGC [26].

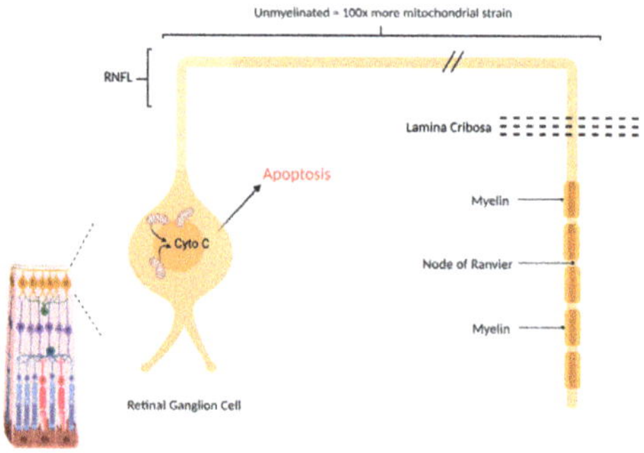

Figure 2. The Retinal Ganglion Cell (RGC) is particularly vulnerable to mitochondrial impairment. Like other neurons, it consumes a great deal of ATP in keeping its membrane potential, that is depleted after every axon potential. Unlike other neurons, it does not fully benefit from the economy of myelin that restricts the membrane changes to the Nodes of Ranvier. The long retinal nerve fiber layer (RNFL) is unmyelinated due to the need for retinal optical transparency, creating a great deal of extra metabolic strain on RGCs.

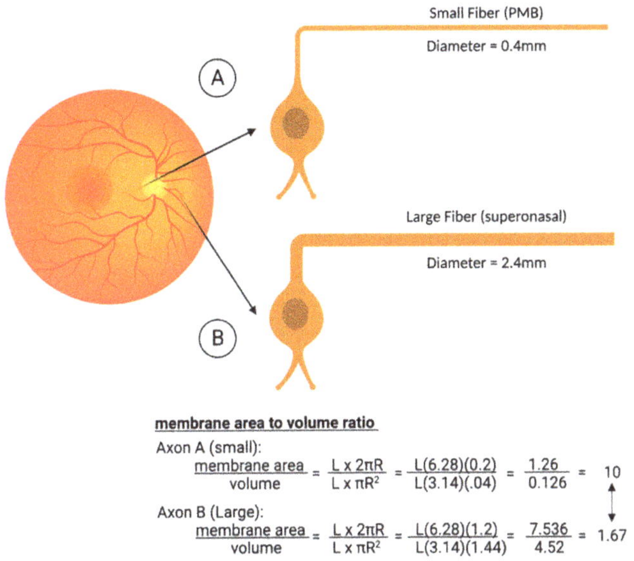

Figure 3. Comparison of the metabolic strain in smaller axons that are concentrated in the papillomacular bundle (PMB). The smaller fiber (**A**) typically has a diameter of only 0.4 microns. Compared to the larger fibers of the nasal retina (**B**), the PMB fiber has a much-reduced volume and hence fewer mitochondria. Although its surface area is a little less as well, the area/volume ratios are six times worse in the smaller fibers, explaining why they are the first to die in LHON. Figures created with biorender.com.

4. Unaffected Carriers and Pre-Symptomatic/Pre-Clinical

Currently, there is no recommended treatment for those individuals who are known carriers of the LHON mutation [2]. That being said, there are important factors to consider in these individuals based on the newest insights we have available regarding LHON. Genetic counseling and lifestyle modification are the current focus of neuro-ophthalmologic consensus statements, but other factors are under investigation for potentially mitigating risk of vision loss.

4.1. Genetics and Counselling

As LHON is a maternally inherited, a male (affected or unaffected) with a known pathogenic mtDNA mutation cannot transmit this to any of his offspring, and a female with a similar mutation will transmit it to all her offspring. As LHON exhibits incomplete penetrance the appearance of disease may vary widely within each family or between families with the same mtDNA mutation. 60% of families will have a history of visual loss affecting maternal relatives. Incomplete penetrance further complicates genetic counseling because it is unknown when or if an LHON mutation carrier will become symptomatic. Unaffected family members should be cautioned that finding the mutation in relatives in maternal line is very likely, and the results will not aide in prognosis. The current international consensus statement released in 2021 is that all maternally related family member do not currently need to be tested. It is generally agreed upon however that they should be screened [2].

If individuals do receive genetic testing, the large majority of positive individuals will be homoplasmic. Heteroplasmy is well documented and genetic testing results documenting heteroplasmy must be carefully interpreted as mtDNA in peripheral blood may not reflect the heteroplasmic load in the RGCs [22]. Along similar lines, preimplantation or prenatal testing for a pregnancy may be done, but there is variability in the mtDNA in amniocyte and chorionic villi and results may not correspond to levels found in RGCs [22]. Therefore, its interpretation should be done cautiously and by experienced providers. In addition, because of non-life-threatening nature of LHON and its highly variable penetrance there are clinical and ethical considerations on if preimplantation or prenatal testing is warranted. Newer genetic developments propose alternative future potential options for genetic modifications. For example, mitochondrial donation from a donated egg or zygote with healthy mitochondria or removing the nucleus and replacing it with the nucleus from the egg or zygote from the affected mother has been done, but again this is a developing field with many ethical considerations [27,28].

Lastly, haplotype J is now well documented as leading to a higher conversion and therefore increases the penetrance of LHON mutations. The phenomena is felt to be due to lower mtDNA and mtDNA-encoded polypeptides This is currently of less importance in regard to genetic counselling clinically, but if known for a carrier may lead to some prognostic value [22,29].

4.2. Neurotoxins

The incomplete penetrance seen in LHON lends to the classic hypothesis and well accepted statement that mtDNA mutations are necessary for an individual to be affected but alone are insufficient to cause vision loss. It is the addition of environmental factors which allows for conversion from asymptomatic individuals (pre-clinical) to affected individuals (clinical). A growing body of data is now available on mitochondrial toxicity, in particular increases in oxidative stress induced by tobacco smoke, other smoke, and alcohol.

Multiple studies have shown that alcohol consumption at high levels, especially binge-drinking, and smoking tobacco have a strong association with more severe symptoms and prognosis in LHON carriers [12,30]. Affected smokers have demonstrated a lower mtDNA copy number as compared with affected non-smokers and with unaffected mutation carriers. Tobacco smoking directly affects the compensatory mechanism counteracting the pathogenic effects of LHON mutations. This regulation of mitochondrial biogenesis and mtDNA copy number has been proven to be crucial in development of vision loss in LHON, having a direct impact on the disease penetrance [31]. These molecular effects have been demonstrated in clinical patients as well. Subgroups of LHON patients who present with delayed onset are found to have increased use of tobacco products. It is hypothesized that these patients are a unique subset that may have been unaffected carriers and became affected later in life after many years of smoking [12]. More recently during the recent COVID-19 pandemic, significant increase in substance abuse, specifically EtOH intake and cigarette smoke, has led to reported conversion of LHON carrier to affected individuals. One case series recently published reported 3 LHON patients all of which were atypical onset > 50 yrs old who had dramatically increased their exposure to EtOH during the COVID 19 pandemic [32]. It is more than just cigarette smoke but exposure to smoke in general that is felt to be associated with disease conversion. There are case reported instances of individuals becoming affected after other forms of smoke inhalation, such as a woodburning stove or rubber tire fires. (Sanchez, JNO 2006) Therefore, it is recommended to not only avoid tobacco related smoke but all smoke inhalations.

4.3. Mitochondrial Biogenesis, Autophagy, and Transmitophagy

Increasing in the mitochondrial quantity and mtDNA copy number to increase total ATP production is a theorized method in which one may prevent disease conversion in pre-symptomatic individuals. This compensatory mechanism has been highlighted in LHON and it has been postulated that increased mitochondrial biogenesis may be a responsible driving factor in its incomplete penetrance [33]. Although there is currently little known in regard to clinical effectiveness in this field it poses an extremely interesting and targetable mechanism of therapeutic intervention. Systemic mitobiogenesis, occurring mainly near the cellular soma is currently being further elucidated. Optic nerve and RCGs pose further challenges given the length of their axons and distance mitochondria would need to be transported. Local mitochondrial biogenesis is likely important in LHON but is currently not well defined in RCGs [34]. Specifically, a quantitative increase of the mitochondrial mass has been attempted to overcome mitochondrial functional deficiencies [34,35].

Additionally, dysfunctional mitochondria are implicated in the triggering of apoptosis. The quality control of mitochondria requires a complex balance of mitobiogenesis and autophagy. Autophagy involves lysosomal degradation and elimination of dysfunctional and damaged proteins and organelles. Autophagy may be significantly compromised in cells with LHON mtDNA mutations. This results in reduced clearance of dysfunctional mitochondria (mitophagy) and is a contributing factor to cellular impairment and death. Pharmacologic activation of mitophagy in LHON cell models has been shown to selectively clear damaged mitochondria and improves overall cellular survival [36]. Transmitophagy is a process unique to RGCs in whichdamaged mitochondria in RCGs coalesce and are exocytosed from the myelinated portion of these axons. They are taken up by surrounding astrocytes and degraded. This helps regulate the mitochondrial number and quality. It is this quality control mitophagy that may become a new therapeutic approach that restores the balance of functional and dysfunctional mitochondria [36].

Many drugs have been studied, among them metformin, rosiglitazone, resveratrol, vitamin B3 and NAD+ precursors which have shown promising results; but no studies specifically relate to vision loss or optic nerve tissues [37–39]. Sets of drugs has been associated with an increased mtDNA amount. Lipoic acid, lipamide, thiazolidinediones and polyphenols have been shown to increase mtDNA copy number in animal models which can be associated with increased mitochondrial proteins, quantity, activity of OXPHOS complexes and ATP amount [34,40]. By targeting these three mechanisms: mtDNA copy, mitobiogenesis, and transmitophagy we may be able to create a new cellular homeostasis that is less predisposed to cellular damage and eventual vision loss in patients with LHON mutations.

4.4. Estrogens

In relation to the section above, estrogens should be discussed during the pre-symptomatic stage of LHON, particularly when it comes to prevention in female patients, as this has one of the largest bodies of literature in relation to potential neuroprotection in LHON. Reduced prevalence of LHON affected women is well established, but there is also an increased incidence of disease seen with patients that may correlate with a decline in estrogens (menopausal patients). It has been found that estradiol levels increase mtDNA content, oxygen consumption and ATP levels in human cybrids with LHON mutations [41]. In vitro studies have shown that specific estrogen receptors localize to the mitochondrial networks of RGCs. Through activation of estrogen receptors, there is increased antioxidant enzyme production (e.g., Superoxide dismutase 2), promotion of mitochondrial biogenesis, and increased mtDNA copy. This in turn enhances cellular viability, ameliorating ROS production and reducing the rate of apoptosis [42]. Although not currently standard of practice there is discussion on the benefits of estrogen therapy in patient who are known unaffected carriers and nearing the age of menopausal onset and is currently an evolving area within the field.

5. Symptomatic Phase

5.1. Antioxidants

Oxidative stress and its modulation is a focal point in mitochondrial disease. The potential benefit in using antioxidants to help reduce the neurotoxic strain imposed on RGCs by ROS is quite a desirable theoretical avenue of treatment. The hypothesized mechanism of reducing the neurotoxic stress from multiple supplements (e.g., vitamins B2, 3, 9, 12, C, ubiquinone, carnitine, L arginine, alpha-lipoic acid amongst others) and their combinations have been attempted to help reduce this ROS imposed stress. None so far have been shown to have any significant benefit in LHON and currently there is not enough scientific evidence to support their use clinically.

5.2. Coenzyme Q_{10} (Coq10)

Of the various over the counter options, the ubiquinone family seemed the most promising for effective treatment. This coenzyme shuttles electrons between complex I and II to complex III of the ETC. The reduced CoQ10 therefore also has antioxidant properties, minimizing ROS generation. Additionally, CoQ10 might deliver the electron as needed to complex III thus restoring energy production. However, the major hindrance to its effect is its inability to cross cell membranes, the mitochondrial membrane, and blood–brain barrier due to its long lipophilic tail and therefore low bioavailability. It has been shown to be partly effective in other mitochondrial related disorders but has not panned out for LHON [43,44]. In order to overcome the issues of drug delivery with CoQ10, Idebenone was developed.

5.3. Idebenone

Idebenone is a synthetically derived molecule which similarly facilitates electron transfer between ETC complexes allowing for improved ATP production and minimized ROS generation [45]. This soluble analog was first shown to be protective in disorders affecting complex I (such as LHON) in both animal and human subjects. Idebenone is activated in the cytoplasm to its oxidized form by NAD(P)H:quinone oxidoreductase (NQO1) thus allowing for conversion into its reduced form to shuttle electrons directly to complex III, bypassing the complex I dysfunction seen in LHON. The formation of Idebenone to its oxidized form therefore appears essential to its therapeutic efficacy, but this oxidized form also has been shown to have potential inhibitory and adverse effects on complex I. Variable expression of NQO1has been postulated to contribute to cases in which Idebenone is ineffective [46–48]. Preclinical studies did confirm a cell specific increase in ATP production and reduced ROS levels in fibroblasts of LHON patients and prevention of RGC loss in LHON mouse models [49,50]. Since the first human case reports in 1992 it has developed a tremendous body of literature.

In 2011 a randomized clinical trial "Rescue of Hereditary Optic Disease Outpatient Study" (RHODOS) presented evidence that idebenone can be beneficial to preserve and/or restore vision [51]. This prospective, placebo-controlled trial evaluated patients with <5 years of visual loss and a trend was noticed in favor of idebenone when the authors analyzed changes in best visual acuity and excluded patients with the 14,484 mutation (higher rate of spontaneous recovery). Patients with more recent onset of vision loss were more likely to demonstrate improvement. Shortly after this, Carelli et al. published a retrospective study showing that the proportion of patients treated with idebenone within 1 year after visual loss in the second eye at varying doses showed demonstratable improvement compared to untreated patients [52]. Additionally, earlier visual improvement was associated with prompt start and longer duration of therapy [52].

These results then triggered a seminal event in LHON treatment, the European Union's authorization of the use of Idebenone in patients with LHON in 2015. This was then followed by the 2017 consensus conference to address therapeutic issues in the treatment of LHON. The consensus statement and most current recommendation is that Idebenone should be started as soon as possible in patients with disease onset of less than 1 year. Additionally, in these subacute/dynamic patients, treatment should be continued for at least 1 year to assess the start of therapeutic response or until a plateau in terms of improvement is reached [2]. With this medication available, the therapeutic window should not be lost by a delay of diagnosis [52,53].

Since then, the previously reported beneficial effect of idebenone on recovery and preservation of vision has been confirmed by multiple other major studies, including the expanded access program (EAP) [54], a Japanese prospective, interventional study [55], and a Netherlands national cohort study [56], and the soon to be published LEROS study—(NCT02774005).

5.4. Elampritide

Elamipretide (MTP-131) is an antioxidant peptide which has been found to increase ATP synthesis as well as reduce ROS production [57]. It targets cardiolipin selectively within the inner membrane of mitochondria and prevents conversion of cytochrome c into peroxidase. Sadun et al. conducted a Phase II Clinical Study (ReSIGHT) of which the results are not yet published but results have been updated as of November 2021—(NCT02693119). In total 12 LHON patients were recruited and treated for 52 weeks. No difference in BCVA was observed, but because of a trend towards improvement, all 12 patients completed an open-label extension with bilateral treatment for a total of at least 84 weeks [47].

5.5. EPI-743

Alpha-tocotrienol quinone (EPI-734) is a third generation quinone molecule that has been studied in depth in vitro and needs further investigation to determine benefit in LHON patients. It has been used and studied in other inherited mitochondrial diseases and has been found to be approximately 1000 to 10,000 fold more potent than coenzyme Q10 (because of drug delivery) or idebenone (because of electron delivery) in protecting mitochondria. It is an antioxidant para-benzoquinone that also replenishes glutathione, acting on oxidoreductase enzymes. Case reports or case series support its benefit in LHON; the largest to date being a small open-label trial, in which EPI-743 arrested disease progression and reversed vision loss in 4 of 5 treated patients with LHON [58,59].

5.6. Cyclosporine

Drugs or molecules developed for use in other pathologic processes which play a role in the modulation of the cellar intrinsic pathway or apoptosis may lead to promising therapy. Cyclosporine A inhibits opening of the mitochondrial permeability transition pore and is one of the anti-apoptotic drugs that has been studied in LHON. Oral cyclosporine (2.5 mg/kg/day) was given to patients in the hope of preventing second-eye involvement in patients with strictly unilateral Leber's hereditary optic neuropathy. Despite cyclosporine treatment, second-eye involvement occurred in all five patients included in the study, resulting in severe loss of vision, down to 20/200 or less. In addition, there was also a worsening of the visual acuity, the mean visual field defect, and the average thickness of the GC-IPL in the first eye affected [60]. Other molecules targeting different signals along the apoptotic pathways remain good candidates for future consideration.

5.7. Light Therapy and Electrical Stimulation

Photons from Near Infrared Light (NIR) light can penetrate diseased retina, be absorbed by mitochondrial photoreceptors, such as cytochrome c oxidase, and potentially promote mitochondrial energy production. Evidence has suggested that NIR light may restore biological function of damaged mitochondria, upregulate cytoprotective factors and inhibit apoptosis [61]. NIR light can also inhibit cell degeneration of retinal ganglion cells caused by inhibitor rotenone to the mitochondrial complex [62,63]. This has been postulated as a potential therapeutic option in LHON. Others, however, are concerns that upregulating OXPHOS with NIR may, by increasing mitochondrial metabolism also increase ROS, worsening the clinic outcome in LHON. The FDA approved the usage of this in patients and a clinical trial was initiated; however, it failed to recruit enough patients. An unpublished study in the Brazilian pedigree failed to show any benefit from NIR.

Electrical stimulation techniques may have shown potential benefits for treatment in diseases which affect the retina and optic nerve. Non-invasive electrical stimulation has been evaluated in traumatic non-arteritis optic neuropathies as well as retinal disease [64]. Recent small preliminary studies have looked at safety and efficacy of skin electrical stimulation in patients with chronic phase LHON with some promising results. Current studies have a lack of randomization and/or control arm, therefore further research is needed [65,66].

5.8. Gene Therapy

The current therapies discussed thus have focused on prevention and compensation. These pharmacologic mechanisms have been ones which ameliorate mitochondrial dysfunction at the cellular level by reducing, or attempting to reduce, ROS generation and the impact of mtDNA mutations on cellular homeostasis. Gene therapy, which alternatively targets replacement and repair of dysfunctional or damaged cellular pathways, poses an exciting new approach in the field.

In order to deliver a gene product to a mitochondrion there are several steps. The vector must endocytose within the cell, internalize within the mitochondria, and affect mitochondrial metabolism. This is very problematic, given that many DNA molecules do not cross mitochondrial membranes unaided. Additionally, mitochondrial genes require allotopic expression. Allotopic expression of mitochondrial genes is the deliberate relocation of mitochondrial gene into the nucleus followed by the importation of the genetically encoded polypeptide from the cytoplasm into mitochondria. The most studied mechanism to date for replacement of dysfunctional mtDNA is via intravitreal (IVT) injection of viral vectors.

The currently most established gene therapy consists of a wild-type of ND4 subunit packaged into an adeno-associated-virus 2 (AAV2) which is injected into the vitreous and targets the closest cells which are RGCs near the macula. In theory, upon cellular transfection, the wild-type ND4 gene is allotopically expressed. The AAV2 gene therapy vector carrying the wild-type ND4 gene gets transported to the nucleus where it is transcribed into messenger RNA which is later transcribed by ribosomes. The genetic sequences encoded also optimize translocation into the inner mitochondrial matrix and allow its integration within complex I to restore function [67]. Preclinical studies have demonstrated that recombinant AAV2 with wild type ND4 can rescue ATP production in cultured fibroblasts isolated from ND4-LHON patients, and that the therapeutic ND4 protein could successfully integrate into complex I in induced LHON models, preventing RGC apoptosis and optic nerve atrophy [68].

To date, there have been several phase I, II and III studies for LHON gene therapy. RESCUE and REVERSE are two randomized, double-blind, sham-controlled, multi-center, phase III clinical studies in which an intravitreal injection administered AAV recombinant wild type ND4 in one eye and an intravitreal administration of sham injection was delivered in the fellow eye [69]. In 2017, these phase III clinical trials studied the effects of single eye injection with GS010, a recombinant, AAV, containing a modified cDNA encoding the human wildtype ND4. They only differed in the duration of vision loss ($\leq$6 months for RESCUE, and >6 months to 1 year for REVERSE). 37 patients with visual acuity loss were included in the RESCUE study and 39 patients were included in the REVERSE study. On average, patients experienced an improvement in their visual acuity of about three lines. The surprising outcome from these trials was that a similar improvement occurred in the contralateral (sham treated) eye [70]. A non-clinical trial on primates suggested a possible retrograde, trans-chiasmatic transit of the vector from the treated eye to the sham-treated eye as an explanation for the unexpected bilateral visual improvement found in the RESCUE and REVERSE studies; however, this is a hotly debated topic in the neuro-ophthalmologic community. Some experts doubt that the number of virions that would make it to the contralateral eye is sufficient to infect enough RCGs for a clinical benefit. In 2019, the enrollment of 98 patients in a new Phase III clinical trial (REFLECT) was completed. The REFLECT study evaluated the efficacy and safety of bilateral intravitreal injections in subjects with 11,778 LHON mutation and follow up has shown that the statistically significant improvement of BCVA from baseline and the nadir reported at 1.5 years post administration was maintained at 2 years [71]. The improvement observed in placebo-treated eyes is consistent with the contralateral effect of a unilateral injection which was previously reported in RESCUE and REVERSE [71].

6. Chronic Phase

Currently there is not enough evidence to recommend treatment in patients in the later chronic stage who have experienced vision loss bilaterally, and there is no evidence to recommend treatment beyond 5 years from onset [2]. Overall, treatment in these individuals remains mostly supportive. Although there is no treatment that can stimulate optic nerve regeneration and repair, prevention of further visual loss by mitigation of risk factors, and supportive assistance for the patients, has great value.

6.1. Supportive Therapy

Currently, with limited available treatment options, the majority of patients with symptomatic LHON will progress to legal blindness (best corrected visual acuity of less than 20/200). As previously mentioned, many will have central scotomas with residual peripheral vision and are good candidates for low vision therapy and rehabilitation services. Additionally, those patients with a fenestration through which they have improved acuity, may be able to maximize this through assistive devices to maintain independence. Ample digital devises, such as smart phones or iPads, can be very helpful. Evidence supporting low vision rehabilitation is less robust, and a recent 2020 Cochrane review found that there was low-certainty evidence that some rehabilitation interventions improved vision related quality of life compared to usual care. Particularly, psychological therapy and methods of enhancing vision had the best evidence [72]. Overall, therapy should consist of a multifaceted approach including methods of enhancing vision, such as magnifying devices, electronic devices, or other technologies to improve remaining vision in combination with multidisciplinary rehabilitation programs such as balance training, occupational therapy, and home safety assessments. Most recently, qualitative data from LHON focus group interviews found that patients were hopeful that therapy would restore autonomy and improve their ability to enjoy a fulfilling life, while alleviating financial demands and demands placed on relatives [73].

6.2. Psychological Counseling

The impact of LHON extends beyond visual and activity related limitations. An important aspect of care for patients with LHON is the psychologic impact it has on both patients and carriers [74,75]. As LHON exhibits incomplete penetrance there may be multiple siblings or family members which are at various disease categories—carrier, pre-symptomatic, or symptomatic. It is important to be sensitive to the interfamilial dynamics and aware of the anxiety it may provoke. Vision-related quality of life is significantly reduced in LHON patients who also have higher levels of depressive symptoms compared to unaffected carriers [74,76]. LHON patients are at increased risk of anxiety and depression. Vision-related quality of life and depressive symptoms correlate with disease duration, suggesting that both may improve as patients adapt to chronic disability [76]. Addressing mental health concerns and promoting the development of skills through personal or therapy engaging strategies may help to overcome limitations thereby improving mood and quality of life in LHON patients.

6.3. Induced Pluripotent Stem Cells

As stated, the chronic phase has particularly challenging limitations in treatment. Once optic atrophy has occurred there is currently no avenue to reverse this process or regrow damaged fibers. The intention of the previously discussed therapies was maximizing remaining vision and prevention of further loss. Induced pluripotent stem cells (iPSCs) present a potential remarkable and spectacular avenue for reversal of vision loss. This field of research could in theory be effective for such a broad scope of etiologies of vision that it would revolutionize the field. At this time, however, it is an extremely challenging option with many hurdles to overcome before becoming clinically feasible. Unlike other cellular derived lines which are more amenable to stem cell related therapy, the neuronal pathway a RCG must travel the re-establish cerebral connections is exceedingly difficult.

In 2006, technology to reprogram somatic cells from patients to human iPSCs was developed [77]. Since then, development of this methodology has been revolutionized to allow for differentiation of iPSCs into RCGs [78–80]. Even if this technology does not evolve into an intervenable clinical therapeutic option, it serves as excellent mechanism of in vitro research. In relation to LHON differentiated RGCs and mini eye organoids have been created as disease models for study [81]. A few studies have been able to identify ways to stimulate RGC axons part way through the optic nerve and even beyond the chiasm. Mechanisms by which this has been accomplished include enhancement of mTOR, augmentation of adenosine 3′,5′-monophosphate (cAMP), and injections of oncomodulin [82]. Additionally, there is exciting advancement in the field of electrical field application to promote RGC survival and direct axon regeneration [83]. For iPSCs to be effective they would need to be appropriately differentiated, safely delivered to the right retinal location, and have the ability to form connections with the other retinal cells. Then, even if this can be accomplished, their axons would have to traverse to the optic nerve, decussate at the chiasm, and travel to the LGN to establish appropriate synaptic connections. Currently, the use of iPSCs is not yet feasible for vision loss related to optic nerve damage; however, the field has shown tremendous growth. The ultimate goal of this method would be to determine how to combine iPSC protocols with molecular pathway activation and RGC support to allow for their survival and regrowth.

6.4. Mitochondrial Gene Editing

Given the limitations in current therapeutics in patients with LHON, the concept of mitochondrial genetic engineering presents a novel and exciting focus. Gene editing tools such as zinc-finger nucleases (mitoZFN) and transcription activator-like effector nucleases (MitoTALENs) have been shown to eliminate mutant mtDNA and shift heteroplasmy [84]. Recent advancements within the field have led to a new approach, mitochondrial base editing. An appropriate mitochondrial targeted DNA base editor might allow for the direct revision of the mutation of interest to wildtype mtDNA. One such example, TALE-linked adenine deaminases (TALEDs), has been tested in human cell lines and was able to edit A-to-G conversion at different target sites within the mitochondrial genome [85,86]. Although still far from clinical use, improvements in these methodologies are making it increasing possible to create targeted therapy against pathogenic mtDNA mutations. This innovative approach adds another potential field of interest in LHON therapy.

7. Conclusions

In conclusion, the field of therapeutic options for LHON is still limited but has recently shown a dramatic expansion in scientific research and potential. This article reviewed supportive, preventative, and interventional therapeutics, how they are currently applied to clinical disease stages, and future promising areas within the field.

The novel insights in molecular mechanism and cellular pathology found in LHON has created multiple new approaches for a deeper understanding of LHON and other mitochondrial optic neuropathies and related diseases. Presently, Idebenone remains the cornerstone of treatment and the only currently licensed therapy; however, the vast arsenal of potential therapies spans everything from repurposing established drugs, creation of novel molecules and gene therapy. The future of the field holds the promise of more efficacious treatment options for the treatment of LHON optic neuropathy.

Funding: This research received no external funding.

Institutional Review Board Statement: Not applicable for studies not involving humans or animals.

Informed Consent Statement: Not applicable.

Data Availability Statement: Not applicable.

Conflicts of Interest: The authors declare no conflict of interest.

References

1. Man, P.; Griffiths, P.; Brown, D.; Howell, N.; Turnbull, D.; Chinnery, P. The Epidemiology of Leber Hereditary Optic Neuropathy in the North East of England. *Am. J. Hum. Genet.* **2003**, *72*, 333–339. [CrossRef] [PubMed]
2. Carelli, V.; Carbonelli, M.; Irenaeus, F.; Kawasaki, A.; Klopstock, T.; Lagrèze, W.A.; La Morgia, C.; Newman, N.J.; Orssaud, C.; Pott, J.W.R. International Consensus Statement on the Clinical and Therapeutic Management of Leber Hereditary Optic Neuropathy. *J. Neuro-Ophthalmol.* **2017**, *37*, 371–381. [CrossRef] [PubMed]
3. Huoponen, K.; Vilkki, J.; Aula, P.; Nikoskelainen, E.K.; Savontaus, M. A New MtDNA Mutation Associated with Leber Hereditary Optic Neuroretinopathy. *Am. J. Hum. Genet.* **1991**, *48*, 1147. [PubMed]
4. Johns, D.R.; Neufeld, M.J.; Park, R.D. An ND-6 Mitochondrial DNA Mutation Associated with Leber Hereditary Optic Neuropathy. *Biochem. Biophys. Res. Commun.* **1992**, *187*, 1551–1557. [CrossRef]
5. Wallace, D.C.; Singh, G.; Lott, M.T.; Hodge, J.A.; Schurr, T.G.; Lezza, A.M.; Elsas, L.J.; Nikoskelainen, E.K. Mitochondrial DNA Mutation Associated with Leber's Hereditary Optic Neuropathy. *Science* **1988**, *242*, 1427–1430. [CrossRef]
6. Sadun, A.A.; Salomao, S.R.; Berezovsky, A.; Sadun, F.; DeNegri, A.M.; Quiros, P.A.; Chicani, F.; Ventura, D.; Barboni, P.; Sherman, J. Subclinical Carriers and Conversions in Leber Hereditary Optic Neuropathy: A Prospective Psychophysical Study. *Trans. Am. Ophthalmol. Soc.* **2006**, *104*, 51.
7. Savini, G.; Barboni, P.; Valentino, M.L.; Montagna, P.; Cortelli, P.; De Negri, A.M.; Sadun, F.; Bianchi, S.; Longanesi, L.; Zanini, M. Retinal Nerve Fiber Layer Evaluation by Optical Coherence Tomography in Unaffected Carriers with Leber's Hereditary Optic Neuropathy Mutations. *Ophthalmology* **2005**, *112*, 127–131. [CrossRef]
8. Balducci, N.; Cascavilla, M.L.; Ciardella, A.; La Morgia, C.; Triolo, G.; Parisi, V.; Bandello, F.; Sadun, A.A.; Carelli, V.; Barboni, P. Peripapillary Vessel Density Changes in Leber's Hereditary Optic Neuropathy: A New Biomarker. *Clin. Exp. Ophthalmol.* **2018**, *46*, 1055–1062. [CrossRef]
9. Jia, Y.; Simonett, J.M.; Wang, J.; Hua, X.; Liu, L.; Hwang, T.S.; Huang, D. Wide-Field OCT Angiography Investigation of the Relationship between Radial Peripapillary Capillary Plexus Density and Nerve Fiber Layer Thickness. *Investig. Ophthalmol. Vis. Sci.* **2017**, *58*, 5188–5194. [CrossRef]
10. Silva, M.; Llòria, X.; Catarino, C.; Klopstock, T. Natural History Findings from a Large Cohort of Patients with Lebers Hereditary Optic Neuropathy (LHON): New Insights into the Natural Disease Course. *Acta Ophthalmol.* **2018**, *96*, 117.
11. Man, P.Y.W.; Turnbull, D.; Chinnery, P. Leber Hereditary Optic Neuropathy. *J. Med. Genet.* **2002**, *39*, 162–169. [CrossRef] [PubMed]
12. Carelli, V.; d'Adamo, P.; Valentino, M.L.; La Morgia, C.; Ross-Cisneros, F.N.; Caporali, L.; Maresca, A.; Loguercio Polosa, P.; Barboni, P.; De Negri, A. Parsing the Differences in Affected with LHON: Genetic versus Environmental Triggers of Disease Conversion. *Brain* **2016**, *139*, e17. [CrossRef] [PubMed]
13. Newman, N.J.; Carelli, V.; Taiel, M.; Yu-Wai-Man, P. Visual Outcomes in Leber Hereditary Optic Neuropathy Patients with the m. 11778G>A (MTND4) Mitochondrial DNA Mutation. *J. Neuro-Ophthalmol.* **2020**, *40*, 547–557. [CrossRef] [PubMed]
14. do VF Ramos, C.; Bellusci, C.; Savini, G.; Carbonelli, M.; Berezovsky, A.; Tamaki, C.; Cinoto, R.; Sacai, P.Y.; Moraes-Filho, M.N.; Miura, H.M. Association of Optic Disc Size with Development and Prognosis of Leber's Hereditary Optic Neuropathy. *Investig. Ophthalmol. Vis. Sci.* **2009**, *50*, 1666–1674. [CrossRef] [PubMed]
15. Pan, B.X.; Ross-Cisneros, F.N.; Carelli, V.; Rue, K.S.; Salomao, S.R.; Moraes-Filho, M.N.; Moraes, M.N.; Berezovsky, A.; Belfort, R.; Sadun, A.A. Mathematically Modeling the Involvement of Axons in Leber's Hereditary Optic Neuropathy. *Investig. Ophthalmol. Vis. Sci.* **2012**, *53*, 7608–7617. [CrossRef] [PubMed]
16. Sadun, A.A.; La Morgia, C.; Carelli, V. Mitochondrial Optic Neuropathies: Our Travels from Bench to Bedside and Back Again. *Clin. Exp. Ophthalmol.* **2013**, *41*, 702–712. [CrossRef]
17. Sadun, A.A.; Win, P.H.; Ross-Cisneros, F.; Walker, S.; Carelli, V. Leber's Hereditary Optic Neuropathy Differentially Affects Smaller Axons in the Optic Nerve. *Trans. Am. Ophthalmol. Soc.* **2000**, *98*, 223.
18. Yu-Wai-Man, P.; Newman, N.J.; Carelli, V.; La Morgia, C.; Biousse, V.; Bandello, F.M.; Clermont, C.V.; Campillo, L.C.; Leruez, S.; Moster, M.L. Natural History of Patients with Leber Hereditary Optic Neuropathy—Results from the REALITY Study. *Eye* **2022**, *36*, 818–826. [CrossRef]
19. Yu-Wai-Man, P.; Chinnery, P.F. Leber Hereditary Optic Neuropathy. In *GeneReviews®*; Adam, M.P., Mirzaa, G.M., Pagon, R.A., Wallace, S.E., Bean, L.J., Gripp, K.W., Amemiya, A., Eds.; University of Washington: Seattle, WA, USA, 1993.
20. Spruijt, L.; Kolbach, D.N.; Rene, F.; Plomp, A.S.; Bauer, N.J.; Smeets, H.J.; de Die-Smulders, C.E. Influence of Mutation Type on Clinical Expression of Leber Hereditary Optic Neuropathy. *Am. J. Ophthalmol.* **2006**, *141*, 676. [CrossRef]
21. Majander, A.; Bowman, R.; Poulton, J.; Antcliff, R.J.; Reddy, M.A.; Michaelides, M.; Webster, A.R.; Chinnery, P.F.; Votruba, M.; Moore, A.T. Childhood-Onset Leber Hereditary Optic Neuropathy. *Br. J. Ophthalmol.* **2017**, *101*, 1505–1509. [CrossRef]
22. Caporali, L.; Maresca, A.; Capristo, M.; Del Dotto, V.; Tagliavini, F.; Valentino, M.L.; La Morgia, C.; Carelli, V. Incomplete Penetrance in Mitochondrial Optic Neuropathies. *Mitochondrion* **2017**, *36*, 130–137. [CrossRef] [PubMed]
23. Carroll, J.; Fearnley, I.M.; Shannon, R.J.; Hirst, J.; Walker, J.E. Analysis of the Subunit Composition of Complex I from Bovine Heart Mitochondria* S. *Mol. Cell. Proteom.* **2003**, *2*, 117–126. [CrossRef] [PubMed]
24. Carelli, V.; Ross-Cisneros, F.N.; Sadun, A.A. Mitochondrial Dysfunction as a Cause of Optic Neuropathies. *Prog. Retin. Eye Res.* **2004**, *23*, 53–89. [CrossRef] [PubMed]
25. Yu, D.-Y.; Cringle, S.J. Oxygen Distribution and Consumption within the Retina in Vascularised and Avascular Retinas and in Animal Models of Retinal Disease. *Prog. Retin. Eye Res.* **2001**, *20*, 175–208. [CrossRef]

26. Adapted from "Electron Transport Chain". by BioRender.Com. 2022. Available online: https://app.biorender.com/biorender-templates (accessed on 1 September 2022).
27. Kang, E.; Wu, J.; Gutierrez, N.M.; Koski, A.; Tippner-Hedges, R.; Agaronyan, K.; Platero-Luengo, A.; Martinez-Redondo, P.; Ma, H.; Lee, Y. Mitochondrial Replacement in Human Oocytes Carrying Pathogenic Mitochondrial DNA Mutations. *Nature* **2016**, *540*, 270–275. [CrossRef] [PubMed]
28. Silva-Pinheiro, P.; Minczuk, M. The Potential of Mitochondrial Genome Engineering. *Nat. Rev. Genet.* **2022**, *23*, 199–214. [CrossRef]
29. Gómez-Durán, A.; Pacheu-Grau, D.; Martínez-Romero, Í.; López-Gallardo, E.; López-Pérez, M.J.; Montoya, J.; Ruiz-Pesini, E. Oxidative Phosphorylation Differences between Mitochondrial DNA Haplogroups Modify the Risk of Leber's Hereditary Optic Neuropathy. *Biochim. Biophys. Acta Mol. Basis Dis.* **2012**, *1822*, 1216–1222. [CrossRef]
30. Yu-Wai-Man, P.; Hudson, G.; Klopstock, T.; Chinnery, P.F. Reply: Parsing the Differences in Affected with LHON: Genetic versus Environmental Triggers of Disease Conversion. *Brain* **2016**, *139*, e18. [CrossRef]
31. Giordano, L.; Deceglie, S.; d'Adamo, P.; Valentino, M.; La Morgia, C.; Fracasso, F.; Roberti, M.; Cappellari, M.; Petrosillo, G.; Ciaravolo, S. Cigarette Toxicity Triggers Leber's Hereditary Optic Neuropathy by Affecting MtDNA Copy Number, Oxidative Phosphorylation and ROS Detoxification Pathways. *Cell Death Dis.* **2015**, *6*, e2021. [CrossRef]
32. Zaslavsky, K.; Margolin, E.A. Leber's Hereditary Optic Neuropathy in Older Individuals Because of Increased Alcohol Consumption During the COVID-19 Pandemic. *J. Neuro-Ophthalmol.* **2021**, *41*, 316–320. [CrossRef]
33. Giordano, C.; Iommarini, L.; Giordano, L.; Maresca, A.; Pisano, A.; Valentino, M.L.; Caporali, L.; Liguori, R.; Deceglie, S.; Roberti, M. Efficient Mitochondrial Biogenesis Drives Incomplete Penetrance in Leber's Hereditary Optic Neuropathy. *Brain* **2014**, *137*, 335–353. [CrossRef] [PubMed]
34. Bahr, T.; Welburn, K.; Donnelly, J.; Bai, Y. Emerging Model Systems and Treatment Approaches for Leber's Hereditary Optic Neuropathy: Challenges and Opportunities. *Biochim. Biophys. Acta Mol. Basis Dis.* **2020**, *1866*, 165743. [CrossRef] [PubMed]
35. Uittenbogaard, M.; Chiaramello, A. Mitochondrial Biogenesis: A Therapeutic Target for Neurodevelopmental Disorders and Neurodegenerative Diseases. *Curr. Pharm. Des.* **2014**, *20*, 5574–5593. [CrossRef]
36. Danese, A.; Patergnani, S.; Maresca, A.; Peron, C.; Raimondi, A.; Caporali, L.; Marchi, S.; La Morgia, C.; Del Dotto, V.; Zanna, C. Pathological Mitophagy Disrupts Mitochondrial Homeostasis in Leber's Hereditary Optic Neuropathy. *Cell Rep.* **2022**, *40*, 111124. [CrossRef] [PubMed]
37. Cerutti, R.; Pirinen, E.; Lamperti, C.; Marchet, S.; Sauve, A.A.; Li, W.; Leoni, V.; Schon, E.A.; Dantzer, F.; Auwerx, J. NAD+-Dependent Activation of Sirt1 Corrects the Phenotype in a Mouse Model of Mitochondrial Disease. *Cell. Metab.* **2014**, *19*, 1042–1049. [CrossRef] [PubMed]
38. Garone, C.; Viscomi, C. Towards a Therapy for Mitochondrial Disease: An Update. *Biochem. Soc. Trans.* **2018**, *46*, 1247–1261. [CrossRef]
39. Pirinen, E.; Auranen, M.; Khan, N.A.; Brilhante, V.; Urho, N.; Pessia, A.; Hakkarainen, A.; Kuula, J.; Heinonen, U.; Schmidt, M.S. Niacin Cures Systemic NAD+ Deficiency and Improves Muscle Performance in Adult-Onset Mitochondrial Myopathy. *Cell Metab.* **2020**, *31*, 1078–1090. [CrossRef]
40. Ruiz-Pesini, E.; Emperador, S.; López-Gallardo, E.; Hernández-Ainsa, C.; Montoya, J. Increasing MtDNA Levels as Therapy for Mitochondrial Optic Neuropathies. *Drug Discov. Today* **2018**, *23*, 493–498. [CrossRef]
41. Giordano, C.; Montopoli, M.; Perli, E.; Orlandi, M.; Fantin, M.; Ross-Cisneros, F.N.; Caparrotta, L.; Martinuzzi, A.; Ragazzi, E.; Ghelli, A. Oestrogens Ameliorate Mitochondrial Dysfunction in Leber's Hereditary Optic Neuropathy. *Brain* **2011**, *134*, 220–234. [CrossRef]
42. Pisano, A.; Preziuso, C.; Iommarini, L.; Perli, E.; Grazioli, P.; Campese, A.F.; Maresca, A.; Montopoli, M.; Masuelli, L.; Sadun, A.A. Targeting Estrogen Receptor β as Preventive Therapeutic Strategy for Leber's Hereditary Optic Neuropathy. *Hum. Mol. Genet.* **2015**, *24*, 6921–6931. [CrossRef]
43. Sun, J.; Zhu, H.; Wang, X.; Gao, Q.; Li, Z.; Huang, H. CoQ10 Ameliorates Mitochondrial Dysfunction in Diabetic Nephropathy through Mitophagy. *J. Endocrinol.* **2019**, *240*, 445–465. [CrossRef] [PubMed]
44. Zhao, L. Protective Effects of Trimetazidine and Coenzyme Q10 on Cisplatin-Induced Cardiotoxicity by Alleviating Oxidative Stress and Mitochondrial Dysfunction. *Anatol. J. Cardiol.* **2019**, *22*, 232. [CrossRef] [PubMed]
45. Lyseng-Williamson, K.A. Idebenone: A Review in Leber's Hereditary Optic Neuropathy. *Drugs* **2016**, *76*, 805–813. [CrossRef] [PubMed]
46. Jaber, S.M.; Shealinna, X.G.; Milstein, J.L.; VanRyzin, J.W.; Waddell, J.; Polster, B.M. Idebenone Has Distinct Effects on Mitochondrial Respiration in Cortical Astrocytes Compared to Cortical Neurons Due to Differential NQO1 Activity. *J. Neurosci.* **2020**, *40*, 4609–4619. [CrossRef] [PubMed]
47. Amore, G.; Romagnoli, M.; Carbonelli, M.; Barboni, P.; Carelli, V.; La Morgia, C. Therapeutic Options in Hereditary Optic Neuropathies. *Drugs* **2021**, *81*, 57–86. [CrossRef]
48. Varricchio, C.; Beirne, K.; Heard, C.; Newland, B.; Rozanowska, M.; Brancale, A.; Votruba, M. The Ying and Yang of Idebenone: Not Too Little, Not Too Much–Cell Death in NQO1 Deficient Cells and the Mouse Retina. *Free Radic. Biol. Med.* **2020**, *152*, 551–560. [CrossRef]
49. Yu-Wai-Man, P.; Soiferman, D.; Moore, D.G.; Burté, F.; Saada, A. Evaluating the Therapeutic Potential of Idebenone and Related Quinone Analogues in Leber Hereditary Optic Neuropathy. *Mitochondrion* **2017**, *36*, 36–42. [CrossRef]

50. Heitz, F.D.; Erb, M.; Anklin, C.; Robay, D.; Pernet, V.; Gueven, N. Idebenone Protects against Retinal Damage and Loss of Vision in a Mouse Model of Leber's Hereditary Optic Neuropathy. *PLoS ONE* **2012**, *7*, e45182. [CrossRef]
51. Klopstock, T.; Yu-Wai-Man, P.; Dimitriadis, K.; Rouleau, J.; Heck, S.; Bailie, M.; Atawan, A.; Chattopadhyay, S.; Schubert, M.; Garip, A. A Randomized Placebo-Controlled Trial of Idebenone in Leber's Hereditary Optic Neuropathy. *Brain* **2011**, *134*, 2677–2686. [CrossRef]
52. Carelli, V.; La Morgia, C.; Valentino, M.L.; Rizzo, G.; Carbonelli, M.; De Negri, A.M.; Sadun, F.; Carta, A.; Guerriero, S.; Simonelli, F. Idebenone Treatment in Leber's Hereditary Optic Neuropathy. *Brain* **2011**, *134*, e188. [CrossRef]
53. Van Everdingen, J.A.; Tjon-Fo-Sang, M.; van den Born, L.; Pott, J.W.R. New Treatment Option for Leber Hereditary Optic Neuropathy: Early Diagnosis Is Required. *Ned. Tijdschr. Voor Geneeskd.* **2021**, *165*, D5444.
54. Catarino, C.B.; von Livonius, B.; Priglinger, C.; Banik, R.; Matloob, S.; Tamhankar, M.A.; Castillo, L.; Friedburg, C.; Halfpenny, C.A.; Lincoln, J.A. Real-World Clinical Experience with Idebenone in the Treatment of Leber Hereditary Optic Neuropathy. *J. Neuro-Ophthalmol.* **2020**, *40*, 558. [CrossRef] [PubMed]
55. Ishikawa, H.; Masuda, Y.; Ishikawa, H.; Shikisima, K.; Goseki, T.; Kezuka, T.; Terao, M.; Miyazaki, A.; Matsumoto, K.; Nishikawa, H. Characteristics of Japanese Patients with Leber's Hereditary Optic Neuropathy and Idebenone Trial: A Prospective, Interventional, Non-Comparative Study. *Jpn. J. Ophthalmol.* **2021**, *65*, 133–142. [CrossRef]
56. Van Everdingen, J.A.; Pott, J.W.R.; Bauer, N.J.; Krijnen, A.M.; Lushchyk, T.; Wubbels, R.J. Clinical Outcomes of Treatment with Idebenone in Leber's Hereditary Optic Neuropathy in the Netherlands: A National Cohort Study. *Acta Ophthalmol.* **2022**, *100*, 700–706. [CrossRef] [PubMed]
57. Szeto, H.H. First-in-class Cardiolipin-protective Compound as a Therapeutic Agent to Restore Mitochondrial Bioenergetics. *Br. J. Pharmacol.* **2014**, *171*, 2029–2050. [CrossRef] [PubMed]
58. Enns, G.M.; Cohen, B.H. Clinical Trials in Mitochondrial Disease: An Update on EPI-743 and RP103. *J. Inborn Errors Metab. Screen.* **2019**, *5*. [CrossRef]
59. Sadun, A.A.; Chicani, C.F.; Ross-Cisneros, F.N.; Barboni, P.; Thoolen, M.; Shrader, W.D.; Kubis, K.; Carelli, V.; Miller, G. Effect of EPI-743 on the Clinical Course of the Mitochondrial Disease Leber Hereditary Optic Neuropathy. *Arch. Neurol.* **2012**, *69*, 331–338. [CrossRef]
60. Leruez, S.; Verny, C.; Bonneau, D.; Procaccio, V.; Lenaers, G.; Amati-Bonneau, P.; Reynier, P.; Scherer, C.; Prundean, A.; Orssaud, C. Cyclosporine A Does Not Prevent Second-Eye Involvement in Leber's Hereditary Optic Neuropathy. *Orphanet J. Rare Dis.* **2018**, *13*, 1–9. [CrossRef]
61. Eells, J.T.; Wong-Riley, M.T.; VerHoeve, J.; Henry, M.; Buchman, E.V.; Kane, M.P.; Gould, L.J.; Das, R.; Jett, M.; Hodgson, B.D. Mitochondrial Signal Transduction in Accelerated Wound and Retinal Healing by Near-Infrared Light Therapy. *Mitochondrion* **2004**, *4*, 559–567. [CrossRef]
62. Rojas, J.C.; Lee, J.; John, J.M.; Gonzalez-Lima, F. Neuroprotective Effects of Near-Infrared Light in an in Vivo Model of Mitochondrial Optic Neuropathy. *J. Neurosci.* **2008**, *28*, 13511–13521. [CrossRef] [PubMed]
63. Zhu, Q.; Xiao, S.; Hua, Z.; Yang, D.; Hu, M.; Zhu, Y.-T.; Zhong, H. Near Infrared (NIR) Light Therapy of Eye Diseases: A Review. *Int. J. Med. Sci.* **2021**, *18*, 109. [CrossRef] [PubMed]
64. Sehic, A.; Guo, S.; Cho, K.-S.; Corraya, R.M.; Chen, D.F.; Utheim, T.P. Electrical Stimulation as a Means for Improving Vision. *Am. J. Pathol.* **2016**, *186*, 2783–2797. [CrossRef] [PubMed]
65. Perin, C.; Viganò, B.; Piscitelli, D.; Matteo, B.M.; Meroni, R.; Cerri, C.G. Non-Invasive Current Stimulation in Vision Recovery: A Review of the Literature. *Restor. Neurol. Neurosci.* **2020**, *38*, 239–250. [CrossRef]
66. Kurimoto, T.; Ueda, K.; Mori, S.; Kamada, S.; Sakamoto, M.; Yamada-Nakanishi, Y.; Matsumiya, W.; Nakamura, M. A Single-Arm, Prospective, Exploratory Study to Preliminarily Test Effectiveness and Safety of Skin Electrical Stimulation for Leber Hereditary Optic Neuropathy. *J. Clin. Med.* **2020**, *9*, 1359. [CrossRef]
67. Bykov, Y.S.; Rapaport, D.; Herrmann, J.M.; Schuldiner, M. Cytosolic Events in the Biogenesis of Mitochondrial Proteins. *Trends Biochem. Sci.* **2020**, *45*, 650–667. [CrossRef] [PubMed]
68. Bonnet, C.; Augustin, S.; Ellouze, S.; Bénit, P.; Bouaita, A.; Rustin, P.; Sahel, J.-A.; Corral-Debrinski, M. The Optimized Allotopic Expression of ND1 or ND4 Genes Restores Respiratory Chain Complex I Activity in Fibroblasts Harboring Mutations in These Genes. *Biochim. Biophys. Acta Mol. Cell Res.* **2008**, *1783*, 1707–1717. [CrossRef] [PubMed]
69. Moster, M.; Sadun, A.; Klopstock, T.; Newman, N.; Vignal-Clermont, C.; Carelli, V.; Yu-Wai-Man, P.; Biousse, V.; Sergott, R.; Katz, B. rAAV2/2-ND4 for the Treatment of Leber Hereditary Optic Neuropathy (LHON): Final Results from the RESCUE and REVERSE Phase III Clinical Trials and Experimental Data in Nonhuman Primates to Support a Bilateral Effect. *Neurology* **2020**, *94*, 2339.
70. Yu-Wai-Man, P.; Newman, N.J.; Carelli, V.; Moster, M.L.; Biousse, V.; Sadun, A.A.; Klopstock, T.; Vignal-Clermont, C.; Sergott, R.C.; Rudolph, G. Bilateral Visual Improvement with Unilateral Gene Therapy Injection for Leber Hereditary Optic Neuropathy. *Sci. Transl. Med.* **2020**, *12*, eaaz7423. [CrossRef] [PubMed]
71. Newman, N.; Yu-Wai-Man, P.; Carelli, V.; Subramanian, P.; Moster, M.; Wang, A.-G.; Donahue, S.; Leroy, B.; Biousse, V.; Vignal-Clermont, C. The Phase III REFLECT Trial: Efficacy and Safety of Bilateral Gene Therapy for Leber Hereditary Optic Neuropathy (LHON)(P17-12.002). *Neurology* **2022**, *98*, 928.
72. van Nispen, R.M.; Virgili, G.; Hoeben, M.; Langelaan, M.; Klevering, J.; Keunen, J.E.; van Rens, G.H. Low Vision Rehabilitation for Better Quality of Life in Visually Impaired Adults. *Cochrane Database Syst. Rev.* **2020**. [CrossRef]

73. Chen, B.S.; Holzinger, E.; Taiel, M.; Yu-Wai-Man, P. The Impact of Leber Hereditary Optic Neuropathy on the Quality of Life of Patients and Their Relatives: A Qualitative Study. *J. Neuro-Ophthalmol.* **2022**, *42*, 316–322. [CrossRef]
74. Gale, J.; Khoshnevis, M.; Frousiakis, S.E.; Karanjia, R.; Poincenot, L.; Sadun, A.A.; Baron, D.A. An International Study of Emotional Response to Bilateral Vision Loss Using a Novel Graphical Online Assessment Tool. *Psychosomatics* **2017**, *58*, 38–45. [CrossRef]
75. Garcia, G.A.; Khoshnevis, M.; Gale, J.; Frousiakis, S.E.; Hwang, T.J.; Poincenot, L.; Karanjia, R.; Baron, D.; Sadun, A.A. Profound Vision Loss Impairs Psychological Well-Being in Young and Middle-Aged Individuals. *Clin. Ophthalmol.* **2017**, *11*, 417. [CrossRef]
76. Kurup, M.; Ching, J.; Yu-Wai-Man, P. Vision-Related Quality of Life and Mental Health in Patients with Leber Hereditary Optic Neuropathy. *Investig. Ophthalmol. Vis. Sci.* **2021**, *62*, 2393.
77. Takahashi, K.; Yamanaka, S. Induction of Pluripotent Stem Cells from Mouse Embryonic and Adult Fibroblast Cultures by Defined Factors. *Cell* **2006**, *126*, 663–676. [CrossRef]
78. Cowan, C.S.; Renner, M.; De Gennaro, M.; Gross-Scherf, B.; Goldblum, D.; Hou, Y.; Munz, M.; Rodrigues, T.M.; Krol, J.; Szikra, T. Cell Types of the Human Retina and Its Organoids at Single-Cell Resolution. *Cell* **2020**, *182*, 1623–1640. [CrossRef]
79. Kruczek, K.; Swaroop, A. Pluripotent Stem Cell-Derived Retinal Organoids for Disease Modeling and Development of Therapies. *Stem Cells* **2020**, *38*, 1206–1215. [CrossRef]
80. Laha, B.; Stafford, B.K.; Huberman, A.D. Regenerating Optic Pathways from the Eye to the Brain. *Science* **2017**, *356*, 1031–1034. [CrossRef]
81. Fligor, C.M.; Huang, K.-C.; Lavekar, S.S.; VanderWall, K.B.; Meyer, J.S. Differentiation of Retinal Organoids from Human Pluripotent Stem Cells. In *Methods in Cell Biology*; Elsevier: Amsterdam, The Netherlands, 2020; Volume 159, pp. 279–302. ISBN 0091-679X.
82. De Lima, S.; Koriyama, Y.; Kurimoto, T.; Oliveira, J.T.; Yin, Y.; Li, Y.; Gilbert, H.-Y.; Fagiolini, M.; Martinez, A.M.B.; Benowitz, L. Full-Length Axon Regeneration in the Adult Mouse Optic Nerve and Partial Recovery of Simple Visual Behaviors. *Proc. Natl. Acad. Sci. USA* **2012**, *109*, 9149–9154. [CrossRef]
83. Peng, M.; Lam, P.; Machnoor, M.; Paknahad, J.; Iseri, E.; Shao, X.; Shahidi, M.; Thomas, B.; Lazzi, G.; Gokoffski, K. Electric Fields Direct Full-Length Optic Nerve Regeneration and Partial Restoration of Visual Function. *Investig. Ophthalmol. Vis. Sci.* **2022**, *63*, 1139.
84. Morgan, M.A.; Lange, L.; Schambach, A. Prime Time for Base Editing in the Mitochondria. *Signal Transduct. Target. Ther.* **2022**, *7*, 1–2. [CrossRef]
85. Cho, S.-I.; Lee, S.; Mok, Y.G.; Lim, K.; Lee, J.; Lee, J.M.; Chung, E.; Kim, J.-S. Targeted A-to-G Base Editing in Human Mitochondrial DNA with Programmable Deaminases. *Cell* **2022**, *185*, 1764–1776. [CrossRef]
86. Barrera-Paez, J.D.; Moraes, C.T. Mitochondrial Genome Engineering Coming-of-Age. *Trends Genet.* **2022**, *38*, 869–880. [CrossRef]

International Journal of *Molecular Sciences*

MDPI

Review

Retinal Ganglion Cell Survival and Axon Regeneration after Optic Nerve Injury: Role of Inflammation and Other Factors

Kimberly A. Wong [1,*] and Larry I. Benowitz [1,2,3,*]

[1] Department of Neurosurgery, Boston Children's Hospital and Harvard Medical School, Boston, MA 02115, USA
[2] F.M. Kirby Neurobiology Center, Boston Children's Hospital, Boston, MA 02115, USA
[3] Department of Ophthalmology, Harvard Medical School, Boston, MA 02115, USA
* Correspondence: kimberlywong16@gmail.com (K.A.W.); larry.benowitz@childrens.harvard.edu (L.I.B.)

Abstract: The optic nerve, like most pathways in the mature central nervous system, cannot regenerate if injured, and within days, retinal ganglion cells (RGCs), the neurons that extend axons through the optic nerve, begin to die. Thus, there are few clinical options to improve vision after traumatic or ischemic optic nerve injury or in neurodegenerative diseases such as glaucoma, dominant optic neuropathy, or optic pathway gliomas. Research over the past two decades has identified several strategies to enable RGCs to regenerate axons the entire length of the optic nerve, in some cases leading to modest reinnervation of di- and mesencephalic visual relay centers. This review primarily focuses on the role of the innate immune system in improving RGC survival and axon regeneration, and its synergy with manipulations of signal transduction pathways, transcription factors, and cell-extrinsic suppressors of axon growth. Research in this field provides hope that clinically effective strategies to improve vision in patients with currently untreatable losses could become a reality in 5–10 years.

Keywords: retina; inflammation; transcription; CNS repair; optic nerve; oncomodulin; myeloid cells; regeneration

Citation: Wong, K.A.; Benowitz, L.I. Retinal Ganglion Cell Survival and Axon Regeneration after Optic Nerve Injury: Role of Inflammation and Other Factors. *Int. J. Mol. Sci.* **2022**, *23*, 10179. https://doi.org/10.3390/ijms231710179

Academic Editors: Neil R. Miller and Rongkung Tsai

Received: 4 August 2022
Accepted: 2 September 2022
Published: 5 September 2022

1. Introduction

Restoring vision after optic nerve injury requires maintaining retinal ganglion cell (RGC) survival while enabling these cells to re-extend axons and re-establish connections in appropriate target areas of the brain. Achieving these goals will entail suppressing pathological processes that lead to RGC death, restoring an active growth state to these neurons, and ensuring that growing axons navigate back to visual relay nuclei of the di- and mesencephalon. One area we emphasize here is the surprising role of the innate immune system in modulating RGC survival, axon regrowth, and myelination. Understanding the mechanisms that underlie these phenomena may eventually enable us to regulate the inflammatory response that inevitably accompanies CNS damage to our advantage and/or isolate beneficial immune-derived factors to improve functional recovery after optic neuropathy. We will also briefly review other strategies to promote RGC survival and regeneration that, in many cases, act synergistically with manipulations of the innate immune system. We are not covering important recent developments in replacing lost RGCs with embryonic stem cells or pluripotent stem cells, though these approaches will require the new neurons to extend axons to appropriate brain areas and therefore involve some of the same issues as axon regeneration from injured RGCs.

2. History

Unlike neurons in the peripheral nervous system (PNS), those of the central nervous system (CNS) cannot spontaneously regenerate damaged axons, and, consequently, CNS injuries or various neurodegenerative diseases often result in severe and irreparable functional losses. The seminal studies of Tello and his mentor, Santiago Ramon y Cajal, were the first to show that, under certain experimental conditions, CNS neurons can be induced to regenerate damaged axons. These early 20th century studies showed that, following optic nerve transection, RGCs could regrow axons through a peripheral nerve graft implanted at the site of axotomy [1], implying that, although these neurons remain regeneration-competent, conditions that enable regeneration to occur are not normally present in the CNS environment after injury. Beginning several decades later, the scientific community undertook hundreds of studies to understand the factors that prevent or enable neurons to regenerate injured axons. Here, we first summarize the results of our group and others to understand how inflammation can be harnessed to promote RGC neuroprotection and enable these neurons to regenerate axons, then proceed to describe complementary lines of investigation.

3. Intraocular Inflammation Promotes RGC Survival and Axon Regeneration

Although the retina, like other parts of the CNS, was long thought to be "immune privileged", i.e., resistant to inflammation, many studies now show that neuroinflammation plays a critical role in the pathology of chronic ocular diseases. In glaucoma and ocular auto-immune diseases, chronic activation of tissue-resident cells (microglia, Muller glia, and astrocytes) can augment neurodegeneration by stimulating the adaptive immune system to target ocular tissues [2–4]. Paradoxically, however, inducing sterile inflammation in the eye in animal models augments RGC survival and axon regeneration. Our lab inadvertently discovered that injury to the lens enhances the survival of RGCs after optic nerve injury (ONI) and enables these cells to begin regenerating axons well beyond the injury site. Lens injury (LI) leads to the infiltration of neutrophils and macrophages that express factors that increase RGC survival and cause RGCs to up-regulate genes linked to axon growth and regeneration (Figure 1a,b [5]). These effects can be mimicked by intravitreal injection of Zymosan, a yeast cell wall preparation [6,7] that activates Toll-like receptor 2 (TLR2) and the pattern recognition receptor dectin-1. Accordingly, the effects of LI or Zymosan are suppressed by blocking receptors for the pro-inflammatory chemokines CCL2 [8] or CXCL5 [9], mimicked by the TLR2 agonist Pam3Cys [10] or the Dectin-1 agonist b-glucan [11], and exceeded by injecting a newly defined set of immature neutrophils [12]. These findings raise the possibility that defined signals associated with sterile inflammation might serve as safe biologics to promote neuroprotection and axon regeneration without the deleterious effects of intraocular inflammation.

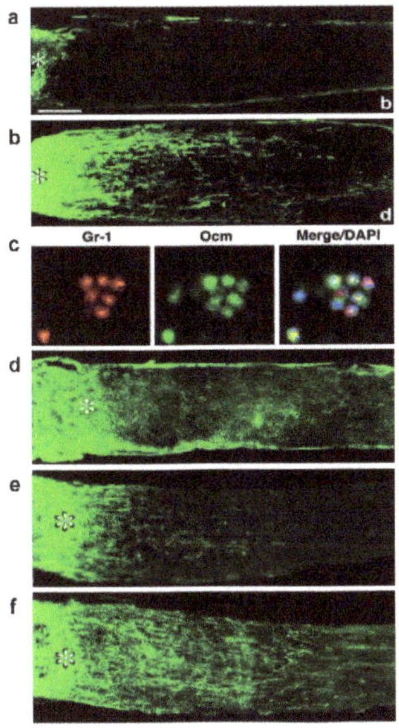

Figure 1. Inflammation-induced optic nerve regeneration and the role of Oncomodulin (Ocm). (**a**) Negative control: Absence of axon regeneration following optic nerve injury (asterisk: site of optic nerve crush injury). (**b**) Intraocular inflammation induced by injury to the lens (shown here) or by other means cited in the text enables retinal ganglion cells (RGCs) to regenerate axons past the injury site. (**c**) Intraocular inflammation is associated with a rapid infiltration of Gr-1-positive neutrophils (red) that express high levels of Ocm (green). (**d**) P1, a peptide antagonist of Ocm based on the N-terminus of the protein, suppresses Zymosan-induced regeneration. (**e**) Slow-release polymer beads containing the cAMP analog CPT-cAMP induce minimal regeneration after optic nerve injury. (**f**) Extensive regeneration with slow-release beads containing Ocm + CPT-cAMP [5,6,13].

4. Oncomodulin: A Key Mediator of Inflammation-Induced Regeneration

The first myeloid cell-derived protein found to play a key role in inflammation-induced regeneration is the 11 kDa Ca^{2+}-binding protein Oncomodulin (Ocm) [13]. Stimulating ocular inflammation via LI or intravitreal Zymosan injection elicits a massive influx of Ocm-expressing neutrophils into the vitreous (Figure 1c) and elevation of Ocm in the inner retina [5,13–15]. Ocm binds with high affinity to a cell-surface receptor on RGCs in a cAMP-dependent manner (Kd ~30 nM) [16] and, in the presence of a cAMP analog (or forskolin) plus D-mannose, enhances neurite outgrowth in cultured RGCs well beyond levels stimulated by well-established growth factors such as brain-derived neurotrophic factor (BDNF), fibroblast growth factor-2 (FGF2), ciliary neurotrophic factor (CNTF), or glial cell-derived neurotrophic factor (GDNF) [13]. In loss-of-function studies, a function-blocking anti-Ocm antibody or peptide antagonist of Ocm nearly eliminates inflammation-induced regeneration (Figure 1d) [5,13,14], while conversely, slow release of Ocm and a cAMP analog from polymer beads stimulates strong regeneration (Figure 1e,f) [15]. However, later studies showed that the beads alone induce some inflammation that contributes to these effects, implying that additional inflammation-associated factors complement the effects of Ocm in vivo.

5. Macrophage-Derived SDF1 Complements the Effects of Ocm

Subsequent studies found that stromal cell-derived factor 1 (SDF1, CXCL12) is highly expressed by infiltrative macrophages following intraocular inflammation (Figure 2a) and complements the effects of Ocm [8]. In cell culture, stimulation with SDF1 induces moderate axon outgrowth from RGCs, and, importantly, is the only factor among many tested (e.g., CNTF, BDNF, FGF2, GDNF, others) that enhances the effects of Ocm (Figure 2b) [8]. In vivo, Zymosan-induced axon regeneration and RGC survival are suppressed by either deleting SDF1 in myeloid cells (LysM-Cre: CXCL12$^{f/f}$ mice), deleting the primary SDF1 receptor, CXCR4, in RGCs (intraocular injection of adeno-associated virus seroform 2 expressing Cre recombinase in CXCR4$^{f/f}$ mice), or inhibiting this pathway with the CXCR4 antagonist, AMD3100 [8]. Conversely, SDF1 combined with Ocm and a cAMP analog induces as much regeneration and neuroprotection as Zymosan (Figure 2c), thus demonstrating the sufficiency of defined molecules in promoting regeneration.

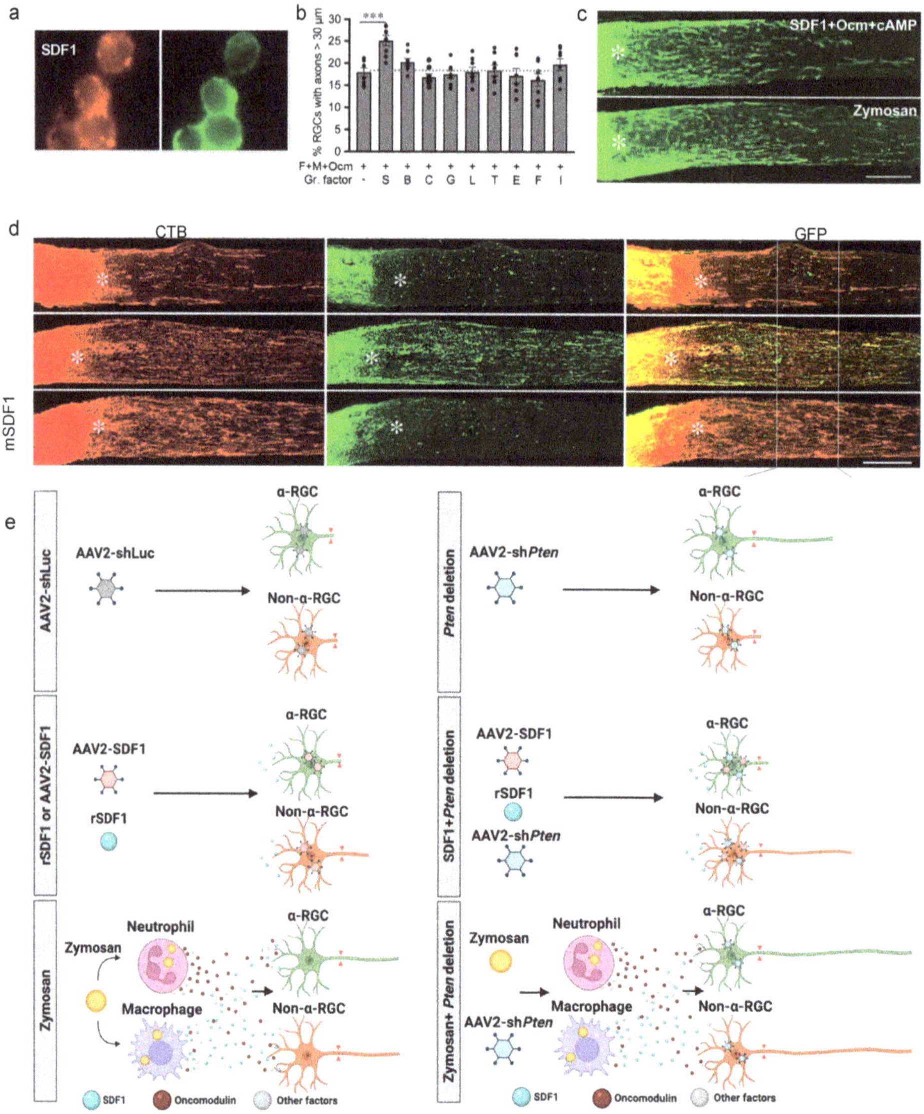

Figure 2. Macrophage-derived SDF1 complements the effects of Ocm (previous page). (**a**) SDF1 (red) is highly expressed in F4/80 macrophages that infiltrate the vitreous by 24 h after intraocular injection of Zymosan. (**b**) Among multiple trophic factors tested in dissociated adult retinal cell cultures,

SDF1 is the only factor that enhances the effects of Ocm (combined with co-factors mannose and CPT-cAMP). B: Brain-derived neurotrophic factor (BDNF); C: ciliary neurotrophic factor (CNTF); G: glial cell-derived trophic factor (GDNF); L: leukemia inhibitory factor (LIF); T: tumor-necrosis factor (TNF); F: fibroblast growth factor-2; I: insulin-like growth factor 2 (IGF2). *** $p < 0.001$. (**c**) SDF1 combined with Ocm and CPT-cAMP induces similar levels of regeneration as Zymosan. (**d**) SDF1 alters the response of different RGC populations to PTEN deletion. aRGCs, the population that extends axons in response to Pten deletion, are identified by virtue of expressing GFP from the Kcng4 promoter. Axons arising from all RGCs, whether aRGCs or non-aRGCs, are labeled with CTB. Top row: In response to SDF1 alone, regenerating GFP-negative axons all arise from non-aRGCs. Middle row: Pten deletion alone induces regeneration primarily from aRGCs (note extensive overlap of GFP and CTB in last panel). Bottom row: Combining SDF1 and Pten deletion suppresses regeneration from aRGCs while strongly increasing overall levels of regeneration from non-αRGCs. (**e**) Schematic illustration showing the response of different RGC populations to various treatments. Top row: AAV2 expressing anti-Pten shRNA (AAV2-shPten) induces axon growth primarily from aRGCs (green cells). AAV2-shLuciferase virus (AAV2-shLuc) has no effects. Middle row: Either recombinant SDF1 (rSDF1) or AAV2 expressing SDF1 (AAV2-SDF1) induces moderate axon growth primarily from non-aRGCs (middle left: orange cells). When combined with Pten deletion, SDF1 induces non-aRGCs to regenerate lengthy axons but prevents aRGCs from responding to Pten deletion (middle right). Bottom row: Zymosan elevates levels of neutrophil-derived Ocm, macrophage-derived SDF1, and other factors, stimulating regeneration from both α- and non-αRGCs (bottom left); Pten deletion combined with Zymosan strongly augments outgrowth from both subtypes (bottom right) [8]. Asterisks show lesion site.

Prior work showed that deleting the tumor-suppressor gene Pten in RGCs induces considerable axon regeneration that primarily arises from aRGC [17]. In contrast, SDF1 stimulates outgrowth in non-aRGCs and enables them to respond strongly to Pten deletion but paradoxically suppresses aRGCs' response to Pten deletion [8]. Zymosan, which elevates levels of both SDF1 and Ocm, stimulates outgrowth from aRGCs and non-aRGCs and amplifies the effects of Pten deletion for multiple RGC classes (Figure 2e).

6. CNTF Gene Therapy, like Zymosan and LI, Promotes Regeneration via Neuroinflammation

CNTF is a leading candidate for neuroprotection in several ocular diseases and has also been of considerable interest for optic nerve regeneration. Although one group has maintained that CNTF (and/or LIF) is the major mediator of inflammation-induced regeneration [18,19], our lab and others found that recombinant CNTF (rCNTF) has little or no effect on optic nerve regeneration (Figure 3a) unless SOCS3, a suppressor of the Jak-STAT signaling pathway, is deleted from RGCs [7,20–23]. On the other hand, many studies have found that CNTF gene therapy (i.e., adeno-associated virus AAV2 expressing CNTF) induces robust regeneration (Figure 3c) [22,24–31]. We discovered that CNTF gene therapy induces far more intraocular inflammation than rCNTF due to baseline inflammation associated with intraocular viral vectors [32] combined with the chemotactic effect of CNTF in amplifying this inflammation [33,34]. The effects of CNTF gene therapy are almost completely lost in mice lacking CCR2, a receptor involved in macrophage recruitment and polarization (Figure 3d,e), and in mice lacking neutrophils [22]. Further work identified the chemokine CCL5 acting on its cognate receptor, CCR5, as the primary mediator of the neuroprotective and pro-regenerative effects of CNTF gene therapy, with Ocm and SDF1 playing lesser roles. Deletion of CCR5 in RGCs or the CCR5 antagonist DAPTA strongly suppress the effects of CNTF gene therapy (Figure 3f,g), whereas recombinant CCL5 mimics these effects (Figure 3h). Thus, these results position CCL5 as another candidate therapy for optic nerve repair and perhaps other optic neuropathies [22].

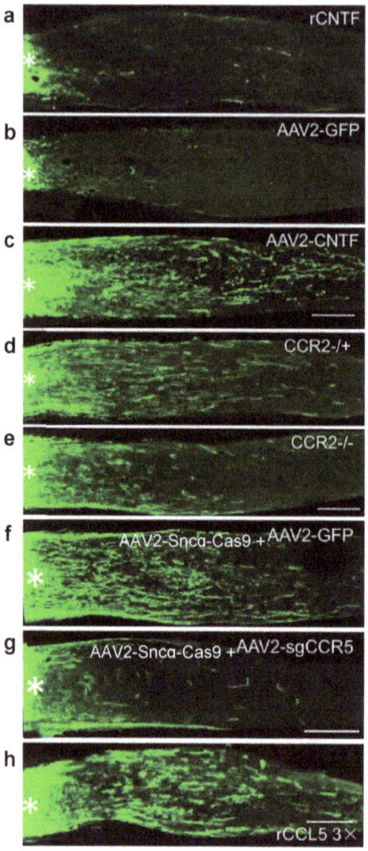

Figure 3. CNTF gene therapy induces optic nerve regeneration by augmenting inflammation and chemokine CCL5. (**a**) Recombinant CNTF protein (1 μg) does not induce appreciable regeneration. (**b**,**c**) Unlike a control adeno-associated protein expressing green fluorescent protein (AAV2-GFP), AAV2 expressing CNTF induces appreciable levels. (**d**,**e**) Whereas mice heterozygous for the chemokine 2 receptor ($CCR2^{+/-}$) regenerate axons in response to CNTF gene therapy (**d**), homozygous null mice show a strongly diminished response (**e**). (**f**,**g**) CRISPR-Cas9 mediated deletion of the chemokine 5 receptor CCR5. Mice received intraocular injection of an adeno-associated virus expressing Cas9 driven by the synuclein-g promoter plus a second virus expressing either GFP ((**f**), control) or a small guide RNA directed to CCR5 (**g**), which nearly eliminated regeneration induced by CNTF gene therapy. (**h**) Recombinant CCL5 induces nearly as much regeneration as CNTF gene therapy. Asterisks indicate lesion site [22].

7. Inflammatory Pre-Conditioning Enables Robust Axon Regeneration

Inducing LI 2 weeks prior to optic nerve injury increases regeneration to a far greater extent than LI or Zymosan applied at the time of nerve injury or by Zymosan preconditioning [35]. Repeated episodes of LI prior to and again after nerve injury transforms neurons into a strong growth state, enabling many RGCs to extend axons the full length of the optic nerve within a few weeks. This effect requires monocyte infiltration into the eye, whereas microglia, neutrophils, and T-cells are not required, nor does it depend upon any of the inflammation-induced growth factors that we have identified to date (Ocm, SDF1, CCL5: Feng et al., in preparation).

8. Synergy between Intraocular Inflammation and Counteracting Cell-Extrinsic Suppressors of Axon Growth

Following nerve injury, myelin debris, the scar that forms at the injury site, and axon-repellant guidance cues all suppress axon regeneration in the optic nerve and elsewhere in the CNS [36–38]. Axon regeneration induced by intraocular inflammation is augmented several-fold by deleting all isoforms of NgR, the receptor expressed on axons and nerve terminals that mediates growth-suppressive effects of the myelin-associated proteins oligodendrocyte-myelin glycoprotein (OMgp), myelin-associated glycoprotein (MAG), and, most potently, isoforms of the protein Nogo (Figure 4). Similarly synergistic effects are seen by combining intraocular inflammation with suppression of signaling through the small GTPase RhoA, which is intracellularly activated by growth-inhibitory signals, or by deleting PTPs, a receptor that mediates growth-suppressive effects of chondroitin sulfate proteoglycans (CSPGs) [39–42], or by enzymatically blocking the effects of chondroitin sulfate proteoglycans (CSPGs) [43]. Combined deletion of two isoforms of NgR plus PTPs results in extraordinary levels of regeneration when coupled with Zymosan-induced inflammation (Figure 4f) [40]. Axon regeneration can also be augmented by increasing inflammation within the optic nerve, presumably by increasing phagocytosis of myelin debris and elements of the fibrotic scar that forms at the injury site [44].

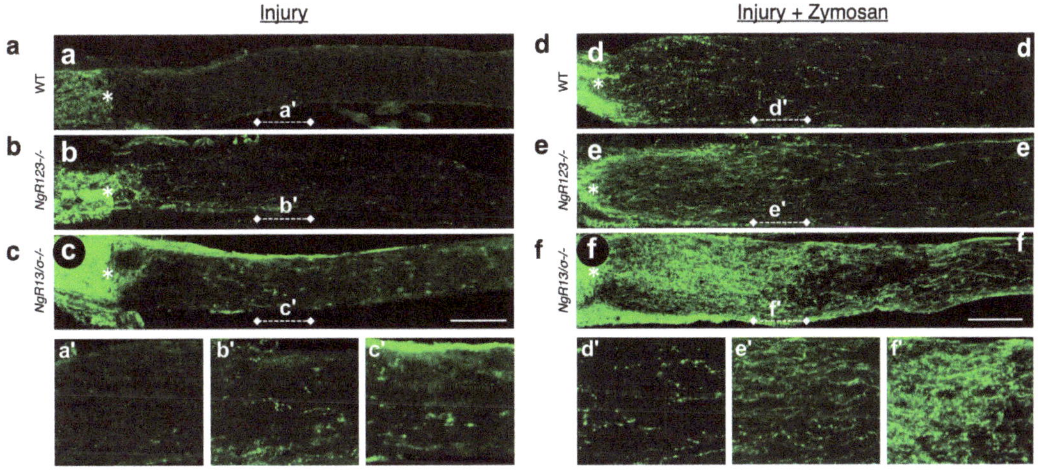

Figure 4. Synergy between intraocular inflammation and deleting receptors for cell-extrinsic suppressors of axon growth. (**a–f**) Longitudinal sections through the optic nerves of wild-type mice (WT) or mice lacking all 3 isoforms of the Nogo receptor (NgR123$^{-/-}$) or of NgR1 and 3 plus PTPs, a receptor that mediates inhibitory effects of chondroitin sulfate proteoglycans (CSPGs). As indicated, mice either underwent optic nerve injury alone or with intraocular inflammation following intraocular injection of zymosan. (**a'–f'**) Regions of optic nerves shown at greater magnification in the corresponding panels below. Note the dramatic increase in regeneration when combining intraocular inflammation with deletion of receptors for the inhibitory molecules associated with myelin and CSPGs. Asterisks show lesion site [40].

9. Role of Microglia in RGC Survival and Axon Regeneration

Microglia are the resident immune cells of the nervous system, and together with Mueller glia and astrocytes, they help maintain retinal homeostasis. Microglia are concentrated in the inner and outer plexiform layers of the retina and throughout the optic nerve, with long ramified processes that interact with and surveil the neural environment and regulate retinal synapses [45,46]. Non-homeostatic (or "reactive") microglia are characteristic of many neurodegenerative diseases, which, in the eye, include glaucoma [46–49], and photoreceptor degeneration [50,51]. It remains unclear whether a chronic microglial response is ultimately beneficial or harmful or whether the microglial response is modulated by other injury-induced signals, including the elevation of zinc or activation of the DLK and LZK kinase cascades in RGCs (Figure 5).

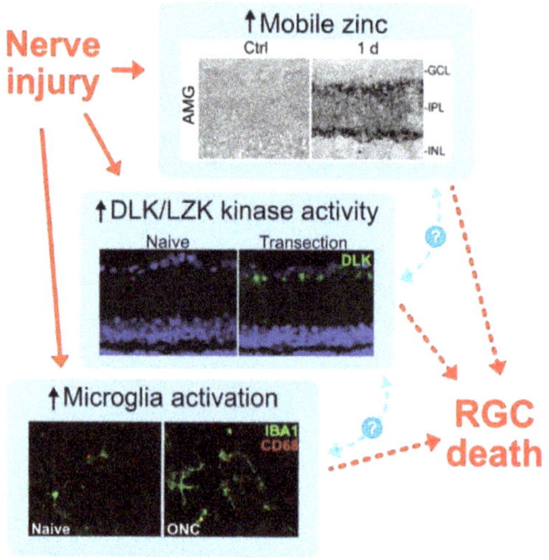

Figure 5. Injury-induced pathways contributing to RGC death after optic nerve injury. Encircled question marks (?) indicate as yet unknown relationships. Up arrows indicate increases.

Elevation of mobile zinc in the inner retina, activation of the DLK and LZK kinase cascades in RGCs, and reaction of resident microglia are hallmarks of optic nerve injury and have all been shown to modulate RGC death. However, mechanistic interactions among these three pathways remain unknown.

Animal studies indicate that reducing microglial activation in glaucoma and other CNS models reduces neuronal cell death and helps resolve neuroinflammation [52–55], supporting the idea that chronic neuroinflammation is harmful in CNS disease. Following optic nerve damage and in glaucoma, one proposed mechanism for RGC death is that reactive microglia express proteins that include tumor necrosis factor-α (TNFα), interleukin 1α (IL-1α), and the complement protein C1q, which together polarize astrocytes to a pro-inflammatory "A1" state [56–59]. A1 astrocytes can in turn promote synapse degradation and induce neuron and oligodendrocyte cell death by secreting long-chain saturated lipids APOE and APOJ-containing lipoparticles [46,56–62]. Although blocking A1 polarization is reported to be strongly neuroprotective after ONI and in mouse glaucoma models [56,58], it is unlikely that microglia are the sole source of A1-inducing proteins. Retinal Tnfa, Il1a, and C1qa expression are all upregulated 3–5 days after optic nerve injury, which correlates with the response timeline of microglia [63]; yet microglial depletion (with the Colony stimulating factor 1 receptor inhibitor PLX5622) does not substantially reduce Tnfa levels. These findings suggest that other cells such as Muller glia or astrocytes may play a role [64–67]. As TNFα signaling mediates RGC and oligodendrocyte death in animal models of glaucoma, likely by increasing the expression of Fas ligand [4,68,69], sustained Tnfa expression provides a plausible explanation for why microglial deletion is insufficient to provide neuroprotection [58,63,70].

One possible contributor to microglial activation in the retina is the elevation of mobile zinc (Zn^{2+}). After ONI, Zn^{2+} accumulates in presynaptic boutons of amacrine cells from which it is exocytosed, contributing to RGC death and repression of regeneration after ONI [71]. In cell culture, the elevation of extracellular Zn^{2+} exacerbates microglial activation to a pro-inflammatory M1 state, resulting in increased nitric oxide (NO) production and altered cytokine expression [72–75]. In vivo, reducing extracellular Zn^{2+} via intraocular Zn^{2+}

chelators or genetic knockout of the vesicular Zn^{2+} transporter ZnT3 reduces microglial activation after ONI [63,71], suggesting that Zn^{2+} elevation in the retina may be one factor contributing to the microglial response after ONI.

Yet, despite the well-documented negative aspects of microglial activation, microglia can play a beneficial role after optic nerve injury. These latter effects are mediated through complement pathway-induced activation of resident microglia and/or by increasing the infiltration of CR3-expressing monocytes/macrophages at the lesion site [44], where these cells phagocytose myelin debris (Figure 6a,b) that would otherwise inhibit axon regeneration [36,76,77]. Interfering with the classical complement pathway by deleting or neutralizing C1q, C3, or CR3 reduces axon regeneration and decreases MBP clearance in the lesion site [44].

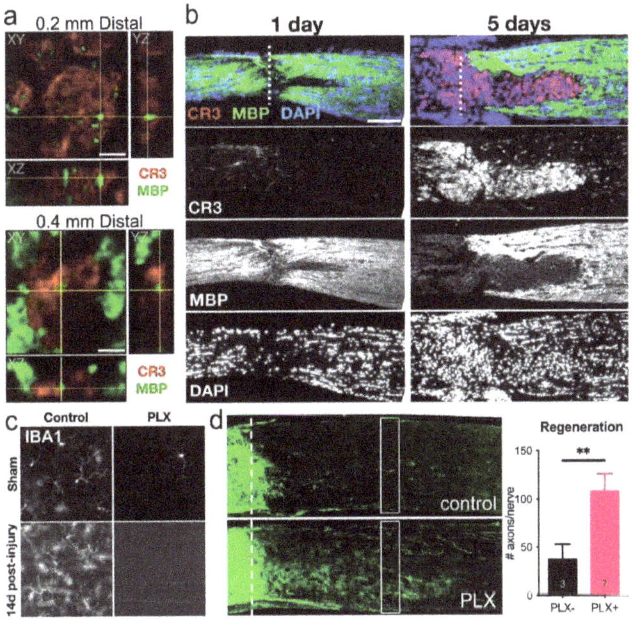

Figure 6. Phagocytic microglia/monocytes alter the local environment of the injury site and modulate axon regeneration. (**a**) Single confocal planes with orthogonal views of myelin basic protein (MBP) debris inside CR3+ cells. Images are from 0.2 and 0.4 mm distal to the injury site at 14 DPI [44]. (**b**) CR3+ microglia and monocytes expand within the site of injury (dotted line) from 1 to 5 days after crush, resulting in a progressive clearance of MBP from the distal optic nerve, allowing for uninhibited axon regeneration [44]. (**c**) Treatment with CSF1R inhibitor, PLX5622 (PLX) results in efficient clearance of IBA1+ microglia from the retina, which is maintained by 14 days after ONI (14d post-ONI). (**d**) Microglia deletion enhances the number of GAP43+ (green) axons regenerating past the crush site (dotted line). Right: Quantitation of regenerating axons 0.5 mm distal to the injury site (□); mean ± s.e.m, n = optic nerves, **, $p \leq 0.01$ by *t*-test [44].

However, in other contexts, ablating microglia can promote optic nerve regeneration (Figure 6c,d) [63]. The CX3CR1 antagonist PLX5622 eliminates ~95% of microglia in the retina, resulting in the loss of retinal Aif1 and C1qa expression within 14 days after ONI [44]. However, we observed only a partial reduction in Aif1 and C1qa and an increase in CR3+ monocytes at the injury site, suggesting a compensatory mechanism by which monocytes may infiltrate into a newly vacant microglial niche [44]. This enhanced CR3+ monocyte infiltration at the injury site is slow to resolve, thereby increasing myelin debris clearance and enhancing axon regeneration in several pro-regenerative treatment paradigms. Together, these results suggest that microglia and immune cells serve multiple and often opposing roles within complex and highly dynamic disease pathologies, highlighting the need for a more thorough understanding of how neuroimmune interactions shape disease pathology and for the development of new tools and therapies to differentially modulate pro-degenerative vs. pro-regenerative subpopulations or signals.

10. Neuroinflammation and RGC-Intrinsic Regulators of Survival and Axon Regeneration: Synergistic Effects

An important advance in the field of CNS repair was the discovery that modulating RGCs' intrinsic response to injury can induce considerable axon regeneration. As noted earlier, deletion of Pten, a lipid- and protein phosphatase that suppresses signaling through the PI3 kinase-Akt pathway, enables aRGCs and a small number of other RGCs to regenerate axons through the injured optic nerve [17,78]. Combining Pten deletion with Zymosan and a cAMP analog induces nearly 10 times the level of optic nerve regeneration as any of the individual treatments alone, and, with time, enables some RGCs to regenerate axons into the brain and form synapses in appropriate target areas (Figure 7) [15,79]. mTOR (mammalian target of rapamycin), a central regulator of cell growth, is an important downstream target of PI3 kinase, and disinhibiting mTOR or upregulating a proximate upstream regulator (cRheb1) also promotes optic nerve regeneration, albeit to a lesser extent than Pten deletion [78]. Manipulating cRheb is reported to synergize with increased RGC activity to enable some RGCs to regenerate axons into central target areas [80].

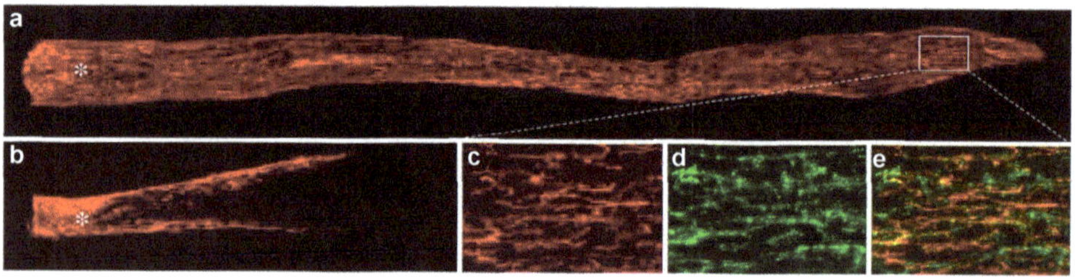

Figure 7. Full-length optic nerve regeneration. (**a**) Intraocular inflammation combined with CPT-cAMP and virally mediated PTEN deletion enables RGCs to regenerate axons the full length of the optic nerve in 8–10 weeks. Axons are labeled by intraocular injection of cholera toxin B fragment (CTB, red). (**b**) Control optic nerve in case treated with intraocular Zymosan and a control virus. (**c**–**e**) Enlargements of area within rectangle show overlap in immunostaining fibers for CTB (**c**, red) and the growth-associated protein GAP43 (**d**, green). Asterisks show lesion site [79].

SOCS3 (Suppressor of cytokine signaling) represses Jak-STAT signaling, the transduction pathway activated by CNTF and related factors (e.g., LIF, IL6), and its deletion in RGCs, like that of Pten, promotes optic nerve regeneration. Socs3 deletion also enables recombinant CNTF, which otherwise has little effect on its own, to augment regeneration beyond the level achieved with SOCS3 deletion alone [23]. Combining double deletion of Pten and Socs3 with CNTF treatment allows many axons to regenerate the full extent of the optic nerve and into the brain, albeit into largely inappropriate areas [81,82]. With long survival times, however, some of these axons become able to drive postsynaptic responses in the suprachiasmatic nucleus [83].

By virtue of regulating cells' program of gene expression, transcription factors represent another key determinant of RGC survival and regenerative capacity. Various members of the Krüppel-like family (KLF) of transcription factors regulate axon outgrowth in RGCs and other neurons [20,84,85]. Deletion of Klf4 promotes a modest level of axon regeneration [84], largely by de-repressing signaling through the Jak-STAT pathway [86]; yet, overexpressing Klf4 along with the transcription factors Oct4 and Sox2 restores immature DNA methylation and transcriptome patterns in RGCs and promotes axon regeneration after optic nerve injury [87]. Deletion of another Krüppel-like TF, Klf9, promotes greater levels of axon regeneration after optic nerve injury than Klf4 deletion [88], an effect that is enhanced even further by combining Klf9 deletion with intraocular Zn^{2+} chelation [89].

One unbiased approach to identifying "master regulators" of the regenerative state is to identify transcription factors that regulate the expression of regeneration-associated genes (RAGs). Using whole-transcriptome RNA sequencing, we identified differentially expressed genes (DEGs) associated with a strong regenerative state in RGCs (Pten deletion combined with the inflammation-associated protein Ocm and a cAMP analog) compared to untreated RGCs. Analysis of cis-regulatory regions of these DEGs predicted the transcriptional and epigenetic repressor REST (NRSF) to be a major repressor of RAGs, a prediction borne out in studies showing that Rest deletion or expression of a dominant-negative Rest mutant promotes considerable axon regeneration and enhances RGC survival after optic nerve injury [90].

Regarding other important cell-intrinsic pathways, Dual leucine zipper kinase (DLK; MAP3K12) and Leucine zipper kinase (LZK; MAP3K13) have been found to be key mediators of RGC cell death after injury [91–93]. DLK/LZK activation by axonal injury triggers a retrograde kinase signaling cascade involving MKK4/7 and JNK1-3 that elevates the expression and/or activation of transcription factors that include cJUN, ATF2, MEF2A, and SOX11 [92]. Yet, while repression of DLK and LZK is highly neuroprotective, their deletion suppresses axon regeneration induced by either Pten deletion [91] or Zymosan plus a cAMP analog [94]. Thus, although inhibition of DLK and LZK greatly prolongs RGC survival, this strategy may be insufficient to halt the visual decline in optic neuropathies. Further investigation into the gene regulatory networks downstream of DLK and LZK may enable us to determine if the networks that regulate cell survival vs. axon regeneration diverge such that more focused manipulations might improve both RGC survival and axon regeneration [94]. Newer research from Welsbie and colleagues shows that, unlike DLK and LZK, germinal cell kinase IV (GCK IV) kinases suppress both RGC survival and axon regeneration, and that their deletion in mice is both neuroprotective and amplifies the effects of Pten deletion in promoting optic nerve regeneration [95].

11. Prospectives

Transcriptomic comparisons of successfully regenerating RGCs and non-regenerating "bystanders", single-cell sequencing, large-scale screening of transcription factors and protein kinases, and other modern methods are steadily identifying new therapeutic candidates to enhance RGC survival and axon regeneration after optic nerve injury [92,93,95–98], lending hope to the possibility that robust RGC neuroprotection and axon regeneration may become a reality in the next 5–10 years. With this goal in sight, the field will also now need to focus on ways to restore at least crude image vision, including the myelination of regenerating axons [99,100] and navigation of regenerating axons to appropriate relay centers in the di- and mesencephalon, where they would need to establish synaptic connections that enable a topographic representation of visual space.

12. Conclusions

Although inflammation can have severely negative effects in certain ocular diseases, sterile inflammation in the eye promotes RGC survival and axon regeneration after optic nerve injury through the expression of immune-derived factors that include Ocm, SDF1, the chemokine CCL5, which mediates most of the effects of CNTF gene therapy, and by enhanced phagocytic activity within the optic nerve. As inflammation is an inevitable feature of neural damage, one important goal will be to learn how to modulate the immune response to optimize outcome; a second goal is to identify additional immune-derived factors that can enhance RGC survival and these cells' ability to form connections with central target areas. Finally, no single approach has yet proven to be a "silver bullet" for restoring visual connections after optic nerve injury, pointing to the likely continuing need for combinatorial treatments to improve functional outcome after optic nerve damage.

Author Contributions: Conceptualization: L.I.B.; Initial draft, editing: K.A.W. and L.I.B.; All authors have read and agreed to the published version of the manuscript.

Funding: This work was supported by the Gilbert Family Foundation Vision Restoration Initiative (to L.I.B.), The Miriam and Sheldon G. Adelson Medical Research Foundation (to L.I.B.), the NIH Intellectual and Developmental Disabilities Research Centers Imaging Core (HD018655) of Boston Children's Hospital, and BrightFocus National Glaucoma Research Postdoctoral Award (to K.A.W.).

Conflicts of Interest: The authors declare no conflict of interest.

References

1. Ramon y Cajal, S. *Degeneration and Regeneration of the Nervous System*; Oxford University Press: New York, NY, USA, 1991; Volume 5.
2. Chen, H.; Cho, K.; Vu, T.; Shen, C.; Kaur, M.; Chen, G.; Mathew, R.; McHam, M.; Fazelat, A.; Lashkari, K.; et al. Commensal microflora-induced T cell responses mediate progressive neurodegeneration in glaucoma. *Nat. Commun.* **2018**, *9*, 3209. [CrossRef] [PubMed]
3. Krishnan, A.; Fei, F.; Jones, A.; Busto, P.; Marshak-Rothstein, A.; Ksander, B.R.; Gregory-Ksander, M. Overexpression of Soluble Fas Ligand following Adeno-Associated Virus Gene Therapy Prevents Retinal Ganglion Cell Death in Chronic and Acute Murine Models of Glaucoma. *J. Immunol.* **2016**, *197*, 4626–4638. [CrossRef] [PubMed]
4. Roh, M.; Zhang, Y.; Murakami, Y.; Thanos, A.; Lee, S.C.; Vavvas, D.G.; Benowitz, L.I.; Miller, J.W. Etanercept, a widely used inhibitor of tumor necrosis factor-alpha (TNF-alpha), prevents retinal ganglion cell loss in a rat model of glaucoma. *PLoS ONE* **2012**, *7*, e40065. [CrossRef]
5. Yin, Y.; Cui, Q.; Gilbert, H.; Yang, Y.; Yang, Z.; Berlinicke, C.; Li, Z.; Zaverucha-do-Valle, C.; He, H.; Petkova, V.; et al. Oncomodulin links inflammation to optic nerve regeneration. *Proc. Natl. Acad. Sci. USA* **2009**, *106*, 19587–19592. [CrossRef]
6. Yin, Y.; Cui, Q.; Li, Y.; Irwin, N.; Fischer, D.; Harvey, A.R.; Benowitz, L.I. Macrophage-derived factors stimulate optic nerve regeneration. *J. Neurosci.* **2003**, *23*, 2284–2293. [CrossRef]
7. Leon, S.; Yin, Y.; Nguyen, J.; Irwin, N.; Benowitz, L. Lens injury stimulates axon regeneration in the mature rat optic nerve. *J. Neurosci.* **2000**, *20*, 4615–4626. [CrossRef]
8. Xie, L.; Cen, L.P.; Li, Y.; Gilbert, H.Y.; Strelko, O.; Berlinicke, C.; Stavarache, M.A.; Ma, M.; Wang, Y.; Cui, Q.; et al. Monocyte-derived SDF1 supports optic nerve regeneration and alters retinal ganglion cells' response to Pten deletion. *Proc. Natl. Acad. Sci. USA* **2022**, *119*, e2113751119. [CrossRef]
9. Liu, Y.F.; Liang, J.J.; Ng, T.K.; Hu, Z.; Xu, C.; Chen, S.; Chen, S.L.; Xu, Y.; Zhuang, X.; Huang, S.; et al. CXCL5/CXCR2 modulates inflammation-mediated neural repair after optic nerve injury. *Exp. Neurol.* **2021**, *341*, 113711. [CrossRef]
10. Hauk, T.G.; Leibinger, M.; Muller, A.; Andreadaki, A.; Knippschild, U.; Fischer, D. Stimulation of axon regeneration in the mature optic nerve by intravitreal application of the toll-like receptor 2 agonist Pam3Cys. *Invest. Ophthalmol. Vis. Sci.* **2010**, *51*, 459–464. [CrossRef]
11. Baldwin, K.T.; Carbajal, K.S.; Segal, B.M.; Giger, R.J. Neuroinflammation triggered by beta-glucan/dectin-1 signaling enables CNS axon regeneration. *Proc. Natl. Acad. Sci. USA* **2015**, *112*, 2581–2586. [CrossRef]
12. Sas, A.R.; Carbajal, K.S.; Jerome, A.D.; Menon, R.; Yoon, C.; Kalinski, A.L.; Giger, R.J.; Segal, B.M. A new neutrophil subset promotes CNS neuron survival and axon regeneration. *Nat. Immunol.* **2020**, *21*, 1496–1505. [CrossRef]
13. Yin, Y.; Henzl, M.; Lorber, B.; Nakazawa, T.; Thomas, T.; Jiang, F.; Langer, R.; Benowitz, L. Oncomodulin is a macrophage-derived signal for axon regeneration in retinal ganglion cells. *Nat. Neurosci.* **2006**, *9*, 843–852. [CrossRef] [PubMed]
14. Kurimoto, T.; Yin, Y.; Habboub, G.; Gilbert, H.; Li, Y.; Nakao, S.; Hafezi-Moghadam, A.; Benowitz, L. Neutrophils express oncomodulin and promote optic nerve regeneration. *J. Neurosci.* **2013**, *33*, 14816–14824. [CrossRef] [PubMed]
15. Kurimoto, T.; Yin, Y.; Omura, K.; Gilbert, H.; Kim, D.; Cen, L.; Moko, L.; Kügler, S.; Benowitz, L. Long-distance axon regeneration in the mature optic nerve: Contributions of oncomodulin, cAMP, and pten gene deletion. *J. Neurosci.* **2010**, *30*, 15654–15663. [CrossRef] [PubMed]
16. Xie, L.; Yin, Y.; Peterson, S.L.; Jayakar, S.; Shi, C.; Lenfers Turnes, B.; Zhang, Z.; Oses-Prieto, J.; Li, J.; Burlingame, A.; et al. The atypical receptor-ligand pair Ocm-R/oncomodulin enables axon regeneration in the central and peripheral nervous systems. In Proceedings of the Society for Neuroscience, San Diego, CA, USA, 12–16 November2022.
17. Duan, X.; Qiao, M.; Bei, F.; Kim, I.J.; He, Z.; Sanes, J.R. Subtype-specific regeneration of retinal ganglion cells following axotomy: Effects of osteopontin and mTOR signaling. *Neuron* **2015**, *85*, 1244–1256. [CrossRef] [PubMed]
18. Leibinger, M.; Muller, A.; Andreadaki, A.; Hauk, T.G.; Kirsch, M.; Fischer, D. Neuroprotective and axon growth-promoting effects following inflammatory stimulation on mature retinal ganglion cells in mice depend on ciliary neurotrophic factor and leukemia inhibitory factor. *J. Neurosci.* **2009**, *29*, 14334–14341. [CrossRef]
19. Leibinger, M.; Andreadaki, A.; Diekmann, H.; Fischer, D. Neuronal STAT3 activation is essential for CNTF- and inflammatory stimulation-induced CNS axon regeneration. *Cell Death Dis.* **2013**, *4*, e805. [CrossRef]
20. Veldman, M.B.; Bemben, M.A.; Goldman, D. Tuba1a gene expression is regulated by KLF6/7 and is necessary for CNS development and regeneration in zebrafish. *Mol. Cell Neurosci.* **2010**, *43*, 370–383. [CrossRef]

21. Pernet, V.; Di Polo, A. Synergistic action of brain-derived neurotrophic factor and lens injury promotes retinal ganglion cell survival, but leads to optic nerve dystrophy in vivo. *Brain* **2006**, *129*, 1014–1026. [CrossRef]
22. Xie, L.; Yin, Y.; Benowitz, L. Chemokine CCL5 promotes robust optic nerve regeneration and mediates many of the effects of CNTF gene therapy. *Proc. Natl. Acad. Sci. USA* **2021**, *118*, e2017282118. [CrossRef]
23. Smith, P.D.; Sun, F.; Park, K.K.; Cai, B.; Wang, C.; Kuwako, K.; Martinez-Carrasco, I.; Connolly, L.; He, Z. SOCS3 deletion promotes optic nerve regeneration in vivo. *Neuron* **2009**, *64*, 617–623. [CrossRef] [PubMed]
24. Bray, E.R.; Yungher, B.J.; Levay, K.; Ribeiro, M.; Dvoryanchikov, G.; Ayupe, A.C.; Thakor, K.; Marks, V.; Randolph, M.; Danzi, M.C.; et al. Thrombospondin-1 Mediates Axon Regeneration in Retinal Ganglion Cells. *Neuron* **2019**, *103*, 642–657.e7. [CrossRef] [PubMed]
25. Leaver, S.G.; Cui, Q.; Plant, G.W.; Arulpragasam, A.; Hisheh, S.; Verhaagen, J.; Harvey, A.R. AAV-mediated expression of CNTF promotes long-term survival and regeneration of adult rat retinal ganglion cells. *Gene Ther.* **2006**, *13*, 1328–1341. [CrossRef]
26. Pernet, V.; Joly, S.; Dalkara, D.; Jordi, N.; Schwarz, O.; Christ, F.; Schaffer, D.V.; Flannery, J.G.; Schwab, M.E. Long-distance axonal regeneration induced by CNTF gene transfer is impaired by axonal misguidance in the injured adult optic nerve. *Neurobiol. Dis.* **2013**, *51*, 202–213. [CrossRef] [PubMed]
27. Yungher, B.J.; Ribeiro, M.; Park, K.K. Regenerative Responses and Axon Pathfinding of Retinal Ganglion Cells in Chronically Injured Mice. *Invest. Ophthalmol. Vis. Sci.* **2017**, *58*, 1743–1750. [CrossRef]
28. Yungher, B.J.; Luo, X.; Salgueiro, Y.; Blackmore, M.G.; Park, K.K. Viral vector-based improvement of optic nerve regeneration: Characterization of individual axons' growth patterns and synaptogenesis in a visual target. *Gene Ther.* **2015**, *22*, 811–821. [CrossRef] [PubMed]
29. Luo, X.; Ribeiro, M.; Bray, E.R.; Lee, D.H.; Yungher, B.J.; Mehta, S.T.; Thakor, K.A.; Diaz, F.; Lee, J.K.; Moraes, C.T.; et al. Enhanced Transcriptional Activity and Mitochondrial Localization of STAT3 Co-induce Axon Regrowth in the Adult Central Nervous System. *Cell Rep.* **2016**, *15*, 398–410. [CrossRef]
30. Bei, F.; Lee, H.H.C.; Liu, X.; Gunner, G.; Jin, H.; Ma, L.; Wang, C.; Hou, L.; Hensch, T.K.; Frank, E.; et al. Restoration of Visual Function by Enhancing Conduction in Regenerated Axons. *Cell* **2016**, *164*, 219–232. [CrossRef]
31. Hellstrom, M.; Pollett, M.A.; Harvey, A.R. Post-injury delivery of rAAV2-CNTF combined with short-term pharmacotherapy is neuroprotective and promotes extensive axonal regeneration after optic nerve trauma. *J. Neurotrauma* **2011**, *28*, 2475–2483. [CrossRef]
32. Liu, Y.F.; Huang, S.; Ng, T.K.; Liang, J.J.; Xu, Y.; Chen, S.L.; Xu, C.; Zhang, M.; Pang, C.P.; Cen, L.P. Longitudinal evaluation of immediate inflammatory responses after intravitreal AAV2 injection in rats by optical coherence tomography. *Exp. Eye Res.* **2020**, *193*, 107955. [CrossRef]
33. Cen, L.P.; Luo, J.M.; Zhang, C.W.; Fan, Y.M.; Song, Y.; So, K.F.; van Rooijen, N.; Pang, C.P.; Lam, D.S.; Cui, Q. Chemotactic effect of ciliary neurotrophic factor on macrophages in retinal ganglion cell survival and axonal regeneration. *Invest. Ophthalmol. Vis. Sci.* **2007**, *48*, 4257–4266. [CrossRef] [PubMed]
34. Kobayashi, H.; Mizisin, A.P. CNTFR alpha alone or in combination with CNTF promotes macrophage chemotaxis in vitro. *Neuropeptides* **2000**, *34*, 338–347. [CrossRef] [PubMed]
35. Feng, Q.; Wong, K.A.; Peterson, S.L.; Benowitz, L. Harnessing neuroinflammation to promote axon regeneration after optic nerve injury. In Proceedings of the Association for Research in Vision and Ophthalmology Annual Meeting, Vancouver, BC, Canada, 28 April–2 May 2019.
36. Schwab, M.E. Nogo and axon regeneration. *Curr. Opin. Neurobiol.* **2004**, *14*, 118–124. [CrossRef] [PubMed]
37. Fawcett, J.W.; Schwab, M.E.; Montani, L.; Brazda, N.; Muller, H.W. Defeating inhibition of regeneration by scar and myelin components. *Handb. Clin. Neurol.* **2012**, *109*, 503–522. [CrossRef]
38. Tran, A.P.; Warren, P.M.; Silver, J. The Biology of Regeneration Failure and Success After Spinal Cord Injury. *Physiol. Rev.* **2018**, *98*, 881–917. [CrossRef]
39. Fischer, D.; He, Z.; Benowitz, L.I. Counteracting the Nogo receptor enhances optic nerve regeneration if retinal ganglion cells are in an active growth state. *J. Neurosci.* **2004**, *24*, 1646–1651. [CrossRef]
40. Dickendesher, T.L.; Baldwin, K.T.; Mironova, Y.A.; Koriyama, Y.; Raiker, S.J.; Askew, K.L.; Wood, A.; Geoffroy, C.G.; Zheng, B.; Liepmann, C.D.; et al. NgR1 and NgR3 are receptors for chondroitin sulfate proteoglycans. *Nat. Neurosci.* **2012**, *15*, 703–712. [CrossRef]
41. Wang, X.; Hasan, O.; Arzeno, A.; Benowitz, L.I.; Cafferty, W.B.; Strittmatter, S.M. Axonal regeneration induced by blockade of glial inhibitors coupled with activation of intrinsic neuronal growth pathways. *Exp. Neurol.* **2012**, *237*, 55–69. [CrossRef]
42. Shen, Y.; Tenney, A.P.; Busch, S.A.; Horn, K.P.; Cuascut, F.X.; Liu, K.; He, Z.; Silver, J.; Flanagan, J.G. PTPsigma is a receptor for chondroitin sulfate proteoglycan, an inhibitor of neural regeneration. *Science* **2009**, *326*, 592–596. [CrossRef]
43. Pearson, C.S.; Mencio, C.P.; Barber, A.C.; Martin, K.R.; Geller, H.M. Identification of a critical sulfation in chondroitin that inhibits axonal regeneration. *eLife* **2018**, *7*, e37139. [CrossRef]
44. Peterson, S.; Li, Y.; Sun, C.; Wong, K.; Leung, K.; de Lima, S.; Hanovice, N.; Yuki, K.; Stevens, B.; Benowitz, L. Retinal Ganglion Cell Axon Regeneration Requires Complement and Myeloid Cell Activity within the Optic Nerve. *J. Neurosci.* **2021**, *41*, 8508–8531. [CrossRef]

45. Schafer, D.; Lehrman, E.; Kautzman, A.; Koyama, R.; Mardinly, A.; Yamasaki, R.; Ransohoff, R.; Greenberg, M.; Barres, B.; Stevens, B. Microglia sculpt postnatal neural circuits in an activity and complement-dependent manner. *Neuron* **2012**, *74*, 691–705. [CrossRef]
46. Stevens, B.; Allen, N.; Vazquez, L.; Howell, G.; Christopherson, K.; Nouri, N.; Micheva, K.; Mehalow, A.; Huberman, A.; Stafford, B.; et al. The classical complement cascade mediates CNS synapse elimination. *Cell* **2007**, *131*, 1164–1178. [CrossRef] [PubMed]
47. Williams, P.A.; Marsh-Armstrong, N.; Howell, G.R.; Bosco, A.; Danias, J.; Simon, J.; Di Polo, A.; Kuehn, M.H.; Przedborski, S.; Raff, M.; et al. Neuroinflammation in glaucoma: A new opportunity. *Exp. Eye Res.* **2017**, *157*, 20–27. [CrossRef] [PubMed]
48. Bosco, A.; Breen, K.; Anderson, S.; Steele, M.; Calkins, D.; Vetter, M. Glial coverage in the optic nerve expands in proportion to optic axon loss in chronic mouse glaucoma. *Exp. Eye Res.* **2016**, *150*, 34–43. [CrossRef]
49. Bosco, A.; Romero, C.; Breen, K.; Chagovetz, A.; Steele, M.; Ambati, B.; Vetter, M. Neurodegeneration severity can be predicted from early microglia alterations monitored in vivo in a mouse model of chronic glaucoma. *Dis. Models Mech.* **2015**, *8*, 443–455. [CrossRef]
50. Ramirez, A.; de Hoz, R.; Salobrar-Garcia, E.; Salazar, J.; Rojas, B.; Ajoy, D.; López-Cuenca, I.; Rojas, P.; Triviño, A.; Ramírez, J. The Role of Microglia in Retinal Neurodegeneration: Alzheimer's Disease, Parkinson, and Glaucoma. *Front. Aging Neurosci.* **2017**, *9*, 214. [CrossRef] [PubMed]
51. Renner, M.; Stute, G.; Alzureiqi, M.; Reinhard, J.; Wiemann, S.; Schmid, H.; Faissner, A.; Dick, H.; Joachim, S. Optic Nerve Degeneration after Retinal Ischemia/Reperfusion in a Rodent Model. *Front. Cell Neurosci.* **2017**, *11*, 254. [CrossRef]
52. Bosco, A.; Inman, D.; Steele, M.; Wu, G.; Soto, I.; Marsh-Armstrong, N.; Hubbard, W.; Calkins, D.; Horner, P.; Vetter, M. Reduced retina microglial activation and improved optic nerve integrity with minocycline treatment in the DBA/2J mouse model of glaucoma. *Invest. Ophthalmol. Vis. Sci.* **2008**, *49*, 1437–1446. [CrossRef]
53. Kumar, V.; Singh, B.; Chauhan, A.; Singh, D.; Patel, D.; Singh, C. Minocycline Rescues from Zinc-Induced Nigrostriatal Dopaminergic Neurodegeneration: Biochemical and Molecular Interventions. *Mol. Neurobiol.* **2016**, *53*, 2761–2777. [CrossRef]
54. Rice, R.; Pham, J.; Lee, R.; Najafi, A.; West, B.; Green, K. Microglial repopulation resolves inflammation and promotes brain recovery after injury. *Glia* **2017**, *65*, 931–944. [CrossRef] [PubMed]
55. Takeda, A.; Shinozaki, Y.; Kashiwagi, K.; Ohno, N.; Eto, K.; Wake, H.; Nabekura, J.; Koizumi, S. Microglia mediate non-cell-autonomous cell death of retinal ganglion cells. *Glia* **2018**, *66*, 2366–2384. [CrossRef] [PubMed]
56. Guttenplan, K.A.; Stafford, B.K.; El-Danaf, R.N.; Adler, D.I.; Münch, A.E.; Weigel, M.K.; Huberman, A.D.; Liddelow, S.A. Neurotoxic Reactive Astrocytes Drive Neuronal Death after Retinal Injury. *Cell Rep.* **2020**, *31*, 107776. [CrossRef] [PubMed]
57. Guttenplan, K.A.; Weigel, M.K.; Prakash, P.; Wijewardhane, P.R.; Hasel, P.; Rufen-Blanchette, U.; Münch, A.E.; Blum, J.A.; Fine, J.; Neal, M.C.; et al. Neurotoxic reactive astrocytes induce cell death via saturated lipids. *Nature* **2021**, *599*, 102–107. [CrossRef]
58. Liddelow, S.; Guttenplan, K.; Clarke, L.; Bennett, F.; Bohlen, C.; Schirmer, L.; Bennett, M.; Münch, A.; Chung, W.; Peterson, T.; et al. Neurotoxic reactive astrocytes are induced by activated microglia. *Nature* **2017**, *541*, 481–487. [CrossRef]
59. Zamanian, J.; Xu, L.; Foo, L.; Nouri, N.; Zhou, L.; Giffard, R.; Barres, B. Genomic analysis of reactive astrogliosis. *J. Neurosci.* **2012**, *32*, 6391–6410. [CrossRef]
60. Bi, F.; Huang, C.; Tong, J.; Qiu, G.; Huang, B.; Wu, Q.; Li, F.; Xu, Z.; Bowser, R.; Xia, X.; et al. Reactive astrocytes secrete lcn2 to promote neuron death. *Proc. Natl. Acad. Sci. USA* **2013**, *110*, 4069–4074. [CrossRef]
61. Lebrun-Julien, F.; Duplan, L.; Pernet, V.; Osswald, I.; Sapieha, P.; Bourgeois, P.; Dickson, K.; Bowie, D.; Barker, P.; Di Polo, A. Excitotoxic death of retinal neurons in vivo occurs via a non-cell-autonomous mechanism. *J. Neurosci.* **2009**, *29*, 5536–5545. [CrossRef]
62. Sofroniew, M. Multiple roles for astrocytes as effectors of cytokines and inflammatory mediators. *Neuroscientist* **2014**, *20*, 160–172. [CrossRef]
63. Wong, K.A.; Peterson, S.; Benowitz, L. Zinc and microglia regulate retinal ganglion cell survival and axon regeneration after optic nerve injury. *Invest. Ophthalmol. Vis. Sci.* **2019**, *60*, 5176.
64. Li, Q.; Cheng, Y.; Zhang, S.; Sun, X.; Wu, J. TRPV4-induced Müller cell gliosis and TNF-α elevation-mediated retinal ganglion cell apoptosis in glaucomatous rats via JAK2/STAT3/NF-κB pathway. *J. Neuroinflammation* **2021**, *18*, 271. [CrossRef] [PubMed]
65. Nelson, C.; Ackerman, K.; O'Hayer, P.; Bailey, T.; Gorsuch, R.; Hyde, D. Tumor necrosis factor-alpha is produced by dying retinal neurons and is required for Muller glia proliferation during zebrafish retinal regeneration. *J. Neurosci.* **2013**, *33*, 6524–6539. [CrossRef] [PubMed]
66. Tezel, G.; Wax, M.B. Increased production of tumor necrosis factor-α by glial cells exposed to simulated ischemia or elevated hydrostatic pressure induces apoptosis in cocultured retinal ganglion cells. *J. Neurosci.* **2000**, *20*, 8693–8700. [CrossRef]
67. Lebrun-Julien, F.; Bertrand, M.J.; De Backer, O.; Stellwagen, D.; Morales, C.R.; Di Polo, A.; Barker, P.A. ProNGF induces TNFalpha-dependent death of retinal ganglion cells through a p75NTR non-cell-autonomous signaling pathway. *Proc. Natl. Acad. Sci. USA* **2010**, *107*, 3817–3822. [CrossRef] [PubMed]
68. Nakazawa, T.; Nakazawa, C.; Matsubara, A.; Noda, K.; Hisatomi, T.; She, H.; Michaud, N.; Hafezi-Moghadam, A.; Miller, J.; Benowitz, L. Tumor necrosis factor-alpha mediates oligodendrocyte death and delayed retinal ganglion cell loss in a mouse model of glaucoma. *J. Neurosci.* **2006**, *26*, 12633–12641. [CrossRef]

69. Krishnan, A.; Kocab, A.J.; Zacks, D.N.; Marshak-Rothstein, A.; Gregory-Ksander, M. A small peptide antagonist of the Fas receptor inhibits neuroinflammation and prevents axon degeneration and retinal ganglion cell death in an inducible mouse model of glaucoma. *J. Neuroinflammation* **2019**, *16*, 184. [CrossRef] [PubMed]
70. Hilla, A.; Diekmann, H.; Fischer, D. Microglia Are Irrelevant for Neuronal Degeneration and Axon Regeneration after Acute Injury. *J. Neurosci.* **2017**, *37*, 6113–6124. [CrossRef] [PubMed]
71. Li, Y.; Andereggen, L.; Yuki, K.; Omura, K.; Yin, Y.; Gilbert, H.; Erdogan, B.; Asdourian, M.; Shrock, C.; de Lima, S.; et al. Mobile zinc increases rapidly in the retina after optic nerve injury and regulates ganglion cell survival and optic nerve regeneration. *Proc. Natl. Acad. Sci. USA* **2017**, *114*, E209–E218. [CrossRef]
72. Higashi, Y.; Aratake, T.; Shimizu, S.; Shimizu, T.; Nakamura, K.; Tsuda, M.; Yawata, T.; Ueba, T.; Saito, M. Influence of extracellular zinc on M1 microglial activation. *Sci Rep.* **2017**, *7*, 43778. [CrossRef]
73. Higashi, Y.; Segawa, S.; Matsuo, T.; Nakamura, S.; Kikkawa, Y.; Nishida, K.; Nagasawa, K. Microglial zinc uptake via zinc transporters induces ATP release and the activation of microglia. *Glia* **2011**, *59*, 1933–1945. [CrossRef]
74. Kauppinen, T.; Higashi, Y.; Suh, S.; Escartin, C.; Nagasawa, K.; Swanson, R. Zinc triggers microglial activation. *J. Neurosci.* **2008**, *28*, 5827–5835. [CrossRef]
75. Ueba, Y.; Aratake, T.; Onodera, K.; Higashi, Y.; Hamada, T.; Shimizu, T.; Shimizu, S.; Yawata, T.; Nakamura, R.; Akizawa, T.; et al. Attenuation of zinc-enhanced inflammatory M1 phenotype of microglia by peridinin protects against short-term spatial-memory impairment following cerebral ischemia in mice. *Biochem. Biophys. Res. Commun.* **2018**, *507*, 476–483. [CrossRef]
76. Brück, W.; Friede, R. The role of complement in myelin phagocytosis during PNS wallerian degeneration. *J. Neurol. Sci.* **1991**, *103*, 182–187. [CrossRef]
77. Neumann, H.; Kotter, M.; Franklin, R. Debris clearance by microglia: An essential link between degeneration and regeneration. *Brain* **2009**, *132*, 288–295. [CrossRef]
78. Park, K.; Liu, K.; Hu, Y.; Smith, P.; Wang, C.; Cai, B.; Xu, B.; Connolly, L.; Kramvis, I.; Sahin, M.; et al. Promoting axon regeneration in the adult CNS by modulation of the PTEN/mTOR pathway. *Science* **2008**, *322*, 963–966. [CrossRef]
79. de Lima, S.; Koriyama, Y.; Kurimoto, T.; Oliveira, J.T.; Yin, Y.; Li, Y.; Gilbert, H.Y.; Fagiolini, M.; Martinez, A.M.; Benowitz, L. Full-length axon regeneration in the adult mouse optic nerve and partial recovery of simple visual behaviors. *Proc. Natl. Acad. Sci. USA* **2012**, *109*, 9149–9154. [CrossRef]
80. Lim, J.H.; Stafford, B.K.; Nguyen, P.L.; Lien, B.V.; Wang, C.; Zukor, K.; He, Z.; Huberman, A.D. Neural activity promotes long-distance, target-specific regeneration of adult retinal axons. *Nat. Neurosci.* **2016**, *19*, 1073–1084. [CrossRef]
81. Sun, F.; Park, K.K.; Belin, S.; Wang, D.; Lu, T.; Chen, G.; Zhang, K.; Yeung, C.; Feng, G.; Yankner, B.A.; et al. Sustained axon regeneration induced by co-deletion of PTEN and SOCS3. *Nature* **2011**, *480*, 372–375. [CrossRef]
82. Luo, X.; Salgueiro, Y.; Beckerman, S.R.; Lemmon, V.P.; Tsoulfas, P.; Park, K.K. Three-dimensional evaluation of retinal ganglion cell axon regeneration and pathfinding in whole mouse tissue after injury. *Exp. Neurol.* **2013**, *247*, 653–662. [CrossRef]
83. Li, S.; He, Q.; Wang, H.; Tang, X.; Ho, K.W.; Gao, X.; Zhang, Q.; Shen, Y.; Cheung, A.; Wong, F.; et al. Injured adult retinal axons with Pten and Socs3 co-deletion reform active synapses with suprachiasmatic neurons. *Neurobiol. Dis.* **2015**, *73*, 366–376. [CrossRef]
84. Moore, D.L.; Blackmore, M.G.; Hu, Y.; Kaestner, K.H.; Bixby, J.L.; Lemmon, V.P.; Goldberg, J.L. KLF family members regulate intrinsic axon regeneration ability. *Science* **2009**, *326*, 298–301. [CrossRef]
85. Blackmore, M.G.; Wang, Z.; Lerch, J.K.; Motti, D.; Zhang, Y.P.; Shields, C.B.; Lee, J.K.; Goldberg, J.L.; Lemmon, V.P.; Bixby, J.L. Krüppel-like Factor 7 engineered for transcriptional activation promotes axon regeneration in the adult corticospinal tract. *Proc. Natl. Acad. Sci. USA* **2012**, *109*, 7517–7522. [CrossRef]
86. Qin, S.; Zou, Y.; Zhang, C.L. Cross-talk between KLF4 and STAT3 regulates axon regeneration. *Nat. Commun.* **2013**, *4*, 2633. [CrossRef]
87. Lu, Y.; Brommer, B.; Tian, X.; Krishnan, A.; Meer, M.; Wang, C.; Vera, D.L.; Zeng, Q.; Yu, D.; Bonkowski, M.S.; et al. Reprogramming to recover youthful epigenetic information and restore vision. *Nature* **2020**, *588*, 124–129. [CrossRef]
88. Apara, A.; Galvao, J.; Wang, Y.; Blackmore, M.; Trillo, A.; Iwao, K.; Brown, D.; Fernandes, K.; Huang, A.; Nguyen, T.; et al. KLF9 and JNK3 Interact to Suppress Axon Regeneration in the Adult CNS. *J. Neurosci.* **2017**, *37*, 9632–9644. [CrossRef]
89. Trakhtenberg, E.; Li, Y.; Feng, Q.; Tso, J.; Rosenberg, P.; Goldberg, J.; Benowitz, L. Zinc chelation and Klf9 knockdown cooperatively promote axon regeneration after optic nerve injury. *Exp. Neurol.* **2018**, *300*, 22–29. [CrossRef]
90. Cheng, Y.; Yin, Y.; Zhang, A.; Bernstein, A.M.; Kawaguchi, R.; Gao, K.; Potter, K.; Gilbert, H.; Ao, Y.; Ou, J.H.; et al. Transcription factor network analysis identifies REST/NRSF as an intrinsic regulator of CNS regeneration in mice. *Nat. Commun.* **2022**, *13*, 4418. [CrossRef]
91. Watkins, T.A.; Wang, B.; Huntwork-Rodriguez, S.; Yang, J.; Jiang, Z.; Eastham-Anderson, J.; Modrusan, Z.; Kaminker, J.S.; Tessier-Lavigne, M.; Lewcock, J.W. DLK initiates a transcriptional program that couples apoptotic and regenerative responses to axonal injury. *Proc. Natl. Acad. Sci. USA* **2013**, *110*, 4039–4044. [CrossRef]
92. Welsbie, D.; Mitchell, K.; Jaskula-Ranga, V.; Sluch, V.; Yang, Z.; Kim, J.; Buehler, E.; Patel, A.; Martin, S.; Zhang, P.; et al. Enhanced Functional Genomic Screening Identifies Novel Mediators of Dual Leucine Zipper Kinase-Dependent Injury Signaling in Neurons. *Neuron* **2017**, *94*, 1142–1154.e6. [CrossRef]

93. Welsbie, D.; Yang, Z.; Ge, Y.; Mitchell, K.; Zhou, X.; Martin, S.; Berlinicke, C.; Hackler, L.; Fuller, J.; Fu, J.; et al. Functional genomic screening identifies dual leucine zipper kinase as a key mediator of retinal ganglion cell death. *Proc. Natl. Acad. Sci. USA* **2013**, *110*, 4045–4050. [CrossRef]
94. Wong, K.A.; Martheswaran, T.; Msaddi, J.; Patel, V.; Li, Y.; Peterson, S.; Benowitz, L. Retinal ganglion cell survival and axon regeneration after optic nerve injury: Crosstalk among early injury signals. *Invest. Ophthalmol. Vis. Sci.* **2021**, *62*, 1661.
95. Patel, A.K.; Broyer, R.M.; Lee, C.D.; Lu, T.; Louie, M.J.; La Torre, A.; Al-Ali, H.; Vu, M.T.; Mitchell, K.L.; Wahlin, K.J.; et al. Inhibition of GCK-IV kinases dissociates cell death and axon regeneration in CNS neurons. *Proc. Natl. Acad. Sci. USA* **2020**, *117*, 33597–33607. [CrossRef]
96. Jacobi, A.; Tran, N.M.; Yan, W.; Benhar, I.; Tian, F.; Schaffer, R.; He, Z.; Sanes, J.R. Overlapping transcriptional programs promote survival and axonal regeneration of injured retinal ganglion cells. *Neuron* **2022**, *110*, 2625–2645.e7. [CrossRef]
97. Tian, F.; Cheng, Y.; Zhou, S.; Wang, Q.; Monavarfeshani, A.; Gao, K.; Jiang, W.; Kawaguchi, R.; Wang, Q.; Tang, M.; et al. Core transcription programs controlling injury-induced neurodegeneration of retinal ganglion cells. *Neuron* **2022**, *110*, 2607–2624.e8. [CrossRef]
98. Guo, L.Y.; Bian, J.; Davis, A.E.; Liu, P.; Kempton, H.R.; Zhang, X.; Chemparathy, A.; Gu, B.; Lin, X.; Rane, D.A.; et al. Multiplexed genome regulation in vivo with hyper-efficient Cas12a. *Nat. Cell Biol.* **2022**, *24*, 590–600. [CrossRef]
99. Marin, M.A.; de Lima, S.; Gilbert, H.Y.; Giger, R.J.; Benowitz, L.; Rasband, M.N. Reassembly of Excitable Domains after CNS Axon Regeneration. *J. Neurosci.* **2016**, *36*, 9148–9160. [CrossRef]
100. Wang, J.; He, X.; Meng, H.; Li, Y.; Dmitriev, P.; Tian, F.; Page, J.C.; Lu, Q.R.; He, Z. Robust Myelination of Regenerated Axons Induced by Combined Manipulations of GPR17 and Microglia. *Neuron* **2020**, *108*, 876–886.e4. [CrossRef]

International Journal of
Molecular Sciences

MDPI

Review

Epigenetic Regulation of Optic Nerve Development, Protection, and Repair

Ajay Ashok [1], Sarita Pooranawattanakul [1], Wai Lydia Tai [1], Kin-Sang Cho [1], Tor P. Utheim [2,3], Dean M. Cestari [1] and Dong Feng Chen [1,*]

1 Department of Ophthalmology, Schepens Eye Research Institute of Massachusetts Eye and Ear, Harvard Medical School, Boston, MA 02114, USA
2 Department of Medical Biochemistry, Oslo University Hospital, 0372 Oslo, Norway
3 Department of Ophthalmology, Oslo University Hospital, 0372 Oslo, Norway
* Correspondence: dongfeng_chen@meei.harvard.edu

Abstract: Epigenetic factors are known to influence tissue development, functionality, and their response to pathophysiology. This review will focus on different types of epigenetic regulators and their associated molecular apparatus that affect the optic nerve. A comprehensive understanding of epigenetic regulation in optic nerve development and homeostasis will help us unravel novel molecular pathways and pave the way to design blueprints for effective therapeutics to address optic nerve protection, repair, and regeneration.

Keywords: optic nerve; epigenetics; myelin; regeneration; oligodendrocytes

Citation: Ashok, A.; Pooranawattanakul, S.; Tai, W.L.; Cho, K.-S.; Utheim, T.P.; Cestari, D.M.; Chen, D.F. Epigenetic Regulation of Optic Nerve Development, Protection, and Repair. *Int. J. Mol. Sci.* **2022**, *23*, 8927. https://doi.org/10.3390/ijms23168927

Academic Editors: Rongkung Tsai and Neil R. Miller

Received: 20 July 2022
Accepted: 8 August 2022
Published: 10 August 2022

1. Introduction

Waddington, in 1942, coined the term 'epigenetics,' which was defined as evident inheritable phenotypic alterations with no variations in genotype [1]. In the past two decades, the field of epigenetics has received immense attention owing to the discovery of several integral epigenetic factors that dictate gene transcription without any alterations to the DNA sequence but by adjusting the configuration of chromatin structure. The functionality of enzymes responsible for DNA and histone modifications eventually translates to altered transcriptional activity [2]. Epigenetics chiefly encompasses the events involving nuclear materials, namely chromatin accessibility, nucleosome positioning, histone modification, DNA methylation/demethylation, and enhancer-promoter interactions [2]. All these phenomena modulate the availability of DNA structure to the polymerase-mediated transcriptional activity resulting in gene expression or repression. In recent years, epigenetics has gained importance due to its proven role in development and pathophysiology [3,4]. Therefore, the current review aims at discussing the research around epigenetics in tissue protection, damage, and repair with a prime focus on the optic nerve—a vital tissue that connects the eye and brain to convey visual information and is essential for supporting visual functionality.

The optic nerve includes millions of nerve fibers originating from retinal ganglion cells (RGCs) that relay visual signals from the posterior eye segment to the brain. Incidents that attenuate the development or injury to the optic nerve and RGCs can lead to irreversible vision loss [5]. RGC axons channel from the retina to congregate and make up the optic nerve fibers. Embryonic RGCs are capable of undergoing axonal regeneration following injury [6]. However, this desirable characteristic is lost swiftly post-birth in almost all mammals. One possible explanation is the switch-off in the epigenetic program that controls optic nerve growth [7]. However, many attempts to restore the regenerative capabilities of the optic nerve in adults using epigenetic modification have been only moderately successful. Conditions affecting the optic nerve, including glaucoma [8], optic nerve atrophy [9], etc., have all been associated with epigenetic dysregulation. Moreover, the eye is considered a window for understanding complex brain functions and disorders [10,11], a phenomenon also linked to plausible epigenetic machinery and malfunction, which makes it even more important to gain knowledge related to these interlinked disorders.

Advancement in technology has led researchers to use novel state-of-the-art technologies to study epigenetic modifications during disease progression and in drug development. Some of these cutting-edge techniques that have been a useful tool in understanding optic nerve pathologies and related mechanisms include chromatin immunoprecipitation (ChIP) assay (DNA-protein interactions-chromatin structure analysis) [3], bisulfite sequencing (De novo DNA methylation exploration) [12]. Assay for Transposase-Accessible Chromatin (ATAC) with high-throughput sequencing (analyze chromatin accessibility across the genome) [13]. However, other advanced techniques such as Hi-C (epigenetic landscapes in 3D chromatin architecture analysis) and Nanopore sequencing have not yet been employed extensively in optic nerve research.

2. Epigenetic Modifications of DNAs and Histones

Epigenetic mechanisms are undoubtedly involved in neuronal differentiation, maturation, and synaptic network formation [14,15]. DNA methylation is pivotal in epigenetic modification that has the potential to tighten up the chromatin structure (Figure 1), thereby limiting the transcription ability of the cell. It involves the methyl group converting onto the C5 position of 5′-CpG-3′ dinucleotides, which results in the formation of 5-methylcytosine (5mC) [16]. This process is fueled by DNA methyltransferase (DNMTs), including DNMT1, DNMT2, DNMT3A, and DNMT3B, and the methyl group is actively contributed by S-adenosyl methionine (SAM). The complicated mechanism of DNA demethylation is mainly propelled by the ten-eleven translocation (TET) protein family. TET hydroxylases convert 5mC into 5-hydroxymethylcytosine (5hmC), thereby adjusting the methylation levels, which occur prior to cell division and multiplication [16]. This is vital because the newly formed cells are required to accumulate their own methylation marks for having their own specific characteristics and for optimal functionality. In humans, the three members of the TET protein family include TET1, TET2, and TET3, which are chiefly classified based on their structure and expression during development. Alternatively, histone can also undergo methylation and demethylation to regulate gene expression. Methylation takes place at different basic residues on histones and based on the magnitude of methylation and its location, it can lead to varying outcomes. The two main categories of histone methyltransferases are lysine-specific (SET (Su (var)3-9, Enhancer of Zeste, Trithorax) domain-containing or non-SET domain containing) and arginine-specific [17]. In both these types of histone methyltransferases, S-Adenosyl methionine (SAM) acts as the methyl donor group. Histone demethylases are categorized into two as well, namely amino oxidase homolog lysine demethylase (KDM) and JmjC domain-containing histone demethylases [18]. Histone methylation is in general associated with transcriptional repression, but methylation of certain lysine and arginine residues in histones leads to transcriptional activation.

These interdependent machineries of DNA and histone methyltransferases and demethylases work in synchrony to preserve the genomic methylation pattern (Figure 1). This critical balance of the methylation status significantly contributes to the induction and progression of various diseases, including vision loss due to optic nerve damage [8,19].

Histone acetylation is another epigenetic event that is unambiguously linked with amplified gene transcription [20]. During this process, histone acetyltransferases (HATs) will add a negatively charged acetyl group to lysine residues on histone proteins. The acetyl groups are removed by histone deacetylases (HDACs). Histone acetylation reduces the electrostatic affinity between histone proteins and DNA, which subsequently endorses a chromatin structure that is pro-gene transcription. HATs and HDACs are characterized based on their cellular localization and substrate preference. All these major epigenetic modifications regulate optic nerve development [21] and recent studies have unraveled their important role in optic nerve protection, regeneration, and repair [22–25].

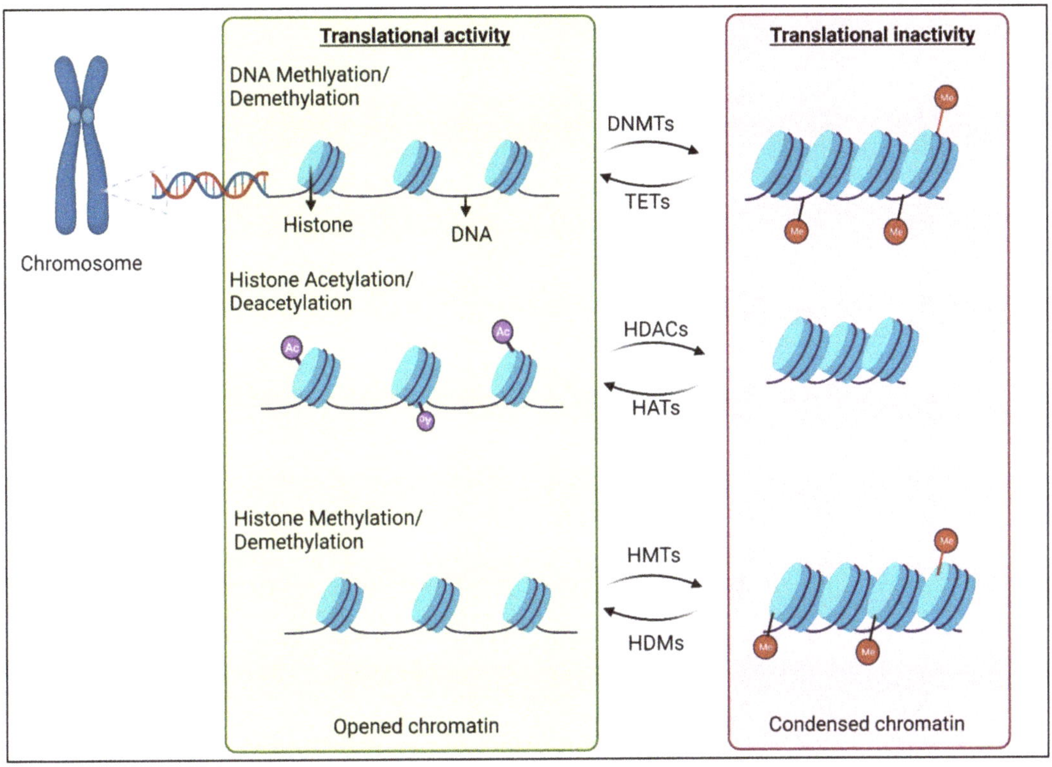

Figure 1. Epigenetic regulation of gene expression. Enhanced translational activity occurs after chromatin structure attains an open configuration, generally following DNA and histone demethylation and histone acetylation. This dynamic epigenetic mechanism is fueled by a group of enzymes that are categorized by their characteristic of presenting or reverting the methyl and acetyl groups on the histone or DNA structure. DNMT: DNA methyltransferase; TET: Ten-eleven translocation enzymes; HDAC: histone deacetylase; HAT: histone acetylase; HMT: histone methyl transferase; HDM: histone demethylase; Me: methyl group; Ac: acetyl group.

3. Epigenetics in Optic Nerve and Retinal Development

During DNA replication, DNA methylation in the developing daughter DNA strand is maintained by DNMT1. DNMT3A and DNMT3B are responsible for "de novo" DNA methylation patterns in certain differentiating cell types [26,27]. Downregulating DNMT1 in cells has been shown to lead to a partial loss of DNA methylation [28], while DNMT3A and DNMT3B [29] are reported to co-express in the eye and have overlapping functions. DNMT2 is a multisubstrate tRNA methyltransferase and has been shown to support multi-tissue development, including the retina [30]. A retina-specific triple knockout mice model showed defective retinal development, validating the vitality of the three DNMTs in the eye [31].

DNA demethylation participates in the development and aging processes of the retina. A significant study aiming at safely reversing the senescence progression and restoring biological function using the eye as a model presented evidence that the ectopic expression of *Oct4* (also known as *Pou5f1*), *Sox2*, and *Klf4* genes (OSK), all of which are transcription factors, promote the re-establishment of the epigenetic scenario of aging neurons in the CNS [12]. The study validates that active demethylation and associated activity of transcriptional factors regulate the course of senescence and its functional reversal. Myelination is an established and comprehensively studied process. OPCs in neonates have several epigenomic regulators actively functioning for this process to occur, including histone deacetylation and repressive histone methyltransferase action [32]. On the contrary, in adults, OPCs retain the property of remyelination during injury or any biological insult. This beneficial property of remyelination becomes less efficient owing to aging. External factors, including extracellular matrix alteration and declining growth factor levels, have all been implicated in the age-dependent failure of the efficient remyelination process.

Myelin is the dedicated membrane sheet spread out from oligodendrocytes (OLs) that cover the optic nerve fibers. OLs, undergo differentiation from oligodendrocyte progenitor cells (OPCs), a process controlled through the interplay between transcription factors and epigenetic regulators [33,34]. This relationship can be modulated by various external stimuli that affect age and disease. OPCs differentiate at the end stage of CNS development and a major hallmark of their maturation is the accumulation of repressive histone K9 and K27 methylation marks [35]. Whilst the differentiation and proliferation of OPCs in neonates are regulated by DNMT 1, it only has minor effects during myelin repair in adult OPCs. However, ablation of DNMT1 in OL blocks the growth of OL progenitors [36]. Moreover, DNMT 1 deletion is known to be lethal in mammals [37] since proliferating cells require a stable epigenetic environment maintained by DNMT 1. The absence of DNMT 1 triggers cell apoptosis [38,39]. DNMT 3A ablation in transgenic mice induced OL differentiation defects and a reduced functionality to remyelinate axons following injury [40]. DNA methylation and hydroxymethylation were detected at a higher level in adult OLs compared to adult OPCs. Amplified hydroxymethylation is required for spinal cord myelin repair in young mice [32]. On the contrary, senescence-dependent mitigation of hydroxymethylation resulted in irregular gene expression causing ineffective myelin repair, proven by the incidents of abnormal swellings at the axon–myelin interface.

In neuronal progenitor cells, the DNA demethylases TETs are necessary for differentiation, axonal growth, and functional neuronal network formation [41]. TET expression in glial cells has been well established, but a lot remains to be unraveled as to what the underlying epigenetic status is. TET1 is a major enzyme propelling DNA hydroxymethylation in oligodendroglia cells in the spinal cord and its level declines with aging [32]. Other enzymes, including TET2 and TET3, though expressed, do not play a significant role. A major reason as to how and why TET1 controls this major phenomenon in the optic nerve could be the presence of a "CXXC" domain, enabling the protein to bind directly with DNA and that is absent in other TETs [42]. An alternative cause could be the distinct protein binding partners of TETs that triggers enzymatic activity. TET1 and TET2 mutant models exhibit faulty developmental myelination, but it is imperative for adult OPCs to activate hydroxymethylation catalyzed by TET1 and subsequent downstream gene expression for a successful differentiation process. In TET2 and TET3 deficient (KO) mice, early-born retinal cell types—RGCs and amacrine cells (AC)—were affected in development [43]. RGCs in TET2 and TET3 KO mice expressed *Zn8*, a marker of cell terminal differentiation but were restricted to the central retina, and the optic nerve in these zebrafish groups was deformed and even absent in a subset [43]. Reduced numbers of Amacrine cells and differentiated red/green double cones were also noted in TET2 and TET3 KO mice and localized only in the central retina. Together, the presence of the DNA demethylation mechanism is a vital phenomenon in normal retinal development and this knowledge can be useful for understanding the altered state of epigenetics during adulthood and disease.

Epigenetic changes are not only limited to the nucleus but can also mediate the functioning of other cellular organelles, such as proteins in the cytoplasm [44] and mitochondria [45]. This in turn affects common cellular events such as apoptosis [46], autophagy [47], inflammation [48] etc. However, to date, very limited groups have studied the relationship between epigenetic modifications, mitochondrial function, and cytoplasmic epigenetic modification in relation to optic nerve development, regeneration, and repair. It is a topic of research whose therapeutic potential remains untapped. A recent comprehensive review discusses in detail the role, interdependency, and localization of epigenetics events in eukaryotic cells [49]. One key study shows lutein endorses neural differentiation, possibly in a PI3K-AKT-dependent manner accompanied by enhanced glycolysis and mitochondrial function [50]. This fuels the synthesis of Acetyl-CoA (an essential ingredient for epigenetic modulation) consistent with epigenetic-based changes in the transcriptome that facilitates neuronal differentiation. Another study understanding myopia discusses plausible cytoplasmic proteins and pathways (Wnt signaling, protein kinase/growth factor signaling, and IGF-1 signaling) regulated by DNA methylation in relation to various ocular cells/tissues [44].

Apart from the addition and removal of a methyl group to the nuclear content, the addition and removal of the acetyl group in histones play a vital role in reconfiguring the chromatin structure and resulting gene expression profile. As described in the previous section (Section 2), HDACs are a major regulator of gene expression, and they act by removing the acetyl group from the histone structure and the family of HDACs has been extensively studied for optic nerve repair and regeneration.

HDACs are known to regulate glial cell development and pathologies of the CNS; however, research studying the developmental expression and functionalities of HDACs in the developing optic nerve and retina are limited. HDACs 1, 2, 3, 5, 6, 8, and 11 are all locally situated to the nuclei of glia during the development and maturation of the optic nerve [21]. HDACs 1 and 2 localize primarily in the nucleus, HDACs 3, 5, 6, 8, and 11 are detected mainly in the cytoplasm and nuclear region during more than one stage of development, and HDACs 4, 9, and 10 are cytoplasmic in all stages of development [21]. These data are the critical initial step in identifying HDAC-associated functions that may plausibly modulate chromatin reconfirmation during differentiation and regeneration of the optic nerve in development and disease processes and pave the way in understanding optic nerve pathologies where localization of HDACs is integral in disease progression.

Other glial cells in the optic nerve are immensely critical for the maintenance of neuronal functioning in the CNS, including astrocytes and microglia. Not much has been conducted directly linking the modulation of these cells and their epigenetic changes in optic nerve pathologies. However, earlier reports using alternative models have established the role of epigenetic factors such as HDACs in these cells. In response to inflammatory conditions, HDAC activity is heightened in the astrocytes. Conjointly, glial inflammatory responses in microglia and astrocytes are mitigated following HDAC activity inhibition [51,52]. In primary human astrocytes, glial fibrillary acidic protein (GFAP) is upregulated in reactive astrocytosis but reduced after HDAC inhibition [53] without affecting astrocyte activation [54]. HDAC inhibition in various CNS injuries reduces the upregulation of IL-1β, cyclooxygenase (COX)-2, iNOS, and TNF-α in reactive astrocytes [54]. Production of glycosaminoglycans like chondroitin sulfate proteoglycan (CSPG) can be increased by reactive astrocytes, thereby lowering acetylation levels in neighboring cells, as they can act as HAT inhibitors [55]. A study by Kuboyama showed that HDAC3 was highly upregulated in a contusion spinal cord injury (SCI) model in microglia/macrophages [56]. Up to date, there has been no report directly examining the behavior of glial cells in the optic nerve following epigenetic alterations, and this topic remains to be explored comprehensively.

Rao et al. showed that histone lysine methylation (e.g., H3K9me2 and H3K27me3) and associated expression of the respective histone methyl transferases, G9a, and enhancer of zeste homolog 2 (Ezh2), occurs in RGCs during retinal development [22]. Moreover, the study also showed inhibition of Ezh2 or G9a is associated with RGC death, thereby cementing the importance of histone methylation patterns in parts of the optic nerve. A recent study also showed that upregulation of Ezh2 is necessary for spontaneous axon regeneration of sensory neurons in different models [25]. Ezh2 does so by downregulating synaptic function-related genes, including *Slc6a13*, which encodes GABA transporter 2. Expression patterns of basic helix-loop-helix (bHLH) transcription factors such as atonal homolog 5 (*ATH5*) and *NeuroM*, *NeuroD*, and *β3* genes, rely heavily upon histone methylation as methylation of histone H3 at *NeuroM* and *NeuroD* promoters regulates RGC development [57].

4. DNA Modification in Optic Nerve Repair and Protection

Several recent studies are trying to shed light on integral epigenetic mechanisms during optic nerve damage and diseases. These findings hold the key to understanding the early events that trigger disease progression and limit the optic nerve's abilities to regenerate following trauma or disease. Some of the most prominent models that are used to comprehend optic nerve damage and related epigenetic modifications include optic nerve crush (ONC) [12], microbead model induced glaucoma [12], streptozotocin (STZ) induced diabetic insult [58], etc. DNA methylation and histone acetylation levels have been abundantly investigated in these studies. The data obtained can help researchers design targeted and efficient therapeutic tools and a recipe for tailoring the epigenetic system in the tissue for successful regeneration and protection.

In lower vertebrates, CNS neurons, including RGCs, regenerate axons throughout their lifetime; however, other neuronal types, such as hindbrain neurons in tadpoles, lose the capacity to regenerate post spinal cord injury [59]. This model offers a unique opportunity to explore genes involved that are responsible for regenerative or non-regenerative responses after CNS injury [59]. Whole genome bisulfite sequencing (WGBS) from animals during optimal axon regeneration time point demonstrated that DNA of regenerative CNS is more accessible. Reduced DNA methylation status was observed in regenerating tadpole hindbrain and frog eye relative to the non-regenerative state [59]. However, a very paradoxical observation was also made in the study where in regenerative CNS of these models, many genes displayed augmented, promoter-associated CpG-methylation following injury and exhibited increased RNA expression and association histone markers for active promoters and enhancers. This might be due to varying upcoming mechanisms that have been studied recently, such as altered connection with activating or repressive transcription factors and histone modifications and augmented association of genes with the nuclear lamina to facilitate an open chromatin structure [60,61]. In both the CNS and PNS, neuronal gene expression is altered following axonal injury. Transcriptional factors such as neurotrophin Bdnf and Sox11 promote efficient axon regeneration in the PNS, in which nerves regenerate after injury, but not in the CNS of mammals [62]. Both these factors are highly influenced by DNA methylation.

Streptozotocin (STZ) is a known inducer of diabetes-related pathologies, including diabetic retinopathy. Multiple administration of STZ increased global DNA methylation in the retina, resulting in RGC damage [63]. Six weeks post-STZ injection, the levels of DNMT 1 and DNMT 3B increased notably relative to control vehicle-injected mice. In RGCs of diabetic retinopathy, DNMT 1 was found to be intensely upregulated, and DNMT 1 modulated DNA methylation was also associated with diabetic retinopathy progression. Mice subjected to ONC displayed an overall reduction in histone acetylation in the RGC layer as early as 24 h post-crush, which is reflective of the decreased expression of several associated genes.

The study mentioned earlier studied the roles of *Oct4, Sox2, and Klf4* (OSK) co-expression in reversing the aging process demonstrated in a glaucomatous animal model of increased axonal density relative to control mice that received no OSK [12]. It suggests a regenerative event mediated after DNA demethylation. OSK-mediated increase in Stat3 mRNA levels in promoting RGC survival and axon regeneration depends on the activities of TET1 and TET2. However, DNA demethylation is not the only factor required for RGC protection and axon regeneration, as overexpressing the TET1 catalytic domain by itself was not successful in promoting axon regeneration. These data indicate a complex intertwined and time-dependent epigenetic machinery that controls DNA methylation during optic nerve growth and homeostasis.

5. Histone Modifications in Optic Nerve Repair and Protection

The histone acetylase (HAT) and HDAC interdependency appear to tilt the balance toward deacetylation in retinal degenerative diseases [64], and hence the effects of HDAC inhibitor (HDACi) treatment have been studied comprehensively in recent years for restoring equilibrium. HDACi is shown to have a neuroprotective effect when treating damaged retinas or differentiated neurons (Figure 2). HDACs are also known to mediate the deacetylation of non-histone proteins, including microtubules, transcription factors, and even enzymes. For instance, axonal injury causes tubulin deacetylation that is mediated by HDAC5 in DRGs and serves as a prerequisite for regenerative growth [65]. Additionally, blocking HDAC5 promoted the acetylation of microtubules and enhanced DRG growth. The data suggest that finely balanced DNA acetylation of cytoskeletal and structural protein-related genes is critical for successful axonal regeneration. Pan inhibition of HDACs can prove to be deleterious and, therefore, selective inhibition of HDACs can prove useful, as shown in a study where targeted inhibition of HDAC6 ameliorated CNS injury characterized by oxidative stress-induced neurodegeneration and insufficient axonal regeneration [66].

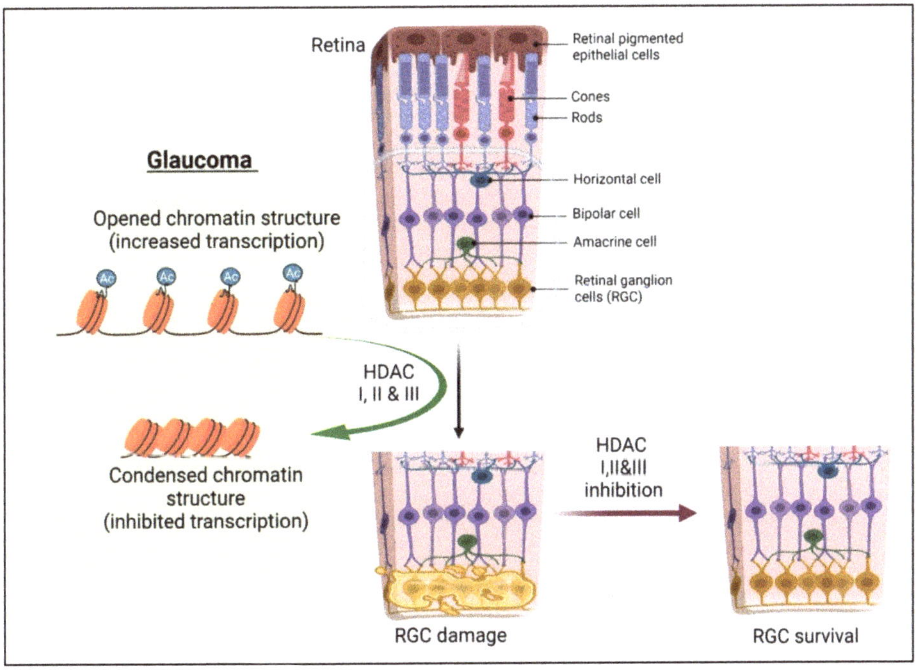

Figure 2. HDAC inhibitors rescue RGCs by modulating the histone acetylation levels. HDAC families I, II, and III are known to upregulate significantly in glaucoma models [64]. Blocking HDAC activity using inhibitors offers significant neuroprotection, including enhanced RGC protection. HDAC activity inhibition reprograms the chromatin structure to a pro-translational configuration which occurs through modulation of factors such as p53, CREB-binding protein/p300 (CBP/p300), and the p300-CBP-associated factor (P/CAF), which facilitate neuroprotection, etc. [67,68]. Ac: acetyl group.

Following ONC, HDAC3 translocated to the nuclei in injured RGCs as a consequence of axonal injury and caused extensive H4 deacetylation and transcriptional dysregulation that resulted in RGC death. In another study, following an acute optic nerve injury, the mRNA levels of class I HDACs, such as HDAC2 and HDAC3, were upregulated and peaked at 72 h in RGCs post-ONC. HDAC3 translocated from the cytoplasm to the nuclei by day 5; an observation consistent with the earlier research where HDAC3 localized to the nuclei in dying cortical neurons in an in vivo Huntington's disease model. Conditional knockout of HDAC3 or pharmacological administration of RGFP966 blocked HDAC3 activity and improved RGC survival in a dose-dependent manner by preventing nuclear atrophy and apoptosis [24,46]. Mere targeted removal of HDAC3 was not potent enough to provide RGCs protection from axonal degeneration or somatic cell death in a glaucoma mouse model. Studies in aged or chronic glaucoma mouse models further demonstrated that using RGFP966 to inhibit HDAC3 activity provided limited protection against somatic cell loss in the ganglion cell layer. A single intravitreal injection of RGFP966 followed by selective blocking of HDAC3 ceased histone deacetylation, heterochromatin formation, apoptosis, and DNA damage post-ONC [46]. Repeated IP administration of RFGP966 prevented RGC loss, proving the importance of DNA acetylation in retinal pathology.

On the other hand, a detailed investigation of epigenetic regulation of oligodendrocytes in the optic nerve remains vague. In an adult zebrafish optic nerve transection model, the process of olig2 positive cells stays undamaged and the total number of olig2 + cells in NFL is not significantly altered [69]. Moreover, HDAC inhibitors (MS-275, M334, and suberoylanilide hydroxamic acid) are known to improve neuronal differentiation and inhibit oligodendrocytes production [70]. In a few reports, they are shown to cause cytotoxic in oligodendrocyte precursor cells [71]. Therefore, the use of these compounds must be carefully regulated as they may present a double-edged sword.

Apart from direct inhibition using synthetic HDAC inhibitors, there are other factors that modulate HDAC activities. Therapeutic effects of mood stabilizers, lithium [72] and valproic acid (VPA), were reported in retinal and optic nerve injury models [73,74]. VPA functions by directly inhibiting the activity of HDAC and causing histone hyperacetylation. Some of the earlier reports revealed that abnormal histone acetylation/deacetylation might relate to RGC damage in glaucoma. Trichostatin A (TSA), a broad-spectrum HDAC inhibitor, promotes neurite outgrowth and neuroprotection along with neuronal differentiation and neurite branching [64]. The same effect was reported in RGCs through histone H3K9 acetylation. SNC-121, a selective ligand that activates the δ-opioid receptor, has shown RGC neuroprotective effect in glaucoma mice model by regulating the expression and activity of HDACs, increasing acetylation of histone (H3, H4, and H2B), and reducing the activity of class I and class IIb HDAC [75]. HDAC 1 & 2, and SIRT1 (a member of the Class III family of HDACs), are plausible p53 deacetylases [76–78]. This entire interplay is acetylation-site and cell-type specific. Double knock out of HDAC 1 & 2 in RGCs in an optic nerve transfection model exhibited a neuroprotective effect [68]. *PUMA*, a novel proapoptotic gene induced by p53, is strongly activated in axotomized RGCs and is also inhibited following HDACI/II ablation, making HDACI&II specific targets for designing the blueprint of neuroprotective therapies [68]. "CREB Binding Protein" (CREBBP, CBP or KAT3A) and "Adenovirus E1A-associated 300-kD Protein" (p300 or KAT3B) are both KAT3 family members that are well recognized for catalyzing acetylation of all core histones. P300 in RGCs are developmentally controlled and their expression remains downregulated post optic nerve injury [23]. It was reported that the regeneration programming after an optic nerve injury relied on the expression of p300, which upregulates acetylation of both histone and non-histone target genes. The Bromodomain and Extra-Terminal Domain (BET) family of proteins is identified by the presence of two tandem bromodomains and an extra-terminal domain. BET family of proteins are encoded by paralogous genes and are made of BRD2, BRD3, BRD4, and BRDT. Bromodomains have the potential to precisely bind acetylated lysine residues in histones and serve as chromatin-targeting modules that decode the histone acetylation code [79]. Hence BET proteins have a pivotal role in modulating gene transcription by altering interactions between bromodomains and acetylated histones during different cell stages of proliferation and differentiation. JQ1, a highly specific blocker of BET proteins, was tested on an acutely damaged RGC model induced by NMDA excitotoxicity [48]. Intravitreal JQ1 administration maintained RGC number, gene expression (including inflammatory genes- *MCP-1*, *TNF*α, *RANTES*, *IL-1*β), and decreased NMDA-induced TUNEL-positive cells in the RGC layer in an animal model.

Another aspect related to post-translational modifications of histone is histone methylation, which mainly occurs on the side chains of lysine. Gene transcription heavily relies on the methylation of histone polypeptides contingent on whether it is mono- di- and tri-methylated. The dimethylation of histone 3 at lysine 9 (H3K9Me2) has been recognized as a chromatin silencer, and it is specifically catalyzed by G9a, a histone methyltransferase [80]. Increased H3K9Me2 has been demonstrated to limit the binding of transcription factors to the promoters of their downstream genes and thus diminishes their further expression [81]. Moreover, G9a has also been found to be significantly expressed in adult mouse retinas and throughout the development. In a traumatic brain injury (TBI) model, increased expression of G9a and H3K9Me2 were noted in RGCs and optic nerves which underwent cell death and oxidative stress [80]. Administration of G9a inhibitor (UNC0638) attenuated H3K9Me2 activity in both optic nerve and RGC and subsequently activated Nrf2 to block oxidative stress. This leaves no doubt that epigenetic regulation plays a pivotal role in retrograde transportation of axons and providing neuroprotection post TBI. The histone methyltransferase catalyzes the tri-methylation of histone H3 at lysine 27 (H3K27me3) to establish a repressive chromatin structure, enhancer of zeste homolog 2 (Ezh2), which is transitorily expressed in the perinatal retina, especially in the RGCs [22,82]. Though Ezh2 does not mediate retinal ganglion cell homeostasis or their susceptibility to injury [82], progressive photoreceptor degeneration was found to be associated with the deletion of Ezh2 from retinal progenitors at the embryonic stage [83]. Cell death in RGC and NMDA-induced inner nuclear layer (INL) was significantly prevented by 3-deazaneplanocin A (DZNep), an inhibitor of transcription of Ezh2 [84]. Moreover, it conserved RGC functionality as shown by maintaining the ERG b/a wave ratio and the b and a-wave amplitudes in NMDA-treated mice. H3K27me3 affects the survival of RGCs at specific transcriptional and epigenetic levels. The absence of H3K27me3 was found to be neuroprotective, as demonstrated by the upregulation of neuroprotective genes in RGCs. Therefore, DZNep, which inhibits Ezh2 activity, could hold the key to novel therapeutic treatment for ocular neurodegenerative diseases. One study looked at lysine-specific demethylase 1 (LSD1-transcription repressor) and its role in the removal of a methyl group from methylated lysine 4 of histone H3 [85]. Tranylcypromine, a major LSD1 inhibitor, repressed neuron cell death post glutamate neurotoxicity and oxidative stress exposure in an NMDA-induced toxicity model. Tranylcypromine overturned the significant glutamate suppression of p38 MAPKc, presenting neuroprotection. Intravitreal administration of tranylcypromine rescued a significant number of RGC in the same model, indicating epigenetic regulation dictating the survival of RGC via the up-regulation of p38 MAPKc activity.

The interaction of transcriptional factor and chromatin accessibility controls the expression levels of several downstream molecular players, such as Gap43 [86] and Tubb3 [87], which localize and function effectively at the growth cone [13]. Most of these downstream genes mediate signaling pathways that control cell metabolism. Several influential pathways that propel cell growth and axon regeneration include deletion of *PTEN*, *IL22*, or *SOCS3* to activate mTOR and *STAT3* pathways [88–90]. Additionally, JAK/STAT pathway, an established molecular event in optic nerve hemostasis and regeneration, is also known to be influenced by epigenetic modifications [91]. However, a lot of research still needs to be done to establish a concrete relationship between these cellular mechanisms in the optic nerve.

6. Conclusions

Epigenetic modifications are critical for all biological mechanisms driving development, homeostasis, and repair of the optic nerve (Table 1). Designing novel therapeutics which can modify the epigenetic setting for modulating the expression and transcriptional activities of vital genes in the optic nerve is the need of the hour. Since epigenetic modifications occur far upstream during the pathological molecular incidents, any adjustment to its characteristics holds the potential to define and alter the entire downstream and ultimate consequence of the pathological event. Therefore, discovering and understanding its machinery in optic nerve regulation must be carried out with high accuracy before coming to any conclusions and pitching novel epigenetic inhibitors as drug options. For instance, HDAC inhibitors seem to be an optimal treatment for RGC rescuing; however, one must realize multiple substrates of HDACs are involved in various biological events, including differentiation, proliferation, and apoptosis; their expression varies at different stages of development and disease progression. In line with these recommendations, earlier reports exploring HDAC inhibitors have also reported side effects like thrombocytopenia, neutropenia, anemia, fatigue, and diarrhea [92,93]. Therefore, the use of HDAC inhibitors to rescue and regenerate optic nerve must be carried out with optimal precision. Moreover, over 14 different HDAC inhibitors are involved in clinical trials for cancer treatment, but there is a risk of cells gaining resistance to these drugs, and these are drawbacks that might translate to optic nerve research as well. A lot of studies and research still need to be conducted as newer epigenetic factors and players are still being discovered in recent times. Epigenetics may hold the key to successful therapeutic options to address optic nerve-associated diseases.

Table 1. Epigenetic Studies in Optic Nerve Tissues.

Cell Type	Epigenetic Player	Experimental Model	Effect	References
RGCs (Retinal ganglion cells)	TET1-dependent deletion of PTEN	Optic nerve crush model	Optic nerve regeneration	[94]
	Class I HDACs and HDAC 2 & 3 upregulation and HDAC3 nuclear localization in RGCs	Optic nerve crush model	Optic nerve degeneration/RGC apoptosis	[64]
	Increased G9a expression and H3K9Me2 activity in the retina (RGC) and optic nerve	Traumatic brain injury (TBI) model	TBI causes apoptosis and oxidative stress in the retina (RGC) and optic nerve	[80]
	Inhibition of retinal HDAC activity (post valproic acid treatment)	- RGCs purified from new-born (postnatal day P0–P2) rat retinas - HeLa cells	Neuroprotection and histone hyperacetylation	[73,74]
	Inhibition of HDAC3 activity (RGFP966 activity)	Optic nerve crush model	RGC survival and repression of the apoptotic gene in RGCs post optic nerve injury	[24,64]
	Double knock out of HDAC1&2	Optic nerve axotomy	Anti-apoptosis and neuroprotection effect	[68]
	3-deazaneplanocin (DZNep) inhibits Ezh2 inhibition using 3-deazaneplanocin (DZNep) -reduces the trimethylation of histone 3 lysine 27 (H3K27me3) or activity	Retinal/RGC damage caused by intravitreal injection of N-methyl-D-aspartate (NMDA)	Prevent cell death and inner nuclear layer thinning induced by NMDA and improved visual function	[84]
	Increased Histone H3K9 acetylation using Trichostatin A (TSA)	Lead-induced neurotoxicity	Promotes neurite outgrowth and branching, neuroprotection, neuronal differentiation, and neurite branching	[95]
	Intravitreal JQ1 (BET inhibitor) administration	RGC damage induced by NMDA excitotoxicity	Sustained RGC number and gene expression and decreased TUNEL-positive cells in the ganglion cell layer	[48]
	Promotion of p38 MAPKc activity and intravitreal administration of tranylcypromine (lysine-specific demethylase 1 (LSD1) inhibitor)	NMDA-induced excitotoxicity	Enhanced RGC survival	[85]
	OSK-mediated vision restoration is TET1/2 dependent ectopic expression of Oct4 (also known as Pou5f1), Sox2, and Klf4 genes (OSK) in RGC	Optic nerve crush model	Axon regeneration	[12]

Table 1. *Cont.*

Cell Type	Epigenetic Player	Experimental Model	Effect	References
OPCs (Oligodendrocyte progenitor cells)	Increased levels of H3K27me3 from NSCs (neural stem cells) to immature OL and significantly decreased levels of histone acetylation (i.e., H3K9ac) at the early stages of OPC differentiation associated with increasing levels of H3K9me3 during OPC maturation	Human pluripotent stem cell culture	Differentiation of OPCs into OLs	[96]
	DNMT1 downregulation in oligodendrocytes	- Conditional mutation in the mouse DNMT1 gene in embryonic stem (ES) cells. - T24, a human bladder transitional carcinoma-derived cell line; A549, a human non-small-cell lung carcinoma cell line, and NIH 3T3, a mouse fibroblast cell line	- Inhibition of OPC growth - Cell apoptosis - Mild impact on myelin reparation process	[38,39]
Myelin	Downregulation of TET1	- TET1 KO mice model	- inefficient myelin repair and axo-myelinic swellings	[32]
			- alters astrocyte morphology and impairs neuronal function	[97]

Disclaimer: All illustrations were created using Biorender (biorender.com).

Author Contributions: A.A. and D.F.C.: conceived the idea, conducted the literature search, and wrote the manuscript; S.P.: modified and edited the figures; W.L.T.: prepared figures and revised the manuscript; K.-S.C., T.P.U. and D.M.C.: edited the manuscript. All authors have read and agreed to the published version of the manuscript.

Funding: This work was supported by grants from Massachusetts Eye and Ear Summit Fund, National Institutes of Health/National Eye Institute: R21 EY033882, R01 EY031696, and R01 EY025250 (D.F.C.).

Institutional Review Board Statement: Not applicable.

Informed Consent Statement: Not applicable.

Data Availability Statement: Not applicable.

Conflicts of Interest: The authors declare no conflict of interest.

References

1. Waddington, C.H. The epigenotype. *Int. J. Epidemiol.* **1942**, *1*, 18–20. [CrossRef] [PubMed]
2. Allis, C.D.; Jenuwein, T. The molecular hallmarks of epigenetic control. *Nat. Rev. Genet.* **2016**, *17*, 487–500. [CrossRef] [PubMed]
3. Pelzel, H.R.; Nickells, R.W. A role for epigenetic changes in the development of retinal neurodegenerative conditions. *J. Ocul. Biol. Dis. Inform.* **2011**, *4*, 104–110. [CrossRef] [PubMed]
4. Pennington, K.L.; DeAngelis, M.M. Epigenetic mechanisms of the aging human retina. *J. Exp. Neurosci.* **2015**, *9*, 51–79. [CrossRef]
5. Yohannan, J.; Boland, M.V. The evolving role of the relationship between optic nerve structure and function in glaucoma. *Ophthalmology* **2017**, *124*, S66–S70. [CrossRef]
6. Fawcett, J.W. The struggle to make CNS axons regenerate: Why has it been so difficult? *Neurochem. Res.* **2020**, *45*, 144–158. [CrossRef]
7. Yun, M.H. Changes in regenerative capacity through lifespan. *Int. J. Mol. Sci.* **2015**, *16*, 25392–25432. [CrossRef]
8. Gauthier, A.C.; Liu, J. Epigenetics and signaling pathways in glaucoma. *BioMed Res. Int.* **2017**, *2017*, 1–12. [CrossRef]

9. Schmitt, H.M.; Schlamp, C.L.; Nickells, R.W. Role of HDACs in optic nerve damage-induced nuclear atrophy of retinal ganglion cells. *Neurosci. Lett.* **2016**, *625*, 11–15. [CrossRef]
10. Mancino, R.; Cesareo, M.; Martucci, A.; Di Carlo, E.; Ciuffoletti, E.; Giannini, C.; Morrone, L.A.; Nucci, C.; Garaci, F. Neurodegenerative process linking the eye and the brain. *Curr. Med. Chem.* **2019**, *26*, 3754–3763. [CrossRef]
11. Ashok, A.; Singh, N.; Chaudhary, S.; Bellamkonda, V.; Kritikos, A.E.; Wise, A.S.; Rana, N.; McDonald, D.; Ayyagari, R. Retinal degeneration and Alzheimer's disease: An evolving link. *Int. J. Mol. Sci.* **2020**, *21*, 7290. [CrossRef]
12. Lu, Y.; Brommer, B.; Tian, X.; Krishnan, A.; Meer, M.; Wang, C.; Vera, D.L.; Zeng, Q.; Yu, D.; Bonkowski, M.S. Reprogramming to recover youthful epigenetic information and restore vision. *Nature* **2020**, *588*, 124–129. [CrossRef]
13. Pita-Thomas, W.; Gonçalves, T.M.; Kumar, A.; Zhao, G.; Cavalli, V. Genome-wide chromatin accessibility analyses provide a map for enhancing optic nerve regeneration. *Sci. Rep.* **2021**, *11*, 1–17. [CrossRef]
14. Yao, B.; Christian, K.M.; He, C.; Jin, P.; Ming, G.-l.; Song, H. Epigenetic mechanisms in neurogenesis. *Nat. Rev. Neurosci.* **2016**, *17*, 537–549. [CrossRef]
15. VandenBosch, L.S.; Reh, T.A. Seminars in cell & developmental bioloy. In *Epigenetics in Neuronal Regeneration*; Elsevier: Amsterdam, The Netherlands, 2020; pp. 63–73.
16. Liu, W.; Wu, G.; Xiong, F.; Chen, Y. Advances in the DNA methylation hydroxylase TET1. *Biomark. Res.* **2021**, *9*, 1–12. [CrossRef]
17. Greer, E.L.; Shi, Y. Histone methylation: A dynamic mark in health, disease and inheritance. *Nat. Rev. Genet.* **2012**, *13*, 343–357. [CrossRef]
18. D'Oto, A.; Tian, Q.W.; Davidoff, A.M.; Yang, J. Histone demethylases and their roles in cancer epigenetics. *J. Med. Oncol. Ther.* **2016**, *1*, 34–40. [CrossRef]
19. Lopez, N.; Clark, A.F.; Tovar-Vidales, T. Epigenetic regulation of optic nerve head fibrosis in glaucoma. *Investig. Ophthalmol. Vis. Sci.* **2019**, *60*, 5668.
20. Ramaiah, M.J.; Tangutur, A.D.; Manyam, R.R. Epigenetic modulation and understanding of HDAC inhibitors in cancer therapy. *Life Sci.* **2021**, *277*, 119504. [CrossRef]
21. Tiwari, S.; Dharmarajan, S.; Shivanna, M.; Otteson, D.C.; Belecky-Adams, T.L. Histone deacetylase expression patterns in developing murine optic nerve. *BMC Dev. Biol.* **2014**, *14*, 30. [CrossRef]
22. Rao, R.C.; Tchedre, K.T.; Malik, M.T.A.; Coleman, N.; Fang, Y.; Marquez, V.E.; Chen, D.F. Dynamic patterns of histone lysine methylation in the developing retina. *Investig. Ophthalmol. Vis. Sci.* **2010**, *51*, 6784–6792. [CrossRef]
23. Gaub, P.; Joshi, Y.; Wuttke, A.; Naumann, U.; Schnichels, S.; Heiduschka, P.; Di Giovanni, S. The histone acetyltransferase p300 promotes intrinsic axonal regeneration. *Brain* **2011**, *134*, 2134–2148. [CrossRef]
24. Schmitt, H.M.; Pelzel, H.R.; Schlamp, C.L.; Nickells, R.W. Histone deacetylase 3 (HDAC3) plays an important role in retinal ganglion cell death after acute optic nerve injury. *Mol. Neurodegener.* **2014**, *9*, 1–15. [CrossRef]
25. Wang, X.-W.; Yang, S.-G.; Hu, M.-W.; Wang, R.-Y.; Zhang, C.; Kosanam, A.R.; Ochuba, A.J.; Jiang, J.-J.; Luo, X.; Qian, J. Histone methyltransferase Ezh2 coordinates mammalian axon regeneration via epigenetic regulation of key regenerative pathways. *BioRxiv* **2022**. [CrossRef]
26. Bradley, M.C.; Markenscoff-Papadimitriou, E.; Duffié, R.; Lomvardas, S. Dnmt3a regulates global gene expression in olfactory sensory neurons and enables odorant-induced transcription. *Neuron* **2014**, *83*, 823–838.
27. Hamidi, T.; Singh, A.K.; Chen, T. Genetic alterations of DNA methylation machinery in human diseases. *Epigenomics* **2015**, *7*, 247–265. [CrossRef]
28. Angileri, K.M.; Gross, J.M. Dnmt1 function is required to maintain retinal stem cells within the ciliary marginal zone of the zebrafish eye. *Sci. Rep.* **2020**, *10*, 11293. [CrossRef]
29. Zhu, X.; Li, D.; Du, Y.; He, W.; Lu, Y. DNA hypermethylation-mediated downregulation of antioxidant genes contributes to the early onset of cataracts in highly myopic eyes. *Redox Biol.* **2018**, *19*, 179–189. [CrossRef]
30. Rai, K.; Chidester, S.; Zavala, C.V.; Manos, E.J.; James, S.R.; Karpf, A.R.; Jones, D.A.; Cairns, B.R. Dnmt2 functions in the cytoplasm to promote liver, brain, and retina development in zebrafish. *Genes Dev.* **2007**, *21*, 261–266. [CrossRef]
31. Singh, R.K.; Mallela, R.K.; Hayes, A.; Dunham, N.R.; Hedden, M.E.; Enke, R.A.; Fariss, R.N.; Sternberg, H.; West, M.D.; Nasonkin, I.O. Dnmt1, Dnmt3a and Dnmt3b cooperate in photoreceptor and outer plexiform layer development in the mammalian retina. *Exp. Eye Res.* **2017**, *159*, 132–146. [CrossRef]
32. Moyon, S.; Frawley, R.; Marechal, D.; Huang, D.; Marshall-Phelps, K.L.; Kegel, L.; Bøstrand, S.M.; Sadowski, B.; Jiang, Y.H.; Lyons, D.A.; et al. TET1-mediated DNA hydroxymethylation regulates adult remyelination in mice. *Nat. Commun.* **2021**, *12*, 3359. [CrossRef]
33. Bergles, D.E.; Richardson, W.D. Oligodendrocyte development and plasticity. *Cold Spring Harb. Perspect. Biol.* **2015**, *8*, a020453. [CrossRef]
34. Emery, B.; Lu, Q.R. Transcriptional and epigenetic regulation of oligodendrocyte development and myelination in the central nervous system. *Cold Spring Harb. Perspect. Biol.* **2015**, *7*, a020461. [CrossRef]
35. Liu, J.; Magri, L.; Zhang, F.; Marsh, N.O.; Albrecht, S.; Huynh, J.L.; Kaur, J.; Kuhlmann, T.; Zhang, W.; Slesinger, P.A. Chromatin landscape defined by repressive histone methylation during oligodendrocyte differentiation. *J. Neurosci.* **2015**, *35*, 352–365. [CrossRef]
36. Moyon, S.; Huynh, J.L.; Dutta, D.; Zhang, F.; Ma, D.; Yoo, S.; Lawrence, R.; Wegner, M.; John, G.R.; Emery, B.; et al. Functional characterization of DNA methylation in the oligodendrocyte lineage. *Cell Rep.* **2016**, *15*, 748–760. [CrossRef]

37. Li, E.; Bestor, T.H.; Jaenisch, R. Targeted mutation of the DNA methyltransferase gene results in embryonic lethality. *Cell* **1992**, *69*, 915–926. [CrossRef]
38. Jackson-Grusby, L.; Beard, C.; Possemato, R.; Tudor, M.; Fambrough, D.; Csankovszki, G.; Dausman, J.; Lee, P.; Wilson, C.; Lander, E. Loss of genomic methylation causes p53-dependent apoptosis and epigenetic deregulation. *Nat. Genet.* **2001**, *27*, 31–39. [CrossRef]
39. Unterberger, A.; Andrews, S.D.; Weaver, I.C.; Szyf, M. DNA methyltransferase 1 knockdown activates a replication stress checkpoint. *Mol. Cell. Biol.* **2006**, *26*, 7575–7586. [CrossRef]
40. Moyon, S.; Ma, D.; Huynh, J.L.; Coutts, D.J.; Zhao, C.; Casaccia, P.; Franklin, R.J. Efficient remyelination requires DNA methylation. *Eneuro* **2017**, *4*. [CrossRef]
41. MacArthur, I.C.; Dawlaty, M.M. TET enzymes and 5-hydroxymethylcytosine in neural progenitor cell biology and neurodevelopment. *Front. Cell Dev. Biol.* **2021**, *9*, 645335. [CrossRef]
42. Zhang, W.; Xia, W.; Wang, Q.; Towers, A.J.; Chen, J.; Gao, R.; Zhang, Y.; Yen, C.-a.; Lee, A.Y.; Li, Y. Isoform switch of TET1 regulates DNA demethylation and mouse development. *Mol. Cell* **2016**, *64*, 1062–1073. [CrossRef]
43. Seritrakul, P.; Gross, J.M. Tet-mediated DNA hydroxymethylation regulates retinal neurogenesis by modulating cell-extrinsic signaling pathways. *PLoS Genet.* **2017**, *13*, e1006987. [CrossRef]
44. Vishweswaraiah, S.; Swierkowska, J.; Ratnamala, U.; Mishra, N.K.; Guda, C.; Chettiar, S.S.; Johar, K.R.; Mrugacz, M.; Karolak, J.A.; Gajecka, M.; et al. Epigenetically dysregulated genes and pathways implicated in the pathogenesis of non-syndromic high myopia. *Sci. Rep.* **2019**, *9*, 4145. [CrossRef]
45. Calió, M.L.; Henriques, E.; Siena, A.; Bertoncini, C.R.A.; Gil-Mohapel, J.; Rosenstock, T.R. Mitochondrial dysfunction, neurogenesis, and epigenetics: Putative implications for amyotrophic lateral sclerosis neurodegeneration and treatment. *Front. Neurosci.* **2020**, *14*, 679. [CrossRef]
46. Schmitt, H.M.; Schlamp, C.L.; Nickells, R.W. Targeting HDAC3 activity with RGFP966 protects against retinal ganglion cell nuclear atrophy and apoptosis after optic nerve injury. *J. Ocul. Pharmacol. Ther.* **2018**, *34*, 260–273. [CrossRef]
47. Li, P.; Ma, Y.; Yu, C.; Wu, S.; Wang, K.; Yi, H.; Liang, W. Autophagy and aging: Roles in skeletal muscle, eye, brain and hepatic tissue. *Front. Cell Dev. Biol.* **2021**, *9*, 752962. [CrossRef]
48. Li, J.; Zhao, L.; Urabe, G.; Fu, Y.; Guo, L.-W. Epigenetic intervention with a BET inhibitor ameliorates acute retinal ganglion cell death in mice. *Mol. Vis.* **2017**, *23*, 149.
49. Wiese, M.; Bannister, A.J. Two genomes, one cell: Mitochondrial-nuclear coordination via epigenetic pathways. *Mol. Metab.* **2020**, *38*, 100942. [CrossRef]
50. Xie, K.; Ngo, S.; Rong, J.; Sheppard, A. Modulation of mitochondrial respiration underpins neuronal differentiation enhanced by lutein. *Neural Regen. Res.* **2019**, *14*, 87. [CrossRef]
51. Faraco, G.; Pittelli, M.; Cavone, L.; Fossati, S.; Porcu, M.; Mascagni, P.; Fossati, G.; Moroni, F.; Chiarugi, A. Histone deacetylase (HDAC) inhibitors reduce the glial inflammatory response in vitro and in vivo. *Neurobiol. Dis.* **2009**, *36*, 269–279. [CrossRef]
52. Suh, H.-S.; Choi, S.; Khattar, P.; Choi, N.; Lee, S.C. Histone deacetylase inhibitors suppress the expression of inflammatory and innate immune response genes in human microglia and astrocytes. *J. Neuroimmune Pharmacol.* **2010**, *5*, 521–532. [CrossRef]
53. Kanski, R.; Sneeboer, M.A.; van Bodegraven, E.J.; Sluijs, J.A.; Kropff, W.; Vermunt, M.W.; Creyghton, M.P.; De Filippis, L.; Vescovi, A.; Aronica, E. Histone acetylation in astrocytes suppresses GFAP and stimulates a reorganization of the intermediate filament network. *J. Cell Sci.* **2014**, *127*, 4368–4380. [CrossRef]
54. Xuan, A.; Long, D.; Li, J.; Ji, W.; Hong, L.; Zhang, M.; Zhang, W. Neuroprotective effects of valproic acid following transient global ischemia in rats. *Life Sci.* **2012**, *90*, 463–468. [CrossRef]
55. Buczek-Thomas, J.A.; Hsia, E.; Rich, C.B.; Foster, J.A.; Nugent, M.A. Inhibition of histone acetyltransferase by glycosaminoglycans. *J. Cell. Biochem.* **2008**, *105*, 108–120. [CrossRef]
56. Kuboyama, T.; Wahane, S.; Huang, Y.; Zhou, X.; Wong, J.K.; Koemeter-Cox, A.; Martini, M.; Friedel, R.H.; Zou, H. HDAC3 inhibition ameliorates spinal cord injury by immunomodulation. *Sci. Rep.* **2017**, *7*, 1–13. [CrossRef]
57. Skowronska-Krawczyk, D.; Ballivet, M.; Dynlacht, B.; Matter, J.-M. Highly specific interactions between bHLH transcription factors and chromatin during retina development. *Development* **2004**, *131*, 4447–4454. [CrossRef]
58. Li, Y.; Du, Z.; Xie, X.; Zhang, Y.; Liu, H.; Zhou, Z.; Zhao, J.; Lee, R.S.; Xiao, Y.; Ivanoviski, S.; et al. Epigenetic changes caused by diabetes and their potential role in the development of periodontitis. *J. Diabetes Investig.* **2021**, *12*, 1326–1335. [CrossRef]
59. Reverdatto, S.; Prasad, A.; Belrose, J.L.; Zhang, X.; Sammons, M.A.; Gibbs, K.M.; Szaro, B.G. Developmental and injury-induced changes in DNA methylation in regenerative versus non-regenerative regions of the vertebrate central nervous system. *BMC Genom.* **2022**, *23*, 2. [CrossRef] [PubMed]
60. Smith, J.; Sen, S.; Weeks, R.J.; Eccles, M.R.; Chatterjee, A. Promoter DNA hypermethylation and paradoxical gene activation. *Trends Cancer* **2020**, *6*, 392–406. [CrossRef] [PubMed]
61. Takasawa, K.; Arai, Y.; Yamazaki-Inoue, M.; Toyoda, M.; Akutsu, H.; Umezawa, A.; Nishino, K. DNA hypermethylation enhanced telomerase reverse transcriptase expression in human-induced pluripotent stem cells. *Hum. Cell* **2018**, *31*, 78–86. [CrossRef] [PubMed]
62. Struebing, F.L.; Wang, J.; Li, Y.; King, R.; Mistretta, O.C.; English, A.W.; Geisert, E.E. Differential expression of Sox11 and Bdnf mRNA isoforms in the injured and regenerating nervous systems. *Front. Mol. Neurosci.* **2017**, *10*, 354. [CrossRef]

63. Wang, X.; Zhang, J.; Liao, Y.; Jin, Y.; Yu, X.; Li, H.; Yang, Q.; Li, X.; Chen, R.; Wu, D. DNMT1-mediated DNA methylation targets CDKN2B to promote the repair of retinal ganglion cells in streptozotocin-induced mongolian gerbils during diabetic retinopathy. *Comput. Math. Methods Med.* **2022**, *2022*, 1–9. [CrossRef]
64. Pelzel, H.R.; Schlamp, C.L.; Nickells, R.W. Histone H4 deacetylation plays a critical role in early gene silencing during neuronal apoptosis. *BMC Neurosci.* **2010**, *11*, 1–20. [CrossRef]
65. Cho, Y.; Cavalli, V. HDAC5 is a novel injury-regulated tubulin deacetylase controlling axon regeneration. *EMBO J.* **2012**, *31*, 3063–3078. [CrossRef]
66. Rivieccio, M.A.; Brochier, C.; Willis, D.E.; Walker, B.A.; D'Annibale, M.A.; McLaughlin, K.; Siddiq, A.; Kozikowski, A.P.; Jaffrey, S.R.; Twiss, J.L.; et al. HDAC6 is a target for protection and regeneration following injury in the nervous system. *Proc. Natl. Acad. Sci. USA* **2009**, *106*, 19599–19604. [CrossRef]
67. Gaub, P.; Tedeschi, A.; Puttagunta, R.; Nguyen, T.; Schmandke, A.; Di Giovanni, S. HDAC inhibition promotes neuronal outgrowth and counteracts growth cone collapse through CBP/p300 and P/CAF-dependent p53 acetylation. *Cell Death Differ.* **2010**, *17*, 1392–1408. [CrossRef]
68. Lebrun-Julien, F.; Suter, U. Combined HDAC1 and HDAC2 depletion promotes retinal ganglion cell survival after injury through reduction of p53 target gene expression. *ASN Neuro* **2015**, *7*, 1759091415593066. [CrossRef]
69. Zou, S.; Tian, C.; Ge, S.; Hu, B. Neurogenesis of retinal ganglion cells is not essential to visual functional recovery after optic nerve injury in adult zebrafish. *PLoS ONE* **2013**, *8*, e57280. [CrossRef]
70. Siebzehnrubl, F.A.; Buslei, R.; Eyupoglu, I.Y.; Seufert, S.; Hahnen, E.; Blumcke, I. Histone deacetylase inhibitors increase neuronal differentiation in adult forebrain precursor cells. *Exp. Brain Res.* **2007**, *176*, 672–678. [CrossRef]
71. Dincman, T.A.; Beare, J.E.; Ohri, S.S.; Gallo, V.; Hetman, M.; Whittemore, S.R. Histone deacetylase inhibition is cytotoxic to oligodendrocyte precursor cells in vitro and in vivo. *Int. J. Dev. Neurosci.* **2016**, *54*, 53–61. [CrossRef]
72. Huang, X.; Wu, D.-Y.; Chen, G.; Manji, H.; Chen, D.F. Support of retinal ganglion cell survival and axon regeneration by lithium through a Bcl-2-dependent mechanism. *Investig. Ophthalmol. Vis. Sci.* **2003**, *44*, 347–354. [CrossRef] [PubMed]
73. Biermann, J.; Boyle, J.; Pielen, A.; Lagrèze, W.A. Histone deacetylase inhibitors sodium butyrate and valproic acid delay spontaneous cell death in purified rat retinal ganglion cells. *Mol. Vis.* **2011**, *17*, 395–403. [PubMed]
74. Phiel, C.J.; Zhang, F.; Huang, E.Y.; Guenther, M.G.; Lazar, M.A.; Klein, P.S. Histone deacetylase is a direct target of valproic acid, a potent anticonvulsant, mood stabilizer, and teratogen. *J. Biol. Chem.* **2001**, *276*, 36734–36741. [CrossRef] [PubMed]
75. Zaidi, S.A.H.; Guzman, W.; Singh, S.; Mehrotra, S.; Husain, S. Changes in class I and IIb HDACs by δ-opioid in chronic rat glaucoma model. *Investig. Ophthalmol. Vis. Sci.* **2020**, *61*, 4. [CrossRef]
76. Luo, J.; Su, F.; Chen, D.; Shiloh, A.; Gu, W. Deacetylation of p53 modulates its effect on cell growth and apoptosis. *Nature* **2000**, *408*, 377–381. [CrossRef]
77. Vaziri, H.; Dessain, S.K.; Eaton, E.N.; Imai, S.-I.; Frye, R.A.; Pandita, T.K.; Guarente, L.; Weinberg, R.A. hSIR2SIRT1 functions as an NAD-dependent p53 deacetylase. *Cell* **2001**, *107*, 149–159. [CrossRef]
78. Mrakovcic, M.; Kleinheinz, J.; Fröhlich, L.F. p53 at the crossroads between different types of HDAC inhibitor-mediated cancer cell death. *Int. J. Mol. Sci.* **2019**, *20*, 2415. [CrossRef]
79. Shi, J.; Vakoc, C.R. The mechanisms behind the therapeutic activity of BET bromodomain inhibition. *Mol. Cell* **2014**, *54*, 728–736. [CrossRef]
80. Gupta, R.; Saha, P.; Sen, T.; Sen, N. An augmentation in histone dimethylation at lysine nine residues elicits vision impairment following traumatic brain injury. *Free. Radic. Biol. Med.* **2019**, *134*, 630–643. [CrossRef]
81. Chase, K.; Feiner, B.; Ramaker, M.; Hu, E.; Rosen, C.; Sharma, R. Examining the effects of the histone methyltransferase inhibitor BIX-01294 on histone modifications and gene expression in both a clinical population and mouse models. *PLoS ONE* **2019**, *14*, e0216463. [CrossRef]
82. Cheng, L.; Wong, L.J.; Yan, N.; Han, R.C.; Yu, H.; Guo, C.; Batsuuri, K.; Zinzuwadia, A.; Guan, R.; Cho, K.-S. Ezh2 does not mediate retinal ganglion cell homeostasis or their susceptibility to injury. *PLoS ONE* **2018**, *13*, e0191853. [CrossRef]
83. Yan, N.; Cheng, L.; Cho, K.; Malik, M.T.A.; Xiao, L.; Guo, C.; Yu, H.; Zhu, R.; Rao, R.C.; Chen, D.F. Postnatal onset of retinal degeneration by loss of embryonic Ezh2 repression of Six1. *Sci. Rep.* **2016**, *6*, 33887. [CrossRef]
84. Xiao, L.; Hou, C.; Cheng, L.; Zheng, S.; Zhao, L.; Yan, N. DZNep protects against retinal ganglion cell death in an NMDA-induced mouse model of retinal degeneration. *Exp. Eye Res.* **2021**, *212*, 108785. [CrossRef]
85. Tsutsumi, T.; Iwao, K.; Hayashi, H.; Kirihara, T.; Kawaji, T.; Inoue, T.; Hino, S.; Nakao, M.; Tanihara, H. Potential neuroprotective effects of an LSD1 inhibitor in retinal ganglion cells via p38 mapk activity. *Investig. Ophthalmol. Vis. Sci.* **2016**, *57*, 6461–6473. [CrossRef]
86. Chung, D.; Shum, A.; Caraveo, G. GAP-43 and BASP1 in axon regeneration: Implications for the treatment of neurodegenerative diseases. *Front. Cell Dev. Biol.* **2020**, *8*, 567537. [CrossRef]
87. Latremoliere, A.; Cheng, L.; DeLisle, M.; Wu, C.; Chew, S.; Hutchinson, E.B.; Sheridan, A.; Alexandre, C.; Latremoliere, F.; Sheu, S.-H. Neuronal-specific TUBB3 is not required for normal neuronal function but is essential for timely axon regeneration. *Cell Rep.* **2018**, *24*, 1865–1879. [CrossRef]
88. Smith, P.D.; Sun, F.; Park, K.K.; Cai, B.; Wang, C.; Kuwako, K.; Martinez-Carrasco, I.; Connolly, L.; He, Z. *SOCS3* Deletion Promotes Optic Nerve Regeneration In Vivo. *Neuron* **2009**, *64*, 617–623. [CrossRef]

89. Lindborg, J.A.; Tran, N.M.; Chenette, D.M.; DeLuca, K.; Foli, Y.; Kannan, R.; Sekine, Y.; Wang, X.; Wollan, M.; Kim, I.-J.; et al. Optic nerve regeneration screen identifies multiple genes restricting adult neural repair. *Cell Reports* **2021**, *34*, 108777. [CrossRef]
90. Park, K.K.; Liu, K.; Hu, Y.; Smith, P.D.; Wang, C.; Cai, B.; Xu, B.; Connolly, L.; Kramvis, I.; Sahin, M. Promoting axon regeneration in the adult CNS by modulation of the *PTEN*/mTOR pathway. *Science* **2008**, *322*, 963–966. [CrossRef]
91. Wang, Y.H.; Huang, M.L. Organogenesis and tumorigenesis: Insight from the JAK/STAT pathway in the Drosophila eye. *Dev. Dyn.* **2010**, *239*, 2522–2533. [CrossRef]
92. Madsen, A.S.; Kristensen, H.M.; Lanz, G.; Olsen, C.A. The effect of various zinc binding groups on inhibition of histone deacetylases 1–11. *ChemMedChem* **2014**, *9*, 614–626. [CrossRef]
93. Younes, A.; Oki, Y.; Bociek, R.G.; Kuruvilla, J.; Fanale, M.; Neelapu, S.; Copeland, A.; Buglio, D.; Galal, A.; Besterman, J. Mocetinostat for relapsed classical Hodgkin's lymphoma: An open-label, single-arm, phase 2 trial. *Lancet Oncol.* **2011**, *12*, 1222–1228. [CrossRef]
94. Weng, Y.-L.; An, R.; Cassin, J.; Joseph, J.; Mi, R.; Wang, C.; Zhong, C.; Jin, S.-G.; Pfeifer, G.P.; Bellacosa, A. An intrinsic epigenetic barrier for functional axon regeneration. *Neuron* **2017**, *94*, 337–346. [CrossRef] [PubMed]
95. Wu, Y.; Xu, Y.; Huang, X.; Ye, D.; Han, M.; Wang, H.-L. Regulatory roles of histone deacetylases 1 and 2 in Pb-induced neurotoxicity. *Toxicol. Sci.* **2018**, *162*, 688–701. [CrossRef] [PubMed]
96. Douvaras, P.; Rusielewicz, T.; Kim, K.H.; Haines, J.D.; Casaccia, P.; Fossati, V. Epigenetic modulation of human induced pluripotent stem cell differentiation to oligodendrocytes. *Int. J. Mol. Sci.* **2016**, *17*, 614. [CrossRef] [PubMed]
97. Xu, W.; Zhang, X.; Liang, F.; Cao, Y.; Li, Z.; Qu, W.; Zhang, J.; Bi, Y.; Sun, C.; Zhang, J.; et al. Tet1 regulates astrocyte development and cognition of mice through modulating GluA1. *Front. Cell Dev. Biol.* **2021**, *9*, 644375. [CrossRef] [PubMed]

International Journal of
Molecular Sciences

MDPI

Review

Treatment and Relapse Prevention of Typical and Atypical Optic Neuritis

George Saitakis [1,2] and Bart K. Chwalisz [1,3,*]

1 Division of Neuro-Ophthalmology, Department of Ophthalmology, Massachusetts Eye & Ear Infirmary, Harvard Medical School, Boston, MA 02115, USA
2 Athens Eye Hospital, 166 75 Athens, Greece
3 Department of Neurology, Massachusetts General Hospital, Harvard Medical School, 15 Parkman Street, Suite 835, Boston, MA 02114, USA
* Correspondence: bchwalisz@mgh.harvard.edu; Tel.: +1-617-724-3646

Abstract: Optic neuritis (ON) is an inflammatory condition involving the optic nerve. Several important typical and atypical ON variants are now recognized. Typical ON has a more favorable prognosis; it can be idiopathic or represent an early manifestation of demyelinating diseases, mostly multiple sclerosis (MS). The atypical spectrum includes entities such as antibody-driven ON associated with neuromyelitis optica spectrum disorder (NMOSD) and myelin oligodendrocyte glycoprotein antibody disease (MOGAD), chronic/relapsing inflammatory optic neuropathy (CRION), and sarcoidosis-associated ON. Appropriate and timely diagnosis is essential to rapidly decide on the appropriate treatment, maximize visual recovery, and minimize recurrences. This review paper aims at presenting the currently available state-of-the-art treatment strategies for typical and atypical ON, both in the acute phase and in the long-term. Moreover, emerging therapeutic approaches and novel steps in the direction of achieving remyelination are discussed.

Keywords: atypical optic neuritis treatment; typical optic neuritis; MOG; NMO; MS prevention

Citation: Saitakis, G.; Chwalisz, B.K. Treatment and Relapse Prevention of Typical and Atypical Optic Neuritis. *Int. J. Mol. Sci.* **2022**, *23*, 9769. https://doi.org/10.3390/ijms23179769

Academic Editors: Neil R. Miller and Rongkung Tsai

Received: 22 July 2022
Accepted: 18 August 2022
Published: 29 August 2022

1. Introduction

Optic neuritis (ON) is an inflammatory condition involving the optic nerve but is far from being a uniform condition, and several important variants are now recognized that can be stratified into typical and atypical forms. Typical, ON usually manifests in young adults, especially women, between 18 and 45 years of age, and can be idiopathic or represent an early manifestation of demyelinating diseases, mostly multiple sclerosis (MS). The atypical spectrum includes entities such as neuromyelitis optica spectrum disorder (NMOSD), myelin oligodendrocyte glycoprotein antibody disease (MOGAD), chronic/relapsing inflammatory optic neuropathy (CRION), and sarcoidosis-associated ON, and in all of these, the clinical presentation, visual prognosis, and recurrence risk differ from typical ON. Importantly, optimal treatment approaches are also not uniform, making it essential to more accurately differentiate these entities based not only on their clinical presentation but also their pathogenesis. We will discuss currently available state-of-the art therapeutic strategies for typical and atypical ON, both in terms of acute treatment with regard to long-term relapse prevention. Moreover, emerging therapeutic approaches and novel steps in the direction of achieving remyelination are discussed.

2. Typical Optic Neuritis

Optic neuritis (ON) is an inflammatory condition involving the optic nerve, manifested usually in young adults, especially women, between 18 and 45 years of age [1]. The majority of the cases are idiopathic, but ON can be associated with demyelinating diseases, most commonly multiple sclerosis (MS). Optic neuritis represents one of the most frequent phenotypes of MS relapse, and occurs as the first demyelinating event in about one out of three MS patients [2]. MS is characterized by the presence of plaques that form in the CNS in combination with inflammation, demyelination, axonal injury, and axonal loss. The plaques are located primarily in the white matter of the brain, spinal cord, and optic pathways, but there is also involvement in the gray matter [3,4]. Depending on their stage of development, they contain varying proportions of immune cells and immunoreactive substances [5]. Plaques are expressed in all forms of MS, but vary over time quantitatively and qualitatively, showing a profound heterogeneity in the structure and immunopathological patterns of demyelination and oligodendrocyte pathology between relapsing-remitting and progressive forms of MS [6]. MS likely represents a T-cell-mediated autoimmune disorder with a predominance of $CD8^+$ cells. The dominant theory is that inflammatory lesions in MS consist mainly of $CD8^+$ and $CD4^+$ T cells, and activated microglia and macrophages [7,8]. There is evidence regarding the suppression of functions that restricts $CD4^+$ T-cell responses, and the tissue-damaging role of $CD8^+$ T cells is reported to co-localize with axonal pathology [9,10]. Experiments in humanized transgenic mice showed that the specific interaction of $CD8^+$ T cells with target cells requires MHC-I expression, which is tightly regulated in neurons and MHC-I molecules, only in response to danger signals such as pro-inflammatory cytokines IFN-γ or TNF-α [9]. However, the role of B cells has also become apparent, as evidenced, for instance, by the effectiveness of B cell inhibition as an MS disease-modifying therapy (DMT).

3. Pathophysiology of ON

In the acute phase, ON pathology is characterized by optic nerve abnormalities and inflammatory demyelination. More specifically, predominant T cell, B cell, and glial cell activation within the nerve increases pro-inflammatory cytokines, leading to the activation of microglia and monocyte-derived macrophages, and further recruitment of $CD4^-$ and $CD8^+$ T cells [11]. The subsequent inflammation leads to demyelination, reactive gliosis, and axonal death [12]. Pro-inflammatory cytokines and cytotoxic factors target myelin-producing oligodendrocytes (OLGs) and oligodendrocyte precursor cells (OPCs), causing apoptosis and exacerbating axonal demyelination [13–16]. Mature OLGs that survive demyelination are unable to produce new myelin sheaths. Remyelination, therefore, requires the migration and regeneration of oligodendrocytes from OPCs [17].

It is worth noting that the acute inflammatory lesions of the afferent visual pathway cause retrograde degeneration of retinal ganglion cells (RGCs). It has been demonstrated that RGC loss is associated with a reduction in post-synaptic proteins and neurite projections, and with persistent microglia and astroglia activation in the inner retina with high levels of iNOS (inducible nitric oxide synthase), IL (interleukin)-1α, TNF (tumor necrosis factor)-α, and C1q (complement component 1q) [15]. Thus, the development of therapeutic agents should focus on anti-inflammatory, anti-apoptotic, and remyelinating mechanisms to achieve neuroprotection and neuro-regeneration in the optic nerve and retina.

4. Acute Treatment of Typical Optic Neuritis/Clinically Isolated Syndrome

In general, MS is characterized by its tendency for recurrence in proximity to a previously affected site, as has been observed radiologically [18,19] and confirmed in post-mortem pathological studies [20]. Lotan et al. showed that in MS, recurrent episodes of ON tend to attack the same optic nerve that was affected before [21]. Similar findings come from a 2011 study [22]. Potential explanations for the recurrent nature of ON in MS is the disruption of the blood–brain barrier during the initial insult and antigenic change and expansion, leading to epitope spreading as a pathogenic event leading to a chronic CNS demyelinating disease [23].

Based on the presence of prominent immunologic activity in the pathologic samples of MS patients and oligoclonal bands in the CSF of most MS patients, it has been suggested that the disease is an immune-mediated disorder [6,24–26]. However, there are alternative theories claiming that MS is not a homogenous condition, thus not fulfilling the criteria of an autoimmune disease [27–29]. Much effort has been invested in identifying the autoantigen(s) against which the oligoclonal bands are directed, so far without success. It is believed that the inflammatory attack is not an outcome of an immune response directed against a specific auto-antigen. Thus, in MS, unlike NMOSD and MOG antibody disease, the immune response may be nonspecific and triggered by tissue changes induced by the previous attack.

Corticosteroid use has traditionally been the common approach for the treatment of ON, with the first implementation dating back to the 1950s [30]. Data from the United States demonstrate that the majority of ophthalmologists and neurologists in the 1980s used to treat their patients with optic neuritis with standard oral doses of corticosteroids, despite the lack of convincing evidence of efficacy [30,31]. The Optic Neuritis Treatment Trial (ONTT) was the first multicenter, randomized, collaborative clinical trial of ON [30,31]. Fifteen centers in the United States participated in the ONTT, recruiting 457 patients between 1 July 1988 and 30 June 1991. Patients were enrolled who had acute unilateral optic neuritis with visual symptoms lasting 8 days or less, aged between 18 and 45 years, with no previous history of optic neuritis in the affected eye, no evidence of associated systemic disease other than MS, and no previous treatment with corticosteroids for MS or optic neuritis [31]. The mean age of patients at study entry was 32 years, 77% of patients were women, and 85% identified as white. The participants were randomized either to be treated with oral prednisone (1 mg/kg daily for 14 days), intravenous methylprednisolone (250 mg every 6 h for 3 days) followed by oral prednisone (1 mg/kg daily for 11 days), or oral placebo. Each regimen was followed by a short oral dosage taper consisting of 20 mg of prednisone (or placebo) on day 15 and 10 mg of prednisone (or placebo) on days 16 and 18 [29,30]. In general, steroid treatment was well tolerated, with only minor adverse effects (sleep disturbance, mild mood change, upset stomach, facial flushing, mild weight gain), except for a case of acute transient depression and another patient that suffered from acute pancreatitis. Patients were evaluated in seven follow-up visits during the first 6 months, at 1 year, then yearly through 1997, in 2001 through 2002, and finally in 2006. According to the study design, the primary outcome for the treatment group comparison was set at 6 months.

The study findings demonstrated that the natural course of visual functions after an episode of typical optic neuritis, either treated or untreated, is one of a rapid visual recovery beginning within 2 weeks after the onset of symptoms, with most of the recovery often taking place after 4 to 6 weeks, and further slow recovery over several months, even up to 1 year [2]. In almost all patients, regardless of the treatment group and initial severity of visual losses, some improvement began within the first 30 days [2,30]. Of clinical relevance, recurrences of optic neuritis occurred more commonly in patients treated with oral prednisolone alone; within 2 years from diagnosis, the probability of recurrence in either eye was almost 2-fold higher in the low-dose prednisone group (30%) than in either the placebo group (14%) or the high-dose intravenous group (16%) [30–33]. The ONTT showed that vision recovered faster in the intravenous group than in the other groups, although the difference among the three groups had faded by 30 days. However, at 6 months, qualitative features such as contrast sensitivity, visual field, and color vision were still slightly better in the intravenous group. By contrast, the prednisone group compared with the placebo group demonstrated no significant differences in the rate of recovery or the 6-month outcome for any aspect of the visual function. At the 6-month point, patients in all three treatment groups had a median visual acuity of 20/16, and fewer than 1 out of 10 patients had a visual outcome of 20/50 or worse. At the 1-year follow-up, there was no statistically significant difference in visual function among the groups. Visual acuity was 20/40 or better in 95% of the placebo group, 94% of the intravenous steroid group, and 91% of the oral steroid group at 1 year. After 15 years, 72% of the eyes affected with optic neuritis had visual acuity of $\geq$20/20, and 66% of the patients had $\geq$20/20 acuity in both eyes [1]. A 2015 Cochrane Systematic Review also reported the failure of intravenous steroids to improve vision outcomes in ON [34]. The ONTT also found that among the 389 patients without a diagnosis of clinically probable or definite MS at study entry, the intravenous steroid group showed a lower rate of development of clinically definite MS within the first 2 years (7.5%) than did the placebo (16.7%) or prednisone (14.7%) groups, but this apparent protective effect was not sustained at 3 years [30]. By 5 years, the treatment had no significant effect on the development of MS. Most of the aforementioned intravenous treatment group benefits on the development of MS were observed in patients with brain findings on the magnetic resonance imaging (MRI) at baseline, because the rate of MS among patients without baseline MRI lesions was so low that therapeutic efficacy could not be determined.

Some potential limitations of the trial include the definition of symptom onset (timed from the visual loss but not from the onset of pain), inclusion of possible MOG cases, the validity of the primary outcome measure of high-contrast visual acuity, and the lack of pharmacokinetic data (making it difficult to develop a plausible biological explanation for as to why oral vs. intravenous corticosteroids should be harmful compared with intravenous corticosteroids). In addition, the long interval between the onset of symptoms and initiation of treatment in ONTT (up to 8 days) leaves open the possibility that a "critical time window" may have been missed, and that more vision loss could be prevented if treatment was initiated in the early inflammatory phase (within 48 h) [35,36]. Experimental evidence supports such a critical time window for treatment initiation in optic neuritis, as it has been shown that inflammation of the optic nerve precedes demyelination and axonal degeneration by about 2 days, and irreversible damage to the axonal cytoskeleton occurs within 5–7 days [35,37]. Indeed, a retrospective study demonstrates significant improvement in both functional and structural outcomes in patients with relapsing ON when treatment is initiated early [38].

The current standard of care for typical optic neuritis, still based on the results of the ONTT, is either no treatment in mild cases or the administration of intravenous steroids to accelerate visual recovery [30,39,40]. A proton pump inhibitor may also be given to prevent peptic ulcers. There is no role for low-dose oral prednisone [31]. This reasoning is consistent with a Cochrane meta-analysis as well [41].

Since the publication of the ONTT, other studies have shown that high-dose oral corticosteroids and high-dose IV methylprednisolone are bioequivalent, and have similar effects on MRI outcomes and clinical MS relapse [2]. Morrow et al., in 2018, showed in a single-blind randomized clinical trial that the efficacy of high-dose oral steroids is bioequivalent to and shows no inferiority to intravenous steroids. More specifically, 55 participants were randomized to either methylprednisolone sodium succinate (1000 mg, IV) daily for 3 days or oral prednisone (1250 mg) daily for 3 days. Improvements in vision were noticed at 1 month and at 6 months [2]. Compliance with this oral regimen has been previously shown to be very high [2]. Similar results were cited by the COPOUSEP trial in France [42]. In addition, a Cochrane review in 2008 compared the efficacy of the two forms of steroid administration and found them to be equally effective. Studies have also shown that intravenous dexamethasone in a dose of 200 mg/day had comparable efficacy to 1 g/day of intravenous methylprednisolone, and has the advantage of low costs and fewer side effects [39]. Intramuscular or subcutaneous adrenocorticotropic hormones are also approved for the treatment of ON- and MS-related relapses [40].

Intravenous immunoglobulin (IVIg) has a potential role in the management of acute optic neuritis, though evidence is limited, and the agent is typically reserved for the treatment of patients with steroid-refractory ON. IVIg may cause rash, fever, and, rarely, aseptic meningitis, thrombosis, hemolysis, and renal dysfunction [39]. In general, plasma exchange (PLEX) is typically favored over IVIg to manage MS relapses that are not responsive to steroid treatments. PLEX is associated with a number of potential side effects including myocardial infarction, arrhythmia, hemolysis, central line placement risk, and death in a small percentage of patients [43]. More recently, high-dose cyclophosphamide (50 mg/kg per day for 4 consecutive days, followed by a granulocyte-colony-stimulating factor 6 days after completion) was evaluated in nine patients with aggressive RRMS as a rescue treatment for acute fulminant relapses. Potential side effects of the short-term high-dose cyclophosphamide monotherapy in patients with MS include neutropenia and infection [40,44].

5. Long-Term Treatment: Immune Prophylaxis against Optic Neuritis Relapses/Progression to Multiple Sclerosis

5.1. Mechanisms of Action in Interferon β in MS and Optic Neuritis

Interferons (IFNs) have been recruited as a potential therapeutic option for MS based on their immunomodulatory and antiproliferative properties [45]. It is believed that IFNs act via several overlapping mechanisms such as the down-regulation of the major histocompatibility complex (MHC) class II expression present on the antigen-presenting cells, the induction of T-cell production of interleukin 10 (IL-10), and thus a shift in the balance toward anti-inflammatory T helper (Th)-2 cells, and the inhibition of T-cell migration as a result of a blockade of metalloproteases and adhesion molecules [46] (Figure 1: a synopsis of IFN mechanisms of action).

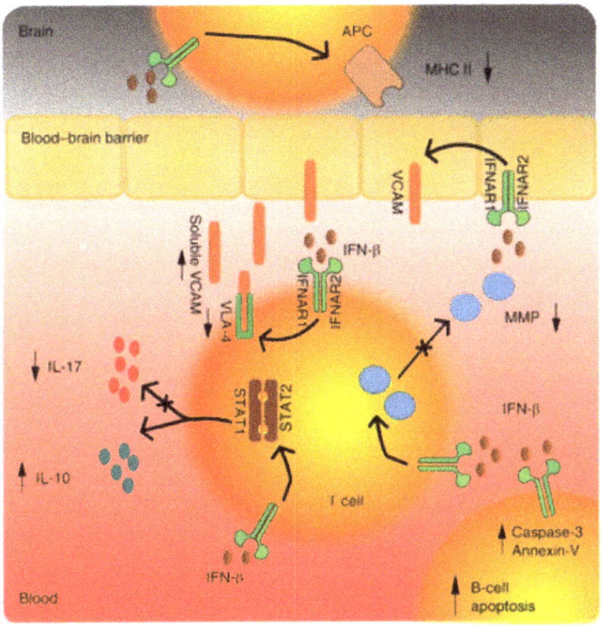

Molecular mechanisms of action of interferon β (IFN-β). Decrease of cellular expression of adhesion molecules (VLA-4) and cleavage of endothelial vascular cell adhesion protein (VCAM) results in decrease in cell sequestration through the blood-brain barrier. Additional decrease of matrix metalloproteinase (MMP) diminishes the ability for lymphocyte penetration. Activation of IFNAR1/2 receptors results in phosphorylation of signal transducers and activators of transcription (STAT)1-STAT2 factors that further results in secretion of anti-inflammatory cytokine profiles. Activation of IFNAR1/2 also results in decrease of major histocompatibility complex II (MHC II) expression and diminishes lymphocyte activation. IFN-β also increases apoptotic markers like Annexin-V and active caspase-3 via Fas-receptor/transmembrane activator and CAML interactor (TACI) signaling, resulting in specific depletion of memory B cells. IL, interleukin.

Figure 1. Molecular Mechanisms of Action of Interferon β [45].

The actions of IFNs are mediated through transcriptional factors and subsequent gene regulation. The major route in which IFN-β produces its effect is by activating the Janus kinase (JAK) signal transducers and activators of the transcription (STAT) pathway. More specifically, IFN-β binding to the type I IFN receptor causes phosphorylation of STAT1 and STAT2 and the formation of STAT1-STAT2 heterodimers, which translocate to the nucleus, bind the IFN-stimulated response element (ISRE), and modulate the expression of ISRE-regulated genes [47]. It has been demonstrated that the cellular response to IFNs is complex and results in changes in the expression of more than 500 genes representing ~0.5% of the human genome [48]. Rizzo et al., focusing on the pivotal role of B cells in MS immunopathology, investigated the mechanism of B-cell apoptosis. The up-regulation of mechanisms that require FAS-receptor/TACI (transmembrane activator and CAML interactor) signaling and the production of apoptotic markers such as Annexin-V and caspase-3 were shown as specific inducers of B-cell apoptosis [49].

5.2. Glatiramer Acetate (GA)

The mechanism of action of GA has long been an enigma. GA has well-established immunomodulatory properties, promoting the expansion of anti-inflammatory and regulatory Th2 and Treg cells and inducing the release of neurotrophic factors. Using various genetically modified mouse strains, as well as human monocytes, Molnarfi et al. showed that GA inhibited the TRIF-dependent pathway, resulting in a reduction in IFN-β production [50] (Figure 2). This observation is consistent with the earlier demonstration that STAT1 phosphorylation is reduced upon activation in type II monocytes [51]. These findings provide a key anti-inflammatory mechanism connecting innate and adaptive immune modulation in GA therapy. Animal studies have also shown that GA-reactive Th2 cells migrate to the CNS and accumulate at the site of active lesions. Thus, GA-reactive T cells provide the effector arm in treatment. However, GA treatment influences both innate and adaptive immune compartments, and it is now recognized that antigen-presenting cells (APCs) are the initial cellular targets for GA, and it is the modulation of the APC compartment to anti-inflammatory (M2) phenotypes that leads to an expansion in regulatory Th2 and Treg cells. In addition, the anti-inflammatory (M2) APCs induced following treatment with GA are responsible for the induction of anti-inflammatory T cells that contribute to its therapeutic benefit [52]. Mechanisms of action of GA that promote immunomodulation and neuroprotection are not mutually exclusive, and several may contribute to the efficacy of the drug (Figure 3).

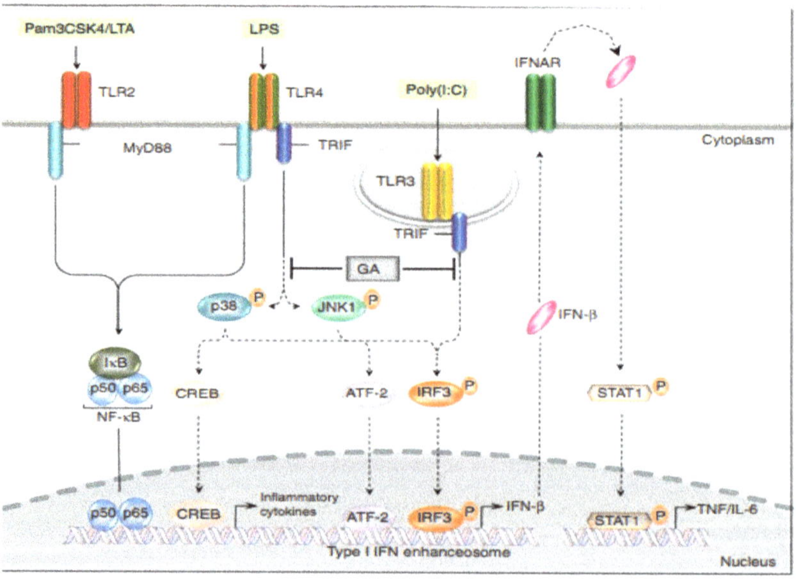

Figure 2. *Cont.*

Glatiramer acetate (GA) treatment modulates type I interferon (IFN) production. GA treatment down-regulates Toll-IL-1 receptor domain-containing adaptor-inducing IFN-β (TRIF) signaling on antigen-presenting cells (APCs), leading to decreased activation of IFN regulatory factor 3 (IRF3) and ATF-2, and subsequent DNA binding of the type I IFN enhanceosome (Molnarfi et al. 2015). Reduction of IFN-β production results in decreased signal transducers and activators of transcription (STAT)1 phosphorylation and activation of proinflammatory cytokines. LPS, Lipid peroxidation; IFNAR, interferon-receptor; TLR, Toll-like receptor; MyD88, myeloid differentiation primary response gene 88; TNF, tumor necrosis factor.

Figure 2. Glatiramer Acetate Modulates Type I Interferon production [50].

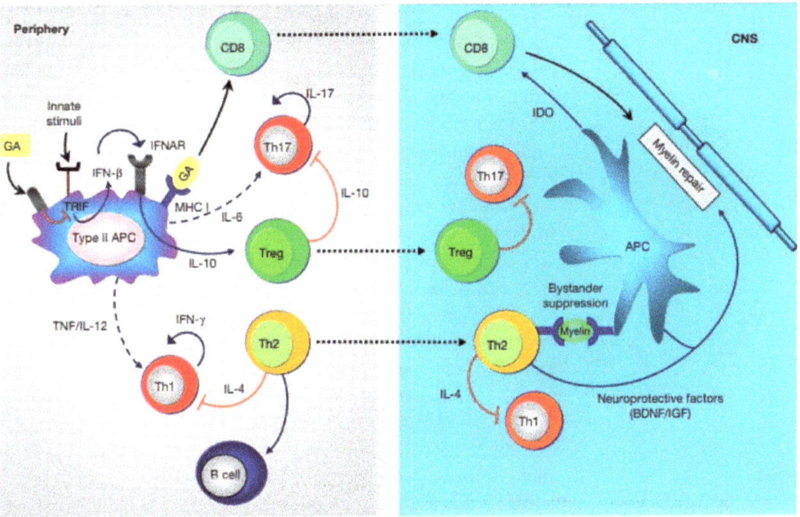

Anti-inflammatory mechanisms induced by glatiramer acetate (GA). GA treatment on antigen-presenting cells (APCs) leads to anti-inflammatory differentiation. Treatment modulates innate stimuli and is associated with down-regulation of type I interferon (IFN), increased T helper (Th)2, and regulatory T (Treg) cell differentiation. Reactivation of GA-reactive Th2 cells in periphery through presentation of myelin antigens is associated with bystander suppression. Th2 cells also modulate B-cell activation. Treg cells down-regulate secretion of proinflammatory cytokines by effector T (Teff) cells both in periphery and in the central nervous system (CNS). $CD8^+$ T cells are generated by antigen presentation of GA in periphery and migrate to the CNS where they contribute to inhibiting myelin degradation. IL, Interleukin; TNF, tumor necrosis factor; IFNAR, interferon-receptor; MHC, major histocompatibility complex; BDNF, brain-derived neurotrophic factor; IGF, insulin-like growth factor; IDO, indoleamine-2,3-dioxygenase; solid lines, cytokines produced by the representative cells; dashed lines, reduced production of cytokines; red lines: inhibitory cytokines.

Figure 3. Anti-inflammatory Mechanisms Induced by Glatiramer Acetate [52].

5.3. Treatment of Clinically Isolated Syndromes

In this article, we are reviewing some of the trials that specifically addressed clinically isolated syndromes such as optic neuritis. These are mostly older trials. We will not cover all multiple sclerosis treatments in detail, but acknowledge that several newer DMTs for MS have class I evidence for MS, and have approval for treatment of both MS and CIS. This evidence (and the FDA approval of these medications) is based on MS trials, not specifically CIS/optic neuritis trials, and will not be reviewed in detail. Thus, in clinical practice, a number of additional MS medicines may be used for high-risk CIS patients, likely with good efficacy, although they were not specifically investigated in the CIS situation. It is beyond the scope of this review to discuss all such treatment options.

The goal of MS treatment is to delay the onset of additional clinical relapses and possibly long-term disability. The first opportunity to initiate disease-modifying therapy in patients with MS may actually be when they are in the clinically isolated syndrome (CIS) stage, i.e., before conversion to clinically definite MS (CDMS). Since 1993, when interferon beta-1b was approved for MS, a growing number of disease-modifying therapies (DMTs) have become available. The goal of DMTs is to decrease the frequency of clinical relapses, lessen the number of new and active multiple sclerosis lesions on MRI, and, in the long term, to slow the progression of neurologic impairment. Since the approval of natalizumab as the first highly active DMT, the ultimate goal of "no evidence of disease activity" (NEDA) has become attainable for many patients. While the treatment of MS is beyond the scope of this review, the evidence for initiating MS DMTs after CIS is discussed.

Most DMTs approved for MS are also approved for the treatment of CIS. However, only a few DMTs have specifically been evaluated in clinical trials to treat CIS (including ON) and to delay the onset of clinically definite MS, including interferons and glatiramer acetate [53–58]. In all trials, the patients who received the active drug developed a second neurologic manifestation (definite multiple sclerosis) less frequently, and (if at all) at a later time, than those given the placebo. Even after a second episode, treated patients had a significantly lower annual rate of relapse for the duration of the follow-up period. Neurologic impairment was generally relatively mild and not significantly different between the two groups.

Interferons and glatiramer acetate have been approved for the treatment of CIS, including ON with two or more inactive typical lesions of multiple sclerosis on MRI. CHAMPS (Controlled High-Risk Subjects Avonex Multiple Sclerosis Prevention Study) was a randomized, double-blind trial involving 383 patients with an initial, acute monosymptomatic demyelinating event—unilateral ON, incomplete transverse myelitis (TM), or brainstem/cerebellar—and at least 2 silent T2 lesions on brain MRI [59]. The patients were randomized to weekly intramuscular interferon β-1a (IFN-b1a) or a placebo. The treatment group experienced a 44% reduction in the rate of development of CDMS compared with the placebo group over 3 years of follow-ups. There were statistically significant beneficial effects on all MRI parameters for the treatment group, including a decrease in T2 lesion development, gadolinium-enhancing lesions, and T2 lesion volume. The 10-year follow-up showed that patients treated immediately after their first episode had a significantly lesser chance of experiencing a second attack compared to those who had delayed treatment. Based on these results, FDA extended its approval of intramuscular IFN-b1a to include patients with CIS deemed to be at high risk for MS. The most common side effects associated with interferons are flu-like symptoms, including myalgia, fever, fatigue, headache, chills, nausea, vomiting, pain, and asthenia [59].

The PRISM (Prevention of Relapses and Disability by Interferon β-1a Subcutaneously in Multiple Sclerosis) trial assessed the efficacy of interferon (IFN)-β1a compared to the placebo, in dosages of 22 μg and 44 μg given subcutaneously in relapsing-remitting MS patients; both treatment groups had fewer relapses [60]. The Early Treatment of Multiple Sclerosis (ETOMS) trial showed that weekly subcutaneous IFN-β1a reduced the conversion to CDMS over 2 years to 34% vs. 45% for the placebo; a post hoc analysis found that the treatment group had a reduced rate of brain atrophy compared with those on the placebo [61]. The BENEFIT (Betaseron in Newly Emerging Multiple Sclerosis for Initial Treatment) study included patients with a single neurologic event and at least 2 clinically silent MRI lesions; in a 24-month study period, the standard dose of IFN-β1 was seen to reduce the risk of MS by 50%. Furthermore, open-label extension studies from the original CHAMPS and BENEFIT cohorts have suggested a possible long-term benefit from the early initiation of disease modifying treatments [62]. The CHAMPIONS (Controlled High-Risk Avonex Multiple Sclerosis Prevention Study in Ongoing Neurologic Surveillance) trial concluded that a delay in treatment by up to 3 years after a first clinical demyelinating attack could lead to an earlier time for CDMS but did not show a long-term effect on the development of new MRI T2-weighted lesions or long-term disability [63]. The REFLEX (REbif FLEXible dosing in early MS) trial evaluated 517 patients with CIS and at least two clinically silent T2 lesions on brain MRI. At two years, the probability of MS diagnosed by the McDonald criteria was significantly lower with subcutaneous interferon β-1a 44 mcg dosed either three times a week or once a week (63 and 76 percent, vs. 86 percent for the placebo). In the subsequent extension phase of the trial, all patients (n = 403) received interferon β-1a. At five years, the group assigned to interferon β-1a treatment in the placebo-controlled phase (i.e., early treatment) continued to have a reduced probability of conversion to MS and fewer new MRI lesions compared with the group whose treatment was delayed for up to two years [64–66].

Glatiramer acetate is an immunomodulator used to reduce relapse frequency in relapsing–remitting multiple sclerosis [39]. The PreCISe (Early GA Treatment in Delaying Conversion to CDMS in Participants Presenting with a Clinically Isolated Syndrome) trial showed a reduced conversion to CDMS (25%) in patients treated with 20 mg of glatiramer acetate subcutaneously daily compared to 43% for the placebo [63].

Teriflunomide also reduces the risk of progression to multiple sclerosis, as has been shown in the TOPIC (Teriflunomide Vs. Placebo in Patients With First Clinical Symptom of Multiple Sclerosis) trial, where 618 adults with a CIS were randomly assigned in a 1:1:1 ratio for treatment with 14 mg of oral teriflunomide daily, 7 mg of teriflunomide daily, or the placebo for up to 108 weeks, with a median treatment duration of over 70 weeks. The agent reduced the risk of relapse-defining CDMS at both the 14 mg dose and the 7 mg dose. The exact mechanisms by which teriflunomide works in MS are not established; it is an oral dihydroorotate dehydrogenase inhibitor that interferes with de novo synthesis of pyrimidines and thus inhibits the proliferation of rapidly dividing cells such as autoreactive T and B cells [64]. The most common adverse effects of teriflunomide were elevated alanine aminotransferase (ALT) levels, diarrhea, hair thinning, paresthesia, and upper respiratory tract infections. Teriflunomide is associated with increased risk for hepatotoxicity and teratogenicity and should not be given to patients with liver disease or women who are pregnant. Full immunization coverage is required prior to treatment initiation [53–55,67]. In addition, intravenous immune globulin and minocycline have been studied for the treatment of CIS or the first demyelinating event, but are not established as effective [56–58].

The early treatment of CIS is not favored by all experts. The decision whether to initiate treatment for CIS has to consider that not all patients go on to develop any additional relapses or lesions, and that the evidence base showing that the early treatment of CIS will prevent long-term disability is very limited. Patients should be informed of the potential benefits, risks, and uncertainties, and participate in decision making [62]. However, once a diagnosis of CDMS is made, the early initiation of treatment is recommended.

6. Emerging Therapeutic Approaches

6.1. *Remyelination/Recovery from Optic Neuritis*

After an acute episode of optic neuritis, GCL complex loss may start as early as 8 days after onset, and RNFL thinning has been reported as early as after 1 month, predicting optic atrophy at month 6. Recovery from relapses in MS patients involves remyelination of white matter and optic nerve lesions after the recruitment and differentiation of oligodendrocyte precursors from the lesion perimeter, but it is limited by axonal degeneration and glial scarring, which are observed even at the earliest stages of the disease. The currently available DMTs have neither neuroprotective effects nor the potential to enhance remyelination; thus, a crucial therapeutic gap exists. Recently, the effectiveness of the sphingosine-1 phosphate receptor (S1PR) modulator fingolimod in promoting remyelination after a first unilateral episode of acute optic neuritis was evaluated in a phase 2 study [68]. Since S1PR are required for lymphocytes to exit lymphatic follicular structures, fingolimod exerts immune modulation by sequestering pathogenic T- and B-cells from the blood stream. Importantly, S1PR are also present on neurons, astrocytes, and oligodendrocytes, as well as resident and CNS-invading myeloid cells, where they were shown to mediate neuroprotective and pro-regenerative effects in preclinical studies [68]. Fingolimod readily crosses the blood–brain barrier. Fingolimod was associated with a better recovery from unilateral optic neuritis compared to treatment with IFN-β 1b, and could have a role as an early treatment by promoting remyelination, preventing astrogliosis, and preserving axons [68].

Recent prospective studies have evaluated novel therapeutic approaches for neuroprotection and remyelination in acute optic neuritis. In 2017, opicinumab, a human monoclonal antibody against leucine-rich repeat and immunoglobulin domain-containing neurite outgrowth inhibitor receptor-interacting protein-1 (anti-LINGO-1), was investigated in the RENEW trial as a potential remyelinative therapy in acute ON [69,70]. It was hypothesized that the agent would enhance remyelination by directly promoting the proliferation and differentiation of oligodendrocyte precursors. LINGO-1 blockade has no detectable immunomodulatory effects. Treatment with opicinumab produced no significant change in the visual evoked potential (VEP) latency at 24 weeks (a measure of remyelination) in the intention-to-treat population; however, significant improvements in VEP latency delay were observed at 24 and 32 weeks in the prespecified per-protocol patient population. Since anti-LINGO-1 treatment had no differential effect on anatomic measures of optic nerve fiber loss, i.e., retinal nerve fiber layer (RNFL) or ganglion cell complex (GCC) thickness in either the intention-to-treat or per-protocol patient population at 24 weeks (with a mean delay of 24 days between ON onset and the start of treatment), the authors suggested that therapeutic windows may be longer for remyelination compared to axonal neuroprotection. The antiepileptic and proposed neuroprotectant phenytoin, studied in a Phase 2 randomized controlled trial, was shown to decrease RNFL loss in acute ON; however, no effect on visual outcomes or VEPs was found [69,70].

As a promising emerging therapy, mesenchymal stem cell (MSC) therapy has been suggested to be capable of stimulating both the remyelination and neuroprotection of axons in other neuro-degenerative diseases and in animal models of ON. In addition, cell-free approaches utilizing extracellular vesicles (EVs) produced by MSCs are considered to be a viable alternative to the transplantation of stem cells. EVs secreted by living cells mainly include exosomes and microvesicles. MSCs are amongst the largest cellular producers of EVs. Recent studies have shown that EVs can accommodate intracellular communication and act as modulators of cellular immunity, cancer biology, and regeneration/remyelination. Importantly, EVs can pass through the blood–brain barrier (BBB), making them suitable for CNS treatment. EVs exhibit anti-inflammatory and neuroprotective effects in multiple animal models of neuro-degenerative diseases and in rodent models of MS [1,71–73]. In particular, MSC-derived EVs are involved in a wide variety of physiological processes including the inhibition of natural killer cells, B cells, and mitogen-activated T cells, moderating microglia and macrophage polarization and reducing oxidative stress. In addition, they show the potential of tissue regeneration and myelin membrane biogenesis [74]. Studies in experimental autoimmune encephalomyelitis (EAE) mice have yielded evidence that EVs attenuate neuroinflammation and demyelination by reducing and downregulating T-cells (Tregs, CD4+), macrophages, astrocytes, and microglia. The immunomodulatory effect may be mediated by promoting a shift in microglial phenotypes from M1 (pro-inflammatory) to M2 (anti-inflammatory) [75]. MSC-EVs may also promote axon remyelination by protecting oligodendrocytes and their precursor cells from damage caused by immune cells [76].

MicroRNAs appear to mediate most EV effects. The pathology of MS is influenced by histone modifications and gene regulation via microRNAs [77,78]. MicroRNAs mediate post-transcriptional gene silencing and are involved in cellular activities including proliferation, differentiation, and migration, as well as disease initiation and disease progression [77,78], Figure 4. A series of studies in MS patients and animal models demonstrate that various types of microRNA (microRNA-219, microRNA-125a-3p, mir-27a) may be involved in the regulation of oligodendrocytes [79]. Exosomes or viral vectors can play a role as carriers of miRNAs to therapeutically regulate MS pathology. In addition, the overexpression of proteins that modulate exosomal miRNA gene expression profiles have the potential to improve the therapeutic effects of exosomes [77,78].

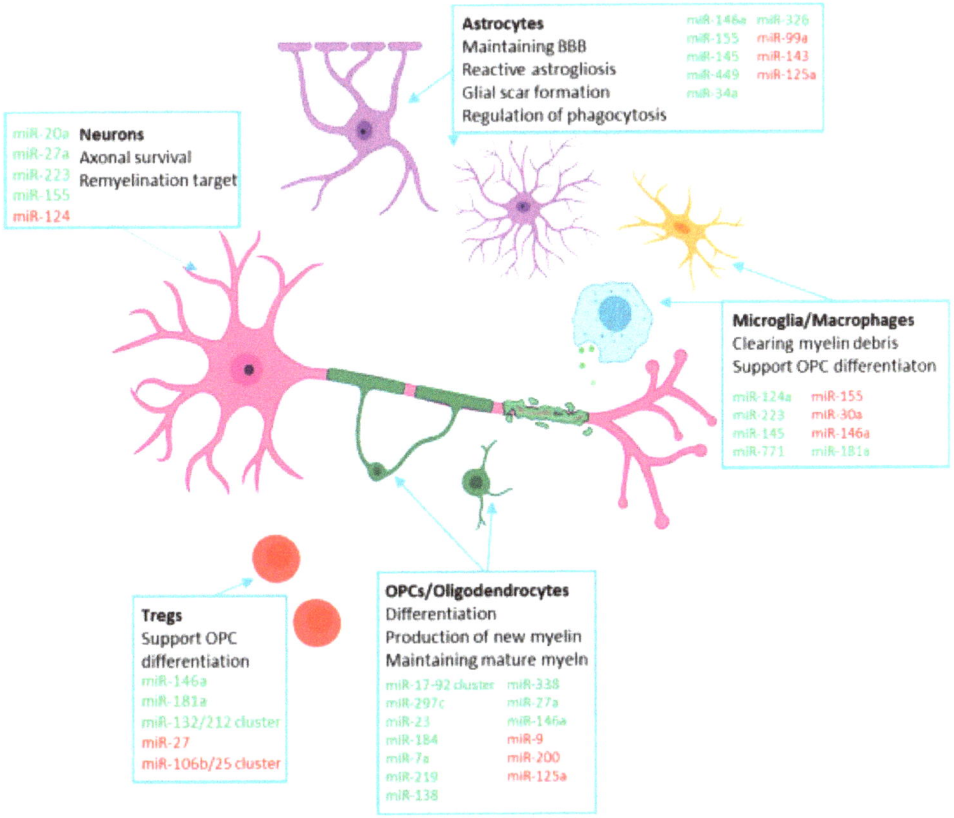

Schematic of key cells involved in remyelination and relevant miRNAs that regulate the process. miRNAs and miRNA clusters that are broadly positive regulators of remyelination are listed in green, and those that are broadly negative regulators of remyelination are listed in red (created with BioRender.com).

Figure 4. Key Cells involved in Remyelination and relevant miRNAs [77].

6.2. Atypical Optic Neuritis

Atypical Optic Neuritis includes entities in the demyelination diseases' spectrum such as ON associated with neuromyelitis optica spectrum disorder (NMOSD), which is associated with aquaporin 4 antibodies (AQP4), and myelin oligodendrocyte glycoprotein antibody disease (MOGAD), which is associated with myelin oligodendrocyte glycoprotein (MOG) antibodies. These diseases differ from typical and MS-related ON in clinical features, visual morbidity, and therapeutic approaches.

6.3. NMOSD

In 2004, the discovery of a pathogenic NMO-associated IgG antibody, targeting the water channel membrane protein aquaporin-4 (AQP4), was an important milestone in differentiating NMO from MS [80]. AQP4 is highly concentrated on astrocyte end feet in the CNS. All NMO lesions show a widespread and early loss of AQP4 immunoreactivity, in contrast to MS lesions, where AQP4 immunoreactivity is often increased [81,82]. The binding of AQP4-ab to astrocyte AQP4 channels triggers classical complement cascade activation, followed by granulocyte, eosinophil, and lymphocyte infiltration, culminating in injury first to astrocytes then to oligodendrocytes, and demyelination, neuronal loss, and neurodegeneration [83]. In humans, AQP4 monomers are expressed in astrocytes in two isoforms: M1-AQP4 and M23-AQP4. Both isoforms have identical extracellular domain residues, but M1-AQP4 has 22 more amino acids at the cytoplasmic N terminus. However, AQP4-ab binding to the ectodomain of astrocytic AQP4 has isoform-specific outcomes. M1-AQP4 is completely internalized, whereas M23-AQP4 resists internalization and is aggregated into larger-order orthogonal arrays of particles (OAPs), a process facilitated by M1-AQP4 deficiency [84]. Alterations in OAPs are required for NMO-IgG to recognize conformational AQP4 epitopes, as well as for the binding of the complement component C1q to clustered AQP4-ab [85,86]. CNS lesions in NMOSD patients are characterized by IgG, IgM, and complement deposits with a rosette pattern, most prominent around vessels, as well as cellular infiltrates of granulocytes (neutrophils and eosinophils) macrophages/microglia and T cells. The key feature is AQP4 loss on astrocytes. In certain lesions however, other typical astrocytic markers, such as glial fibrillary acidic protein (GFAP) and S-100β, are still detectable, indicating AQP4 loss precedes astrocyte death. Ultimately, the preservation or secondary loss of neurons and the associated demyelination will depend on disease severity. Demyelination affects both gray and white matter, sometimes with necrosis, cavitation, and thickened, hyalinized vessels. Thus, the autoimmune response in NMOSD primarily affects astrocytes and is initiated by the autoantibody-mediated loss of AQP4 [87].

The visual outcome after NMOSD-ON is less favorable compared to MS-ON and MOGAD, supported by an increased thinning of RNFL and GCL complex in NMOSD cases [44,88]. Therefore, early and aggressive treatment is appropriate in the acute phase of NMOSD-ON. The ONTT did not enroll any NMOSD patients, and its findings are not applicable to NMOSD-ON. Given the devastating nature of NMOSD-ON, no treatment is not an option, and steroids alone may be insufficient in many cases [88]. Given the recurrent nature and devastating morbidity of relapses, disease-modifying therapy should be instituted early after the diagnosis of NMOSD is established [88,89].

6.4. Acute NMOSD Relapses

Relapses are usually treated with 1 g of high-dose **IV methylprednisolone (IVMP)** daily for 3–7 days, followed by oral steroid tapering. The likelihood of complete visual recovery increases when IVMP is administered within 5 days of the onset of NMOSD ON [36]. However, Kleiter et al. demonstrated, in their analysis of NMOSD optic neuritis, an incomplete efficacy of IVMP, as only 33% of patients achieved complete remission [90]. Furthermore, repeated courses of IV steroids only reduced the number of non-responders. Patients with optic neuritis and concurrent myelitis had an even worse prognosis [90].

IVIg and **PLEX** are immunomodulatory therapies that may offer additional benefits for acute optic neuritis treatment in NMOSD. Clinical trials have suggested a range of potential improvements in visual functions from 45–55%; however, due to their retrospective design, they failed to define criteria for the optimal use or timing of PLEX [46]. There was also mostly no distinct interval between the completion of IVMP and the institution of PLEX, rendering debatable whether clinical improvement results from PLEX induction or from delayed IVMP effects. Features such as male sex, lower baseline disability, rapid initiation of treatments, and shorter relapse durations have been associated with a greater response to PLEX. According to one study, 50% of patients with poor visual recovery after high-dose intravenous steroids (<20/200 or less) recovered a visual acuity of at least 20/30, with a mean time to PLEX initiation of 30 days [91]. The reasoning for this treatment in NMOSD is based on the fact that most of the astrocyte and neural destruction is caused by the deposition of AQP4-IgG and the subsequent complement activation. PLEX removes circulating antibodies, complements, and cytokines from the blood, which may shorten the action of antibodies and lessen further inflammation and necrosis [92]. Some retrospective studies of NMOSD have shown that the very early concurrent initiation of PLEX or immunoadsorption with corticosteroids during acute relapses may improve outcomes [90,93–95]. However, even delayed PLEX therapy may still be a reasonable treatment option for patients with acute refractory ON [89]. PLEX may be accompanied by serious side effects such as hypotension, infection, hypocalcemia, and coagulopathy [93]. In addition, several authors have described the use of monthly or yearly PLEX sessions to avoid relapses in NMOSD patients. It seems that the removal of the humoral autoimmunity, in addition to the modulation of cellular inflammation by IVMP, may increase the interval between relapses [96–98].

Immunoadsorption represents an alternative form of therapeutic apheresis, currently not approved in the United States. It uses modified membranes to achieve the selective removal of antibodies from plasma, allowing for the removal of the pathogenic autoantibodies while sparing other plasma proteins, therefore eliminating the need for protein replacement and potentially minimizing complications. Immunoadsorption has been reported to benefit steroid refractory ON and NMOSD-ON [93].

As an additional therapeutic solution, in a retrospective study of 10 NMOSD patients unresponsive to IVMP, IVIg was effective in 50% of patients [87]. Recently, a retrospective study demonstrated the superiority of high-dose IVMP plus IVIgG treatment compared to a high dose of IVMP alone [99].

When the aforementioned interventions fail to salvage visual functions, immunosuppression with intravenous cyclophosphamide may represent an avenue of final resort. A subset of NMSOD patients with acute TM seem to have benefited from this treatment [100]. Outside of case reports, no clinical studies have been published on the response of severe ON to intravenous cyclophosphamide, and the treatment is not without risk.

6.5. NMOSD Relapse Prevention

In contrast to MS, in NMOSD, functional decline and the development of disability are related primarily to relapses [101]. After acute stabilization, the early institution of long-term preventative and maintenance immunosuppressive therapies is needed to minimize permanent visual and neurologic disability [101]. So far, no standard management has been agreed upon for first-line treatment or treatment switching [87]. Since June 2019, there are now three new monoclonal antibodies FDA-approved for treating AQP4-Ab-seropositive NMOSD patients, targeting three different disease pathways, based on efficacy in phase III randomized controlled trials. Prior to this, the most commonly used conventional maintenance/disease modifying therapies were rituximab, azathioprine, and mycophenolate mofetil (MMF) used off label. Immunosuppressive therapies such as methotrexate, mitoxantrone, and cyclophosphamide have been shown to be beneficial in highly active NMOSD, but are infrequently used due to their less favorable risk–benefit profiles [102]. Low-dose corticosteroids have not been systematically studied but are frequently used, either as maintenance therapy or as an add-on to conventional immunosuppressants [103]. There is also a level 2 recommendation for hematopoietic stem cell transplantation (HSCT) in refractory courses (106, 107, CAMPUS; NCT04064944).

Azathioprine and **MMF** are agents with broad immunosuppressive properties which have been used, based on retrospective studies or uncontrolled case series published before 2019, as effective first-line treatments for NMOSD, either as a monotherapy or in conjunction with low-dose corticosteroids [103]. The agents have demonstrated efficacy, with a significant reduction in the annual relapse rate and the stabilization or improvement of EDSS scores [87]. For full biologic effects to be observed, AZA and MMF require at least 4–6 months of treatment, rendering oral steroid co-administration advisable to provide an immunosuppressive bridge from treatment onset [101]. In contrast to rituximab, the immunomodulatory effects of AZA and MMF are mediated by the rather unselective suppression of fast-dividing immune cells [104]. Retrospective comparisons among these agents are subject to confounding by indication and other biases and have produced mixed results.

MMF is a noncompetitive inhibitor of inosine monophosphate dehydrogenase, an enzyme essential for de novo synthesis of the purine nucleotide guanosine-5′-monophosphate, which inhibits the proliferation of lymphocytes [105–107]. MMF is a semi-synthetic derivative of mycophenolic acid (MPA), which is the active metabolite of MMF. MPA acts as a selective noncompetitive inhibitor of inosine 5-monophosphate dehydrogenase type II, which is a rate-limiting enzyme in the de novo synthesis of guanine ribo- and 2-deoxyribonucleotides. MPA has a mean terminal half-life of 17 h and has been shown to prevent the production of interferon gamma (INF-γ), lipopolysaccharide-induced interleukin-6 (IL-6), and oxidative stress [108]. At a cellular level, MPA depletes the guanosine pool in lymphocytes and inhibits T- and B-cell proliferation/transendothelial migration, macrophage activation, dendritic cell functioning, and immunoglobulin production [109].

AZA is a prodrug form of 6-mercaptopurine (6-MP), which was first introduced in clinical practice in the 1960s for kidney transplantation to prevent immunological rejection. The agent is converted non-enzymatically to 6-MP, which is metabolized in the liver to the active metabolite 6-thioinosinic acid and works as a purine antagonist that gives negative feedback on purine metabolism and inhibits DNA and RNA synthesis. Its action results in the inhibition of T-cell activation, a reduction in antibody production, and a decrease in the levels of circulating monocytes and granulocytes [110].

Among the benefits of AZA treatment are the convenient oral administration and the affordability of the agent compared to rituximab [106]. Recently, data from 150 NMOSD patients treated with AZA showed that 69% had no accumulation of disability after a 5-year follow-up [111]. A retrospective study evaluating 103 AQP4-IgG-seropositive NMOSD patients demonstrated that 89% of patients had a significant reduction in median ARR from 1.5 to 0, 61%, remained relapse-free at a median follow-up of 18 months, and neurological functions improved or stabilized in 78% of patients with azathioprine treatment [106]. Unfortunately, treatment was discontinued in the last follow-up for 46% of patients due to side effects in 62% (increased liver enzymes and pancytopenia). Many patients discontinue AZA over time, raising the concern of poor tolerability [106]. Common side effects include bone marrow suppression with consequent pancytopenia and hepatitis, and viral infections. Intolerance is not uncommon as well. More rarely, pancreatitis and severe gastrointestinal disturbances can occur [106]. An increased risk of malignancies has been shown, with lymphoma development in 3% of patients in a large NMOSD series [107]. Patients on AZA should be monitored regularly with complete blood count, liver, and renal function tests [106].

MMF seems effective in doses of 1750 mg to 2000 mg per day and may be used in conjunction with prednisone [107]. In 2009, Jacob et al. showed in a case series of 24 patients with NMOSD the effectiveness of the agent. The median dose of MMF was set at 2000 mg per day for a median duration of 27 months. A total of 79% had an improvement in ARR, and disability was stabilized or improved in 91%. One died of disease complication during follow-up, and 25% had to discontinue MMF treatment due to side effects including headache, constipation, easy bruising, anxiety, hair loss, diarrhea, abdominal pain, and leukopenia [112]. More recently, a study reported 50.7% of patients experience a relapse on MMF, 59.7% continued on MMF, and 83% showed a stabilization or improvement in their disability at the most recent follow-up [113]. In addition, among 28 patients treated at the Mayo Clinic and the Johns Hopkins Hospital with MMF, failure rate was 36%, similar to that of rituximab and better than for azathioprine [114]. Case series and a meta-analysis suggest that the efficacy of mycophenolate mofetil is comparable to rituximab, and mycophenolate mofetil was more tolerable in meta-analyses [107,114]. Known adverse effects of MMF include an increased risk of lymphoma in transplanted patients and nonmelanoma skin carcinomas, infections (viral and bacterial), gastrointestinal symptoms (ulcers, hemorrhages), and cytopenia [106,114]. Teratogenicity represents a major concern with the need for contraception in young female patients in their reproductive age, as congenital malformations have been reported in 26% of live births, and the risk of first-trimester pregnancy loss is 45% in exposed patients [114]. Figures 5 and 6 demonstrate the mechanisms of action of agents utilized in the treatment of NMOSD.

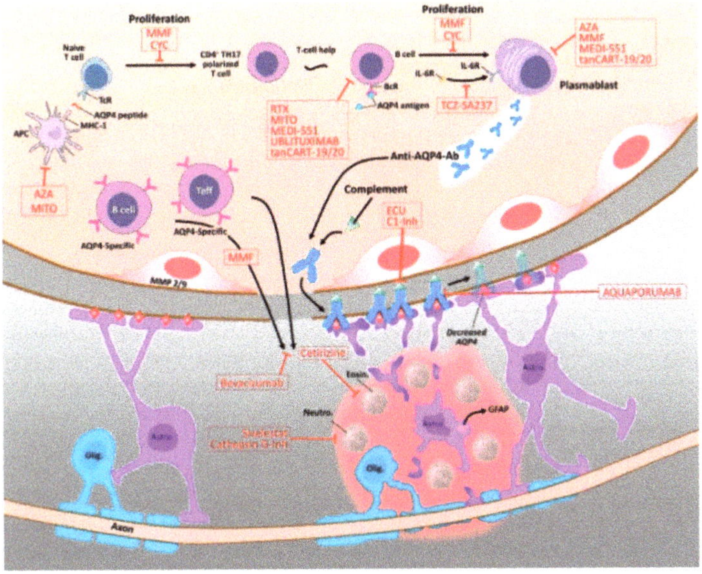

Pharmacological effects of the drugs currently used or assessed in neuromyelitis optica spectrum disorders, especially when AQP4 antibodies are presents. *Ab* antibody, *APC* antigen-presenting cell, *AQP4* aquaporin-4, *Astro* astrocyte, *AZA* azathioprine, *BcR* B-cell receptor, *Cathepsin G-Inh* Cathepsin G-Inhibitor, *CYC* cyclophosphamide, *C1-Inh* C1-esterase inhibitor, *ECU* Eculizumab, *Eosin* Eosinophil, *GFAP* glial fibrillary acidic protein, *IL-6R* interleukin-6 receptor, *MEDI-551* inebilizumab, *MHC-1* major histocompatibility complex class 1, *MITO* mitoxantrone, *MMF* mycophenolate mofetil, *MMP* matrix metalloproteinases, *Neutro* Neutrophil, *Olig* oligodendrocyte, *RTX* rituximab, *SA237* satralizumab, *tanCART-19/20* tandem chimeric antigen receptor T cells transduced with the anti-CD19/CD20 vector, *TCR* T-cell receptor, *TCZ* tocilizumab, *TH* T helper

Figure 5. Pharmacological Effects of the drugs used in NMOSD [115].

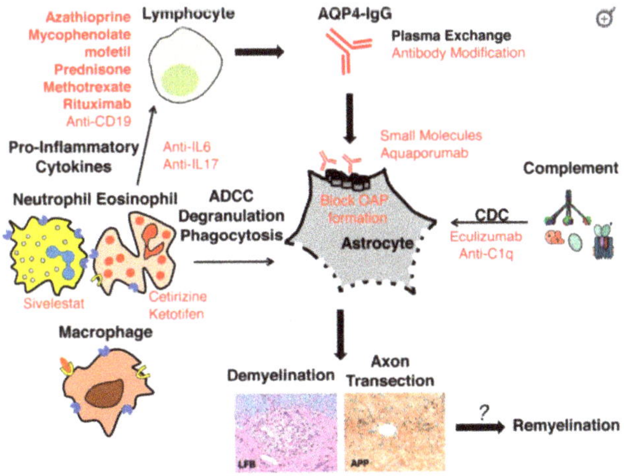

Figure 6. *Cont.*

Current and emerging therapeutic strategies for NMO. Therapeutics (red) that are current (bold) and novel are listed individually next to the process that they inhibit. Immunosuppressant medications are designed to decrease the activity of antibody-producing B cells and pro-inflammatory T cells. Aquaporin-4 immunoglobulin G (AQP4-IgG) modulation may block the pathogenic action of autoantibodies. Blocking therapies are designed to prevent the binding of pathogenic autoantibodies to their astrocytic target. Reducing orthogonal array of particle (OAP) formation is intended to modify the assembly of AQP4 target to decrease antibody binding. Neutrophil and eosinophil inhibitors are intended to limit Fc receptor-mediated destructive mechanisms. Complement inhibition is designed to limit complement-dependent cytotoxicity (CDC) and membrane attack complex formation. Definitive therapies to promote remyelination in lesioned tissue remain to be developed. ADCC, antibody-dependent cell-mediated toxicity; APP, amyloid precursor protein; LFB, luxol fast blue.

Figure 6. Current and Emerging Therapeutic Strategies for NMO [116].

Methotrexate is a folate derivative which inhibits dihydrofolate reductase and nucleotide synthesis. Traditionally, it has been used in weekly oral doses in the treatment of autoimmune diseases such as rheumatoid arthritis and Crohn's disease. The evidence for methotrexate in NMOSD comes from small observational studies, the largest of which included 14 AQP4-IgG-seropositive patients followed for a median of 21.5 months, demonstrating an improvement in ARR ranging from 64% to 100%, and a relapse freedom in 22% to 75% of patients [108,114]. Patients should be monitored for bone marrow suppression and liver functioning. The most common side effects are bone marrow suppression and impaired liver functions, while rare, serious complications include pneumonitis, aplastic anemia, and opportunistic infections. Methotrexate is a teratogen.

Alternative broad-spectrum immunosuppressive agents include mitoxantrone, cyclophosphamide, cyclosporine A, and tacrolimus. A systematic review in 2019 identified 8 studies with 117 NMOSD patients treated with the agents [117]. The majority of the studies reported a significant improvement 6 months to 5 years following treatment in terms of ARR [117]. **Mitoxantrone** is a topoisomerase II inhibitor impairing DNA repair, resulting in a drop in B and T cells. A comparison study of NMOSD treatments demonstrated the inferiority of mitoxantrone to rituximab and azathioprine/prednisolone with regard to the relapse rate [118]. Mitoxantrone has been associated with severe adverse events, such as dose-limiting cardiotoxicity and an increased risk of acute myeloid leukemia, especially in patients having received a cumulative dose greater than 60 mg/m^2 [107]. **Cyclophosphamide** is an alkylating agent that crosslinks guanine bases in DNA. There is controversy with regard to its effectivity in NMOSD patients. Data from Brazil showed relapses in six out of seven patients treated with pulse doses of cyclophosphamide [119]. In contrast, a recent retrospective study of 41 patients treated for a median of 13.6 months reported a median ARR drop from 0.7 to 0.0 [120]. Mitoxantrone and cyclophosphamide are teratogenic. A report in 2013 of nine seropositive NMOSD patients treated with **Cyclosporine A** showed a decrease in ARR from 2.7 to 0.4 [113]. Cyclosporine A is a calcineurin inhibitor that binds to cyclophilins, resulting in the inhibition of the translocation of transcription factors, leading to a reduced transcriptional activation of several cytokines and ultimately to reduced T cell proliferation [106]. Potential side effects include hypertension, nephrotoxicity, tremor, opportunistic infections, and increased hair growth. **Tacrolimus** is also a calcineurin inhibitor, which reduces peptidyl-prolyl isomerase activity by binding to immunophilin FKBP-12 and leads to the inhibition of T lymphocyte signal transduction and IL-2 transcription. It is an orally administered agent, widely used in organ transplantation and systemic autoimmune diseases. A Chinese retrospective study of 25 patients with NMOSD treated with 2 to 3 mg/d of tacrolimus, and concomitant prednisone in 60% of patients, found that tacrolimus decreased the ARR by 86% and improved the EDSS from 4.5 pretreatment to 2.3 at the last follow-up [121]. In addition, another study in Japan of patients with NMOSD showed that the initiation of prednisolone followed by tapering doses of prednisolone and tacrolimus in 25 patients, dosed with 1 to 6 mg/d, achieved relapse freedom in 92%, with relapses only seen in patients with subtherapeutic serum concentrations [107]. Serious side effects associated with the use of the agent include severe infections and malignancies. Hyperglycemia, diabetes mellitus, hyperkalemia, nephrotoxicity, and tremors have been also described [107,121].

A potential role for **long-term intermittent IVIg** in preventing relapses in NMOSD has been suggested, as there is evidence that IVIg is effective in reducing the relapse rate and improving neurological disability in NMOSD patients. One case series treated 8 NMOSD patients (2 seropositive) with IVIg (0.7 g/kg/day for 3 days, 4–21 infusions per patient) for a mean duration of 19 months, demonstrating a remarkable decrease in the mean ARR and the EDSS score as well. In addition, a study where IVIg (0.4 g/kg/day for 5 days, then 0.4–1.0 g/kg/day every 2 to 3 months) was given to six NMOSD patients (4 seropositive) for an extended mean duration of 4 years confirmed the favorable results in terms of median ARR improvement, while 50% of the patients were relapse-free at a 4-year-follow-up. In conclusion, IVIg could be considered a safe alternative in NMOSD patients with repeated infections from immunosuppressant therapy; however, controlled trials are required to confirm efficacy [106].

Rituximab has been used to prevent relapse in NMOSD on an off-label basis for more than 15 years [102]. The agent is recommended as a first-line maintenance treatment of NMOSD in the 2010 guidelines from the European Federation of Neurological Societies and the 2014 recommendations of the Neuromyelitis Optica Study Group [122]. It is a chimeric monoclonal antibody that rapidly leads to marked CD20+ B cell depletion via complement-mediated and cell-mediated cytotoxicity. In addition, there is evidence that rituximab in AQP4-IgG-seropositive patients leads to a predominance of B regulatory cells after therapy [58]. B cell depletion lasts, on average, 6–9 months [106]. A meta-analysis in 2016 on 25 studies re-demonstrated the efficacy and safety of Rituximab in NMOSD patients regarding the annual relapse rate (ARR) and qualitative indices [102]. Importantly, a prospective study of 100 NMOSD with a long follow up of 7 years showed that 94% of patients experienced a significant reduction in ARR, and 70% were relapse-free while on rituximab [123]. In comparative studies, rituximab has shown its superiority to AZA and MMF in decreasing annual relapse rates and relapse severity as well as preventing new relapses [87,103]. A common therapeutic approach is the administration of an induction dose of 1000 mg of rituximab once or repeated twice 2 weeks apart, followed by a fixed a fixed regimen of 1000 mg of rituximab every 6 months [124]. Alternative approaches include a dosing regimen based on body mass index, administering 375 mg/m^2 per week for 4 weeks, or an individualized dosing scheme on the basis of CD19+ lymphocytes reemergence [102].

It is worth noting that in Japan, rituximab for NMOSD has been covered by insurance from June 2022. Recently, Tahara et al. conducted the RIN-1 study in Japan, the first multicenter, randomized double-blind placebo-controlled Phase III time-to-event clinical trial of rituximab in NMOSD [125]. AQP4-antibody-positive patients with an EDSS of 7.0 or less were randomized 1:1 to receive either rituximab intravenously (375 mg/m^2 of body surface for week 1 to 4, then 1000 mg i.v. at week 24, 26, 48, and 50) or with a matching placebo and concomitant oral prednisolone, which was tapered over the study's duration of 72 weeks. No other immunosuppressants were allowed. None of the patients treated with rituximab relapsed, in contrast to 37% on the placebo [125].

In long-term rituximab therapy, however, 15–45% of patients continue to have relapses. This may potentially be related to the early repopulation of B cells, or to the sequestration of tissue-resident B cells outside the blood stream [126]. Alternative theories include the presence of neutralizing antibodies against rituximab, polymorphisms in the FCGR3A-F allele, and CNS compartmentalization of pathogenic B cells that may also interfere with effective B cell depletion by the agent [102].

Rituximab use can result in the development of hypogammaglobulinemia in a significant portion of patients (20–65%), especially with prolonged therapy, and an increased risk for severe infections, including herpes zoster, tuberculosis, and recurrent sino-pulmonary and urinary tract infections [127]. Hepatitis B, active tuberculosis, and other severe infections need to be excluded or treated before the initiation of treatment. In cases of severe hypogammaglobulinemia, an inadequate response to vaccines, and/or frequent or severe infections, the supplementation of IVIG 400 mg/kg every 4 weeks targeting a serum level 9 of 800–1000 is recommended [127,128]. Infusion reactions are common and can usually be managed by pretreatment with intravenous steroids, antihistamine, and slow infusion [107]. In addition, there have been rare cases of progressive multifocal leukoencephalopathy (PML) following rituximab therapy in rheumatoid arthritis, but none has been reported in NMOSD [129].

Tocilizumab is a humanized monoclonal antibody against the IL-6 receptor, which has been approved for the treatment of rheumatoid arthritis, giant cell arteritis, juvenile idiopathic arthritis, and cytokine release syndrome; however, it is not FDA licensed for NMOSD [130]. The rationale for tocilizumab use in NMOSD is based on the involvement of IL-6 in the pathophysiology of disease [130,131]. IL-6 promotes an increased bloodbrain barrier permeability with the infiltration of proinflammatory cytokines and antibodies into the CNS and the survival of a plasmablast population responsible for secreting anti-AQP4 antibodies, leading to increased AQP4-IgG production in vitro and ex vivo [130,131]. IL-6 represents the only cytokine that is found in higher levels in the serum and the cerebrospinal fluid of patients with NMOSD compared with MS controls [107,130].

A series of case reports has documented the effectiveness of tocilizumab in NMOSD, including patients refractory to rituximab, since 2013 [107]. For example, three patients with aggressive AQP4-IgG-seropositive NMOSD uncontrolled by other immunosuppressants and completely CD19-depleted by rituximab, when switched to tocilizumab, showed an ARR decrease from 3.0 to 0.6, though without improvement in clinical disability [106]. In addition, a pilot study with seven NMOSD patients who had experienced multiple relapses in the preceding year on immunosuppressants and corticosteroids, and were treated consequently with intravenous tocilizumab, reported a fall in mean ARR from 2.9 to 0.4, with five of seven participants achieving relapse freedom for at least 1 year. In another observational study of eight patients treated with tocilizumab as an add-on therapy for NMOSD, it showed remarkable effectivity in reducing the relapses by 90% compared with the baseline [107,130]. In 2019, a study of 12 NMOSD patients treated with subcutaneous tocilizumab also demonstrated the effectiveness of agent 37. Potential side effects of tocilizumab include a modest increase in lipoproteins, bowel perforation, and a higher risk of neutropenia and infections, such as tuberculosis, invasive fungal infections, and bacterial infections, the latter mainly with concomitant methotrexate. However, opportunistic infections are less likely to occur in NMOSD compared to rheumatoid arthritis [107,130].

In 2020, the TANGO trial was the first head-to-head prospective, randomized comparison study between an established and new therapeutic agent in NMOSD. It was a phase 2, open label, time-to-event study in China that compared the safety and efficacy of tocilizumab and azathioprine in NMOSD patients [132]. The tocilizumab group included 59 patients (85% AQP4 seropositive), and the azathioprine group 59 patients (90% AQP4 seropositive). Tocilizumab was administered at 8 mg/kg IV every 4 weeks, with concomitant immunosuppressive coverage for the first 12 weeks of treatment. Azathioprine was given initially, at an oral dose of 25 mg daily and increased by 25 mg per day to a target of 2–3 mg/kg/day, with immunosuppressives for the first 6 months of treatment. Analysis of the primary outcome of the time to first relapse favored tocilizumab over azathioprine, with a median of 78.9 weeks for tocilizumab vs. 56.7 weeks for azathioprine. Relapse occurred in 14% of the tocilizumab group and 47% of the azathioprine group. In the subgroup analysis of patients with concomitant autoimmune diseases, 9% in the tocilizumab group and 35% in the azathioprine group relapsed. In contrast, no differences were noticed in the risk of relapse among patients without concomitant autoimmune diseases. Regarding disability progression at 3 months, tocilizumab demonstrated a more favorable profile compared to azathioprine (8% vs. 25%) [132]. Furthermore, AQP4-IgG levels dropped by 50% in the tocilizumab group and remained unchanged in the azathioprine group. In seronegative patients, relapse occurred in 22% with tocilizumab and 50% of patients on azathioprine. Overall, adverse events were equally frequent, but some serious adverse events including the elevation of alanine transferase and upper respiratory and urinary tract infections were more common in the azathioprine group compared to tocilizumab. There was one death in each group, but neither death was treatment-related [132]. The authors concluded that tocilizumab significantly reduced the risk of relapse compared with azathioprine in NMOSD, proposing the agent as a potentially effective and safe treatment for relapse prevention in NMOSD [107,132].

MS Therapies. It is worth noting that some agents used in MS such as interferon, natalizumab, and fingolimod have been shown to not benefit or have a detrimental impact in AQP4-antibody-positive NMOSD. More specifically, IFN-β increases the relapse rate and promotes severe exacerbations, possibly by increasing the production of BAFF and IL-17 [133]—Figure 7. In addition, natalizumab, an antibody against very late antigen 4, has been reported to have no effect or to worsen disease activity in NMOSD patients either seropositive or seronegative. The proposed mechanisms of exacerbation involve florid active demyelination, severe neutrophilic and eosinophilic infiltrates, and severe astrocyte loss. The increase in the numbers of peripheral proinflammatory T cells or eosinophils can lead to eosinophil migration to the CNS, resulting in a surge in lesion formation or the stabilization of AQP4-specific bone marrow plasma cells. Furthermore, oral fingolimod has the potential to accelerate NMO disease activity; fulminant disease may develop early on after the initiation of therapy. A theory similar to natalizumab has been suggested, with fingolimod promoting bone marrow egress of eosinophils, triggering enhanced lesion activity and AQP4-IgG production.

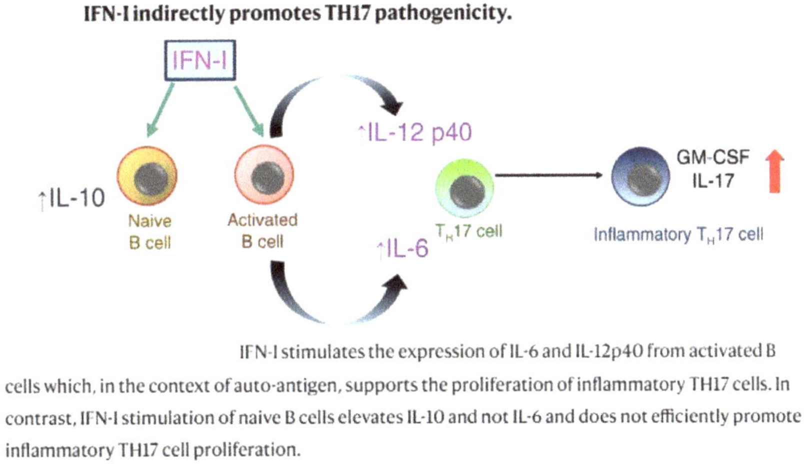
IFN-I indirectly promotes TH17 pathogenicity.
IFN-I
↑IL-12 p40
GM-CSF
IL-17
↑IL-10
Naive B cell
Activated B cell
↑IL-6
T_H17 cell
Inflammatory T_H17 cell
IFN-I stimulates the expression of IL-6 and IL-12p40 from activated B cells which, in the context of auto-antigen, supports the proliferation of inflammatory TH17 cells. In contrast, IFN-I stimulation of naive B cells elevates IL-10 and not IL-6 and does not efficiently promote inflammatory TH17 cell proliferation.

Figure 7. INF-I and TH17 pathogenicity [133].

6.6. FDA-Approved Disease-Modifying Therapies for NMOSD

Eculizumab is a humanized monoclonal IgG2/IgG4-hybrid antibody targeting C5, which inhibits cleavage and thus prevents the release of pro-inflammatory C5a and the involvement of C5b (the terminal complement component) in the membrane attack complex (MAC). Consequently, eculizumab could have dual action downregulating adaptive and innate immune responses either through C5a in the periphery (decreasing the chemotaxis of leukocytes to the inflammatory sites) or through C5b on astrocytes in the CNS [134]. Pathological analyses in NMOSD patients with acute lesions have shown both the early and specific involvement of the CNS vasculature and the crucial role of the complement in pathogenesis, demonstrating extensive, perivascular complement activation [130]. Eculizumab has been approved by the FDA as a treatment to prevent relapse in AQP4-IgG-seropositive adults with NMOSD since 2019, followed by the European Union and Japan. Of note, all patients who are to start eculizumab must receive the meningococcal vaccination at least 2 weeks before the first dose, since blocking the complement system increases the risk of infection with encapsulated bacteria. However, meningococcal vaccines do not fully protect against meningococcal disease, and concomitant antibiotic therapy can be considered [87,135]. Additional limitations on the widespread use of the agent include the frequent dosage scheme of bimonthly intravenous infusions and the high cost [87].

The efficacy of eculizumab in the prevention of relapse in NMOSD was initially suggested in 2013 by an open-label phase II trial of 14 AQP4-IgG-seropositive NMOSD patients with a highly active disease (55 attacks in 2 previous years in total). A total of 12 patients were relapse-free, and none progressed, 2 patients had possible attacks during twelve months on eculizumab, whereas 5 relapsed within five months after withdrawal. One patient who had received prior immunization suffered meningococcal sepsis and sterile meningitis during the treatment, and another one a fatal myocardial infarction (deemed unrelated) during follow-up. The PREVENT trial in 2019 was a phase 3, randomized, double-blind, placebo-controlled, time-to-event study of 143 AQP4-seropositive patients with NMOSD with EDSS less than or equal to 7 and a highly active disease (at least two relapses in the prior year or three in the prior 24 months) who were randomized 2:1 to eculizumab 900 mg, IV weekly × 4 doses followed by 1200 mg every 2 weeks or a placebo [136]. Patients were allowed to continue their prior immunosuppressive therapies, which occurred in 76% of cases. Patients who had been recently treated with rituximab, mitoxantrone, IVIg, and prednisone >20 mg per day, or were suffering from active bacterial infections, were excluded from the trial. Forty-six patients had previously used rituximab, which was stopped within three months before inclusion. In addition, all of the participants were vaccinated against Neisseria meningitidis before receiving treatment. The primary endpoint was the first adjudicated relapse. Given the uncertainty of when the final relapse would occur, the sponsor terminated the trial after 23 of the predefined 24 adjudicated relapses. Clinical relapse occurred in 3% of patients in the eculizumab group and 43% of patients in the non-eculizumab group, resulting in a 94% relative-risk reduction. In a subset analysis of patients who were on concomitant immunosuppression, 4% of the eculizumab group and 54% of the non-eculizumab group of patients experienced a relapse. However, there was no significant difference in disability progression. One patient on eculizumab and azathioprine died from pulmonary empyema, with cultures yielding Peptostreptococcus micros and Streptococcus intermedius [137]. During the open-label extension trial involving 137 patients, serious adverse events were reported in 36% of treated patients, including two cases of sepsis and one case of Neisseria gonorrheae infection, but no deaths. Furthermore, there was a higher rate of upper respiratory tract infections and headache in the eculizumab arm, but there were no cases of meningococcal infection [107].

Inebilizumab was the first B-cell-depleting agent to be approved by the FDA for the treatment of AQP4-IgG-seropositive NMOSD patients in June 2020. Prior to this, B cell depletion with the anti-CD20 agent rituximab had been used for off-label NMOSD treatment. However, rituximab does not deplete plasmablasts, which do not express CD20 [102,124]. Inebilizumab is an afucosylated humanized IgG1κ, anti-CD19 monoclonal antibody that directly binds CD19 with high affinity on the surface of B cells, which demonstrates dual action on B cell depletion through antibody-dependent cellular cytotoxicity and antibody-dependent cellular phagocytosis. Cytotoxicity specifically is enhanced via the process of afucosylation, which leads to a dramatic increase in the affinity of inebilizumab for FcγRIIIA, a receptor that mediates antibody-dependent cytotoxicity. CD19 expression on B cells begins at the pro-B stage. The wider expression of CD19 compared to CD20 on cells that constitute the B-cell lineage allows inebilizumab to target a broader range of pathogenic B cells not being targeted by anti-CD20 agents. Additionally, CD19-positive plasmablasts circulating in the peripheral blood of individuals with NMOSD may produce AQP4-IgG antibodies [138].

The N-Momentum trial (2019) was a phase 2/3, randomized, double-blind, placebo-controlled, time-to-event study of AQP4-seropositive and AQP4-seronegative patients with NMOSD. A total of 230 adults with active NMOSD were enrolled, defined as at least one attack requiring treatment the year before enrollment or two attacks in 2 years and an EDSS of 8 or less [139]. A total of 91% of the participants were women with a mean age of 43, and 92% of the patients were seropositive for AQP4 antibody. Exclusion criteria included treatment with rituximab or other B-cell-depleting agents within the previous 6 months, previously receiving a bone marrow transplant or T cell vaccination therapy, IVIg within the previous 1 month, natalizumab, cyclosporin, methotrexate, mitoxantrone, cyclophosphamide, tocilizumab, or eculizumab within the previous 3 months, or previous alemtuzumab or total lymphoid irradiation. About 70% of participants had had prior exposure to disease-modifying therapies. Patients were randomized 3:1 into the inebilizumab group (74–92% seropositive) or placebo group (56–93% seropositive). Interestingly, of the 17 AQP4-seronegative patients, 7 had antibodies against MOG. The patients were treated with 300 mg of inebilizumab IV or a placebo on days 1 and 15. Furthermore, all participants were given 20 mg of prednisone daily or an equivalent dose of other glucocorticoids between days 1 and 14, and then tapered through day 21 to minimize the risk of relapse at treatment initiation. Patients were not concomitantly treated with other immunosuppressive therapies. In the active group, a maintenance dose of 300 mg of inebilizumab was administered every 26 weeks. The double-blinded period lasted up to 197 days, until a new NMOSD attack, or until the termination of enrollment. All patients were thereafter offered open-label therapy. Because of a clear demonstration of efficacy, enrollment was stopped before reaching the target of 252 patients and 67 adjudicated attacks. Relapse occurred in 12% in the inebilizumab arm and in 39% in the placebo group (73% relative risk reduction). In the subgroup analysis of patients who were AQP4 seropositive, relapse occurred in 11% in the inebilizumab group and in 42% in the placebo group (hazard ratio 0.23). Due to the sample's inequality regarding seronegative patients among groups (only four participants were randomized to the placebo arm), efficacy could not be interpreted in the seronegative subset. Of note, the trial also confirmed that the efficacy of inebulizumab was consistent across the clinical presentations of myelitis and optic neuritis domains [138–140].

The secondary endpoints remarkably showed that patients treated with inebilizumab had a significantly reduced likelihood to experience optic neuritis compared to the placebo arm (10 patients in each group); however, there were no differences in changes in the low-contrast visual acuity binocular score from the baseline among the groups. Additionally, the treated arm demonstrated a considerable reduction in the numbers of B cells (less than 10% of baseline) and the maintenance of low counts during the trial. The immunological effects of inebulizumab were observed within 4 weeks after the initiation of treatment. Furthermore, among AQP4-seropositive patients, fewer had a statistically significant worsening of their EDSS score. The inebilizumab arm also had lower numbers of cumulative active MRI lesions and NMOSD-related hospitalizations compared with the placebo [139–141]. Serious adverse events were similar among both the inebulizumab (9%) and placebo groups (5%); however, 2% of patients on the agent developed transient grade 3 neutropenia. There were no malignancies observed during the study. No death occurred during the placebo-controlled phase, but two patients died during the open-label phase. The first one was initially randomized on the placebo and passed away by respiratory insufficiency after a severe NMOSD attack preceded by pneumonia, and his death was considered unrelated to the treatment. The second patient, originally receiving inebilizumab, developed new neurological symptoms (weakness, aphasia, neurological decline, seizures) 9 days after receiving the maintenance dose. MRI showed new large lesions in white and grey matter, considered not representative for progressive multifocal leukoencephalopathy (PML), although one of three PCR tests on CSF was positive for JC virus, and brain biopsy was not performed; ultimately, the possibility that the death was treatment-related could not be excluded [140,141].

Inebilizumab is contraindicated for patients with active hepatitis B and active or untreated latent tuberculosis. Inebilizumab can also cause hypogammaglobulinemia, resulting in recurrent or serious opportunistic infections, which may require the discontinuation of the treatment or IVIg administration. Additionally, B-cell-depleting therapies in general are associated with an increased risk for malignancy and infection, including PML [107,138].

Satralizumab is a humanized IgG2 monoclonal antibody which binds membrane-bound or soluble interleukin 6-receptors, preventing the IL-6-induced inflammatory cascade. The pharmacokinetics of the agent have been optimized compared to its predecessor via an enhanced "antibody-recycling" process allowing for a longer half-life than tocilizumab. Satralizumab is designed to dissociate, pH-dependently, from the satralizumab-IL6-R complex within the endosome and to be recycled for repeated antigen binding in the peripheral blood, extending the interval of re-administration. Satralizumab is the third and most recent agent (2020) approved by the FDA for the treatment of adult patients with AQP4-IgG-seropositive NMOSD, including by self-injection [103,142,143]. In Japan, the agents are licensed for the treatment of both adults and children. Satralizumab is administered subcutaneously at weeks 0, 2, and 4, and then monthly, with instructions on withholding treatment in the event of an active infection, elevated liver enzymes, or neutropenia, and is contraindicated in patients with hepatitis B and active or untreated latent tuberculosis [107,144].

The safety and efficacy of satralizumab were evaluated in the SAkuraSky and SAkuraStar trials, phase III, randomized, double-blind, placebo-controlled, time-to-event studies of AQP4-seropositive (70%) and AQP4-seronegative patients (30%) with NMOSD [142,143]. In the SAkuraSky trial, patients on prior immunosuppressive therapies continued these treatments at stable doses (rituximab was excluded). In the SAkuraStar trial, the investigators compared only satralizumab monotherapy to the placebo without the use of concomitant immunosuppressive therapies. The therapeutical approach was either 120 mg of satralizumab subcutaneously or the placebo at weeks 0, 2, and 4, and then every 4 weeks. Inclusion criteria for the SAkuraSky trial included adolescents (age of at least 12 years) and adults, diagnosis of NMOSD by the 2006 criteria, history of at least two relapses in the previous 2 years with at least one relapse in the previous 12 months, and an EDSS score of 6.5 or less. In contrast, the SAkuraStar trial only included adults with the same prerequisites needed to be met. For both trials participants were excluded if they had received treatment with rituximab within the previous 6 months, eculizumab or multiple sclerosis disease-modifying therapies within the previous 6 months, anti-CD4 agents, cladribine, or mitoxantrone within 2 years, or IL-6 targets, alemtuzumab, total-body irradiation, or bone marrow transplantation in the past [142,143].

In the SakuraSky trial, a total of 83 patients were recruited (7 adolescents), randomized 1:1 to the satralizumab (41 patients) and to the placebo (42 patients) arms, with a median treatment duration of 107.4 weeks and 32.5 weeks, respectively. The primary endpoint was the first protocol-defined relapse in a time-to-event analysis. The major secondary endpoints were the change from the baseline to week 24 in the visual analogue scale (VAS) pain score and the Functional Assessment of Chronic Illness Therapy-Fatigue (FACITF) score. Relapse occurred in 20% in the satralizumab group and 43% in the placebo group; the percentages of patients free from relapse at 48 weeks was 89% and 66% in the satralizumab and placebo groups, respectively, and 78% and 59% at 96 weeks. In addition, the subgroup analysis revealed that 11% of AQP4-seropositive NMOSD patients (55 cases) in the satralizumab arm experienced relapses compared to 43% in the placebo group, while among 28 seronegative patients, relapse occurred in 36% and 43% in the satralizumab and placebo groups, respectively. Based on the subgroup analysis, it has been suggested that satralizumab reduces the risk of relapse compared to the placebo in AQP4-IgG-seropositive patients, but there was insufficient evidence to prove the agent's effectivity in the seronegative participants. Regarding the secondary outcomes, no significant differences were found in either the VAS pain score or the FACIT-F score. Of note, in the satralizumab and the placebo arms, serious side effects occurred at similar percentages (17–21%). Injection-related reactions were more frequent in the satralizumab group (12% vs. 5%).

In the SAkuraStar trial, patients were randomized 2:1 to the satralizumab monotherapy or placebo. A similar efficacy was demonstrated, with a significant reduction in the time to the first relapse and relapse risk in AQP4-IgG-seropositive NMOSD patients with an active disease. Relapse occurred in 30% of the satralizumab group and 50% of the placebo arm, with subgroup analysis showing 22% of seropositive patients treated with satralizumab relapsing compared to 57% in the placebo group. In the AQP4-seronegative subgroup, the percentages of relapse were 46% and 33%, respectively. No significant benefit was found on secondary outcome measures of pain or fatigue. Comparably to SAkuraSky, 19% of satralizumab-treated and 16% of placebo-treated NMOSD patients experienced adverse events, with injection reactions in 5% and 16%, respectively. In general, satralizumab showed a favorable safety profile in both studies, as no anaphylactic reactions, opportunistic infections, or deaths occurred. Only one patient in the SAkuraStar trial discontinued treatment due to pneumonia.

6.7. Emerging Therapeutic Strategies

A series of agents are currently under investigation for the prevention of disease activity in NMOSD.

Ublituximab is a third-generation chimeric IgG1 monoclonal antibody with high affinity to the Fcγ receptor IIIa (FCγRIIIA), an epitope on CD20-positive B-cells which is not targeted by rituximab, and a depleting larger number of B-cells [103,145]. Ublituximab allows for shortening the infusion duration and lowering doses compared to other anti- CD20 monoclonal antibodies and demonstrates enhanced antibody-dependent cellular cytotoxicity (ADCC) activity, while complement-dependent cytotoxicity (CDC) is retained [87,146]. In 2019, ublituximab was investigated in five AQP4-seropositive patients in a pilot safety study, phase Ib, as a novel add-on therapy in acute relapses of NMOSD (ON or TM) [92]. The agent was administered once in a 450 mg dose intravenously within 5 days of relapse onset as a concomitant treatment to high-dose intravenous corticosteroids (1000 mg per day on days 1–5). There were no severe adverse effects, and in three patients, EDSS improved at a 90 d follow-up. Two patients exhibited relapses within three months due to an insufficient depletion of B-cells [146].

Furthermore, **BAT4406F** is another potentially effective agent that is a fully humanized anti-CD20 monoclonal antibody to be investigated in a phase I RCT on safety, tolerability, and pharmacokinetics in NMOSD patients (NCT04146285). It will be administered via intravenous infusions, following an open-label dose escalation [37]. Additional potential B-cell-mediated therapeutic approaches that could be leveraged in the treatment of NMOSD include **chimeric antigen receptor (CAR) T cell therapy**, **belimumab** (an inhibitor of B lymphocyte stimulator (BLyS)), and several anti-CD20 monoclonal antibodies, such as **ocrelizumab**, **ofatumumab**, and **obinutuzumab** [104,147]. **Telitacicept** is a recombinant transmembrane activator and calcium modulator and cyclophilin ligand interactor fusion antibody acting by inhibiting both BLyS and proliferation-inducing ligands. In 2021, the agent was approved for the treatment of systemic lupus erythematosus, subcutaneously given weekly (160 mg), after showing efficacy and safety in a pivotal phase 2b trial (NCT02885610). An ongoing phase 3 randomized, placebo-controlled study is currently evaluating telitacicept in AQP4-ab-positive NMOSD patients without recent immunosuppressive treatment (NCT03330418, [107,148]).

Bortezomib is a 26S proteasome inhibitor, FDA-approved for the treatment of multiple myeloma. The agent depletes plasma cells and is being evaluated in a range of autoantibody-driven neurologic autoimmune diseases, including myasthenia gravis and anti-NMDA-receptor encephalitis. Bortezomib was investigated in patients with highly relapsing NMOSD as an add-on medication in a small open-label study of five AQP4-Ab-positive Chinese women who had at least two relapses in the previous 6 months or three relapses throughout their life despite treatment with various immunosuppressants including prednisolone, azathioprine, rituximab, or cyclophosphamide (NCT02893111). The participants received four cycles of subcutaneous bortezomib at a dosage of 1 mg/m^2

of body surface area on days 1, 4, 8, and 11 per cycle, followed by a 10-day treatment-free interval with concomitant oral steroid or azathioprine. Four out of five patients were relapse-free during a one-year follow-up. Side effects were mild and transient; however, long-term outcome and safety profiles were not reported. No patient experienced further neurological deterioration at the end of the study, and the median EDSS scores reduced from 5.5 at baseline to 3.5 after a 1-year follow-up, associated with an improvement in the pain scale. Furthermore, treatment significantly decreased serum AQP4 antibody titers, precursor B cell counts, peripheral blood CD19+ B cells, and mainly, CD138+ plasma cells. The findings suggest a promising role of bortezomib as an escalating approach in highly active NMOSD cases refractory to or intolerant of current immunosuppressants by depleting long-lived plasma cells. Phase 2 has been completed, but results are not yet available [87]. Importantly, the potentially unfavorable side effect profile of the agent is a matter of concern, as bortezomib is possibly associated with a rebound in plasma cell activity with an overshooting production of autoantibodies after cessation of the drug. In addition, it frequently induces peripheral neuropathy [103,149].

Subcutaneous injection of **batoclimab** (**HBM9161**) is being evaluated in NMOSD. It is a human monoclonal antibody that targets FcRn and accelerates the degradation of IgG, reducing total IgG levels in the blood (including pathological IgG). Based on its suggested anti-lgG properties, it is expected to rapidly reduce AQP4-IgG levels when administered with IVMP. The agent is injected subcutaneously at a dose of 340 mg or 680 mg weekly for a period of 4 weeks, and is being evaluated in a phase 1, open-label dose exploration study of NMOSD patients experiencing relapses (NCT04227470). Furthermore, a new study comparing thw efficacy and safety of immunoadsorption and PLEX for acute relapses of refractory NMOSD (CAMPUS; NCT04064944) has been announced, but is not recruiting yet [87].

Imlifidase, an IgG-degrading bacterial enzyme, is another agent that could be effective in AQP4-seropositive NMOSD. It mediates the cleavage of IgG molecules into Fab and Fc segments. The concept was conceived based on promising results from animal models of NMOSD, which have demonstrated that the transformation of AQP4 antibodies into inactive antibodies by the microbial-mediated deglycosylation of IgG heavy chains may have a role in NMOSD therapeutic armamentarium. Leveraging the same strategy of downregulating pathogenic autoantibodies, the potential effectivity of **rozanolixizumab** and **efgartigimod** could be suggested. These agents constitute inhibitors of neonatal Fc receptors (FcRn), crucial for antibody stability [150].

Bruton's tyrosine kinase (BTK) is an enzyme that plays a crucial role both in B cell development by transmitting intracellular signals from the pre-B cell receptor, and in the Fc-receptor-mediated activation of myeloid cells. It promotes antigen recognition via antibody-mediated opsonization. In contrast to the typical CD20 monoclonal antibodies, BTK inhibitors inactivate B cells without causing prolonged and repeated B cell depletion, thus lowering the risk for serious opportunistic infections. BTK inhibitors are being developed as therapeutic agents for MS, with promising findings from phase 2 clinical trials, while phase 3 trials are underway. An open-label phase 2 trial will be starting soon to evaluate the efficacy and safety of the agent **SHR1459 (Bruton's Tyrosine Kinase Inhibitor)**, orally administered, in preventing relapses in NMOSD (NCT04670770) [87,151].

Bevacizumab is an anti-angiogenic compound, and more specifically, a monoclonal immunoglobulin that targets vascular endothelial growth factor (VEGF), that has been widely used for the treatment of retinal diseases. VEGF-neutralizing antibodies such as bevacizumab have the potential to restore BBB integrity, as antibodies targeting brain microvascular endothelial cells (BMEC) are believed to induce disruption of the BBB mediated by VEGF, leading to pathogenic AQP4 antibodies entering into the central nervous system. Of note, anti-BMEC antibodies were found in the sera of 10/14 NMO patients, but were absent in MS and healthy controls [102,152]. Data on its efficacy as an add-on agent for treatment of ON and/or TM in NMOSD come from a phase 1b trial where bevacizumab proved to be effective and safe in 10 patients, with none requiring escalation to PLEX after high-dose IVMP plus IV bevacizumab. The suggested approach is the infusion of 10 mg/kg intravenously at the onset of exacerbation and, if needed, a subsequent dose during the plasma exchange phase [107].

Ravulizumab is a second-generation monoclonal antibody targeting C5 and blocking its activation, thus inhibiting C5 cleavaging into fragments C5a and C5b. It is derived from eculizumab and was designed to provide prolonged therapy intervals by utilizing the "Ab-recycling" approach. The agents show increased affinity for the neonatal receptor FcRn, and rapid endosomal dissociation of the ravulizumab-C5 complex allows lysosomal degradation of C5 while recycling ravulizumab to the vascular space through the FcRn 66. Ravulizumab has an extended serum half-life (3 to 4 folds) compared to its predecessor. Based on evidence of non-inferiority to eculizumab derived from two large phase III trials in patients with paroxysmal nocturnal hemoglobinuria, the agent was approved by the FDA and EMA for use in adult patients. Ravulizumab is administered every 2 months. Since December 2019, a phase 3, external, placebo-controlled, open-label, multicenter study of ravulizumab efficacy and safety in AQP4-Ab-positive NMOSD patients has been underway (NCT04201262) [153–155].

Alternative ways to target the complement cascade are being explored based on evidence that blockage of the C1 component prevents the formation of proinflammatory anaphylatoxins C3a and C3b while preserving the lectin pathway, which is important for neutralizing encapsulated bacteria. Indeed, in animal models, **C1qmab**, a monoclonal antibody against C1q components, effectively reduced complement-dependent cytotoxicity. In addition, an open label, phase 1b trial which investigated the **C1 esterase inhibitor** as a concomitant therapy to steroids for the management of acute NMOSD relapses showed favorable results regarding safety and effectivity, with 90% of patients returning to their baseline EDSS score [102].

Granulocyte-targeting strategies have also been considered in NMOSD treatment, as animal models suggest that granulocytes mediate NMO pathogenesis, and neutrophils and eosinophils are highly prevalent in NMOSD lesions. It is suggested that neutrophil entry into the CNS is an early step in the formation of NMOSD lesions. Blocking neutrophil elastase, a proteolytic, highly destructive enzyme that triggers the production of inflammatory cytokines, helps reduce neutrophil entrance into the brain. **Sivelestat** is a neutrophil elastase inhibitor which is being investigated in acute NMO relapses. In a mouse model of experimental autoimmune encephalomyelitis, the agent reduced ADCC. Phase I/II clinical trials were discontinued for various reasons. Sivelestat has already been approved in Japan and Korea for ARDS treatment [156].

NPB-01 IVIg (400 mg/kg/day for 5 consecutive days) is being investigated for its potential role in NMOSD mediated by the inactivation of auto-reactive T-cells. However, a phase 2 RCT in AQP4-ab-positive NMOSD patients did not improve responses when added to IVMP, but detailed results are not available.

Cetirizine, a second-generation H1 antagonist that stabilizes eosinophil degranulation, was investigated in a small open label add-on pilot study and showed a decrease in ARR in NMO patients at a 1-year follow-up; however, no significant difference in EDSS scores were observed [157]. Cetirizine was administered orally at 10 mg each day. Another potential consideration for use in NMOSD is anti-IL-5 agents, which deplete eosinophils [158].

Aquaporumab is a recombinant monoclonal antibody derived from clonally expanded mouse CSF plasma cells with a point mutation in the area that codes for effector Fc IgG functioning. The agent constitutes a targeted non-immunosuppressive therapy that binds AQP4 with high-affinity cells, displacing AQP4-Ab from binding. The Fc portion of aquaporumab specifically aims at disabling AQP4-Ab from triggering CDC or ADCC downstream mechanisms. A study in a mouse model of NMO has showed that aquaporumab prevented the formation of new NMO lesions through steric competition with pathologic AQP4 antibodies [159]. Recently, Duan et al. described **AQmab**, which has an eightfold increased binding affinity to the AQP4 receptor compared to aquaporumab [147].

Another idea worth noting would be the induction of **immune tolerance** to the autoantigen by vaccination, as the majority of NMOSD patients have underlying AQP4 autoimmunity with the autoantigen clearly defined.

6.8. Cell-Based Therapies

Cell-based therapies are gaining momentum as promising treatments in the armamentarium against severe autoimmune diseases, such as refractory NMOSD and MOGAD, aiming at either the depletion of autoreactive effector cells or the modulation of autoreactive T and B cell responses, resulting in the restoration of tolerance. Various cellular treatment approaches have been investigated in NMOSD and occasionally in MOGAD as well, including autologous hematopoietic stem cell transplantation (HSCT) and chimeric antigen receptors (CAR)-T cell, tolerogenic dendritic cell, and mesenchymal stem cell treatment. The therapies have entered early-stage clinical trials or have been used as a rescue treatment in treatment-refractory or highly aggressive cases. Progress in the field is slowed down by the rarity of the diseases, the shortage of biomarkers able to predict long term outcomes and effectiveness, challenges in the manufacturing of cellular products, and the lack of adequate animal models that mirror the human disease [160].

Hematopoietic Stem Cell Transplantation (HSCT) in NMOSD and MOGAD is aimed at achieving the elimination of the dysfunctional immune system with high-dose chemotherapy and rebuilding through hematopoietic stem cell infusion in order for long-term remission to be achieved. **Autologous Stem Cell Transplantation (AHSCT)** is preferred as it avoids graft-versus-host reactions. Complications of AHSCT include neutropenic fever, serious infections, electrolyte abnormalities, blood pressure fluctuations, and the emergence of new autoimmune diseases, including myasthenia gravis and hyperthyroidism. Mortality associated with the therapy has improved significantly over the last several decades and is now around 0.2% [160]. The first case report of an autologous stem cell transplantation in a 23-year-old severely affected patient with refractory NMOSD was published in 2010. In a 12-month follow-up, the patient remained blind, but paraparesis and dysesthesia remitted [161].

Results of the two largest studies of AHSCT in NMOSD patients were discrepant, possibly due to the choice of conditioning regimen [162,163]. The European Registry retrospective AHSCT study included 16 patients with NMOSD refractory to immunosuppressants, with 10% remaining relapse-free and 48% with progression-free survival at 5 years, but the study did not use rituximab. Eighty percent of initially seropositive patients remained seropositive throughout the study. In contrast, in a US-based clinical trial that included 13 patients (11 AQP4-IgG-seropositive and 1 with neuropsychiatric SLE), all participants followed the same therapeutic approach treatment, consisting of cyclophosphamide, rituximab, anti-thymocyte globulin, and plasmapheresis. Eighty-three percent of patients were relapse free at 5 years off all immunosuppressants. Furthermore, at 1 and 5 years after transplant, improved scores in the EDSS and in the Neurological Rating scale were recorded. Interestingly and importantly, 9 of 11 AQP4-seropositive patients in the US study seroconverted to being AQP4-seronegative after HSCT, and all of them remained relapse-free at the last follow-up despite the fact that two regained AQP4-seropositive status within 2 years of transplant. The two patients who remained AQP4-seropositive throughout the study were the ones who had clinical relapses. In addition, complement-activating and cell-killing ability was lost in six of seven patients. The possibility of prolonged drug-free remission with conversion to AQP4-IgG seronegativity following nonmyeloablative hematopoietic stem cell transplantation warrants further study. Each study recorded one death (patient with coexisting SLE in the US trial due to SLE complications) [162,163].

A recent meta-analysis in 2020 including the aforementioned three studies evaluated 31 NMOSD patients in total who underwent AHSCT [164]. Cumulative progression-free survival was 76% during a follow-up period between 2 and 13 years. Treatment-related mortality was 0%. Despite the promising results, a number of patients had persisting AQP4 antibodies and relapsed within 5, and the optimal conditioning regimen remains to be determined as well [110] Based on these findings, the European Bone Marrow Transplantation (EBMT) Autoimmune Diseases Working Party (ADWP) issued guidelines recommending the use of AHSCT in NMOSD as a clinical option, with grade II evidence, in therapy-refractory patients [104].

Only a few patients treated with **allogeneic HSCT (alloHSCT)** have been reported [105,165]. AlloHSCT has the potential for a more profound immunotherapeutic effect, eliminating all autoreactive lymphocytes by allogeneic donor T lymphocytes. In addition to the increased risk of morbidity and mortality after alloHSCT, there are reports of the development of immune-mediated peripheral and central nervous system diseases, including a case of MOGAD after alloHSCT in haematological patients [105,165]. Due to limited clinical evidence, alloHSCT in NMO was classified as developmental by the EBMT-ADWP and is currently not recommended as a clinical option [104].

One phase Ib, open-label, multiple-ascending-doses, single-center clinical trial was conducted recently in Spain, evaluating the efficacy and safety autologous of **tolerogenic peptide-loaded dendritic cells (DC)** in 4 AQP4+ NMOSD patients [166]. The tolerogenic phenotype of DC was induced by the addition of dexamethasone; DC from NMOSD patients were stimulated with seven myelin peptides and AQP4. Three doses of tolerogenic DC were administered intravenously at week 0, 2, and 4 at progressively increasing doses, and all patients received concomitant treatment with rituximab [3] or mycophenolate [1]. All patients remained clinically stable, no relapses occurred, and the tolerogenic DC-based therapy proved to be safe. Immunological analysis demonstrated a trend of decreased T cell proliferation, a significant increase in Interleukin-10 production, and an upregulation of type 1 regulatory T (Tr1) cells, findings confirmatory of tolerance induction [166].

Another cell-based therapeutic approach is the employment of **chimeric antigen receptors (CAR)**, proteins carrying both an antigen-binding and a T-cell-activating function, allowing T cells to target a specific protein. B cell targeting using **CAR-T cell** therapy is being investigated mainly in the treatment of hematological malignancies, but there is also an emerging interest in the field of autoimmunity, where dysregulated B cell activation leads to an antibody-mediated targeting of healthy body tissue. Breaking the immune tolerance towards autoreactive immune cells induces the cytotoxic death of these specific cells, which may downregulate the immune overactivation driving autoimmunity. Indeed, recent promising results come from a murine model of SLE [160]. In the field of NMOSD, an open-label phase I clinical trial is currently underway, utilizing B cell maturation antigen **(BCMA) CAR-T cell** therapy in patients with refractory AQP4-IgG-seropositive NMOSD (ClinicalTrials.gov NCT04561557). Twelve NMOSD patients will be enrolled and receive BCMA CAR-T cells following lymphodepletion with cyclophosphamide and fludarabine. Primary outcome measures include the incidence of dose-limiting toxicities and adverse events. The concentration of AQP4-IgG titers in the serum 3 months after infusion and the CAR-T cell proliferation 2 years after infusion will be studied as secondary outcome measures, together with clinical and radiological outcomes, including the annualized relapse rate and active MRI lesions. The first results of this clinical trial are expected by the end of 2023 [160].

Mesenchymal stem cells (MSCs) constitute multipotent stromal progenitor cells, derived from allogeneic human-umbilical-cord-derived tissue (hUC-MSC), autologous bone marrow (bMSC), or autologous adipose tissue. Among the beneficial effects of MSC treatment are their regenerative potential, immunomodulatory properties inhibiting pro-inflammatory cytokines, and a neuroprotective action by the secretion of neurotrophic and survival-promoting growth factors. In the field of NMOSD, clinical trials with both bMSC and hUC-MSC have been conducted. Compared to bMSC, hUC-MSC are easily collectable, and although not autologous, these MSCs have a low risk for the induction of allogeneic immune responses and consequently transplant rejection [106,118]. In a pilot study, 15 AQP4-seropositive NMOSD patients were treated with a single intravenous infusion of autologous bMSC, and at 2 years follow-up, favorable results were observed regarding relapses (87% relapse-free) and disability (improvement in 40%). HUC-MSC in the treatment of AQP4 IgG+ NMOSD patients was first investigated in 2012 in five cases, when the cells were administered by an intravenous and intrathecal route combined, divided over four infusions; favorable results were found following transplantation in terms of relapses, EDSS score, and peripheral blood B lymphocyte counts. Interestingly, the 10-year follow up in 2020 demonstrated that four out of five treated NMOSD patients showed reduced annual relapse occurrence compared to before treatment, with only two patients completing the 10-year follow-up period due to the death of two patients (attributed to rapid disease progression) and failure to follow up with one patient. The safety profile was promising, with no observed long-term tumor formation or peripheral organ disorders. The investigators concluded that hUC-MSC transplantation warrants further clinical trials [160,167].

6.9. Remyelination

Therapeutic approaches aimed at improving regeneration and restoring functionality are still missing. A future treatment pathway inducing remyelination or myelin repair would be beneficial. Promoting the differentiation and proliferation of oligodendrocyte precursor cells (OPC) to mature oligodendrocytes capable of myelination might be a key component of the concept. **Clobetasol** has been shown to promote OPC differentiation in cultured cells and to induce remyelination in mouse brains with AQP-IgG and complement-induced injury [168].

7. Therapeutic Approach to AQP4-IgG-Seronegative NMOSD Patients

Although AQP4-ab-negative patients are considered in the 2015 NMOSD diagnostic criteria, a large diagnostic disagreement has been reported in this subgroup of patients, even among experts in this field, owing to the inconsistent use of the criteria. Consequently, the diagnosis of patients who fulfil the 2015 diagnostic criteria for AQP4-IgG seronegative NMOSD patients requires caution, and seronegative status should be confirmed with cell-based assays, with repeat blood work at least two to three times in a period of 6–9 months. In addition, AQP4-IgG-seronegative patients should be assayed for MOG-IgG by cell-based assays.

There are therapeutic challenges for double-seronegative NMOSD patients (seronegative for both AQP4-IgG and MOG-IgG), as the recent randomized placebo-controlled clinical trials of eculizumab, inebulizumab, and satralizumab either did not include such patients (eculizumab) or failed to provide evidence that the newer agents are effective for relapse prevention (inebulizumab and satralizumab) in this group. In the N-MOmentum and SAkuraStar trials, which compared a placebo to inebilizumab and satralizumab, respectively, AQP4-seronegative patients were included, but these trials were not sufficiently powered to evaluate the response in this subgroup, rendering the results primarily applicable to AQP4-seropositive patients.

Recently, the Spanish NMO Study Group reported that double-seronegative and AQP4-IgG-seropositive NMOSD patients had a similar clinical outcome, while those seropositive for MOG-IgG had a more favorable prognosis [169]. Moreover, a study in France that included 67 patient and employed MMF as a first-line therapy concluded that the agent was effective in relapse prevention and disability stabilization/improvement in NMOSD patients (based on 2015 diagnostic criteria), irrespective of the seropositivity status (AQP4-IgG seropositive, MOG-IgG seropositive, or double-seronegative) [113]. In addition, another recent multicenter retrospective study of 245 NMOSD patients found a similar efficacy of rituximab and MMF both in AQP4-IgG-seropositive and double-seronegative NMOSD patients [170].

7.1. MOG

The myelin oligodendrocyte glycoprotein is one of several proteins produced by oligodendrocytes, the myelin-forming cells of the CNS. Together with other proteins such as myelin basic protein (MBP), proteolipid protein (PLP), and myelin-associated glycoprotein

(MAG), MOG is an essential component of oligodendrocyte surface membranes. These glycoproteins have fundamental roles in the formation, maintenance, and disintegration of myelin sheaths [171]. Compared to other glycoproteins MOG is only found in relatively small amounts within myelin; however, its structure (extracellular IgV domain) and the outmost external location on myelin sheaths make it easily accessible to the potential antibodies and T-cell response involvement. MOG expression starts when myelination begins and is thus a possible differentiation marker for oligodendrocyte maturation. Several essential functions of MOG are suggested: the regulation of oligodendrocyte microtubule stability, maintaining the structural integrity of the myelin sheath by its adhesion features, and the mediation of interactions between myelin and the immune system [172]. In humans and rodents, the MOG gene is located in the major histocompatibility complex (MHC) locus. Molecules encoded by this region are found on the surfaces of cells and are involved in antigen presentation, inflammation regulation, the complement system, and the innate and adaptive immune responses. In addition, the gene has a certain structural similarity to the B7-CD28 superfamily—encoded proteins are expressed on the surface of antigen-presenting cells (APC) [173]. In addition, MOG can directly activate the classical pathway of the complement cascade; reports from experimental studies suggest that the binding of MOG to the C1q and C3d components can activate the complement system.

Neuropathological evidence has shown that the inflammatory infiltration in MOGAD consists mainly of CD4+ T cells and granulocytes, in contrast to MS, where CD8+ T cells predominate. Compared to MS, intracortical rather than leukocortical demyelinated lesions were more common. Importantly, AQP-4 was preserved, as MOGAD is not an astrocytopathy. Complement deposition within active lesions was observed, but not on astrocytes or glia limitans. Contrary to expectations, MOG was not preferentially lost [174].

NMOSD and MOGAD are two antibody-mediated entities; however, both have different targets. AQP4-ab-positive NMOSD is characterized by AQP4 loss, dystrophic astrocytes, and the absence of cortical demyelination [87]. By contrast, MOGAD pathology is characterized by the coexistence of perivenous and confluent primary demyelination, with partial axonal preservation and reactive gliosis in the white and gray matter, and with a particular abundance of intracortical demyelinating lesions [174]. This occurs on the background of CD4-dominated T cells and granulocytic inflammatory infiltrates [87]. In addition, contrary to classical AQP4-ab-positive NMOSD, in MOGAD, the expression of AQP4 is preserved [174].

The phenotype of MOGAD is broad and includes ON, TM, and acute demyelinating encephalomyelitis (ADEM). ON is the most common presentation in adults, whereas ADEM is in children [175]. In MOGAD, disability appears to depend on relapses, with severe disability being reported in 47% of adult MOGAD patients, in >70% of whom it results from the first attack [176]. Clinical characteristics suggestive of MOGAD-ON include recurrent ON, bilateral involvement, prominent disc edema, and longitudinally extensive ON and/or perineural enhancement of the optic nerve on MRI [96]. Although the nadir of vision loss is severe with MOGAD-ON, the recovery is typically better than with AQP4-IgG ON, and, in general, MOGAD-associated demyelination has been suggested to have a more favorable prognosis compared with AQP4-seropositive NMOSD, featuring a lower EDSS and reduced risk of visual and motor disability. The clinical course of MOGAD can be monophasic; however, approximately 50% of patients with MOGAD will experience a recurrent demyelinating attack, most commonly ON [177].

Disability from both AQP4- and MOG-associated ON is accumulated by poor recovery from attacks. Interestingly, when serum samples from 177 of 448 patients enrolled in the ONTT were assayed for AQP4- and MOG-IgG, only four MOG-IgG-seropositive patients were identified. Therefore, the results of the ONTT are not informative regarding the impact of high-dose corticosteroids on visual recovery in NMOSD-ON and MOG-ON. Importantly, the clinical course of MOGAD-ON, as in NMOSD-ON, differs from idiopathic and MS-associated ON (where steroids do not affect the ultimate visual outcome) by being typically briskly steroid-responsive and sometimes steroid-dependent [38].

Treatment with corticosteroids is almost always used in acute MOGAD-ON to aid in visual recovery, and there are limited data on the natural history without treatment. As such, new onset diseases or acute relapses are typically treated with high-dose IV methylprednisolone for 3–5 days. According to a European cohort, a number of patients had an extremely rapid return to baseline within 48 h following steroid initiation [175].

Acute attacks that respond poorly to steroids can be treated with PLEX or immunoadsorption. Observational studies have shown that, similarly to NMOSD, a shorter time to treatment correlated with less retinal nerve fiber layer losses and better visual outcomes [36]. Similarly to NMOSD, "time equals vision". The optimal treatment initiation may be by day 4, but treatment even before day 7 still offers an opportunity for very good visual outcomes in MOGAD [36].

Typically, MOGAD-ON neuritis relapses respond well to steroids, but patients are often vulnerable to relapses on tapering or withdrawal of steroids [177]. A recurrent course is associated with higher titers of MOG-IgG during the first months and/or maintenance of seropositive status despite treatment [175]. In contrast, low titers or seroconversion to negativity in the early course represent a reliable predictor of a monophasic course.

The treatment of MOGAD has been largely extrapolated from AQP4-IgG NMOSD and is currently understandardized, still based on clinical experience and observational studies (Class IV evidence), with no approved drugs, to date, for long-term relapse prevention in adult patients. No phase III multicenter randomized clinical trials have been performed to assess treatment effectiveness in MOGAD, due to difficulties related to the recent recognition and low prevalence of this disease, the wide age range, and broad clinical spectrum. MOGAD-ON frequently recurs when patients are on no-maintenance long-term treatment, with 80% of patients having two or more attacks over a median time of 2.9 years [176]. Prior retrospective studies suggest that long-term immunosuppressant therapy may reduce the frequency of recurrent attacks, while most DMTs used to treat MS have not demonstrated usefulness in preventing relapses in MOGAD. Compared to pediatric patients, adult MOGAD patients may have a higher risk of relapses and a worse functional recovery as well as a shorter median time until a second attack, supporting the use of long-term relapse prevention treatments in adult seropositive patients with ON and/or TM.

Maintenance oral steroids at the lowest possible dose are an effective treatment strategy in MOGAD. The Australasian and New Zealand MOG Study Group recently showed that relapses commonly occurred with doses of <20 mg prednisone per day in adults, and that a duration of treatment or less than 3 months was associated with a 2-fold higher risk of relapses, compared to patients treated for a longer time [175]. In addition, the concomitant use of oral steroids as an adjunct to immunosuppressive drugs was accompanied b ay reduced risk for relapses (5% vs. 38% on immunosuppressive monotherapy). Some patients on maintenance low-dose prednisone alone had a relapse-free course, indicating the efficacy of steroids in sustaining remission, but the significant long-term metabolic and bone health-related adverse effects warrant caution. Interestingly, a subgroup of MOGAD patients remained relapse free on no immunotherapy for a long time after the initial treatment with steroids, to only experience a relapse after many years [175]. Another group in China demonstrated that the early tapering or discontinuation of oral steroids within 30 days had as an outcome a relapse in 59% of patients [178]. In conclusion, a prolonged steroid taper may reduce the chance of early relapses and provide an acceptable maintenance option, with close monitoring during and after steroid cessation.

Based on data from a recent, large multicenter cohort of MOG-IgG-positive patients conducted by Mayo Clinic, **maintenance IVIg**, at 3- or 4-week intervals, applied in 10 patients (5 pediatrics), demonstrated the lowest relapse rate (only 20% had a relapse) compared to alternative immunosuppressives with a relapse rate >50% (59% for AZA, 73% for MMF, 62% for RTX) [177]. Chen et al. suggested that IVIg effectivity in suppressing future attacks was independent of a bias toward using IVIg in patients with a more benign disease, and that long-term IVIg is an effective maintenance immunotherapy for patients with MOGAD [123]. Previous small retrospective studies support these results, especially in children [126]. By contrast, the Australian cohort showed a higher relapse rate in three out of seven patients receiving long-term IVIg; however, the median ARR for the cohort was 0, and the highest relapse rate in patients treated with IVIg was the lowest among the treatments evaluated (range 0–0.75) [175,177]. Furthermore, IVIg treatment efficacy was shown in a large European retrospective cohort of MOG-IgG-positive patients with ON and/or TM as a therapeutic approach after an acute relapse showing favorable results, as 50% of patients experienced complete (or almost complete) recovery and 44% partial recovery (measured by visual acuity and EDSS) [175].

Azathioprine and **MMF** seem to be effective and safe therapeutic strategies for long-term immunosuppression in adult MOGAD patients, with failure and intolerance being the most frequent causes for the agents' discontinuation. The agents can be used as a monotherapy or in combination with oral steroids.

Based on a systematic review that included 17 articles, azathioprine (2–3 mg/kg/day divided into 2–3 doses) achieves a reduction in the mean and median ARR, as well as the stabilization or improvement of the EDSS [179]. Azathioprine was found to have the second lowest post-treatment ARR after IVIG, although the slightly lower pretreatment ARR for recipients of azathioprine compared to patients receiving the other therapies could have led to a bias. Patients on AZA were also more frequently on concomitant maintenance prednisone. The interval between the initiation of azathioprine and the first relapse ranged from 3 to 9 months (median of 6 months) [179,180].

Cobo-Calvo et al. recently reported a significant reduction in relapses in patients treated with MMF in a cohort of Spanish and French adult patients with relapsing MOGAD [128]. Furthermore, the systematic analysis in adult MOGAD patients, showed the efficacy of MMF (1500–3000 mg/day divided into two doses) in a total sample of 96 treated patients with the agent, regarding ARR and EDSS indices [179]. Similar promising results come from a more recent prospective study, especially in a subset of patients with isolated ON or high MOG-IgG titers. Eighty-six percent of patients had a reduced risk for relapse after 400 days of follow up [181]. In the Australian cohort, MMF also appeared to be effective, but treatment failure rates were higher, and relapses were often associated with steroid tapering, suggesting the steroid was producing the benefit in these patients [175]. Consistent findings were derived from the Mayo Clinic as well, where MMF use in 13 patients documented a more modest reduction in relapse rates compared to the other immunosuppressive agents [177].

Limited data about the potential use of cyclophosphamide in MOGAD are available. Similar to the Australian cohort, which reported 50% failure [177], in the Mayo Clinic cohort, two of three patients had relapses during treatment with the agent [177]. Chen et al. commented that even though the lack of apparent efficacy could be attributed to the small total number of patients treated with IV cyclophosphamide or to the reservation of this potent agent for the most severe and refractory cases, the findings may indicate that cytotoxic CD8 T cells are not key effectors of MOGAD pathogenesis. Confirmatory of the potential lack of the agent's efficacy in MOGAD patients is the fact that when the two patients who relapsed early on cyclophosphamide switched to rituximab, they stabilized without further relapse [177].

Whittam et al. showed in a multicenter study of 98 patients treated with rituximab that the agent reduces the relapse rate for MOGAD, but the benefit did not appear to be as great as for AQP4-IgG-positive NMOSD [182]. Recently, the same group demonstrated in a study of 71 adult MOGAD patients on rituximab a relapse rate of 42%, with a median follow-up time of 12.7 months [183]. Interestingly, the investigators found that MOG-specific B cells were only detected in about 60% of these patients, indicating that MOG-specific B cells are not linked to levels of serum MOG-Abs, casting doubt on whether B-cell-depleting treatments should be used in MOG-seropositive patients. The findings of the aforementioned studies concur with the data derived from the systematic review, which concluded that, similar to AQP4-ab-positive NMOSD patients, new relapses within the few weeks after the first rituximab infusion occurred in about 30% of MOGAD patients despite B cell depletion, with a median time from the most recent infusion to the first relapse of 2.6 (range: 0.6–5.8) months [183]. It has been also suggested, that in relapsing MOG-seropositive patients needing rituximab, regular CD19 monitoring and proactively redosing a brittle patient in the event of B-cell repopulation might reduce the incidence of repopulation relapses, as this has been demonstrated in NMOSD [175].

Emerging therapeutic approaches which have been used successfully in the treatment of NMOSD could also be evaluated in MOGAD. To date, tocilizumab has been used with varied effectivity in some patients with rituximab-refractory MOGAD. Furthermore, the NMOmetum trial, which compared inebelizumab vs. placebo administration in NMOSD patients, also enrolled seven adult MOGAD patients, but separate outcomes for the MOGAD subgroup were not specifically reported [184]. Novel, future, potential treatments, also being investigated in NMOSD include: efgartigimod, a synthetic IgG1 Fc analog, which has shown efficacy as a substitute for IVIG in treating the IgG-mediated neuromuscular disorder myasthenia gravis; rozalixizumab, an inhibitor of the neonatal Fc receptor; and Bruton's tyrosine kinase inhibitors.

7.2. Chronic Relapsing Inflammatory Optic Neuropathy

The main characteristic of patients with chronic relapsing inflammatory optic neuropathy (CRION) is the rapid and excellent response to corticosteroid therapy, as well steroid dependence, with relapses within weeks or months after the withdrawal of or a decrease in corticosteroids [185]. CRION requires careful consideration and differentiation from typical, demyelinating optic neuritis, since the treatment is entirely different, and the outcome without treatment is likely to be very poor. Furthermore, the standard treatment of typical ON is not adequate for CRION [186].

Already when CRION was first described by Kidd in 2003, the authors concluded that treatment with corticosteroids was able to induce an abrupt and prompt relief of pain and, at times, a complete restoration of normal visual acuity and color vision even months after the onset of symptoms [186]. There was evidence that following steroid withdrawal, patients tended to relapse, necessitating long-term immunosuppression, which appears to arrest progression of the disease in the majority of cases [186]. Since then, the clinical experience has evolved, and although CRION patients generally tend to respond well to steroids, cumulative damage can lead to poor visual outcomes and structural changes in RNFL and GCL complexes permanently. Indeed, a recent study showed that up to 25% of patients can end up with a final visual acuity <20/40 [187]. Consequently, early diagnosis and timely management are key for restoring as well as preserving vision.

For the time being, treatment recommendations are based on the activity of the disease and the clinical experience with related disorders, as no CRION-specific formal guidelines have been established yet. The general approach in the acute phase of the disease is the administration of IV methylprednisolone 1 mg/kg for 3–5 days, possibly with added IVIg or PLEX in severe cases, followed by oral steroids (1 mg/kg) with gradual tapering, as an abrupt withdrawal of treatment may lead to the irreversible worsening of visual acuity [185,188]. Given that relapses are common, the abrupt disruption of treatment should be avoided, and the minimal effective glucocorticoid dose be identified. In addition, the early initiation of a steroid-sparing immunomodulatory agent would be a reasonable consideration given the well-known iatrogenic morbidity of glucocorticoids. Azathioprine, rituximab, IVIg, cyclophosphamide, and methotrexate have been used for long-term and short-term treatment in single reports [136]. Natalizumab has also been employed [185]. Of course, if MOG or AQP4 seropositivity or another connective tissue disease can be identified, the therapeutic approach should be targeted at those disorders [188].

8. Conclusions

Typical and atypical ON follow a different natural history, rendering crucial the timely differentiation between them. Treating typical ON primarily accelerates recovery without any effect on the final visual outcome. However, the diagnosis of CIS such as

ON provides the opportunity to closely monitor a patient clinically, and consider early initiation of MS DMTs. However, more work is needed to find remyelinating and reparative treatment approaches.

Among atypical causes of ON, NMOSD-related ON stands out in its severity. Prompt and aggressive treatment is needed to save vision and CNS functioning. In addition, the early initiation of relapse-prevention strategies is recommended. Slow steroid tapering and the recruitment of additional long-term therapies should be considered for MOGAD-ON and CRION.

Funding: This research received no external funding.

Institutional Review Board Statement: Not applicable.

Informed Consent Statement: Not applicable.

Conflicts of Interest: The authors declare no conflict of interest.

References

1. Menon, V.; Saxena, R.; Misra, R.; Phuljhele, S. Management of optic neuritis. *Indian J. Ophthalmol.* **2011**, *59*, 117–122. [PubMed]
2. Morrow, S.A.; Fraser, J.A.; Day, C.; Bowman, D.; Rosehart, H.; Kremenchutzky, M.; Nicolle, M. Effect of treating acute optic neuritis with bioequivalent oral vs intravenous corticosteroids—A randomized clinical trial. *JAMA Neurol.* **2018**, *75*, 690–696. [CrossRef] [PubMed]
3. Huang, W.J.; Chen, W.W.; Zhang, X. Multiple sclerosis: Pathology, diagnosis and treatments. *Exp. Ther. Med.* **2017**, *13*, 3163–3166. [CrossRef] [PubMed]
4. Compston, A.; Coles, A. Multiple sclerosis. *Lancet* **2008**, *372*, 1502–1517. [CrossRef]
5. Wingerchuk, D.; Lucchinetti, C.; Noseworthy, J. Multiple Sclerosis: Current Pathophysiological Concepts. *Lab. Investig.* **2001**, *81*, 263–281. [CrossRef]
6. Lucchinetti, C.; Brück, W.; Parisi, J.; Scheithauer, B.; Rodriguez, M.; Lassmann, H. Heterogeneity of multiple sclerosis lesions: Implications for the pathogenesis of demyelination. *Ann. Neurol.* **2000**, *47*, 707–717. [CrossRef]
7. Traugott, U.; Reinherz, E.L.; Raine, C.S. Multiple sclerosis. Distribution of T cells, T cell subsets and Ia-positive macrophages in lesions of different ages. *J. Neuroimmunol.* **1983**, *4*, 201–221. [CrossRef]
8. Ferguson, B.; Matyszak, M.K.; Esiri, M.M.; Perry, V.H. Axonal damage in acute multiple sclerosis lesions. *Brain* **1997**, *120*, 393–399. [CrossRef]
9. Bitsch, A.; Schuchardt, J.; Bunkowski, S.; Kuhlmann, T.; Brück, W. Acute axonal injury in multiple sclerosis. Correlation with demyelination and inflammation. *Brain* **2000**, *123*, 1174–1183. [CrossRef]
10. Hu, D.; Ikizawa, K.; Lu, L.; Sanchirico, M.E.; Shinohara, M.L.; Cantor, H. Analysis of regulatory CD8 T cells in Qa-1-deficient mice. *Nat. Immunol.* **2004**, *5*, 516–523. [CrossRef]
11. Toosy, A.T.; Mason, D.F.; Miller, D.H. Optic neuritis. *Lancet Neurol.* **2014**, *13*, 83–99. [CrossRef]
12. Babbe, H.; Roers, A.; Waisman, A.; Lassmann, H.; Goebels, N.; Hohlfeld, R.; Friese, M.; Schröder, R.; Deckert, M.; Schmidt, S.; et al. Clonal expansions of CD8(+) T cells dominate the T cell infiltrate in active multiple sclerosis lesions as shown by micromanipulation and single cell polymerase chain reaction. *J. Exp. Med.* **2000**, *192*, 393–404. [CrossRef]
13. Carlström, K.E.; Zhu, K.; Ewing, E.; Krabbendam, I.E.; Harris, R.A.; Falcão, A.M.; Jagodic, M.; Castelo-Branco, G.; Piehl, F. Gsta4 controls apoptosis of differentiating adult oligodendrocytes during homeostasis and remyelination via the mitochondria-associated Fas-Casp8-Bid-axis. *Nat. Commun.* **2020**, *11*, 4071. [CrossRef]
14. Chamberlain, K.A.; Chapey, K.S.; Nanescu, S.E.; Huang, J.K. Creatine enhances mitochondrial-mediated oligodendrocyte survival after demyelinating injury. *J. Neurosci.* **2017**, *37*, 1479–1492. [CrossRef]
15. Jin, J.; Smith, M.D.; Kersbergen, C.J.; Kam, T.-I.; Viswanathan, M.; Martin, K.; Dawson, T.M.; Dawson, V.L.; Zack, D.J.; Whartenby, K.; et al. Glial pathology and retinal neurotoxicity in the anterior visual pathway in experimental autoimmune encephalomyelitis. *Acta Neuropathol. Commun.* **2019**, *7*, 125. [CrossRef]
16. Cannella, B.; Raine, C.S. The adhesion molecule and cytokine profile of multiple sclerosis lesions. *Ann. Neurol.* **1995**, *37*, 424–435. [CrossRef]
17. Kuhlmann, T.; Miron, V.; Cui, Q.; Wegner, C.; Antel, J.; Brück, W. Differentiation block of oligodendroglial progenitor cells as a cause for remyelination failure in chronic multiple sclerosis. *Brain* **2008**, *131 Pt 7*, 1749–1758. [CrossRef]
18. Goodkin, D.E. The Natural History of Multiple Sclerosis. In *Treatment of Multiple Sclerosis*; Clinical Medicine and the Nervous System; Rudick, R.A., Goodkin, D.E., Eds.; Springer: London, UK, 1992.
19. Koopmans, R.A.; Li, D.K.B.; Oger, J.J.F.; Kastrukoff, L.F.; Jardine, C.; Costley, L.; Hall, S.; Grochowski, E.W.; Paty, D.W. Chronic progressive multiple sclerosis: Serial magnetic resonance brain imaging over six months. *Ann. Neurol.* **1989**, *26*, 248–256. [CrossRef]
20. Prineas, J.W.; Barnard, R.O.; Kwon, E.E.; Sharer, L.R.; Cho, E.S. Multiple sclerosis: Remyelination of nascent lesions. *Ann. Neurol.* **1993**, *33*, 137–151. [CrossRef]

21. Lotan, I.; Hellmann, M.A.; Benninger, F.; Stiebel-Kalish, H.; Steiner, I. Recurrent optic neuritis—Different patterns in multiple sclerosis, neuromyelitis optica spectrum disorders and MOG-antibody disease. *J. Neuroimmunol.* **2018**, *324*, 115–118. [CrossRef]
22. Burman, J.; Raininko, R.; Fagius, J. Bilateral and recurrent optic neuritis in multiple sclerosis. *Acta Neurol. Scand.* **2011**, *123*, 207–210. [CrossRef] [PubMed]
23. Quintana, F.J.; Patel, B.; Yeste, A.; Nyirenda, M.; Kenison, J.; Rahbari, R.; Fetco, D.; Hussain, M.; O'Mahony, J.; Magalhaes, S.; et al. Canadian Pediatric Demyelinating Disease Network. Epitope spreading as an early pathogenic event in pediatric multiple sclerosis. *Neurology* **2014**, *83*, 2219–2226. [CrossRef] [PubMed]
24. Frohman, E.M.; Racke, M.K.; Raine, C.S. Multiple sclerosis—The plaque and its pathogenesis. *N. Engl. J. Med.* **2006**, *354*, 942–955. [CrossRef] [PubMed]
25. Qin, Y.; Duquette, P.; Zhang, Y.; Talbot, P.; Poole, R.; Antel, J. Clonal expansion and somatic hypermutation of V (H) genes of B cells from cerebrospinal fluid in multiple sclerosis. *J. Clin. Investig.* **1998**, *102*, 1045–1050. [CrossRef]
26. Noseworthy, J.H.; Lucchinetti, C.; Rodriguez, M.; Weinshenker, B.G. Multiple sclerosis. *N. Engl. J. Med.* **2000**, *343*, 938–952. [CrossRef]
27. Sriram, S.; Steiner, I. Experimental allergic encephalomyelitis: A misleading model of multiple sclerosis. *Ann. Neurol.* **2005**, *58*, 939–945. [CrossRef]
28. Hellmann, M.A.; Steiner, I.; Mosberg-Galili, R. Sudden sensorineural hearing loss in multiple sclerosis: Clinical course and possible pathogenesis. *Acta Neurol. Scand.* **2011**, *124*, 245–249. [CrossRef]
29. Lemus, H.N.; Warrington, A.E.; Rodriguez, M. Multiple Sclerosis: Mechanisms of Disease and Strategies for Myelin and Axonal Repair. *Neurol. Clin.* **2018**, *36*, 1–11. [CrossRef]
30. Nancy, J.; Newman, M.D. Atlanta, Georgia, the Optic Neuritis Treatment Trial. Commentary, AAO. Available online: https://www.aaojournal.org/article/S0161-6420(19)32364-4/pdf (accessed on 2 February 2022).
31. Beck, R.W.; Gal, R.L. Treatment of acute optic neuritis: A summary of findings from the optic neuritis treatment trial. *Arch. Ophthalmol.* **2008**, *126*, 994–995. [CrossRef]
32. Beck, R.W.; Cleary, P.A.; Anderson, M.M., Jr.; Keltner, J.L.; Shults, W.T.; Kaufman, D.I.; Buckley, E.G.; Corbett, J.J.; Kupersmith, M.J.; Miller, N.R.; et al. A randomized controlled trail of corticosteroids in the treatment of acute optic neuritis. *N. Engl. J. Med.* **1992**, *326*, 581–588. [CrossRef]
33. Optic Neuritis Study Group. Visual function 5 years after optic neuritis: Experience of the Optic Neuritis Treatment Trial. *Arch. Ophthalmol.* **1997**, *115*, 1545–1552. [CrossRef]
34. Gal, R.L.; Vedula, S.S.; Beck, R. Corticosteroids for treating optic neuritis. *Cochrane Database Syst. Rev.* **2015**, *2015*, CD001430.
35. Petzold, A.; Braithwaite, T.; van Oosten, B.W.; Balk, L.; Martinez-Lapiscina, E.H.; Wheeler, R.; Wiegerinck, N.; Waters, C.; Plant, G.T. Case for a new corticosteroid treatment trial in optic neuritis: Review of updated evidence. *J. Neurol. Neurosurg. Psychiatry* **2020**, *91*, 9–14. [CrossRef]
36. Stiebel-Kalish, H.; Hellmann, M.A.; Mimouni, M.; Paul, F.; Bialer, O.; Bach, M.; Lotan, I. Does time equal vision in the acute treatment of a cohort of AQP4 and MOG optic neuritis? *Neurol. Neuroimmunol. Neuroinflamm.* **2019**, *6*, e572. [CrossRef]
37. Bsteh, G.; Berek, K.; Hegen, H.; Teuchner, B.; Buchmann, A.; Voortman, M.M.; Auer, M.; Zinganell, A.; Di Pauli, F.; Deisenhammer, F.; et al. Serum neurofilament levels correlate with retinal nerve fiber layer thinning in multiple sclerosis. *Mult. Scler. J.* **2019**, *26*, 1682–1690. [CrossRef]
38. Osinga, E.; van Oosten, B.; de Vries-Knoppert, W.; Petzold, A. Time is vision in recurrent optic neuritis. *Brain Res.* **2017**, *1673*, 95–101. [CrossRef]
39. Phuljhele, S.; Kedar, S.; Saxena, R. Approach to optic neuritis: An update. *Indian J. Ophthalmol.* **2021**, *69*, 2266–2276.
40. Horton, L.; Bennett, J.L. Acute Management of Optic Neuritis: An Evolving Paradigm. *J. Neuroophthalmol.* **2018**, *38*, 358–367. [CrossRef]
41. Wilhelm, H.; Schabet, M. Continuing medical education the diagnosis and treatment of optic neuritis. *Dtsch. Arztebl. Int.* **2015**, *112*, 616–626.
42. Le Page, E.; Veillard, D.; Laplaud, D.A.; Hamonic, S.; Wardi, R.; Lebrun, C.; Zagnoli, F.; Wiertlewski, S.; Deburghgraeve, V.; Coustans, M.; et al. Oral versus intravenous high-dose methylprednisolone for treatment of relapses inpatients with multiple sclerosis (COPOUSEP): A randomised, controlled, double-blind, non-inferiority trial. *Lancet* **2015**, *386*, 974–981. [CrossRef]
43. Bonnan, M.; Cabre, P. Plasma Exchange in Severe Attacks of Neuromyelitis Optica. *Mult. Scler. Int.* **2012**, *2012*, 787630. [CrossRef]
44. Bennett, J.L. Optic Neuritis. *Continuum* **2019**, *25*, 1236–1264. [CrossRef]
45. Jakimovski, D.; Kolb, C.; Ramanathan, M.; Zivadinov, R.; Weinstock-Guttman, B. Interferon β for Multiple Sclerosis. *Cold Spring Harb. Perspect. Med.* **2018**, *8*, a032003. [CrossRef]
46. Dhib-Jalbut, S.; Marks, S. Interferon-beta mechanisms of action in multiple sclerosis. *Neurology* **2010**, *74* (Suppl. S1), S17–S24. [CrossRef] [PubMed]
47. Rudick, R.A.; Ransohoff, R.M.; Lee, J.C.; Peppler, R.; Yu, M.; Mathisen, P.M.; Tuohy, V.K. In vivo effects of interferon beta-1a on immunosuppressive cytokines in multiple sclerosis. *Neurology* **1998**, *50*, 1294–1300. [CrossRef]
48. Hartrich, L.; Weinstock-Guttman, B.; Hall, D.; Badgett, D.; Baier, M.; Patrick, K.; Feichter, J.; Hong, J.; Ramanathan, M. Dynamics of immune cell trafficking in interferon-β treated multiple sclerosis patients. *J. Neuroimmunol.* **2003**, *139*, 84–92. [CrossRef]

49. Rizzo, F.; Giacomini, E.; Mechelli, R.; Buscarinu, M.C.; Salvetti, M.; Severa, M.; Coccia, E.M. Interferon-β therapy specifically reduces pathogenic memory B cells in multiple sclerosis patients by inducing a FAS-mediated apoptosis. *Immunol. Cell. Biol.* **2016**, *94*, 886–894. [CrossRef]
50. Molnarfi, N.; Prod'homme, T.; Schulze-Topphoff, U.; Spencer, C.M.; Weber, M.S.; Patarroyo, J.C.; Lalive, P.H.; Zamvil, S.S. Glatiramer acetate treatment negatively regulates type I interferon signaling. *Neurol. Neuroimmunol. Neuroinflamm.* **2015**, *2*, e179. [CrossRef] [PubMed]
51. Weber, M.S.; Hohlfeld, R.; Zamvil, S.S. Mechanism of action of glatiramer acetate in treatment of multiple sclerosis. *Neurotherapeutics* **2007**, *4*, 647–653. [CrossRef] [PubMed]
52. Prod'homme, T.; Zamvil, S.S. The Evolving Mechanisms of Action of Glatiramer Acetate. *Cold Spring Harb. Perspect. Med.* **2019**, *9*, a029249.
53. Polman, C.H.; Reingold, S.C.; Banwell, B.; Clanet, M.; Cohen, J.A.; Filippi, M.; Fujihara, K.; Havrdova, E.; Hutchinson, M.; Kappos, L.; et al. Diagnostic criteria for multiple sclerosis: 2010 revisions to the McDonald criteria. *Ann. Neurol.* **2011**, *69*, 292–302. [CrossRef]
54. Kieseier, B.C.; Benamor, M. Pregnancy outcomes following maternal and paternal exposure to teriflunomide during treatment for relapsing-remitting multiple sclerosis. *Neurol. Ther.* **2014**, *3*, 133–138. [CrossRef]
55. Andersen, J.B.; Moberg, J.Y.; Spelman, T.; Magyari, M. Pregnancy Outcomes in Men and Women Treated with Teriflunomide. A Population-Based Nationwide Danish Register Study. *Front. Immunol.* **2018**, *9*, 2706. [CrossRef]
56. Fazekas, F.; Lublin, F.D.; Li, D.; Freedman, M.S.; Hartung, H.P.; Rieckmann, P.; Sørensen, P.S.; Maas-Enriquez, M.; Sommerauer, B.; Hanna, K.; et al. Intravenous immunoglobulin in relapsing-remitting multiple sclerosis: A dose-finding trial. *Neurology* **2008**, *71*, 265–271. [CrossRef]
57. Sørensen, P.S.; Sellebjerg, F.; Lycke, J.; Färkkilä, M.; Créange, A.; Lund, C.G.; Schluep, M.; Frederiksen, J.L.; Stenager, E.; Pfleger, C.; et al. Minocycline added to subcutaneous interferon β-1a in multiple sclerosis: Randomized Recycline study. *Eur. J. Neurol.* **2016**, *23*, 861–870. [CrossRef]
58. Metz, L.M.; Li, D.K.B.; Traboulsee, A.L.; Duquette, P.; Eliasziw, M.; Cerchiaro, G.; Greenfield, J.; Riddehough, A.; Yeung, M.; Kremenchutzky, M.; et al. Trial of Minocycline in a Clinically Isolated Syndrome of Multiple Sclerosis. *N. Engl. J. Med.* **2017**, *376*, 2122–2133. [CrossRef]
59. Jacobs, L.D.; Beck, R.W.; Simon, J.H.; Kinkel, R.P.; Brownscheidle, C.M.; Murray, T.J.; Simonian, N.A.; Slasor, P.J.; Sandrock, A.W.; The CHAMPS Study Group. Intramuscular interferon beta-1a therapy initiated during a first demyelinating event in multiple sclerosis. *N. Engl. J. Med.* **2000**, *343*, 898–904. [CrossRef]
60. Goodin, D.S.; Bates, D. Treatment of early multiple sclerosis: The value of treatment initiation after a first clinical episode. *Mult. Scler.* **2009**, *15*, 1175–1182. [CrossRef]
61. Comi, G.; Filippi, M.; Barkhof, F.; Durelli, L.; Edan, G.; Fernández, O.; Hartung, H.; Seeldrayers, P.; Sørensen, P.S.; Rovaris, M.; et al. Effect of early interferon treatment on conversion to definite multiple sclerosis: A randomised study. *Lancet* **2001**, *357*, 1576–1582. [CrossRef]
62. Efendi, H. Clinically Isolated Syndromes: Clinical Characteristics, Differential Diagnosis, and Management. *Noro Psikiyatr. Ars.* **2015**, *52* (Suppl. S1), S1–S11. [CrossRef]
63. Marcus, J.F.; Waubant, E.L. Updates on Clinically Isolated Syndrome and Diagnostic Criteria for Multiple Sclerosis. *Neurohospitalist* **2013**, *3*, 65–80. [CrossRef]
64. Gold, R.; Wolinsky, J.S. Pathophysiology of multiple sclerosis and the place of teriflunomide. *Acta Neurol. Scand.* **2011**, *124*, 75–84. [CrossRef]
65. Comi, G.; De Stefano, N.; Freedman, M.S.; Barkhof, F.; Polman, C.H.; Uitdehaag, B.M.J.; Casset-Semanaz, F.; Hennessy, B.; Moraga, M.S.; Rocak, S.; et al. Comparison of two dosing frequencies of subcutaneous interferon beta-1a in patients with a first clinical demyelinating event suggestive of multiple sclerosis (REFLEX): A phase 3 randomised controlled trial. *Lancet Neurol.* **2012**, *11*, 33. [CrossRef]
66. Comi, G.; De Stefano, N.; Freedman, M.S.; Barkhof, F.; Uitdehaag, B.M.; de Vos, M.; Marhardt, K.; Chen, L.; Issard, D.; Kappos, L. Subcutaneous interferon β-1a in the treatment of clinically isolated syndromes: 3-year and 5-year results of the phase III dosing frequency-blind multicentre REFLEXION study. *J. Neurol. Neurosurg. Psychiatry* **2017**, *88*, 285–294. [CrossRef]
67. Miller, A.E.; Wolinsky, J.S.; Kappos, L.; Comi, G.; Freedman, M.S.; Olsson, T.P.; Bauer, D.; Benamor, M.; Truffinet, P.; O'Connor, P.W.; et al. Oral teriflunomide for patients with a first clinical episode suggestive of multiple sclerosis (TOPIC): A randomised, double-blind, placebo-controlled, phase 3 trial. *Lancet Neurol.* **2014**, *13*, 977–986. [CrossRef]
68. Albert, C.; Mikolajczak, J.; Liekfeld, A.; Piper, S.K.; Scheel, M.; Zimmermann, H.G.; Nowak, C.; Dörr, J.; Bellmann-Strobl, J.; Chien, C.; et al. Fingolimod after a first unilateral episode of acute optic neuritis (MOVING)—Preliminary results from a randomized, rater-blind, active-controlled, phase 2 trial. *BMC Neurol.* **2020**, *20*, 75. [CrossRef]
69. Cadavid, D.; Balcer, L.; Galetta, S.; Aktas, O.; Ziemssen, T.; Vanopdenbosch, L.; Frederiksen, J.; Skeen, M.; Jaffe, G.J.; Butzkueven, H.; et al. Safety and efficacy of opicinumab in acute optic neuritis (RENEW): A randomised, placebo-controlled, phase 2 trial. *Lancet Neurol.* **2017**, *16*, 189–199. [CrossRef]
70. Ranger, A.; Ray, S.; Szak, S.; Dearth, A.; Allaire, N.; Murray, R.; Gardner, R.; Cadavid, D.; Mi, S. Anti-LINGO-1 has no detectable immunomodulatory effects in preclinical and phase 1 studies. *Neurol. Neuroimmunol. Neuroinflamm.* **2017**, *5*, e417. [CrossRef] [PubMed]

71. Swanson, W.B.; Gong, T.; Zhang, Z.; Eberle, M.; Niemann, D.; Dong, R.; Rambhia, K.J.; Ma, P.X. Controlled release of odontogenic exosomes from a biodegradable vehicle mediates dentinogenesis as a novel biomimetic pulp capping therapy. *J. Control. Release* **2020**, *324*, 679–694. [CrossRef] [PubMed]
72. Mathew, B.; Torres, L.A.; Gamboa Acha, L.; Tran, S.; Liu, A.; Patel, R.; Chennakesavalu, M.; Aneesh, A.; Huang, C.C.; Feinstein, D.L.; et al. Uptake and distribution of administered bone marrow mesenchymal stem cell extracellular vesicles in retina. *Cells* **2021**, *10*, 730. [CrossRef] [PubMed]
73. Mathew, B.; Ravindran, S.; Liu, X.; Torres, L.; Chennakesavalu, M.; Huang, C.C.; Feng, L.; Zelka, R.; Lopez, J.; Sharma, M.; et al. Mesenchymal stem cell-derived extracellular vesicles and retinal ischemia-reperfusion. *Biomaterials* **2019**, *197*, 146–160. [CrossRef]
74. Dai, Y.D.; Sheng, H.; Dias, P.; Jubayer Rahman, M.; Bashratyan, R.; Regn, D.; Marquardt, K. Autoimmune responses to exosomes and candidate antigens contribute to type 1 diabetes in non-obese diabetic mice. *Curr. Diabetes Rep.* **2017**, *17*, 130. [CrossRef]
75. Laso-Garcia, F.; Ramos-Cejudo, J.; Carrillo-Salinas, F.J.; Otero-Ortega, L.; Feliu, A.; Gomez-de Frutos, M.; Mecha, M.; Díez-Tejedor, E.; Guaza, C.; Gutiérrez-Fernández, M. Therapeutic potential of extracellular vesicles derived from human mesenchymal stem cells in a model of progressive multiple sclerosis. *PLoS ONE* **2018**, *13*, e0202590.
76. Thomi, G.; Joerger-Messerli, M.; Haesler, V.; Muri, L.; Surbek, D.; Schoeberlein, A. Intranasally administered exosomes from umbilical cord stem cells have preventive neuroprotective effects and contribute to functional recovery after perinatal brain injury. *Cells* **2019**, *8*, 855. [CrossRef]
77. Duffy, C.P.; McCoy, C.E. The role of MicroRNAs in repair processes in multiple sclerosis. *Cells* **2020**, *9*, 1711. [CrossRef]
78. Ma, Q.; Matsunaga, A.; Ho, B.; Oksenberg, J.R.; Didonna, A. Oligodendrocyte specific Argonaute profiling identifies microRNAs associated with experimental autoimmune encephalomyelitis. *J. Neuroinflamm.* **2020**, *17*, 297. [CrossRef]
79. Marangon, D.; Boda, E.; Parolisi, R.; Negri, C.; Giorgi, C.; Montarolo, F.; Perga, S.; Bertolotto, A.; Buffo, A.; Abbracchio, M.P.; et al. In vivo silencing of miR-125a-3p promotes myelin repair in models of white matter demyelination. *Glia* **2020**, *68*, 2001–2014. [CrossRef]
80. Lennon, V.A.; Wingerchuk, D.M.; Kryzer, T.J.; Pittock, S.J.; Lucchinetti, C.F.; Fujihara, K.; Nakashima, I.; Weinshenker, B.G. A serum autoantibody marker of neuromyelitis optica: Distinction from multiple sclerosis. *Lancet* **2004**, *364*, 2106–2112. [CrossRef]
81. Misu, T.; Fujihara, K.; Kakita, A.; Konno, H.; Nakamura, M.; Watanabe, S.; Takahashi, T.; Nakashima, I.; Takahashi, H.; Itoyama, Y. Loss of aquaporin 4 in lesions of neuromyelitis optica: Distinction from multiple sclerosis. *Brain* **2007**, *130*, 1224–1234. [CrossRef]
82. Roemer, S.F.; Parisi, J.E.; Lennon, V.A.; Benarroch, E.E.; Lassmann, H.; Bruck, W.; Mandler, R.N.; Weinshenker, B.G.; Pittock, S.J.; Wingerchuk, D.M.; et al. Pattern-specific loss of aquaporin-4 immunoreactivity distinguishes neuromyelitis optica from multiple sclerosis. *Brain* **2007**, *130*, 1194–1205. [CrossRef]
83. Kawachi, I.; Lassmann, H. Neurodegeneration in multiple sclerosis and neuromyelitis optica. *J. Neurol. Neurosurg. Psychiatry* **2017**, *88*, 137–145. [CrossRef] [PubMed]
84. Hinson, S.R.; Romero, M.F.; Popescu, B.F.; Lucchinetti, C.F.; Fryer, J.P.; Wolburg, H.; Fallier-Becker, P.; Noell, S.; Lennon, V.A. Molecular outcomes of neuromyelitis optica (NMO)-IgG binding to aquaporin-4 in astrocytes. *Proc. Natl. Acad. Sci. USA* **2012**, *109*, 1245–1250. [CrossRef] [PubMed]
85. Crane, J.M.; Lam, C.; Rossi, A.; Gupta, T.; Bennett, J.L.; Verkman, A.S. Binding affinity and specificity of neuromyelitis optica autoantibodies to aquaporin-4 M1/M23 isoforms and orthogonal arrays. *J. Biol. Chem.* **2011**, *286*, 16516–16524. [CrossRef] [PubMed]
86. Papadopoulos, M.C.; Verkman, A.S. Aquaporin 4 and neuromyelitis optica. *Lancet Neurol.* **2012**, *11*, 535–544. [CrossRef]
87. Contentti, E.C.; Correale, J. Neuromyelitis optica spectrum disorders: From pathophysiology to therapeutic strategies. *J. Neuroinflamm.* **2021**, *18*, 208. [CrossRef]
88. Stiebel-Kalish, H.; Lotan, I.; Brody, J.; Chodick, G.; Bialer, O.; Marignier, R.; Bach, M.; Hellmann, M.A. Retinal nerve fiber layer may be better preserved in MOG-IgG versus AQP4-IgG optic neuritis: A cohort study. *PLoS ONE* **2017**, *12*, e0170847. [CrossRef]
89. Chen, J.J.; Tobin, W.O.; Majed, M.; Jitprapaikulsan, J.; Fryer, J.P.; Leavitt, J.A.; Flanagan, E.P.; McKeon, A.; Pittock, S.J. Prevalence of myelin oligodendrocyte glycoprotein and aquaporin-4-IgG in patients in the optic neuritis treatment trial. *JAMA Ophthalmol.* **2018**, *136*, 419–422. [CrossRef]
90. Kleiter, I.; Gahlen, A.; Borisow, N.; Fischer, K.; Wernecke, K.D.; Wegner, B.; Hellwig, K.; Pache, F.; Ruprecht, K.; Havla, J.; et al. Neuromyelitis optica: Evaluation of 871 attacks and 1,153 treatment courses. *Ann. Neurol.* **2016**, *79*, 206–216. [CrossRef]
91. Deschamps, R.; Gueguen, A.; Parquet, N.; Saheb, S.; Driss, F.; Mesnil, M.; Vignal, C.; Aboab, J.; Depaz, R.; Gout, O. Plasma exchange response in 34 patients with severe optic neuritis. *J. Neurol.* **2016**, *263*, 883–887. [CrossRef]
92. Restrepo-Aristizábal, C.; Giraldo, L.M.; Giraldo, Y.M.; Pino-Pérez, A.M.; Álvarez-Gómez, F.; Franco, C.A.; Tobón, J.V.; Ascencio, J.L.; Zuluaga, M.I. PLEX: The best first-line treatment in nmosd attacks experience at a single center in Colombia. *Heliyon* **2021**, *7*, e06811. [CrossRef]
93. Yasuda, T.; Mikami, T.; Kawase, Y. Efficacy of tryptophan immunoadsorption plasmapheresis for neuromyelitis optica in two cases. *Ther. Apher. Dial.* **2015**, *19*, 411–412. [CrossRef]
94. Bonnan, M.; Valentino, R.; Debeugny, S.; Merle, H.; Fergé, J.L.; Mehdaoui, H.; Cabre, P. Short delay to initiate plasma exchange is the strongest predictor of outcome in severe attacks of NMO spectrum disorders. *J. Neurol. Neurosurg. Psychiatry* **2018**, *89*, 346–351. [CrossRef]

95. Kleiter, I.; Gahlen, A.; Borisow, N.; Fischer, K.; Wernecke, K.D.; Hellwig, K.; Pache, F.; Ruprecht, K.; Havla, J.; Kümpfel, T.; et al. Apheresis therapies for NMOSD attacks. A retrospective study of 207 therapeutic interventions. *Neurol. Neurol. Neuroimmunol. Neuroinflamm.* **2018**, *5*, e504.
96. Oji, S.; Nomura, K. Immunoadsorption in neurological disorders. *Transfus. Apher. Sci.* **2017**, *56*, 671–676. [CrossRef]
97. Schwartz, J. Guidelines on the use of therapeutic apheresis in clinical practice—Evidence-based approach from the writing committee of the American society for apheresis: The seventh special issue. *J. Clin. Apher.* **2016**, *31*, 149–162. [CrossRef]
98. Lipphardt, M.; Wallbach, M.; Koziolek, M.J. Plasma exchange or immunoadsorption in demyelinating diseases: A meta-analysis. *J. Clin. Med.* **2020**, *9*, 1597. [CrossRef]
99. Li, X.; Tian, D.C.; Fan, M.; Xiu, Y.; Wang, X.; Li, T.; Jia, D.; Xu, W.; Song, T.; Shi, F.D.; et al. Intravenous immunoglobulin for acute attacks in neuromyelitis optica spectrum disorders (NMOSD). *Mult. Scler. Relat. Disord.* **2020**, *44*, 102325. [CrossRef]
100. Greenberg, B.M.; Thomas, K.P.; Krishnan, C.; Kaplin, A.I.; Calabresi, P.A.; Kerr, D.A. Idiopathic transverse myelitis: Corticosteroids, plasma exchange, or cyclophosphamide. *Neurology* **2007**, *68*, 1614–1617. [CrossRef]
101. Carnero Contentti, E.; Rojas, J.I.; Cristiano, E.; Daccach Marques, V.; Flores-Rivera, J.; Lana-Peixoto, M.; Carlos, N.; Papais-Alvarenga, R.; Sato, D.K.; de Castillo, I.S.; et al. Latin American consensus recommendations for management and treatment of neuromyelitis optica spectrum disorders in clinical practice. *Mult. Scler. Relat. Disord.* **2020**, *45*, 102428. [CrossRef]
102. Tugizova, M.; Vlahovic, L.; Tomczak, A.; Wetzel, N.S.; Han, M.H. New Therapeutic Landscape in Neuromyelitis Optica. *Curr. Treat Options Neurol.* **2021**, *23*, 13. [CrossRef]
103. Held, F.; Klein, A.-K.; Berthele, A. Drug Treatment of Neuromyelitis Optica Spectrum Disorders: Out with the Old, in with the New? *ImmunoTargets Ther.* **2021**, *10*, 87–101. [CrossRef] [PubMed]
104. Sharrack, B.; Saccardi, R.; Alexander, T.; Badoglio, M.; Burman, J.; Farge, D.; Greco, R.; Jessop, H.; Kazmi, M.; Kirgizov, K.; et al. Autologous haematopoietic stem cell transplantation and other cellular therapy in multiple sclerosis and immune-mediated neurological diseases: Updated guidelines and recommendations from the EBMT Autoimmune Diseases Working Party (ADWP) and the Joint Accreditation Committee of EBMT and ISCT (JACIE). *Bone Marrow Transplant.* **2020**, *55*, 283–306. [PubMed]
105. Ceglie, G.; Papetti, L.; Valeriani, M.; Merli, P. Hematopoietic stem cell transplantation in neuromyelitis optica-spectrum disorders (NMO-SD): State-of-the-art and future perspectives. *Int. J. Mol. Sci.* **2020**, *21*, 5304. [CrossRef] [PubMed]
106. Chan, K.-H.; Lee, C.-Y. Treatment of Neuromyelitis Optica Spectrum Disorders, Review. *Int. J. Mol. Sci.* **2021**, *22*, 8638. [CrossRef]
107. Wallach, A.I.; Tremblay, M.; Kister, I. Advances in the Treatment of Neuromyelitis Optica Spectrum Disorder. *Neurol. Clin.* **2021**, *39*, 35–49. [CrossRef]
108. Miljkovic, D.; Samardzic, T.; Drakulic, D.; Stosic-Grujicic, S.; Trajkovic, V. Immunosuppressants leflunomide and mycophenolic acid inhibit fibroblast IL-6 production by distinct mechanisms. *Cytokine* **2002**, *19*, 181–186. [CrossRef]
109. Allison, A.C.; Eugui, E.M. Mycophenolate mofetil and its mechanisms of action. *Immunopharmacology* **2000**, *47*, 85–118. [CrossRef]
110. Nielsen, O.H.; Vainer, B.; Rask-Madsen, J. Review article: The treatment of inflammatory bowel disease with 6-mercaptopurine or azathioprine. *Aliment. Pharmacol. Ther.* **2001**, *15*, 1699–1708. [CrossRef]
111. Bichuetti, D.B.; Perin, M.M.M.; Souza, N.A.; Oliveira, E.M.L. Treating neuromyelitis optica with azathioprine: 20-year clinical practice. *Mult. Scler.* **2019**, *25*, 1150–1161. [CrossRef]
112. Jacob, A.; Matiello, M., Weinshenker, B.G.; Wingerchuk, D.M.; Lucchinetti, C.; Shuster, E.; Carter, J.; Keegan, B.M.; Kantarci, O.H.; Pittock, S.J. Treatment of neuromyelitis optica with mycophenolate mofetil: Retrospective analysis of 24 patients. *Arch. Neurol.* **2009**, *66*, 1128–1133. [CrossRef]
113. Montcuquet, A.; Collongues, N.; Papeix, C.; Zephir, H.; Audoin, B.; Laplaud, D.; Bourre, B.; Brochet, B.; Camdessanche, J.P.; Labauge, P.; et al. Effectiveness of mycophenolate mofetil as first-line therapy in AQP4-IgG, MOG-IgG, and seronegative neuromyelitis optica spectrum disorders. *Mult. Scler.* **2017**, *23*, 1377–1384. [CrossRef]
114. Songwisit, S.; Kosiyakul, P.; Jitprapaikulsan, J.; Prayoonwiwat, N.; Ungprasert, P.; Siritho, S. Efficacy and safety of mycophenolate mofetil therapy in neuromyelitis optica spectrum disorders: A systematic review and meta-analysis. *Sci. Rep.* **2020**, *10*, 16727.
115. Collongues, N.; Ayme-Dietrich, E.; Monassier, L.; de Seze, J. Pharmacotherapy for Neuromyelitis Optica Spectrum Disorders: Current Management and Future Options. *Drugs* **2019**, *79*, 125–142. [CrossRef]
116. Kowarik, M.C.; Soltys, J.; Bennett, J.L. The treatment of neuromyelitis optica. *J. Neuroophthalmol.* **2014**, *34*, 70–82. [CrossRef]
117. Enriquez, C.A.G.; Espiritu, A.I.; Pasco, P.M.D. Efficacy and tolerability of mitoxantrone for neuromyelitis optica spectrum disorder: A systematic review. *J. Neuroimmunol.* **2019**, *332*, 126–134. [CrossRef]
118. Jarius, S.; Aboul-Enein, F.; Waters, P.; Kuenz, B.; Hauser, A.; Berger, T.; Lang, W.; Reindl, M.; Vincent, A.; Kristoferitsch, W. Antibody to aquaporin-4 in the long-term course of neuromyelitis optica. *Brain* **2008**, *131 Pt 11*, 3072–3080. [CrossRef]
119. Bichuetti, D.B.; Oliveira, E.M.; Boulos Fde, C.; Gabbai, A.A. Lack of response to pulse cyclophosphamide in neuromyelitis optica: Evaluation of 7 patients. *Arch. Neurol.* **2012**, *69*, 938–939. [CrossRef]
120. Xu, Y.; Wang, Q.; Ren, H.T.; Qiao, L.; Zhang, Y.; Fei, Y.Y. Comparison of efficacy and tolerability of azathioprine, mycophenolate mofetil, and cyclophosphamide among patients with neuromyelitis optica spectrum disorder: A prospective cohort study. *J. Neurol. Sci.* **2016**, *370*, 224–228. [CrossRef]
121. Chen, B.; Wu, Q.; Ke, G.; Bu, B. Efficacy and safety of tacrolimus treatment for neuromyelitis optica spectrum disorder. *Sci. Rep.* **2017**, *7*, 831. [CrossRef]

122. Trebst, C.; Jarius, S.; Berthele, A.; Paul, F.; Schippling, S.; Wildemann, B.; Borisow, N.; Kleiter, I.; Aktas, O.; Kümpfel, T. Update on the diagnosis and treatment of neuromyelitis optica: Recommendations of the Neuromyelitis Optica Study Group (NEMOS). *J. Neurol.* **2014**, *261*, 1–16. [CrossRef]
123. Kim, S.H.; Jeong, I.H.; Hyun, J.W.; Joung, A.; Jo, H.J.; Hwang, S.H.; Yun, S.; Joo, J.; Kim, H.J. Treatment outcomes with rituximab in 100 patients with neuromyelitis optica: Influence of FCGR3A polymorphisms on the therapeutic response to rituximab. *JAMA Neurol.* **2015**, *72*, 989–995. [CrossRef]
124. Ellwardt, E.; Ellwardt, L.; Bittner, S.; Zipp, F. Monitoring Bcell repopulation after depletion therapy in neurologic patients. *Neurol. Neuroimmunol. Neuroinflamm.* **2018**, *5*, e463. [CrossRef]
125. Tahara, M.; Oeda, T.; Okada, K.; Kiriyama, T.; Ochi, K.; Maruyama, H.; Fukaura, H.; Nomura, K.; Shimizu, Y.; Mori, M.; et al. Safety and efficacy of rituximab in neuromyelitis optica spectrum disorders (RIN-1 study): A multicentre, randomised, double-blind, placebo-controlled trial. *Lancet Neurol.* **2020**, *19*, 298–306. [CrossRef]
126. Graf, J.; Mares, J.; Barnett, M.; Aktas, O.; Albrecht, P.; Zamvil, S.S.; Hartung, H.P. Targeting B cells to modify MS, NMOSD, and MOGAD: Part 2. *Neurol. Neuroimmunol. Neuroinflamm.* **2020**, *8*, e919.
127. Marcinnò, A.; Marnetto, F.; Valentino, P.; Martire, S.; Balbo, A.; Drago, A.; Leto, M.; Capobianco, M.; Panzica, G.; Bertolotto, A. Rituximab-induced hypogammaglobulinemia in patients with neuromyelitis optica spectrum disorders. *Neurol. Neuroimmunol. Neuroinflamm.* **2018**, *5*, e498. [CrossRef] [PubMed]
128. Wingerchuk, AAN2019. Available online: https://issuu.com/americanacademyofneurology/docs/aan_onsiteguide_web_with_links (accessed on 25 February 2022).
129. Ghrenassia, E.; Mariotte, E.; Azoulay, E. Rituximab-related severe toxicity. *Int. J. Crit. Care Emerg. Med.* **2018**, *2018*, 579–596.
130. Holmøy, T.; Høglund, R.A.; Illes, Z.; Myhr, K.-M.; Torkildsen, Ø. Recent progress in maintenance treatment of neuromyelitis optica spectrum disorder. *J. Neurol.* **2021**, *268*, 4522–4536. [CrossRef] [PubMed]
131. Chihara, N.; Aranami, T.; Sato, W.; Miyazaki, Y.; Miyake, S.; Okamoto, T.; Ogawa, M.; Toda, T.; Yamamura, T. Interleukin 6 signaling promotes anti-aquaporin 4 autoantibody production from plasma blasts in neuromyelitis optica. *Proc. Natl. Acad. Sci. USA* **2011**, *108*, 3701–3706. [CrossRef]
132. Zhang, C.; Zhang, M.; Qiu, W.; Ma, H.; Zhang, X.; Zhu, Z.; Yang, C.S.; Jia, D.; Zhang, T.X.; Yuan, M.; et al. Safety and efficacy of tocilizumab versus azathioprine in highly relapsing neuromyelitis optica spectrum disorder (TANGO): An open-label, multicentre, randomised, phase 2 trial. *Lancet Neurol.* **2020**, *19*, 391–401. [CrossRef]
133. Agasing, A.M.; Wu, Q.; Khatri, B.; Borisow, N.; Ruprecht, K.; Brandt, A.U.; Gawde, S.; Kumar, G.; Quinn, J.L.; Ko, R.M.; et al. Transcriptomics and proteomics reveal a cooperation between interferon and T-helper 17 cells in neuromyelitis optica. *Nat. Commun.* **2020**, *11*, 2856. [CrossRef]
134. Pardo, S.; Giovannoni, G.; Hawkes, C.; Lechner-Scott, J.; Waubant, E.; Levy, M. Editorial on: Eculizumab in aquaporin-4-positive neuromyelitis optica spectrum disorder. *Mult. Scler. Relat. Disord.* **2019**, *33*, A1–A2. [CrossRef]
135. Levy, M.; Fujihara, K.; Palace, J. New therapies for neuromyelitis optica spectrum disorder. *Lancet Neurol.* **2021**, *20*, 60–67. [CrossRef]
136. Fox, E.; Lovett-Racke, A.E.; Gormley, M.; Liu, Y.; Petracca, M.; Cocozza, S.; Shubin, R.; Wray, S.; Weiss, M.S.; Bosco, J.A.; et al. A phase 2 multicenter study of ublituximab, a novel glycoengineered anti-CD20 monoclonal antibody, in patients with relapsing forms of multiple sclerosis. *Mult. Scler.* **2021**, *27*, 420–429. [CrossRef]
137. Pittock, S.J.; Berthele, A.; Fujihara, K.; Nakashima, I.; Kim, H.J.; Levy, M.; Palace, J.; Nakashima, I.; Terzi, M.; Totolyan, N.; et al. Eculizumab in aquaporin-4-positive neuromyelitis optica spectrum disorder. *N. Engl. J. Med.* **2019**, *381*, 614–625. [CrossRef]
138. Tullman, M.J.; Zabeti, A.; Vuocolo, S.; Dinh, Q. Inebilizumab for treatment of neuromyelitis optica spectrum disorder. *Neurodegener. Dis. Manag.* **2021**, *11*, 341–352. [CrossRef]
139. Cree, B.A.C.; Bennett, J.L.; Kim, H.J.; Weinshenker, B.G.; Pittock, S.J.; Wingerchuk, D.M.; Fujihara, K.; Paul, F. Inebilizumab for the treatment of neuromyelitis optica spectrum disorder (N-MOmentum): A double-blind, randomized placebo-controlled phase 2/3 trial. *Lancet* **2019**, *394*, 1352–1363. [CrossRef]
140. Cree, B.A.; Bennett, J.L.; Kim, H.J.; Weinshenker, B.G.; Pittock, S.J.; Wingerchuk, D.; Fujihara, K.; Paul, F.; Cutter, G.R.; Marignier, R.; et al. Sensitivity analysis of the primary endpoint from the N-MOmentum study of inebilizumab in NMOSD. *Mult. Scler.* **2021**, *27*, 2052–2061. [CrossRef]
141. Marignier, R.; Bennett, J.L.; Kim, H.J.; Weinshenker, B.G.; Pittock, S.J.; Wingerchuk, D.; Fujihara, K.; Paul, F.; Cutter, G.R.; Green, A.J.; et al. Disability outcomes in the N-MOmentum trial of inebilizumab in neuromyelitis optica spectrum disorder. *Neurol. Neuroimmunol. Neuroinflamm.* **2021**, *8*, e978. [CrossRef]
142. Traboulsee, A.; Greenberg, B.M.; Bennett, J.L.; Szczechowski, L.; Fox, E.; Shkrobot, S.; Yamamura, T.; Terada, Y.; Kawata, Y.; Wright, P.; et al. Safety and efficacy of satralizumab monotherapy in neuromyelitis optica spectrum disorder: A randomised, double-blind, multicentre, placebo-controlled phase 3 trial. *Lancet Neurol.* **2020**, *19*, 402–412. [CrossRef]
143. Yamamura, T.; Kleiter, I.; Fujihara, K.; Palace, J.; Greenberg, B.; Zakrzewska-Pniewska, B.; Patti, F.; Tsai, C.-P.; Saiz, A.; Yamazaki, H.; et al. Trial of Satralizumab in neuromyelitis optica spectrum disorder. *N. Engl. J. Med.* **2019**, *381*, 2114–2124. [CrossRef]
144. Enspryng Prescribing Information. 2020. Available online: https://www.gene.com/download/pdf/enspryng_prescribing.pdf (accessed on 5 February 2022).
145. Mealy, M.A.; Levy, M. A pilot safety study of ublituximab, a monoclonal antibody against CD20, in acute relapses of neuromyelitis optica spectrum disorder. *Medicine* **2019**, *98*, e15944. [CrossRef]

146. Kim, W.; Kim, H.J. Monoclonal antibody therapies for multiple sclerosis and neuromyelitis optica spectrum disorder. *J. Clin. Neurol.* **2020**, *16*, 355–368. [CrossRef]
147. Tradtrantip, L.; Asavapanumas, N.; Verkman, A.S. Emerging therapeutic targets for neuromyelitis optica spectrum disorder. *Expert Opin. Ther. Targets* **2020**, *24*, 219–229. [CrossRef]
148. Liossis, S.N.; Staveri, C. What's new in the treatment of systemic lupus erythematosus. *Front. Med.* **2021**, *8*, 655100. [CrossRef]
149. Zhang, C.; Tian, D.-C.; Yang, C.-S.; Han, B.; Wang, J.; Yang, L.; Shi, F.-D. Safety and efficacy of bortezomib in patients with highly relapsing neuromyelitis optica spectrum disorder. *JAMA Neurol.* **2017**, *74*, 1010–1012. [CrossRef]
150. Howard, J.F., Jr.; Bril, V.; Burns, T.M.; Mantegazza, R.; Bilinska, M.; Szczudlik, A.; Beydoun, S.; Garrido, F.J.R.R.; Piehl, F.; Rottoli, M.; et al. Randomized phase 2 study of FcRn antagonist efgartigimod in generalized myasthenia gravis. *Neurology* **2019**, *92*, e2661–e2673. [CrossRef]
151. Montalban, X.; Arnold, D.L.; Weber, M.S.; Staikov, I.; Piasecka-Stryczynska, K.; Willmer, J.; Martin, E.C.; Dangond, F.; Syed, S.; Wolinsky, J.S. Placebo-Controlled Trial of an Oral BTK Inhibitor in Multiple Sclerosis. *N. Engl. J. Med.* **2019**, *380*, 2406–2417. [CrossRef] [PubMed]
152. Shimizu, F.; Schaller, K.L.; Owens, G.P.; Cotleur, A.C.; Kellner, D.; Takeshita, Y.; Obermeier, B.; Kryzer, T.J.; Sano, Y.; Kanda, T.; et al. Glucose-regulated protein 78 autoantibody associates with blood-brain barrier disruption in neuromyelitis optica. *Sci. Transl. Med.* **2017**, *9*, eaai9111. [CrossRef] [PubMed]
153. Lee, J.W.; de Fontbrune, F.S.; Lee, L.W.L.; Pessoa, V.; Gualandro, S.; Füreder, W.; Ptushkin, V.; Rottinghaus, S.T.; Volles, L.; Shafner, L.; et al. Ravulizumab (ALXN1210) vs eculizumab in adult patients with PNH naive to complement inhibitors: The 301 study. *Blood* **2019**, *133*, 530–539. [CrossRef] [PubMed]
154. Kulasekararaj, A.G.; Hill, A.; Rottinghaus, S.T.; Langemeijer, S.; Wells, R.; Gonzalez-Fernandez, F.A.; Gaya, A.; Lee, J.W.; Gutierrez, E.O.; Piatek, C.I.; et al. Ravulizumab (ALXN1210) vs eculizumab in C5-inhibitor–experienced adult patients with PNH: The 302 study. *Blood* **2019**, *133*, 540–549. [CrossRef]
155. McKeage, K. Ravulizumab: First global approval. *Drugs* **2019**, *79*, 347–352. [CrossRef]
156. Araki, M.; Yamamura, T. Neuromyelitis optica spectrum disorders: Emerging therapies. *Clin. Exp. Neuroimmunol.* **2017**, *8*, 107–116. [CrossRef]
157. Katz Sand, I.; Fabian, M.T.; Telford, R.; Kraus, T.A.; Chehade, M.; Masilamani, M.; Moran, T.; Farrell, C.; Ebel, S.; Cook, L.J.; et al. Open-label, add-on trial of cetirizine for neuromyelitis optica. *Neurol. Neuroimmunol Neuroinflamm.* **2018**, *5*, e441. [CrossRef]
158. Roufosse, F. Targeting the interleukin-5 pathway for treatment of eosinophilic conditions other than asthma. *Front. Med.* **2018**, *5*, 49. [CrossRef]
159. Tradtrantip, L.; Zhang, H.; Saadoun, S.; Phuan, P.W.; Lam, C.; Papadopoulos, M.C.; Bennett, J.L.; Verkman, A.S. Anti-aquaporin-4 monoclonal antibody blocker therapy for neuromyelitis optica. *Ann. Neurol.* **2012**, *71*, 314–322. [CrossRef]
160. Derdelinckx, J.; Reynders, T.; Wens, I.; Cools, N.; Willekens, B. Cells to the Rescue: Emerging Cell-Based Treatment Approaches for NMOSD and MOGAD. *Int. J. Mol. Sci.* **2021**, *22*, 7925. [CrossRef]
161. Peng, F.; Qiu, W.; Li, J.; Hu, X.; Huang, R.; Lin, D.; Bao, J.; Jiang, Y.; Bian, L. A preliminary result of treatment of neuromyelitis optica with autologous peripheral hematopoietic stem cell transplantation. *Neurologist* **2010**, *16*, 375–378. [CrossRef]
162. Greco, R.; Bondanza, A.; Vago, L.; Moiola, L.; Rossi, P.; Furlan, R.; Martino, G.; Radaelli, M.; Martinelli, V.; Carbone, M.R.; et al. Allogeneic hematopoietic stem cell transplantation for neuromyelitis optica. *Ann. Neurol.* **2014**, *75*, 447–453. [CrossRef]
163. Burt, R.K.; Balabanov, R.; Han, X.; Burns, C.; Gastala, J.; Jovanovic, B.; Helenowski, I.; Jitprapaikulsan, J.; Fryer, J.P.; Pittock, S.J. Autologous nonmyeloablative hematopoietic stem cell transplantation for neuromyelitis optica. *Neurology* **2019**, *93*, E1732–E1741. [CrossRef]
164. Zhang, P.; Liu, B. Effect of autologous hematopoietic stem cell transplantation on multiple sclerosis and neuromyelitis optica spectrum disorder: A PRISMA compliant meta-analysis. *Bone Marrow Transplant.* **2020**, *55*, 1928–1934. [CrossRef]
165. Hau, L.; Kállay, K.; Kertész, G.; Goda, V.; Kassa, C.; Horváth, O.; Liptai, Z.; Constantin, T.; Kriván, G. Allogeneic Haematopoietic Stem Cell Transplantation in a Refractory Case of Neuromyelitis Optica Spectrum Disorder. *Mult. Scler. Relat. Disord.* **2020**, *42*, 102110. [CrossRef]
166. Zubizarreta, I.; Flórez-Grau, G.; Vila, G.; Cabezón, R.; España, C.; Andorra, M.; Saiz, A.; Llufriu, S.; Sepulveda, M.; Sola-Valls, N.; et al. Immune Tolerance in Multiple Sclerosis and Neuromyelitis Optica with Peptide-Loaded Tolerogenic Dendritic Cells in a Phase 1b Trial. *Proc. Natl. Acad. Sci. USA* **2019**, *116*, 8463–8470. [CrossRef]
167. Lu, Z.; Zhu, L.; Liu, Z.; Wu, J.; Xu, Y.; Zhang, C.J. IV/IT hUC-MSCs Infusion in RRMS and NMO: A 10-Year Follow-Up Study. *Front. Neurol.* **2020**, *11*, 967. [CrossRef]
168. Yao, X.; Su, T.; Verkman, A.S. Clobetasol promotes remyelination in a mouse model of neuromyelitis optica. *Acta Neuropathol. Commun.* **2016**, *4*, 42. [CrossRef]
169. Sepúlveda, M.; Armangué, T.; Sola-Valls, N.; Arrambide, G.; Meca-Lallana, J.E.; Oreja-Guevara, C.; Mendibe, M.; De Arcaya, A.A.; Aladro, Y.; Casanova, B.; et al. Neuromyelitis optica spectrum disorders comparison according to the phenotype and serostatus. *Neurol. Neuroimmunol. Neuroinflamm.* **2016**, *3*, e225. [CrossRef]
170. Mealy, M.A.; Kim, S.H.; Schmidt, F.; López, R.; Jimenez Arango, J.A.; Paul, F.; Wingerchuk, D.M.; Greenberg, B.M.; Kim, H.J.; Levy, M. Aquaporin-4 serostatus does not predict response to immunotherapy in neuromyelitis optica spectrum disorders. *Mult. Scler. J.* **2018**, *24*, 1737–1742. [CrossRef]

171. Quarles, R.H. Myelin Sheaths: Glycoproteins Involved in Their Formation, Maintenance and Degeneration. *Cell. Mol. Life Sci.* **2002**, *59*, 1851–1871. [CrossRef]
172. Ambrosius, W.; Michalak, S.; Kozubski, W.; Kalinowska, A. Myelin Oligodendrocyte Glycoprotein Antibody-Associated Disease: Current Insights into the Disease Pathophysiology, Diagnosis and Management. *Int. J. Mol. Sci.* **2020**, *22*, 100. [CrossRef]
173. Sharpe, A.H.; Freeman, G.J. The B7-CD28 Superfamily. *Nat. Rev. Immunol.* **2002**, *1861*, 2455–2461. [CrossRef]
174. Höftberger, R.; Guo, Y.; Flanagan, E.P.; Lopez-Chiriboga, A.S.; Endmayr, V.; Hochmeister, S.; Joldic, D.; Pittock, S.J.; Tillema, J.M.; Gorman, M.; et al. The pathology of central nervous system inflammatory demyelinating disease accompanying myelin oligodendrocyte glycoprotein autoantibody. *Acta Neuropathol.* **2020**, *139*, 875–892. [CrossRef]
175. Ramanathan, S.; Mohammad, S.; Tantsis, E.; Nguyen, T.K.; Merheb, V.; Fung, V.S.C.; White, O.B.; Broadley, S.; Lechner-Scott, J.; Vucic, S.; et al. Clinical course, therapeutic responses and outcomes in relapsing MOG antibody-associated demyelination. *J. Neurol. Neurosurg. Psychiatry* **2018**, *89*, 127–137. [CrossRef] [PubMed]
176. Whittam, D.H.; Karthikeayan, V.; Gibbons, E.; Kneen, R.; Chandratre, S.; Ciccarelli, O.; Hacohen, Y.; de Seze, J.; Deiva, K.; Hintzen, R.Q.; et al. Treatment of MOG antibody associated disorders: Results of an international survey. *J. Neurol.* **2020**, *267*, 3565–3577. [CrossRef] [PubMed]
177. Chen, J.J.; Flanagan, E.P.; Bhatti, M.T.; Jitprapaikulsan, J.; Dubey, D.; Lopez Chiriboga, A.S.S.; Fryer, J.P.; Weinshenker, B.G.; McKeon, A.; Tillema, J.M.; et al. Steroid-sparing maintenance immunotherapy for MOG-IgG associated disorder. *Neurology* **2020**, *95*, e111–e120. [CrossRef] [PubMed]
178. Song, H.; Zhou, H.; Yang, M.; Wang, J.; Liu, H.; Sun, M.; Xu, Q.; Wei, S. Different characteristics of aquaporin-4 and myelin oligodendrocyte glycoprotein antibody-seropositive male optic neuritis in China. *J. Ophthalmol.* **2019**, *2019*, 4015075. [CrossRef]
179. Hacohen, Y.; Wong, Y.Y.; Lechner, C.; Jurynczyk, M.; Wright, S.; Konuskan, B.; Kalser, J.; Poulat, A.L.; Maurey, H.; Ganelin-Cohen, E.; et al. Disease course and treatment responses in children with relapsing myelin oligodendrocyte glycoprotein antibody-associated disease. *JAMA Neurol.* **2018**, *75*, 478–487. [CrossRef]
180. Lu, Q.; Luo, J.; Hao, H.; Liu, R.; Jin, H.; Jin, Y.; Gao, F. Efficacy and safety of long-term immunotherapy in adult patients with MOG antibody disease: A systematic analysis. *J. Neurol.* **2020**, *268*, 4537–4548. [CrossRef]
181. Li, S.; Ren, H.; Yan, X.; Xu, T.; Zhang, Y.; Yin, H.; Zhang, W.; Li, J.; Ren, X.; Fang, F.; et al. Long-term efficacy of mycophenolate mofetil in myelin oligodendrocyte glycoprotein antibody-associated disorders: A prospective study. *Neurol. Neuroimmunol. Neuroinflamm.* **2020**, *7*, e705. [CrossRef]
182. Whittam, D.H.; Cobo-Calvo, A.; Lopez-Chiriboga, A.S.; Pardo, S.; Dodd, J.; Brandt, A.; Berek, K.; Berger, T.; Gombolay, G.; Oliveira, L.M.; et al. Treatment of MOG-IgG associated demyelination with Rituximab: A multinational study of 98 patients. *Neurology* **2018**, *90* (Suppl. S15), S13.
183. Whittam, D.H.; Cobo-Calvo, A.; Lopez-Chiriboga, A.S.; Pardo, S.; Gornall, M.; Cicconi, S.; Brandt, A.; Berek, K.; Berger, T.; Jelcic, I.; et al. Treatment of MOG-IgG-associated disorder with rituximab: An international study of 121 patients. *Mult. Scler. Relat. Disord.* **2020**, *44*, 102251. [CrossRef]
184. Contentti, E.C.; Marrodan, M.; Correale, J. Emerging drugs for the treatment of adult MOGIgG-associated diseases. *Expert Opin. Emerg. Drugs* **2021**, *26*, 75–78. [CrossRef]
185. Renjen, P.N.; Chaudhari, D.M.; Ahmad, K.; Garg, S.; Mishra, A. A review of chronic relapsing inflammatory optic neuropathy. *Apollo Med.* **2020**, *17*, 256–258. [CrossRef]
186. Kidd, D.; Burton, B.; Plant, G.T.; Graham, E.M. Chronic relapsing inflammatory optic neuropathy (CRION). *Brain* **2003**, *126*, 276–284. [CrossRef]
187. Lee, H.-J.; Kim, B.; Waters, P.; Woodhall, M.; Irani, S.; Ahn, S.; Kim, S.-J.; Kim, S.-M. Chronic relapsing inflammatory optic neuropathy (CRION): A manifestation of myelin oligodendrocyte glycoprotein antibodies. *J. Neuroinflamm.* **2018**, *15*, 302. [CrossRef]
188. Mukharesh, L.; Douglas, V.P.; Chwalisz, B.K. Chronic Relapsing Inflammatory Optic Neuropathy (CRION). *Curr. Opin. Ophthalmol.* **2021**, *32*, 521–526. [CrossRef]

International Journal of *Molecular Sciences*

MDPI

Review

Remodeling of the Lamina Cribrosa: Mechanisms and Potential Therapeutic Approaches for Glaucoma

Ryan G. Strickland [1], Mary Anne Garner [1], Alecia K. Gross [1] and Christopher A. Girkin [2,*]

[1] Department of Neurobiology, University of Alabama at Birmingham, Birmingham, AL 35294, USA; rgstrick@uab.edu (R.G.S.); magarner@uab.edu (M.A.G.); agross@uab.edu (A.K.G.)

[2] Department of Ophthalmology and Vision Sciences, University of Alabama at Birmingham, Birmingham, AL 35294, USA

* Correspondence: cgirkin@uabmc.edu; Tel.: +1-205-325-8620

Abstract: Glaucomatous optic neuropathy is the leading cause of irreversible blindness in the world. The chronic disease is characterized by optic nerve degeneration and vision field loss. The reduction of intraocular pressure remains the only proven glaucoma treatment, but it does not prevent further neurodegeneration. There are three major classes of cells in the human optic nerve head (ONH): lamina cribrosa (LC) cells, glial cells, and scleral fibroblasts. These cells provide support for the LC which is essential to maintain healthy retinal ganglion cell (RGC) axons. All these cells demonstrate responses to glaucomatous conditions through extracellular matrix remodeling. Therefore, investigations into alternative therapies that alter the characteristic remodeling response of the ONH to enhance the survival of RGC axons are prevalent. Understanding major remodeling pathways in the ONH may be key to developing targeted therapies that reduce deleterious remodeling.

Keywords: glaucoma; optic nerve head; lamina cribrosa; lamina cribrosa cells; scleral fibroblasts; glial cells; intraocular pressure

Citation: Strickland, R.G.; Garner, M.A.; Gross, A.K.; Girkin, C.A. Remodeling of the Lamina Cribrosa: Mechanisms and Potential Therapeutic Approaches for Glaucoma. *Int. J. Mol. Sci.* **2022**, *23*, 8068. https://doi.org/10.3390/ijms23158068

Academic Editors: Neil R. Miller and Rongkung Tsai

Received: 1 June 2022
Accepted: 19 July 2022
Published: 22 July 2022

1. Introduction

Glaucomatous optic neuropathy (GON) remains the leading cause of irreversible blindness worldwide, and the prevalence is expected to increase in the coming decades [1,2]. Glaucoma is a progressive optic neuropathy which is characterized, in part, by pronounced reorganization of cells in the lamina cribrosa (LC) and peripapillary sclera (ppScl). The variable loading forces imparted on the LC and ppScl by intraocular pressure (IOP), counterbalanced with cerebrospinal fluid (CSF) pressure, result in a region of high strain (tissue stretch) that impacts all ONH cell types and initiates cellular and extracellular matrix (ECM) remodeling. These cellular responses and subsequent ECM remodeling can negatively impact this milieu through which the projecting retinal ganglion cell (RGC) axons must traverse, and this may account for the increased vulnerability to further glaucomatous injury seen in the aged optic nerve or with increasing glaucoma severity (Figure 1).

While IOP lowering remains the only proven treatment, glaucoma can develop and progress even at normal or low levels of IOP. Thus, increasing interest in understanding potential pathways that modulate the pathologic remodeling in the LC and ppScl as a potential approach to develop novel "non-IOP" lowering treatments is emerging, and an abundance of work investigating the mechanisms that underly the ONH remodeling response has been conducted. The aim of this review is to describe the active responses of three major cell populations thought to be most critical to the remodeling response seen in the glaucomatous ONH: LC cells, glial cells, and scleral fibroblasts and to discuss potential therapeutic pathways. While each cell type serves a different purpose, each of these cell populations utilizes similar pathways to respond to the chemical and physical signals presented. Importantly, these responses appear to be consistent between animal models and human tissue culture models of the disease. While therapeutics aims at altering ECM remodeling are a promising potential treatment for glaucoma, it is not the only mechanism that can be exploited clinically.

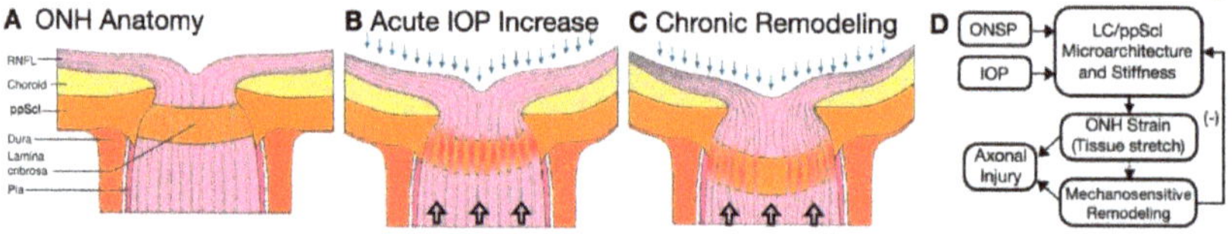

Figure 1. Mechanotransduction and optic nerve head remodeling. (**A**) Healthy optic nerve head (ONH) anatomy detailing key regions. (**B**,**C**) Increased intraocular pressure (IOP, blue arrows) is counterbalanced by optic nerve sheath pressure (ONSP, open arrows) resulting in tissue strain in the optic nerve head (ONH). This can damage axons directly (red) and activates cellular mechanotransduction that drives remodeling of the lamina cribrosa (LC) and peripapillary scleral (ppScl). (**C**) This remodeling alters the material properties and tissue architecture that modulates the stain that drives further remodeling. (**D**) This creates a negative feedback loop (−) that increases the vulnerability of the RGC axons to further glaucomatous injury. Deformation of any mechanical structure under load (strain) is determined by the loading forces (stress) along with its architecture and material properties.

2. Remodeling Response in Aging and Glaucoma

The ONH contains the LC, which is a thin multilayered, reticular load-bearing connective tissue that allows RGC axons and blood vessels to traverse this region of high strain while being supported by glial cells, LC cells, and a load-bearing collagenous matrix. Its unique structure makes it the "weak point" within the sclero-corneal shell where mechanical strain from changes in internal and external pressures on the globe are focused. The LC inserts and anchors itself into the ppScl which provides substantial support to counteract IOP [3–5]. In fact, the ppScl may experience the greatest amount of strain in response to elevated IOP [6,7]. The LC and ppScl also receive counteracting pressure from the post-laminar CSF [8]. Since the LC and overlying peripapillary choroid are perfused via branches of the posterior ciliary arteries that are encased in the ppScl, these vessels are subjected to direct mechanical forces as well. Thus, the classic vascular and mechanical theories of glaucoma pathogenesis are inseparably intertwined with the mechanical behavior of the LC and ppScl directly impacting perfusion and vice versa.

As with any load bearing structure, the amount of deformation (strain) experienced by the LC and ppScl is dependent on the morphology and material properties of these tissues, both of which are altered by both age-related and glaucomatous remodeling. Thus, the mechanocelluar response of the tissues, which is driven by strain, directly modifies the structure and material properties (stiffness) of the LC and ppScl which, in turn, alters the strain driving the remodeling. This dynamic creates a feedforward mechanism that may result in an increasingly pathologic milieu. This mechanism may account for the increased susceptibility to glaucomatous injury seen with aging and with increasing glaucoma severity observed across several prospective glaucoma studies [9–13].

A key pathologic characteristic of the glaucomatous ONH is ECM disorganization [14–16]. The generation of new ECM is an important component of the glaucomatous response and reorganization of the existing ECM is vital to understand for the development of new treatments. Animal models and ex vivo testing of human cadaveric tissues has shown that the sclera is known to stiffen with age and glaucoma, driving increased strain to the ONH [17,18]. In the non-human primate model of glaucoma, LC structure is dramatically disturbed, and collagen density is altered differently depending on the collagen subtype [14,19,20].

The molecular mechanisms of ECM reorganization center largely on the transforming growth factor-β (TGF-β) pathway, although other pathways are likely implicated. TGF-β is typically inactivated by latency associated peptide (LAP) and enzymes that cleave LAP can consequently activate TGF-β, allowing it to bind to a TGF-β receptor complex and activate downstream Smads that control transcription (Figure 2) [21]. In turn, this pathway results in the increased production of ECM molecules and proteins [22–24]. There are several potential mechanisms for TGF-β activation. Interactions with matrix metalloproteinases (MMPs), integrins, and thrombospondin (TSP) can all trigger TGF-β activation [25,26].

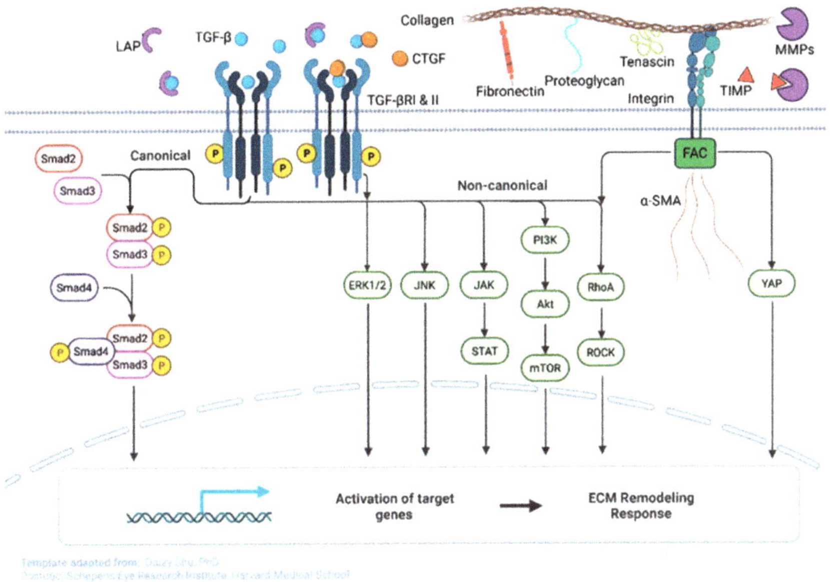

Figure 2. Canonical and non-canonical TGF-β pathways of importance and notable interactions with CTGF and integrin signaling. All pathways ultimately lead to alterations in ECM remodeling responses when activated. Adapted from "Canonical and Non-canonical TGFb Pathways in EMT", by BioRender.com (2022). Available online: https://app.biorender.com/biorender-templates, accessed on 7 June 2022.

There are a multitude of enzymes in the MMP family with various substrate specificity and all contribute to the degradation of ECM components such as collagen, gelatins, laminin, and more [27,28]. In the glaucomatous ONH, MMP-1, -2, -3, and -14 have all demonstrated upregulation [29]. The TSP family has been implicated in a variety of fibrotic pathologies due to its ability to activate TGF-β, and it has implications in ECM remodeling and in IOP levels in knock-out mouse models [30,31]. However, evidence suggests that expression levels of TSP isoforms may vary depending on disease stage, such as low TSP-4 expression in early glaucoma that increases in late stages of the disease [32]. Lastly, integrin signaling-mediated activation of TGF-β may also be more pertinent to glial cells and vascular endothelial cells in the ONH [33]. In total, the elements of this pathway have multiple different implications on the profibrotic responses of the cell types discussed below. Cellular responses include generation of newly synthesized ECM, ECM editing, cellular migration, and cellular contractility. Overall, there are four cell types involved in ONH remodeling including the lamina cribrosa (LC) cells, which are in contact with the laminar beams, astrocytes and microglia cells within the pores of the LC, and scleral fibroblasts within the ppScl.

3. Lamina Cribrosa Cells

LC cells are typically differentiated from regional astrocytes by the lack of GFAP, constitutive expression of α-smooth muscle actin (α-SMA), alternate shape, and localization among other factors [34,35]. While LC cells typically maintain the supportive laminar beams and ECM through production of collagen, elastin, and fibronectin [35], they are also capable of dynamic reactions to external stimuli that can alter the properties of the ECM.

For example, human LC cells in culture exposed to mechanical strain demonstrated altered expression levels of multiple genes that implicate ECM components, cell proliferation, growth factors, and cell surface receptors [36]. In addition to mechanical strain, LC cells can also respond to oxidative stress by upregulating fibrotic genes and production of collagen and α-SMA [37]. Human LC cells cultured in hypoxic conditions also demonstrate increased expression of ECM-related factors such as macrophage migration inhibitory factor and discoidin domain receptor [38–40]. This evidence shows that mechanical strain, oxidative stress, and hypoxia, all potentially relevant to the pathogenesis of primary open-angle glaucoma (POAG), cause LC cells to express and secrete collagen as well as other fibrotic molecules.

LC cells are likely to play a critical role in reorganization and remodeling of the LC in response to mechanical activation also through the TGF-β pathway. Specifically, MMP-2 expression and activity are both increased in response to glaucomatous conditions [24,34,41]. MMP and TSP1 expression is upregulated in LC cells responding to mechanical stress [24,36]. Increased expression and secretion of active MMPs that digest ECM components are likely a major component of ECM disorganization in response to strain. Additionally, LC cells use the ECM matrix as a scaffolding and with localized degradation, LC cells may use the detachment to migrate within the ONH which could underlie the ability of the LC to migrate posteriorly within the ONH [42,43]. There is evidence that application of human TGF-β2 also stimulates MMP activity in porcine LC cells which further supports the role of this pathway in another animal model [44]. Unfortunately, rodent ONHs do not contain LC cells and, though it has been noted previously, there remains no published attempts to culture primate LC cells [45].

As previously mentioned, these notable ECM modifying proteins can also function as activators of latent TGF-β. However, there is also evidence of the reverse: active TGF-β and the subsequent Smad transcriptional regulation pathway controls the expression level of its own activating partners. For instance, application of TGF-β1 to cultured human LC cells induced greater expression of TSP [23]. This evidence suggests that the initial triggers of the TGF-β activation initiate a feed-forward mechanism of ECM remodeling in the LC that has deleterious effects on the axons of the RGCs in the region [26]. This feed-forward signaling mechanism has been demonstrated in the other cell types described below.

TGF-β, as well as mechanical and oxidative stress, can also influence aspects of ECM regulation in LC cells through calcium-dependent pathways. For instance, LC cells cultured from glaucomatous human eyes demonstrated dysregulation of calcium, such as high intracellular levels in response to previously mentioned stimuli and a reduced ability to sequester free cytoplasmic calcium [46,47]. Increased levels of cellular calcium can have a variety of effects on signaling pathways due to the dynamic nature of calcium as a second messenger. Of those pathways, the activation of nuclear factor of activated T-cells (NFAT) may be most relevant to LC cells. In short, calcineurin can bind calcium to calmodulin, which can dephosphorylate NFAT. NFAT then complexes with transcription factors to influence transcription of genes including those that modulate the ECM [48]. While inhibition of this pathway may aid in the treatment of glaucoma, it is not fully understood what precedes the loss of calcium regulation in glaucomatous LC cells. However, one potential preceding factor may be the presence of transient receptor potential canonical (TRPC) channels, a class of voltage-independent channels that preferentially respond to calcium ions and are not necessarily dependent on stimuli such as TGF-β or oxidative and mechanical stresses [49,50]. Interestingly, isoforms of TRPCs, such as 1 and 6, are significantly overexpressed in glaucomatous LC cells cultured from human ONHs [51]. The increased presence of these channels may disturb homeostatic levels of calcium in LC cells, thereby inducing dysregulation. Additionally, these channels modulate transcription of ECM components such as TGF-β, α-SMA, collagen, and MMPs likely through the NFAT pathway described previously [49,51]. Furthermore, TRPC-1 and -6, at least in cancerous cells of the central nervous system, also regulate cell migration [49,52,53]. While these mechanisms of migration have not directly been shown in LC cells, it is possible that glaucomatous LC cells overexpressing these TRPCs may initiate signaling cascades that increase the degree to which LC cells migrate within the LC, potentially contributing to posterior LC migration.

4. Glial Cells

The ONH also contains a resident population of glial cells that create the blood–brain barrier (BBB) and myelinate the RGC axons in the post-laminar region. Dormant microglia are also primed for reactionary responses to local insult or disease [29,54]. Astrocytes, like LC cells, demonstrate mechanosensitive properties and are reactive to glaucomatous conditions in humans and other animal models [55–58]. In the healthy ONH, astrocytes typically support the BBB, but type 1B astrocytes, the dominant subtype in the ONH, can also assist the LC cells in producing the ECM in response to glaucomatous conditions [15,59–61]. Furthermore, astrocytes make connections with other astrocytes and LC cells which could aid in coordinating responses to mechanical strain. Actin reorganization of astrocytes in response to elevated pressure can occur within hours of IOP elevation in rodents and reorganization to baseline may happen over the same time scale, or perhaps even days [62,63]. Reactive astrocytes also produce MMPs which could serve a similar purpose as suggested previously; to sever connections to allow cellular displacement as well as rearrangement of the ECM [29]. As discussed above, MMP function ties in closely with TGF-β, and evidence shows that astrocytes utilize the TGF-β pathway in response to glaucoma as well [22,64,65]. Also prominent to the TGF-β pathway is connective tissue growth factor (CCN2; referred to here as CTGF), a significant binding partner of TGF-β that has been shown to affect the TGF-β pathway, and it is required for Smad1 but not Smad3 activation [66]. CTGF is a mediator of ECM synthesis in the anterior segment as well, as demonstrated by a murine model with increased secretion of CTGF resulting in trabecular meshwork (TM) remodeling and increased IOP [67]. Further evidence in mice shows that the astrocytic levels of CTGF in the ONH increases in glaucomatous animals as a result of elevated IOP and stiffness, which agrees with the observation that there are elevated levels of CTGF in glaucomatous ONHs of humans as well [68]. At least in mice, CTGF seems to be predominantly expressed by astrocytes in the ONH [69], but there is reason to suggest that CTGF may affect other cell types such as LC cells [37].

Integrin signaling in astrocytes may also be involved in the LC cell in detecting tissue strain and inducing cellular migration and reattachment [33]. However, these are not the only molecules involved in astrocytic remodeling as myosin light chain kinase has increased expression in response to mechanical strain of astrocytes and is implicated in cellular migration [70]. Moreover, phosphoinositide 3-kinase, protein kinase C, and tyrosine kinase have also be implicated in migration [71]. Astrocytes also detect mechanical strain with TRPCs which may provide early responses to initial IOP increases. For example, in an induced mouse model, reactive astrocytes respond within one hour of an IOP increase, likely mediated by TRPC isoforms sensitive to stretch [72]. As previously mentioned, this TRPC-NFAT pathway can induce transcriptional changes related to the ECM and can influence cellular migration.

Astrocytic responses are not limited to mechanoreceptors as hypoxia can also trigger responses. Hypoxia-inducible factor-1α (HIF-1α) is a transcriptional factor that is upregulated in response to hypoxic conditions and plays a role in cellular metabolism, proliferation, and angiogenesis [73]. The link between the glaucomatous ONH and HIF-1α was first noted by examining human eye post-mortem, but it has been noted in glaucomatous dogs as well [39,74]. These findings have been replicated in induced rodent models of glaucoma, and the evidence indicates that HIF-1α activation is localized to astrocytes of the retina and ONH [75,76]. There is currently no explanation for why HIF-1α responses are localized to astrocytes and not microglia or RGCs in these models. However, it does indicate that global hypoxic conditions of the ONH, at least on these early timescales, cannot explain RGC dysfunction due to ischemia. Alternatively, PACE4, a subtilisin-like protein convertase, is known to increase expression in response to hypoxia, which may also occur due to vascular compression or primary vascular or vasospastic disease [39,77]. PACE4 also displays constitutive expression and activity in glial cells across the retina, but more so in the ONH [78]. This may be an important factor to consider given the evidence that the PACE family interacts with inhibitors of MMPs, tissue inhibitors of matrix metalloproteinases (TIMPs), as well as TGF-β [79].

Astrocytes at the post-laminar, myelination transition zone (MTZ) are also of interest due to the potential posterior shift of the LC that may be signaled by mechanotransduction of the cells. Specifically, galectin-3 (also known as Lgals3 or Mac-2) has been shown to be upregulated and involved in astrocytic phagocytosis of RGC axons [80]. Additionally, recent evidence in an inducible murine model has shown that astrocytes near the MTZ react by projecting longitudinal processes into the axonal bundles of the ONH, rather than encasing the axons, perhaps contributing to phagocytosis [56]. There is also reason to believe that such phagocytotic absorbance of mitochondria localized to the axons may precede RGC degeneration [81–83].

Microglia are also present in the ONH and are activated in glaucomatous eyes [84]. Similar to LC cells, activated microglia express both TGF-β and MMPs which are not produced in the microglia of healthy ONHs [29]. While microglia are likely incapable of the secretion of ECM molecules, there is mounting evidence that suggests that microglia across the central nervous system are highly active in the maintenance of the ECM through reorganization using MMPs, TSPs, and other similar proteins [85,86]. These processes may be important in the formation of glial scarring, a deposit of new ECM that may not be beneficial to the RGC axons [87]. While this produces a physical obstruction within the ONH that can damage axons, deposits of proteoglycans such as tenascin, which is produced by astrocytes in a mechanically independent model of glaucoma, may provide some initial protection to the axons [88–90]. Furthermore, tenascin is a substrate on which MMPs can act and remodel. Activation of microglia can be dependent on integrin signaling, detection of damaged cells, and growth factors such as TGF-β [33,86,91,92]. While some components of astrocyte activation are necessary for cellular repair and neurotrophic factors, persistent activation can lead to secretion of cytotoxic molecules that are likely further detrimental to the RGC axons [93].

The reactivity of both astrocytes and microglia contributes to the neuroinflammatory conditions of the ONH that may negatively impact the surrounding milieu. This perspective of GON is complex and has generated a rapidly emerging line of work which has recently been adequately reviewed [94–98].

5. Scleral Fibroblasts

The ppScl, or scleral flange, is the portion of sclera immediately surrounding the scleral canal which provides an anchoring point for the LC. It also contains the penetrating branches of the posterior ciliary arteries that perfuse the LC and overlying choroid. The ppScl, as with the remaining sclera, is composed of a dense, collagenous ECM interspersed with resident fibroblasts that maintain the ECM [99]. Similar to the other cell types, the scleral fibroblasts of the ppScl also produce ECM remodeling factors in response to glaucomatous conditions as demonstrated in human tissue and primate, and mouse models [19,100]. A notable characteristic of these cells is that when active and responsive, they differentiate into myofibroblasts consequently expressing α-SMA [101–103]. Differentiation of scleral fibroblasts can be caused by a mechanosensitive response to increased pressure and leads to the secretion of ECM materials, such as collagen, and ECM editors, such as MMPs and TIMPs [104–107]. Myofibroblast differentiation is also partly dependent on Src-kinase pathways as inhibitors of the pathway, such as dasatinib, can restrict the process [108]. Myofibroblast differentiation requires transcriptional changes which can be seen as soon as 30 min after mechanical strain is applied to human tissue culture [109].

Scleral fibroblasts use the collagenous matrix as the point of cell adhesion. This collagenous matrix of the ppScl is morphologically distinct from the rest of the sclera. Specifically, collagen in the ppScl runs in a circumferential pattern around the ONH while collagen in the posterior sclera is arranged in a "basket-woven" pattern [110,111]. Interestingly, this pattern correlates with distribution and alignment of scleral fibroblasts. Fibroblast density increases in proximity to the ONH, and fibroblast projections are highly aligned with collagenous structures [112]. There is also limited evidence to suggest that such fibroblast density gradients may exist in mouse as well [113]. Given this precise alignment of fibroblasts and collagen, these cells likely play a role in the detection of tissue stretch. The reaction of fibroblasts may also differ based on localization as α-SMA expression appears to disrupt fibroblast projection alignment with collagen in the peripheral sclera, but not the ppScl, and fibroblast orientation is most altered when cells detect both strain and TGF-β signaling simultaneously [112]. These synergistic processes likely reinforce chronic glaucomatous remodeling of the ppScl, altering its biomechanical properties.

Properties of scleral fibroblast differentiation and proliferation are partly mediated by both Yes-Associated-Protein (YAP) and Rho-associated protein kinase (ROCK) [114,115]. A notable trait of myofibroblasts is their expression of α-SMA, which may aid in acutely altering scleral stiffness and in cell migration [116]. Furthermore, fibroblast migration is also associated with ROCK and YAP as inhibition of both leads to reduction in rates of migration as well as the contractile abilities associated with α-SMA [114,115]. ROCK inhibitors thus may be a potential treatment that is currently used to increase aqueous outflow in the anterior segment.

Similar to LC cells, TGF-β and Smad-based transcription play a role in fibroblast responses as well. Application of TGF-β to cultured scleral fibroblasts induces higher levels of α-SMA expression and contractility [115] and binding partners of Smad are upregulated in scleral fibroblasts responding to stretch [109]. Additionally, YAP and Smad3 are shown to interact in human scleral fibroblasts which undergo strain [114]. Within an induced mouse model of glaucoma, upregulation in both TSP and integrin expression, both activators of TGF-β, have been demonstrated [104]. Furthermore, an ECM remodeling protein, TGF-β inducible protein (TGF-βip), is known to express in response to TGF-β signaling pathways, especially in collagen rich tissues [117]. There is evidence of the presence and secretion of TGF-βip in human and non-human primate sclera, and TGF-βip has binding properties with integrins at the cell surface in human scleral fibroblasts, which are implicated in stretch detection and in the modulation of the biomechanical properties of the cell [118–120]. TGF-βip can also inhibit fibroblast adhesion to collagen, which likely affects remodeling and cellular migration [119]. Taken together, these results suggest that scleral fibroblasts in glaucomatous conditions use similar signaling pathways to LC cells, such as TGF-β, to differentiate, migrate, and induce extensive remodeling of the sclera and ppScl.

6. Discussion

Glaucoma treatment is difficult due to its complex, incompletely understood, pathophysiology, and while IOP lowering is impactful, it does not universally prevent the progression or development of the disease. These approaches to lower IOP focus on reducing the mechanical stress applied to the optic nerve head. Altering the material properties or morphology of the LC and ppScl by manipulation of the processes involved in ONH remodeling has the potential to increase the resilience of the ONH to the stress induced by changing IOP and promote RGC survival. However, it remains unclear what mechanical properties of the sclera and LC are beneficial and what properties are harmful. For example, there have been hypotheses that increased stiffness could resist elevated IOP levels [17]. However, a stiffer scleral may increase the strain experienced by the OHN by directing stress to the weakest point in the eye wall. Multiple scleral stiffening compounds such as glyceraldehyde, glutaraldehyde, and genipin have failed to demonstrate RGC protection in rodent models or tree shrews thus far [121–123] and may be harmful to the retina as well [124]. Alternatively, perhaps reducing scleral stiffness could alleviate certain cases of glaucoma through the application of collagenase or other compounds that break down glycosaminoglycans [125–127]. Although the evidence is limited, one study showed that rats with experimentally induced glaucoma and subsequently treated with a glycosaminoglycan digesting agent via intravitreal injection demonstrated preservation of RGC dendritic fields [128]. While it is promising that the manipulation of scleral material properties may impact glaucoma development, it is unclear how a collagenous LC may respond to approaches that increase or decrease LC stiffness in terms of RGC survival.

Several therapeutic approaches targeting the cells that create the ECM have been suggested in an attempt to inhibit molecular pathways that trigger ECM secretion (Table 1). Notably, many of the drugs under investigation target some element of the TGF-β pathways referenced previously. For instance, losartan inhibits the G-protein-coupled receptor (GPCR) angiotensin 1 and is a target for the TGF-β ligand [129]. When losartan was administered orally to mice with experimentally induced glaucoma, RGC loss was prevented, likely by inhibiting the degree to which scleral fibroblasts could remodel the ECM [130]. However, a side effect of losartan is decreased blood pressure which could reduce ocular perfusion pressure, a critical risk factor for glaucoma.

Table 1. Potential therapeutic targets to alter glaucomatous remodeling.

Mechanism of Action	Drug(s)	Impact on Optic Nerve Remodeling	Models Tested	References
Prostaglandin F receptor agonist	Bimatoprost, Latanoprost, Fluprostenol, Tafluprost, Travoprost	Upregulation of MMP-1, -3, -9	Mouse, Rat, Rabbit, Guinea Pig, Cat, Dog, Pig, Primate, Human	[131–156]
Hybrid prostaglandin F receptor agonist and nitric oxide donator	Latanoprostene bunod	Upregulation of MMPs and decrease cell contractility	Mouse, Rabbit, Dog, Primate, Human	[157–159]
β-adrenoceptor antagonist	Betaxolol, Timolol	Increased blood flow velocity	Mouse, Rat, Rabbit, Cat, Dog, Pig, Primate, Human	[160–174]
α_2-adrenergic agonist	Apraclonidine, Brimonidine	Anti-apoptotic; RGC survival signal	Mouse, Rat, Guinea Pig, Rabbit, Cat, Dog, Pig, Primate, Human	[139,175–188]
Carbonic anhydrase inhibitor	Acetazolamide, Brinzolamide, Dorzolamide, Methazolamide	Increased blood flow and oxygen tension	Mouse, Rat, Guinea Pig, Rabbit, Dog, Pig, Primate, Human	[189–210]
ROCK Inhibitor	Fasudil, Netarsudil, Ripasudil	Inhibits contractility and migration of fibroblasts; inhibits production of ECM; inhibits cell death pathways	Mouse, Rat, Rabbit, Dog, Primate, Human	[211–226]
Inhibits secretion of TGF-β	Tranilast	Prevents TGF-β mediated fibrotic responses by nearby cells	Rabbit, Human culture	[227–229]
Inhibit transcription of TGF-β	ISTH0036, TbetaRII (RNAi)	Decreased levels of TGF-β expression	Mouse, Human Culture, Human	[230–232]
Direct immunosuppression of TGF-β	Lerdelimumab	Targeted inactivation of TGF-β to prevent receptor binding	Rabbit, Human	[233,234]
Inhibit TSP1 binding to LAP	LSKL	Inhibits TSP1 mediated activation of latent TGF-β	Mouse	[235]
Direct immunosuppression of CTGF	Pamrevlumab	Inhibits CTGF interaction with TGF-β	Human Culture	[37]
Reduce YAP and CTGF expression	Verteporfin (without light activation)	Reduces cell contractility via YAP; reduces CTGF interaction with TGF-β	Mouse, Human Culture, Human	[236–238]
Increased nitric oxide production	Atorvastatin, Lovastatin, Simvastatin	Inhibit RhoA/ROCK pathway and reduce levels of MMP-2 and -9, decrease cell contractility	Mouse, Rat, Rabbit, Dog, Pig, Human Culture	[65,239–249]
Angiotensin 1 receptor (AT1R) inhibitor	Losartan	Inhibits Smad2 phosphorylation	Mice, Rat, Rabbit, Human	[130,250–252]
Glycosaminoglycan degrading enzyme	Chondroitinase ABC	Weakens ECM (reduces stiffness)	Rat, Pig, Primate, Human Culture	[125,128,253, 254]
Inhibit myosin light chain phosphorylation	Src-family tyrosine kinase (SFK) inhibitors (PP2)	Alters cell adhesion, reduces cell contractility, and permeability of cell layers	Rabbit, Human Culture	[108,255]

Additionally, the competitive antagonist LSKL, which can cross the BBB, may be another candidate for the treatment of glaucoma. LSKL prevents TSP1 from binding to LAP which prevents activation of TGF-β and its downstream pathway. The result is that LSKL administration to rodents leads to reduced fibrosis with minimal side effects [26,256,257]. Despite the potential, there has not been any published evidence that LSKL can ameliorate the glaucomatous ONH and preserve RGCs [30]. CTGF, a primary interactor of

TGF-β, is also profibrotic, and inhibition of CTGF in cultured human LC cells using the monoclonal antibody FG-3019 blocked ECM synthesis in these cells [37]. The antibody FG-3019, or pamrevlumab, is currently being evaluated in clinical trials for idiopathic pulmonary fibrosis, but its effectiveness beyond cultured cells in glaucoma has not yet been illustrated [258]. While intriguing, there are also a multitude of other potential therapies or pathway targets of TGF-β that could be beneficial for the treatment of glaucoma [259]. Future therapeutic pathways may further probe the relationship between TGF-β and both bone morphogenic proteins (BMPs) and Wnt signaling; two candidates that may inhibit profibrotic responses [260,261].

Another method to prevent remodeling in the ONH is to prevent the synthesis of collagen by LC cells and astrocytes before it is secreted. The drug tranilast is known to inhibit collagen synthesis and has been shown to work on cultured human LC cells and astrocytes [228]. The inhibition of rho-associated protein kinase (ROCK) has also been shown to prevent scleral fibroblast from exhibiting myofibroblast features, limiting contractility and expression of α-SMA [115]. In fact, ROCK inhibitors, such as K-115 or ripasudil, are currently being investigated in clinical trials for glaucoma treatment [222,262–264].

Some common currently available systemic and topical treatment may also potentially impact glaucoma development. Statins have been shown to prevent TGF-β-mediated activation of MMPs through ROCK pathway inhibition in cultured human eye [65]. Additionally, simvastatin has demonstrated a protective effect on RGC survival in a mouse model of retinal ischemia via elevated IOP [240]. Whether or not statins could be effective at treating human cases of glaucoma with little side effects is unknown [265], but administrative database studies and meta-analyses have suggested a potential protective effect, slowing the development of glaucoma [266–268]. Lastly, prostaglandin analogues, the most common IOP-lowering treatment for glaucoma, work by upregulation of MMPs via the prostaglandin F receptor. These same pathways that alter the ECM of the iris and ciliary body to lower IOP are also involved in glaucomatous remodeling in the posterior pole [269]. While it is unknown whether these compounds would reach therapeutic levels in the posterior pole with topical administration, methods of delivery could be developed to impact the ONH more directly.

In summary, there is intriguing emerging evidence that manipulation of the mechanical properties of the sclera and/or ONH may provide an alternative treatment for glaucoma that is independent of IOP lowering. However, it is possible that implementing a combination of treatments exploiting several mechanisms, such as IOP lowering, ECM remodeling, and neuroprotection, may provide the most effective treatment for patients. The resident cells of the ONH and ppScl that drive remodeling of these critical load-bearing connective tissues can potentially be recruited to improve the resilience of the optic nerve to glaucomatous injury. It is critical that additional research is conducted to clarify how the material properties in the LC and scleral should be adjusted to a beneficial effect and to elucidate the mechanocellular pathways involved in age-related and glaucomatous remodeling.

Author Contributions: R.G.S.: Conceptualization, writing—original draft preparation, writing—review and editing, investigation. M.A.G.: writing—review and editing, A.K.G.: Conceptualization, review and editing, funding acquisition, supervision. C.A.G.: Conceptualization, writing—review and editing, funding acquisition, supervision. All authors have read and agreed to the published version of the manuscript.

Funding: National Eye Institute: R01EY028284 (Girkin), National Eye Institute: 5R01EY030096 (Gross), EyeSight Foundation of Alabama (Girkin), Research to Prevent Blindness (Girkin).

Institutional Review Board Statement: Not applicable.

Informed Consent Statement: Not applicable.

Data Availability Statement: Not applicable.

Conflicts of Interest: The authors declare no conflict of interest.

References

1. Tham, Y.-C.; Li, X.; Wong, T.Y.; Quigley, H.A.; Aung, T.; Cheng, C.-Y. Global prevalence of glaucoma and projections of glaucoma burden through 2040: A systematic review and meta-analysis. *Ophthalmology* **2014**, *121*, 2081–2090. [CrossRef] [PubMed]
2. Quigley, H.A.; Broman, A.T. The number of people with glaucoma worldwide in 2010 and 2020. *Br. J. Ophthalmol.* **2006**, *90*, 262–267. [CrossRef] [PubMed]
3. Downs, J.C.; Girkin, C.A. Lamina cribrosa in glaucoma. *Curr. Opin. Ophthalmol.* **2017**, *28*, 113–119. [CrossRef] [PubMed]
4. Sigal, I.A. Interactions between geometry and mechanical properties on the optic nerve head. *Investig. Ophthalmol. Vis. Sci.* **2009**, *50*, 2785–2795. [CrossRef] [PubMed]
5. Grytz, R.; Fazio, M.A.; Libertiaux, V.; Bruno, L.; Gardiner, S.; Girkin, C.A.; Downs, J.C. Age- and race-related differences in human scleral material properties. *Investig. Ophthalmol. Vis. Sci.* **2014**, *55*, 8163–8172. [CrossRef]
6. Coudrillier, B.; Tian, J.; Alexander, S.; Myers, K.M.; Quigley, H.A.; Nguyen, T.D. Biomechanics of the human posterior sclera: Age- and glaucoma-related changes measured using inflation testing. *Investig. Ophthalmol. Vis. Sci.* **2012**, *53*, 1714–1728. [CrossRef]
7. Safa, B.N.; Wong, C.A.; Ha, J.; Ethier, C.R. Glaucoma and biomechanics. *Curr. Opin. Ophthalmol.* **2022**, *33*, 80–90. [CrossRef]
8. Downs, J.C. Optic nerve head biomechanics in aging and disease. *Exp. Eye Res.* **2015**, *133*, 19–29. [CrossRef]
9. AGIS Investigators. The Advanced Glaucoma Intervention Study (AGIS): 12. Baseline risk factors for sustained loss of visual field and visual acuity in patients with advanced glaucoma. *Am. J. Ophthalmol.* **2002**, *134*, 499–512. [CrossRef]
10. Leske, M.C.; Heijl, A.; Hussein, M.; Bengtsson, B.; Hyman, L.; Komaroff, E.; Early Manifest Glaucoma Trial Group. Factors for glaucoma progression and the effect of treatment: The Early Manifest Glaucoma Trial. *Arch. Ophthalmol.* **2003**, *121*, 48–56. [CrossRef]
11. Musch, D.C.; Gillespie, B.W.; Lichter, P.R.; Niziol, L.M.; Janz, N.K.; CIGTS Study Investigators. Visual field progression in the Collaborative Initial Glaucoma Treatment Study the impact of treatment and other baseline factors. *Ophthalmology* **2009**, *116*, 200–207. [CrossRef] [PubMed]
12. Drance, S.; Anderson, D.R.; Schulzer, M.; Collaborative Normal-Tension Glaucoma Study Group. Risk factors for progression of visual field abnormalities in normal-tension glaucoma. *Am. J. Ophthalmol.* **2001**, *131*, 699–708. [CrossRef]
13. Gordon, M.O.; Beiser, J.A.; Brandt, J.D.; Heuer, D.K.; Higginbotham, E.J.; Johnson, C.A.; Keltner, J.L.; Miller, J.P.; Parrish, R.K.; Wilson, M.R.; et al. The Ocular Hypertension Treatment Study: Baseline factors that predict the onset of primary open-angle glaucoma. *Arch. Ophthalmol.* **2002**, *120*, 714–720, Discussion 829. [CrossRef] [PubMed]
14. Hernandez, M.R.; Andrzejewska, W.M.; Neufeld, A.H. Changes in the extracellular matrix of the human optic nerve head in primary open-angle glaucoma. *Am. J. Ophthalmol.* **1990**, *109*, 180–188. [CrossRef]
15. Hernandez, M.R. Ultrastructural immunocytochemical analysis of elastin in the human lamina cribrosa. Changes in elastic fibers in primary open-angle glaucoma. *Investig. Ophthalmol. Vis. Sci.* **1992**, *33*, 2891–2903.
16. Sawaguchi, S.; Yue, B.Y.; Fukuchi, T.; Abe, H.; Suda, K.; Kaiya, T.; Iwata, K. Collagen fibrillar network in the optic nerve head of normal monkey eyes and monkey eyes with laser-induced glaucoma—A scanning electron microscopic study. *Curr. Eye Res.* **1999**, *18*, 143–149. [CrossRef]
17. Quigley, H.A. The contribution of the sclera and lamina cribrosa to the pathogenesis of glaucoma: Diagnostic and treatment implications. *Prog. Brain Res.* **2015**, *220*, 59–86. [CrossRef]
18. Fazio, M.A.; Grytz, R.; Morris, J.S.; Bruno, L.; Gardiner, S.K.; Girkin, C.A.; Downs, J.C. Age-related changes in human peripapillary scleral strain. *Biomech. Model. Mechanobiol.* **2014**, *13*, 551–563. [CrossRef]
19. Quigley, H.A.; Dorman-Pease, M.E.; Brown, A.E. Quantitative study of collagen and elastin of the optic nerve head and sclera in human and experimental monkey glaucoma. *Curr. Eye Res.* **1991**, *10*, 877–888. [CrossRef]
20. Fukuchi, T.; Sawaguchi, S.; Hara, H.; Shirakashi, M.; Iwata, K. Extracellular matrix changes of the optic nerve lamina cribrosa in monkey eyes with experimentally chronic glaucoma. *Graefe's Arch. Clin. Exp. Ophthalmol.* **1992**, *230*, 421–427. [CrossRef]
21. Prendes, M.A.; Harris, A.; Wirostko, B.M.; Gerber, A.L.; Siesky, B. The role of transforming growth factor β in glaucoma and the therapeutic implications. *Br. J. Ophthalmol.* **2013**, *97*, 680–686. [CrossRef] [PubMed]
22. Zode, G.S.; Sethi, A.; Brun-Zinkernagel, A.-M.; Chang, I.-F.; Clark, A.F.; Wordinger, R.J. Transforming growth factor-β2 increases extracellular matrix proteins in optic nerve head cells via activation of the Smad signaling pathway. *Mol. Vis.* **2011**, *17*, 1745–1758. [PubMed]
23. Kirwan, R.P.; Leonard, M.O.; Murphy, M.; Clark, A.F.; O'Brien, C.J. Transforming growth factor-beta-regulated gene transcription and protein expression in human GFAP-negative lamina cribrosa cells. *Glia* **2005**, *52*, 309–324. [CrossRef] [PubMed]
24. Kirwan, R.P.; Crean, J.K.; Fenerty, C.H.; Clark, A.F.; O'Brien, C.J. Effect of cyclical mechanical stretch and exogenous transforming growth factor-beta1 on matrix metalloproteinase-2 activity in lamina cribrosa cells from the human optic nerve head. *J. Glaucoma* **2004**, *13*, 327–334. [CrossRef]
25. Annes, J.P.; Munger, J.S.; Rifkin, D.B. Making sense of latent TGFbeta activation. *J. Cell Sci.* **2003**, *116*, 217–224. [CrossRef]
26. Murphy-Ullrich, J.E.; Downs, J.C. The Thrombospondin1-TGF-β Pathway and Glaucoma. *J. Ocul. Pharmacol. Ther.* **2015**, *31*, 371–375. [CrossRef]
27. Murphy, G.; Nagase, H. Progress in matrix metalloproteinase research. *Mol. Aspects Med.* **2008**, *29*, 290–308. [CrossRef]
28. Page-McCaw, A.; Ewald, A.J.; Werb, Z. Matrix metalloproteinases and the regulation of tissue remodelling. *Nat. Rev. Mol. Cell Biol.* **2007**, *8*, 221–233. [CrossRef]
29. Yuan, L.; Neufeld, A.H. Activated microglia in the human glaucomatous optic nerve head. *J. Neurosci. Res.* **2001**, *64*, 523–532. [CrossRef]

30. Murphy-Ullrich, J.E.; Suto, M.J. Thrombospondin-1 regulation of latent TGF-β activation: A therapeutic target for fibrotic disease. *Matrix Biol.* **2018**, *68–69*, 28–43. [CrossRef]
31. Haddadin, R.I.; Oh, D.-J.; Kang, M.H.; Villarreal, G.; Kang, J.-H.; Jin, R.; Gong, H.; Rhee, D.J. Thrombospondin-1 (TSP1)-null and TSP2-null mice exhibit lower intraocular pressures. *Investig. Ophthalmol. Vis. Sci.* **2012**, *53*, 6708–6717. [CrossRef] [PubMed]
32. Iomdina, E.N.; Tikhomirova, N.K.; Bessmertny, A.M.; Serebryakova, M.V.; Baksheeva, V.E.; Zalevsky, A.O.; Kotelin, V.I.; Kiseleva, O.A.; Kosakyan, S.M.; Zamyatnin, A.A.; et al. Alterations in proteome of human sclera associated with primary open-angle glaucoma involve proteins participating in regulation of the extracellular matrix. *Mol. Vis.* **2020**, *26*, 623–640. [PubMed]
33. Morrison, J.C. Integrins in the optic nerve head: Potential roles in glaucomatous optic neuropathy (an American Ophthalmological Society thesis). *Trans. Am. Ophthalmol. Soc.* **2006**, *104*, 453–477.
34. Wallace, D.M.; O'Brien, C.J. The role of lamina cribrosa cells in optic nerve head fibrosis in glaucoma. *Exp. Eye Res.* **2016**, *142*, 102–109. [CrossRef]
35. Hernandez, M.R.; Igoe, F.; Neufeld, A.H. Cell culture of the human lamina cribrosa. *Investig. Ophthalmol. Vis. Sci.* **1988**, *29*, 78–89.
36. Kirwan, R.P.; Fenerty, C.H.; Crean, J.; Wordinger, R.J.; Clark, A.F.; O'Brien, C.J. Influence of cyclical mechanical strain on extracellular matrix gene expression in human lamina cribrosa cells in vitro. *Mol. Vis.* **2005**, *11*, 798–810. [PubMed]
37. Wallace, D.M.; Clark, A.F.; Lipson, K.E.; Andrews, D.; Crean, J.K.; O'Brien, C.J. Anti-connective tissue growth factor antibody treatment reduces extracellular matrix production in trabecular meshwork and lamina cribrosa cells. *Investig. Ophthalmol. Vis. Sci.* **2013**, *54*, 7836–7848. [CrossRef] [PubMed]
38. Kirwan, R.P.; Felice, L.; Clark, A.F.; O'Brien, C.J.; Leonard, M.O. Hypoxia regulated gene transcription in human optic nerve lamina cribrosa cells in culture. *Investig. Ophthalmol. Vis. Sci.* **2012**, *53*, 2243–2255. [CrossRef]
39. Tezel, G.; Wax, M.B. Hypoxia-inducible factor 1alpha in the glaucomatous retina and optic nerve head. *Arch. Ophthalmol.* **2004**, *122*, 1348–1356. [CrossRef]
40. McElnea, E.M.; Quill, B.; Docherty, N.G.; Irnaten, M.; Siah, W.F.; Clark, A.F.; O'Brien, C.J.; Wallace, D.M. Oxidative stress, mitochondrial dysfunction and calcium overload in human lamina cribrosa cells from glaucoma donors. *Mol. Vis.* **2011**, *17*, 1182–1191.
41. Yan, X.; Tezel, G.; Wax, M.B.; Edward, D.P. Matrix metalloproteinases and tumor necrosis factor alpha in glaucomatous optic nerve head. *Arch. Ophthalmol.* **2000**, *118*, 666–673. [CrossRef] [PubMed]
42. Yang, H.; Williams, G.; Downs, J.C.; Sigal, I.A.; Roberts, M.D.; Thompson, H.; Burgoyne, C.F. Posterior (outward) migration of the lamina cribrosa and early cupping in monkey experimental glaucoma. *Investig. Ophthalmol. Vis. Sci.* **2011**, *52*, 7109–7121. [CrossRef] [PubMed]
43. Yang, H.; Thompson, H.; Roberts, M.D.; Sigal, I.A.; Downs, J.C.; Burgoyne, C.F. Deformation of the early glaucomatous monkey optic nerve head connective tissue after acute IOP elevation in 3-D histomorphometric reconstructions. *Investig. Ophthalmol. Vis. Sci.* **2011**, *52*, 345–363. [CrossRef] [PubMed]
44. Liou, J.-J.; Geest, J.P.V. Effect of transforming growth factor beta 2 on matrix metalloproteinase activity in porcine lamina cribrosa cells. *Investig. Ophthalmol. Vis. Sci.* **2020**, *61*, 902.
45. Burgoyne, C.F. The non-human primate experimental glaucoma model. *Exp. Eye Res.* **2015**, *141*, 57–73. [CrossRef] [PubMed]
46. Irnaten, M.; Barry, R.C.; Wallace, D.M.; Docherty, N.G.; Quill, B.; Clark, A.F.; O'Brien, C.J. Elevated maxi-K(+) ion channel current in glaucomatous lamina cribrosa cells. *Exp. Eye Res.* **2013**, *115*, 224–229. [CrossRef]
47. Irnaten, M.; Zhdanov, A.; Brennan, D.; Crotty, T.; Clark, A.; Papkovsky, D.; O'Brien, C. Activation of the NFAT-Calcium Signaling Pathway in Human Lamina Cribrosa Cells in Glaucoma. *Investig. Ophthalmol. Vis. Sci.* **2018**, *59*, 831–842. [CrossRef]
48. Tidu, F.; De Zuani, M.; Jose, S.S.; Bendíčková, K.; Kubala, L.; Caruso, F.; Cavalieri, F.; Forte, G.; Frič, J. NFAT signaling in human mesenchymal stromal cells affects extracellular matrix remodeling and antifungal immune responses. *iScience* **2021**, *24*, 102683. [CrossRef]
49. Asghar, M.Y.; Törnquist, K. Transient receptor potential canonical (TRPC) channels as modulators of migration and invasion. *Int. J. Mol. Sci.* **2020**, *21*, 1739. [CrossRef]
50. Sharma, S.; Hopkins, C.R. Review of transient receptor potential canonical (TRPC5) channel modulators and diseases. *J. Med. Chem.* **2019**, *62*, 7589–7602. [CrossRef]
51. Irnaten, M.; O'Malley, G.; Clark, A.F.; O'Brien, C.J. Transient receptor potential channels TRPC1/TRPC6 regulate lamina cribrosa cell extracellular matrix gene transcription and proliferation. *Exp. Eye Res.* **2020**, *193*, 107980. [CrossRef] [PubMed]
52. Chigurupati, S.; Venkataraman, R.; Barrera, D.; Naganathan, A.; Madan, M.; Paul, L.; Pattisapu, J.V.; Kyriazis, G.A.; Sugaya, K.; Bushnev, S.; et al. Receptor channel TRPC6 is a key mediator of Notch-driven glioblastoma growth and invasiveness. *Cancer Res.* **2010**, *70*, 418–427. [CrossRef]
53. Bomben, V.C.; Turner, K.L.; Barclay, T.-T.C.; Sontheimer, H. Transient receptor potential canonical channels are essential for chemotactic migration of human malignant gliomas. *J. Cell. Physiol.* **2011**, *226*, 1879–1888. [CrossRef] [PubMed]
54. Hernandez, M.R. The optic nerve head in glaucoma: Role of astrocytes in tissue remodeling. *Prog. Retin. Eye Res.* **2000**, *19*, 297–321. [CrossRef]
55. Bowman, C.L.; Ding, J.P.; Sachs, F.; Sokabe, M. Mechanotransducing ion channels in astrocytes. *Brain Res.* **1992**, *584*, 272–286. [CrossRef]
56. Wang, R.; Seifert, P.; Jakobs, T.C. Astrocytes in the optic nerve head of glaucomatous mice display a characteristic reactive phenotype. *Investig. Ophthalmol. Vis. Sci.* **2017**, *58*, 924–932. [CrossRef]

57. Pena, J.D.; Agapova, O.; Gabelt, B.T.; Levin, L.A.; Lucarelli, M.J.; Kaufman, P.L.; Hernandez, M.R. Increased elastin expression in astrocytes of the lamina cribrosa in response to elevated intraocular pressure. *Investig. Ophthalmol. Vis. Sci.* **2001**, *42*, 2303–2314.
58. Rogers, R.S.; Dharsee, M.; Ackloo, S.; Sivak, J.M.; Flanagan, J.G. Proteomics analyses of human optic nerve head astrocytes following biomechanical strain. *Mol. Cell. Proteom.* **2012**, *11*, M111.012302. [CrossRef]
59. Hernandez, M.R.; Wang, N.; Hanley, N.M.; Neufeld, A.H. Localization of collagen types I and IV mRNAs in human optic nerve head by in situ hybridization. *Investig. Ophthalmol. Vis. Sci.* **1991**, *32*, 2169–2177.
60. Ye, H.; Yang, J.; Hernandez, M.R. Localization of collagen type III mRNA in normal human optic nerve heads. *Exp. Eye Res.* **1994**, *58*, 53–63. [CrossRef]
61. Pena, J.D.; Roy, S.; Hernandez, M.R. Tropoelastin gene expression in optic nerve heads of normal and glaucomatous subjects. *Matrix Biol.* **1996**, *15*, 323–330. [CrossRef]
62. Tehrani, S.; Davis, L.; Cepurna, W.O.; Choe, T.E.; Lozano, D.C.; Monfared, A.; Cooper, L.; Cheng, J.; Johnson, E.C.; Morrison, J.C. Astrocyte Structural and Molecular Response to Elevated Intraocular Pressure Occurs Rapidly and Precedes Axonal Tubulin Rearrangement within the Optic Nerve Head in a Rat Model. *PLoS ONE* **2016**, *11*, e0167364. [CrossRef] [PubMed]
63. Sun, D.; Qu, J.; Jakobs, T.C. Reversible reactivity by optic nerve astrocytes. *Glia* **2013**, *61*, 1218–1235. [CrossRef] [PubMed]
64. Neumann, C.; Yu, A.; Welge-Lüssen, U.; Lütjen-Drecoll, E.; Birke, M. The effect of TGF-beta2 on elastin, type VI collagen, and components of the proteolytic degradation system in human optic nerve astrocytes. *Investig. Ophthalmol. Vis. Sci.* **2008**, *49*, 1464–1472. [CrossRef] [PubMed]
65. Kim, M.-L.; Sung, K.R.; Kwon, J.; Shin, J.A. Statins Suppress TGF-β2-Mediated MMP-2 and MMP-9 Expression and Activation Through RhoA/ROCK Inhibition in Astrocytes of the Human Optic Nerve Head. *Investig. Ophthalmol. Vis. Sci.* **2020**, *61*, 29. [CrossRef]
66. Nakerakanti, S.S.; Bujor, A.M.; Trojanowska, M. CCN2 is required for the TGF-β induced activation of Smad1-Erk1/2 signaling network. *PLoS ONE* **2011**, *6*, e21911. [CrossRef]
67. Junglas, B.; Kuespert, S.; Seleem, A.A.; Struller, T.; Ullmann, S.; Bösl, M.; Bosserhoff, A.; Köstler, J.; Wagner, R.; Tamm, E.R.; et al. Connective tissue growth factor causes glaucoma by modifying the actin cytoskeleton of the trabecular meshwork. *Am. J. Pathol.* **2012**, *180*, 2386–2403. [CrossRef]
68. Dillinger, A.E.; Weber, G.R.; Mayer, M.; Schneider, M.; Göppner, C.; Ohlmann, A.; Shamonin, M.; Monkman, G.J.; Fuchshofer, R. CCN2/CTGF-A Modulator of the Optic Nerve Head Astrocyte. *Front. Cell Dev. Biol.* **2022**, *10*, 864433. [CrossRef]
69. Dillinger, A.E.; Kuespert, S.; Froemel, F.; Tamm, E.R.; Fuchshofer, R. CCN2/CTGF promotor activity in the developing and adult mouse eye. *Cell Tissue Res.* **2021**, *384*, 625–641. [CrossRef]
70. Miao, H.; Crabb, A.W.; Hernandez, M.R.; Lukas, T.J. Modulation of factors affecting optic nerve head astrocyte migration. *Investig. Ophthalmol. Vis. Sci.* **2010**, *51*, 4096–4103. [CrossRef]
71. Tezel, G.; Hernandez, M.R.; Wax, M.B. In vitro evaluation of reactive astrocyte migration, a component of tissue remodeling in glaucomatous optic nerve head. *Glia* **2001**, *34*, 178–189. [CrossRef] [PubMed]
72. Choi, H.J.; Sun, D.; Jakobs, T.C. Astrocytes in the optic nerve head express putative mechanosensitive channels. *Mol. Vis.* **2015**, *21*, 749–766. [PubMed]
73. Lee, P.; Chandel, N.S.; Simon, M.C. Cellular adaptation to hypoxia through hypoxia inducible factors and beyond. *Nat. Rev. Mol. Cell Biol.* **2020**, *21*, 268–283. [CrossRef] [PubMed]
74. Savagian, C.A.; Dubielzig, R.R.; Nork, T.M. Comparison of the distribution of glial fibrillary acidic protein, heat shock protein 60, and hypoxia-inducible factor-1alpha in retinas from glaucomatous and normal canine eyes. *Am. J. Vet. Res.* **2008**, *69*, 265–272. [CrossRef] [PubMed]
75. Chidlow, G.; Wood, J.P.M.; Casson, R.J. Investigations into Hypoxia and Oxidative Stress at the Optic Nerve Head in a Rat Model of Glaucoma. *Front. Neurosci.* **2017**, *11*, 478. [CrossRef] [PubMed]
76. Ergorul, C.; Ray, A.; Huang, W.; Wang, D.Y.; Ben, Y.; Cantuti-Castelvetri, I.; Grosskreutz, C.L. Hypoxia inducible factor-1α (HIF-1α) and some HIF-1 target genes are elevated in experimental glaucoma. *J. Mol. Neurosci.* **2010**, *42*, 183–191. [CrossRef]
77. Egger, M.; Schgoer, W.; Beer, A.G.E.; Jeschke, J.; Leierer, J.; Theurl, M.; Frauscher, S.; Tepper, O.M.; Niederwanger, A.; Ritsch, A.; et al. Hypoxia up-regulates the angiogenic cytokine secretoneurin via an HIF-1alpha- and basic FGF-dependent pathway in muscle cells. *FASEB J.* **2007**, *21*, 2906–2917. [CrossRef]
78. Fuller, J.A.; Brun-Zinkernagel, A.-M.; Clark, A.F.; Wordinger, R.J. Subtilisin-like proprotein convertase expression, localization, and activity in the human retina and optic nerve head. *Investig. Ophthalmol. Vis. Sci.* **2009**, *50*, 5759–5768. [CrossRef]
79. Nour, N.; Mayer, G.; Mort, J.S.; Salvas, A.; Mbikay, M.; Morrison, C.J.; Overall, C.M.; Seidah, N.G. The cysteine-rich domain of the secreted proprotein convertases PC5A and PACE4 functions as a cell surface anchor and interacts with tissue inhibitors of metalloproteinases. *Mol. Biol. Cell* **2005**, *16*, 5215–5226. [CrossRef]
80. Nguyen, J.V.; Soto, I.; Kim, K.-Y.; Bushong, E.A.; Oglesby, E.; Valiente-Soriano, F.J.; Yang, Z.; Davis, C.O.; Bedont, J.L.; Son, J.L.; et al. Myelination transition zone astrocytes are constitutively phagocytic and have synuclein dependent reactivity in glaucoma. *Proc. Natl. Acad. Sci. USA* **2011**, *108*, 1176–1181. [CrossRef]
81. Cooper, M.L.; Crish, S.D.; Inman, D.M.; Horner, P.J.; Calkins, D.J. Early astrocyte redistribution in the optic nerve precedes axonopathy in the DBA/2J mouse model of glaucoma. *Exp. Eye Res.* **2016**, *150*, 22–33. [CrossRef] [PubMed]
82. Davis, C.O.; Kim, K.-Y.; Bushong, E.A.; Mills, E.A.; Boassa, D.; Shih, T.; Kinebuchi, M.; Phan, S.; Zhou, Y.; Bihlmeyer, N.A.; et al. Transcellular degradation of axonal mitochondria. *Proc. Natl. Acad. Sci. USA* **2014**, *111*, 9633–9638. [CrossRef] [PubMed]

83. Muench, N.A.; Patel, S.; Maes, M.E.; Donahue, R.J.; Ikeda, A.; Nickells, R.W. The influence of mitochondrial dynamics and function on retinal ganglion cell susceptibility in optic nerve disease. *Cells* **2021**, *10*, 1593. [CrossRef] [PubMed]
84. Neufeld, A.H. Microglia in the optic nerve head and the region of parapapillary chorioretinal atrophy in glaucoma. *Arch. Ophthalmol.* **1999**, *117*, 1050–1056. [CrossRef]
85. Crapser, J.D.; Arreola, M.A.; Tsourmas, K.I.; Green, K.N. Microglia as hackers of the matrix: Sculpting synapses and the extracellular space. *Cell. Mol. Immunol.* **2021**, *18*, 2472–2488. [CrossRef] [PubMed]
86. Nayak, D.; Roth, T.L.; McGavern, D.B. Microglia development and function. *Annu. Rev. Immunol.* **2014**, *32*, 367–402. [CrossRef]
87. Hirsch, S.; Bähr, M. Immunocytochemical characterization of reactive optic nerve astrocytes and meningeal cells. *Glia* **1999**, *26*, 36–46. [CrossRef]
88. Pena, J.D.; Varela, H.J.; Ricard, C.S.; Hernandez, M.R. Enhanced tenascin expression associated with reactive astrocytes in human optic nerve heads with primary open angle glaucoma. *Exp. Eye Res.* **1999**, *68*, 29–40. [CrossRef]
89. Pena, J.D.; Taylor, A.W.; Ricard, C.S.; Vidal, I.; Hernandez, M.R. Transforming growth factor beta isoforms in human optic nerve heads. *Br. J. Ophthalmol.* **1999**, *83*, 209–218. [CrossRef]
90. Reinehr, S.; Reinhard, J.; Wiemann, S.; Stute, G.; Kuehn, S.; Woestmann, J.; Dick, H.B.; Faissner, A.; Joachim, S.C. Early remodelling of the extracellular matrix proteins tenascin-C and phosphacan in retina and optic nerve of an experimental autoimmune glaucoma model. *J. Cell. Mol. Med.* **2016**, *20*, 2122–2137. [CrossRef]
91. Hou, L.; Bao, X.; Zang, C.; Yang, H.; Sun, F.; Che, Y.; Wu, X.; Li, S.; Zhang, D.; Wang, Q. Integrin CD11b mediates α-synuclein-induced activation of NADPH oxidase through a Rho-dependent pathway. *Redox Biol.* **2018**, *14*, 600–608. [CrossRef] [PubMed]
92. Hanisch, U.-K.; Kettenmann, H. Microglia: Active sensor and versatile effector cells in the normal and pathologic brain. *Nat. Neurosci.* **2007**, *10*, 1387–1394. [CrossRef] [PubMed]
93. García-Bermúdez, M.Y.; Freude, K.K.; Mouhammad, Z.A.; van Wijngaarden, P.; Martin, K.K.; Kolko, M. Glial cells in glaucoma: Friends, foes, and potential therapeutic targets. *Front. Neurol.* **2021**, *12*, 624983. [CrossRef] [PubMed]
94. Rolle, T.; Ponzetto, A.; Malinverni, L. The role of neuroinflammation in glaucoma: An update on molecular mechanisms and new therapeutic options. *Front. Neurol.* **2020**, *11*, 612422. [CrossRef]
95. Tezel, G. Molecular regulation of neuroinflammation in glaucoma: Current knowledge and the ongoing search for new treatment targets. *Prog. Retin. Eye Res.* **2022**, *87*, 100998. [CrossRef]
96. Mac Nair, C.E.; Nickells, R.W. Neuroinflammation in glaucoma and optic nerve damage. *Prog. Mol. Biol. Transl. Sci.* **2015**, *134*, 343–363. [CrossRef]
97. Soto, I.; Howell, G.R. The complex role of neuroinflammation in glaucoma. *Cold Spring Harb. Perspect. Med.* **2014**, *4*, a017269. [CrossRef]
98. Williams, P.A.; Marsh-Armstrong, N.; Howell, G.R.; Lasker/IRRF Initiative on Astrocytes and Glaucomatous Neurodegeneration Participants. Neuroinflammation in glaucoma: A new opportunity. *Exp. Eye Res.* **2017**, *157*, 20–27. [CrossRef]
99. Watson, P.G.; Young, R.D. Scleral structure, organisation and disease. A review. *Exp. Eye Res.* **2004**, *78*, 609–623. [CrossRef]
100. Cone-Kimball, E.; Nguyen, C.; Oglesby, E.N.; Pease, M.E.; Steinhart, M.R.; Quigley, H.A. Scleral structural alterations associated with chronic experimental intraocular pressure elevation in mice. *Mol. Vis.* **2013**, *19*, 2023–2039.
101. Hinz, B.; Phan, S.H.; Thannickal, V.J.; Prunotto, M.; Desmoulière, A.; Varga, J.; De Wever, O.; Mareel, M.; Gabbiani, G. Recent developments in myofibroblast biology: Paradigms for connective tissue remodeling. *Am. J. Pathol.* **2012**, *180*, 1340–1355. [CrossRef] [PubMed]
102. Hinz, B.; Phan, S.H.; Thannickal, V.J.; Galli, A.; Bochaton-Piallat, M.-L.; Gabbiani, G. The myofibroblast: One function, multiple origins. *Am. J. Pathol.* **2007**, *170*, 1807–1816. [CrossRef] [PubMed]
103. Hinz, B. Myofibroblasts. *Exp. Eye Res.* **2016**, *142*, 56–70. [CrossRef] [PubMed]
104. Oglesby, E.N.; Tezel, G.; Cone-Kimball, E.; Steinhart, M.R.; Jefferys, J.; Pease, M.E.; Quigley, H.A. Scleral fibroblast response to experimental glaucoma in mice. *Mol. Vis.* **2016**, *22*, 82–99.
105. Shelton, L.; Rada, J.S. Effects of cyclic mechanical stretch on extracellular matrix synthesis by human scleral fibroblasts. *Exp. Eye Res.* **2007**, *84*, 314–322. [CrossRef]
106. Fujikura, H.; Seko, Y.; Tokoro, T.; Mochizuki, M.; Shimokawa, H. Involvement of mechanical stretch in the gelatinolytic activity of the fibrous sclera of chicks, in vitro. *JPN J. Ophthalmol.* **2002**, *46*, 24–30. [CrossRef]
107. Yamaoka, A.; Matsuo, T.; Shiraga, F.; Ohtsuki, H. TIMP-1 production by human scleral fibroblast decreases in response to cyclic mechanical stretching. *Ophthalmic Res.* **2001**, *33*, 98–101. [CrossRef]
108. Chow, A.; McCrea, L.; Kimball, E.; Schaub, J.; Quigley, H.; Pitha, I. Dasatinib inhibits peripapillary scleral myofibroblast differentiation. *Exp. Eye Res.* **2020**, *194*, 107999. [CrossRef]
109. Cui, W.; Bryant, M.R.; Sweet, P.M.; McDonnell, P.J. Changes in gene expression in response to mechanical strain in human scleral fibroblasts. *Exp. Eye Res.* **2004**, *78*, 275–284. [CrossRef]
110. Coudrillier, B.; Pijanka, J.; Jefferys, J.; Sorensen, T.; Quigley, H.A.; Boote, C.; Nguyen, T.D. Collagen structure and mechanical properties of the human sclera: Analysis for the effects of age. *J. Biomech. Eng.* **2015**, *137*, 041006. [CrossRef]
111. Voorhees, A.P.; Jan, N.-J.; Hua, Y.; Yang, B.; Sigal, I.A. Peripapillary sclera architecture revisited: A tangential fiber model and its biomechanical implications. *Acta Biomater.* **2018**, *79*, 113–122. [CrossRef] [PubMed]
112. Szeto, J.; Chow, A.; McCrea, L.; Mozzer, A.; Nguyen, T.D.; Quigley, H.A.; Pitha, I. Regional differences and physiologic behaviors in peripapillary scleral fibroblasts. *Investig. Ophthalmol. Vis. Sci.* **2021**, *62*, 27. [CrossRef] [PubMed]

113. Wu, H.; Chen, W.; Zhao, F.; Zhou, Q.; Reinach, P.S.; Deng, L.; Ma, L.; Luo, S.; Srinivasalu, N.; Pan, M.; et al. Scleral hypoxia is a target for myopia control. *Proc. Natl. Acad. Sci. USA* **2018**, *115*, E7091–E7100. [CrossRef] [PubMed]
114. Hu, D.; Jiang, J.; Ding, B.; Xue, K.; Sun, X.; Qian, S. Mechanical strain regulates myofibroblast differentiation of human scleral fibroblasts by YAP. *Front. Physiol.* **2021**, *12*, 712509. [CrossRef]
115. Pitha, I.; Oglesby, E.; Chow, A.; Kimball, E.; Pease, M.E.; Schaub, J.; Quigley, H. Rho-Kinase Inhibition Reduces Myofibroblast Differentiation and Proliferation of Scleral Fibroblasts Induced by Transforming Growth Factor β and Experimental Glaucoma. *Transl. Vis. Sci. Technol.* **2018**, *7*, 6. [CrossRef]
116. Qu, J.; Chen, H.; Zhu, L.; Ambalavanan, N.; Girkin, C.A.; Murphy-Ullrich, J.E.; Downs, J.C.; Zhou, Y. High-Magnitude and/or High-Frequency Mechanical Strain Promotes Peripapillary Scleral Myofibroblast Differentiation. *Investig. Ophthalmol. Vis. Sci.* **2015**, *56*, 7821–7830. [CrossRef]
117. Skonier, J.; Neubauer, M.; Madisen, L.; Bennett, K.; Plowman, G.D.; Purchio, A.F. cDNA cloning and sequence analysis of beta ig-h3, a novel gene induced in a human adenocarcinoma cell line after treatment with transforming growth factor-beta. *DNA Cell Biol.* **1992**, *11*, 511–522. [CrossRef]
118. Shelton, L.; Troilo, D.; Lerner, M.R.; Gusev, Y.; Brackett, D.J.; Rada, J.S. Microarray analysis of choroid/RPE gene expression in marmoset eyes undergoing changes in ocular growth and refraction. *Mol. Vis.* **2008**, *14*, 1465–1479.
119. Shelton, L.; Rada, J.A.S. Inhibition of human scleral fibroblast cell attachment to collagen type I by TGFBIp. *Investig. Ophthalmol. Vis. Sci.* **2009**, *50*, 3542–3552. [CrossRef]
120. Hu, S.; Cui, D.; Yang, X.; Hu, J.; Wan, W.; Zeng, J. The crucial role of collagen-binding integrins in maintaining the mechanical properties of human scleral fibroblasts-seeded collagen matrix. *Mol. Vis.* **2011**, *17*, 1334–1342.
121. Kimball, E.C.; Nguyen, C.; Steinhart, M.R.; Nguyen, T.D.; Pease, M.E.; Oglesby, E.N.; Oveson, B.C.; Quigley, H.A. Experimental scleral cross-linking increases glaucoma damage in a mouse model. *Exp. Eye Res.* **2014**, *128*, 129–140. [CrossRef] [PubMed]
122. Hannon, B.G.; Schwaner, S.A.; Boazak, E.M.; Gerberich, B.G.; Winger, E.J.; Prausnitz, M.R.; Ethier, C.R. Sustained scleral stiffening in rats after a single genipin treatment. *J. R. Soc. Interface* **2019**, *16*, 20190427. [CrossRef] [PubMed]
123. Coudrillier, B.; Campbell, I.C.; Read, A.T.; Geraldes, D.M.; Vo, N.T.; Feola, A.; Mulvihill, J.; Albon, J.; Abel, R.L.; Ethier, C.R. Effects of peripapillary scleral stiffening on the deformation of the lamina cribrosa. *Investig. Ophthalmol. Vis. Sci.* **2016**, *57*, 2666–2677. [CrossRef] [PubMed]
124. Hamdaoui, M.E.; Levy, A.M.; Stuber, A.B.; Girkin, C.A.; Kraft, T.W.; Samuels, B.C.; Grytz, R. Scleral crosslinking using genipin can compromise retinal structure and function in tree shrews. *Exp. Eye Res.* **2022**, *219*, 109039. [CrossRef]
125. Murienne, B.J.; Jefferys, J.L.; Quigley, H.A.; Nguyen, T.D. The effects of glycosaminoglycan degradation on the mechanical behavior of the posterior porcine sclera. *Acta Biomater.* **2015**, *12*, 195–206. [CrossRef]
126. Spoerl, E.; Boehm, A.G.; Pillunat, L.E. The influence of various substances on the biomechanical behavior of lamina cribrosa and peripapillary sclera. *Investig. Ophthalmol. Vis. Sci.* **2005**, *46*, 1286–1290. [CrossRef]
127. Hatami-Marbini, H.; Pachenari, M. Tensile Viscoelastic Properties of the Sclera after Glycosaminoglycan Depletion. *Curr. Eye Res.* **2021**, *46*, 1299–1308. [CrossRef]
128. Tribble, J.R.; Williams, P.A.; Caterson, B.; Sengpiel, F.; Morgan, J.E. Digestion of the glycosaminoglycan extracellular matrix by chondroitinase ABC supports retinal ganglion cell dendritic preservation in a rodent model of experimental glaucoma. *Mol. Brain* **2018**, *11*, 69. [CrossRef]
129. Ehanire, T.; Ren, L.; Bond, J.; Medina, M.; Li, G.; Bashirov, L.; Chen, L.; Kokosis, G.; Ibrahim, M.; Selim, A.; et al. Angiotensin II stimulates canonical TGF-β signaling pathway through angiotensin type 1 receptor to induce granulation tissue contraction. *J. Mol. Med.* **2015**, *93*, 289–302. [CrossRef]
130. Quigley, H.A.; Pitha, I.F.; Welsbie, D.S.; Nguyen, C.; Steinhart, M.R.; Nguyen, T.D.; Pease, M.E.; Oglesby, E.N.; Berlinicke, C.A.; Mitchell, K.L.; et al. Losartan treatment protects retinal ganglion cells and alters scleral remodeling in experimental glaucoma. *PLoS ONE* **2015**, *10*, e0141137. [CrossRef]
131. Ota, T.; Murata, H.; Sugimoto, E.; Aihara, M.; Araie, M. Prostaglandin analogues and mouse intraocular pressure: Effects of tafluprost, latanoprost, travoprost, and unoprostone, considering 24-hour variation. *Investig. Ophthalmol. Vis. Sci.* **2005**, *46*, 2006–2011. [CrossRef] [PubMed]
132. Park, H.Y.L.; Kim, J.H.; Lee, D.E.; Lee, J.H.; Park, C.K. Changes of the Retina and Intrinsic Survival Signals in a Rat Model of Glaucoma following Brinzolamide and Travoprost Treatments. *Ophthalmic Res.* **2011**, *46*, 208–217. [CrossRef] [PubMed]
133. Kurashima, H.; Watabe, H.; Sato, N.; Abe, S.; Ishida, N.; Yoshitomi, T. Effects of prostaglandin F(2α) analogues on endothelin-1-induced impairment of rabbit ocular blood flow: Comparison among tafluprost, travoprost, and latanoprost. *Exp. Eye Res.* **2010**, *91*, 853–859. [CrossRef] [PubMed]
134. Gagliuso, D.J.; Wang, R.-F.; Mittag, T.W.; Podos, S.M. Additivity of bimatoprost or travoprost to latanoprost in glaucomatous monkey eyes. *Arch. Ophthalmol.* **2004**, *122*, 1342–1347. [CrossRef] [PubMed]
135. Netland, P.A.; Landry, T.; Sullivan, E.K.; Andrew, R.; Silver, L.; Weiner, A.; Mallick, S.; Dickerson, J.; Bergamini, M.V.; Robertson, S.M.; et al. Travoprost compared with latanoprost and timolol in patients with open-angle glaucoma or ocular hypertension. *Am. J. Ophthalmol.* **2001**, *132*, 472–484. [CrossRef]
136. Hellberg, M.R.; Sallee, V.L.; McLaughlin, M.A.; Sharif, N.A.; Desantis, L.; Dean, T.R.; Zinke, P.W. Preclinical efficacy of travoprost, a potent and selective FP prostaglandin receptor agonist. *J. Ocul. Pharmacol. Ther.* **2001**, *17*, 421–432. [CrossRef]

137. Carvalho, A.B.; Laus, J.L.; Costa, V.P.; Barros, P.S.M.; Silveira, P.R. Effects of travoprost 0.004% compared with latanoprost 0.005% on the intraocular pressure of normal dogs. *Vet. Ophthalmol.* **2006**, *9*, 121–125. [CrossRef]
138. Schnichels, S.; Hurst, J.; de Vries, J.W.; Ullah, S.; Gruszka, A.; Kwak, M.; Löscher, M.; Dammeier, S.; Bartz-Schmidt, K.-U.; Spitzer, M.S.; et al. Self-assembled DNA nanoparticles loaded with travoprost for glaucoma-treatment. *Nanomedicine* **2020**, *29*, 102260. [CrossRef]
139. Hernández, M.; Urcola, J.H.; Vecino, E. Retinal ganglion cell neuroprotection in a rat model of glaucoma following brimonidine, latanoprost or combined treatments. *Exp. Eye Res.* **2008**, *86*, 798–806. [CrossRef]
140. McDonald, J.E.; Kiland, J.A.; Kaufman, P.L.; Bentley, E.; Ellinwood, N.M.; McLellan, G.J. Effect of topical latanoprost 0.005% on intraocular pressure and pupil diameter in normal and glaucomatous cats. *Vet. Ophthalmol.* **2016**, *19*, 13–23. [CrossRef]
141. El-Nimri, N.W.; Wildsoet, C.F. Effects of topical latanoprost on intraocular pressure and myopia progression in young guinea pigs. *Investig. Ophthalmol. Vis. Sci.* **2018**, *59*, 2644–2651. [CrossRef] [PubMed]
142. Ling, Y.; Hu, Z.; Meng, Q.; Fang, P.; Liu, H. Bimatoprost increases mechanosensitivity of trigeminal ganglion neurons innervating the inner walls of rat anterior chambers via activation of TRPA1. *Investig. Ophthalmol. Vis. Sci.* **2016**, *57*, 567–576. [CrossRef] [PubMed]
143. Crowston, J.G.; Lindsey, J.D.; Morris, C.A.; Wheeler, L.; Medeiros, F.A.; Weinreb, R.N. Effect of bimatoprost on intraocular pressure in prostaglandin FP receptor knockout mice. *Investig. Ophthalmol. Vis. Sci.* **2005**, *46*, 4571–4577. [CrossRef] [PubMed]
144. Chen, J.; Dinh, T.; Woodward, D.F.; Holland, M.; Yuan, Y.-D.; Lin, T.-H.; Wheeler, L.A. Bimatoprost: Mechanism of ocular surface hyperemia associated with topical therapy. *Cardiovasc. Drug Rev.* **2005**, *23*, 231–246. [CrossRef] [PubMed]
145. Stamer, W.D.; Piwnica, D.; Jolas, T.; Carling, R.W.; Cornell, C.L.; Fliri, H.; Martos, J.; Pettit, S.N.; Wang, J.W.; Woodward, D.F. Cellular basis for bimatoprost effects on human conventional outflow. *Investig. Ophthalmol. Vis. Sci.* **2010**, *51*, 5176–5181. [CrossRef]
146. Bartoe, J.T.; Davidson, H.J.; Horton, M.T.; Jung, Y.; Brightman, A.H. The effects of bimatoprost and unoprostone isopropyl on the intraocular pressure of normal cats. *Vet. Ophthalmol.* **2005**, *8*, 247–252. [CrossRef]
147. Ogundele, A.B.; Earnest, D.; McLaughlin, M.A. In vivo comparative study of ocular vasodilation, a relative indicator of hyperemia, in guinea pigs following treatment with bimatoprost ophthalmic solutions 0.01% and 0.03%. *Clin. Ophthalmol.* **2010**, *4*, 649–652. [CrossRef]
148. Lee, S.S.; Burke, J.; Shen, J.; Almazan, A.; Orilla, W.; Hughes, P.; Zhang, J.; Li, H.; Struble, C.; Miller, P.E.; et al. Bimatoprost sustained-release intracameral implant reduces episcleral venous pressure in dogs. *Vet. Ophthalmol.* **2018**, *21*, 376–381. [CrossRef]
149. Fukano, Y.; Kawazu, K. Disposition and metabolism of a novel prostanoid antiglaucoma medication, tafluprost, following ocular administration to rats. *Drug Metab. Dispos.* **2009**, *37*, 1622–1634. [CrossRef]
150. Kanamori, A.; Naka, M.; Fukuda, M.; Nakamura, M.; Negi, A. Tafluprost protects rat retinal ganglion cells from apoptosis in vitro and in vivo. *Graefes Arch. Clin. Exp. Ophthalmol.* **2009**, *247*, 1353–1360. [CrossRef]
151. Mayama, C.; Ishii, K.; Saeki, T.; Ota, T.; Tomidokoro, A.; Araie, M. Effects of topical phenylephrine and tafluprost on optic nerve head circulation in monkeys with unilateral experimental glaucoma. *Investig. Ophthalmol. Vis. Sci.* **2010**, *51*, 4117–4124. [CrossRef] [PubMed]
152. Izumi, N.; Nagaoka, T.; Sato, E.; Mori, F.; Takahashi, A.; Sogawa, K.; Yoshida, A. Short-term effects of topical tafluprost on retinal blood flow in cats. *J. Ocul. Pharmacol. Ther.* **2008**, *24*, 521–526. [CrossRef] [PubMed]
153. Liu, Y.; Mao, W. Tafluprost once daily for treatment of elevated intraocular pressure in patients with open-angle glaucoma. *Clin. Ophthalmol.* **2013**, *7*, 7–14. [CrossRef]
154. Kwak, J.; Kang, S.; Lee, E.R.; Park, S.; Park, S.; Park, E.; Lim, J.; Seo, K. Effect of preservative-free tafluprost on intraocular pressure, pupil diameter, and anterior segment structures in normal canine eyes. *Vet. Ophthalmol.* **2017**, *20*, 34–39. [CrossRef] [PubMed]
155. Arfaee, F.; Armin, A. A comparison between the effect of topical tafluprost and latanoprost on intraocular pressure in healthy male guinea pigs. *J. Exotic Pet Med.* **2021**, *39*, 91–95. [CrossRef]
156. Fuchshofer, R.; Kuespert, S.; Junglas, B.; Tamm, E.R. The prostaglandin f2α analog fluprostenol attenuates the fibrotic effects of connective tissue growth factor on human trabecular meshwork cells. *J. Ocul. Pharmacol. Ther.* **2014**, *30*, 237–245. [CrossRef] [PubMed]
157. Saeki, T.; Tsuruga, H.; Aihara, M.; Araie, M.; Rittenhouse, K. Dose-Response Profile of PF-03187207 (PF-207) and Peak IOP Lowering Response Following Single Topical Administration to FP Receptor Knockout Mice vs. Wild Type Mice. *Investig. Ophthalmol. Vis. Sci.* **2009**, *50*, 4064.
158. Krauss, A.H.P.; Impagnatiello, F.; Toris, C.B.; Gale, D.C.; Prasanna, G.; Borghi, V.; Chiroli, V.; Chong, W.K.M.; Carreiro, S.T.; Ongini, E. Ocular hypotensive activity of BOL-303259-X, a nitric oxide donating prostaglandin F2α agonist, in preclinical models. *Exp. Eye Res.* **2011**, *93*, 250–255. [CrossRef]
159. Mehran, N.A.; Sinha, S.; Razeghinejad, R. New glaucoma medications: Latanoprostene bunod, netarsudil, and fixed combination netarsudil-latanoprost. *Eye* **2020**, *34*, 72–88. [CrossRef]
160. Liu, H.K.; Chiou, G.C.; Garg, L.C. Ocular hypotensive effects of timolol in cat eyes. *Arch. Ophthalmol.* **1980**, *98*, 1467–1469. [CrossRef]
161. Watanabe, K.; Chiou, G.C. Action mechanism of timolol to lower the intraocular pressure in rabbits. *Ophthalmic Res.* **1983**, *15*, 160–167. [CrossRef] [PubMed]
162. Schuettauf, F.; Quinto, K.; Naskar, R.; Zurakowski, D. Effects of anti-glaucoma medications on ganglion cell survival: The DBA/2J mouse model. *Vision Res.* **2002**, *42*, 2333–2337. [CrossRef]
163. Goto, W.; Ota, T.; Morikawa, N.; Otori, Y.; Hara, H.; Kawazu, K.; Miyawaki, N.; Tano, Y. Protective effects of timolol against the neuronal damage induced by glutamate and ischemia in the rat retina. *Brain Res.* **2002**, *958*, 10–19. [CrossRef]

164. Watson, P.; Stjernschantz, J. A six-month, randomized, double-masked study comparing latanoprost with timolol in open-angle glaucoma and ocular hypertension. The Latanoprost Study Group. *Ophthalmology* **1996**, *103*, 126–137. [CrossRef]
165. Bartels, S.P. Aqueous humor flow measured with fluorophotometry in timolol-treated primates. *Investig. Ophthalmol. Vis. Sci.* **1988**, *29*, 1498–1504.
166. Yu, D.Y.; Su, E.N.; Cringle, S.J.; Alder, V.A.; Yu, P.K.; Desantis, L. Effect of betaxolol, timolol and nimodipine on human and pig retinal arterioles. *Exp. Eye Res.* **1998**, *67*, 73–81. [CrossRef] [PubMed]
167. Smith, L.N.; Miller, P.E.; Felchle, L.M. Effects of topical administration of latanoprost, timolol, or a combination of latanoprost and timolol on intraocular pressure, pupil size, and heart rate in clinically normal dogs. *Am. J. Vet. Res.* **2010**, *71*, 1055–1061. [CrossRef]
168. Millar, J.C.; Clark, A.F.; Pang, I.-H. Assessment of aqueous humor dynamics in the mouse by a novel method of constant-flow infusion. *Investig. Ophthalmol. Vis. Sci.* **2011**, *52*, 685–694. [CrossRef]
169. Wood, J.P.; DeSantis, L.; Chao, H.M.; Osborne, N.N. Topically applied betaxolol attenuates ischaemia-induced effects to the rat retina and stimulates BDNF mRNA. *Exp. Eye Res.* **2001**, *72*, 79–86. [CrossRef]
170. Osborne, N.N.; DeSantis, L.; Bae, J.H.; Ugarte, M.; Wood, J.P.; Nash, M.S.; Chidlow, G. Topically applied betaxolol attenuates NMDA-induced toxicity to ganglion cells and the effects of ischaemia to the retina. *Exp. Eye Res.* **1999**, *69*, 331–342. [CrossRef]
171. Uji, Y.; Kuze, M.; Matubara, H.; Doi, M.; Sasoh, M. Effects of the beta1-selective adrenergic antagonist betaxolol on electroretinography in the perfused cat eye. *Doc. Ophthalmol.* **2003**, *106*, 37–41. [CrossRef] [PubMed]
172. Holló, G.; Whitson, J.T.; Faulkner, R.; McCue, B.; Curtis, M.; Wieland, H.; Chastain, J.; Sanders, M.; DeSantis, L.; Przydryga, J.; et al. Concentrations of betaxolol in ocular tissues of patients with glaucoma and normal monkeys after 1 month of topical ocular administration. *Investig. Ophthalmol. Vis. Sci.* **2006**, *47*, 235–240. [CrossRef] [PubMed]
173. Tamaki, Y.; Araie, M.; Tomita, K.; Nagahara, M. Effect of topical betaxolol on tissue circulation in the human optic nerve head. *J. Ocul. Pharmacol. Ther.* **1999**, *15*, 313–321. [CrossRef] [PubMed]
174. Miller, P.E.; Schmidt, G.M.; Vainisi, S.J.; Swanson, J.F.; Herrmann, M.K. The efficacy of topical prophylactic antiglaucoma therapy in primary closed angle glaucoma in dogs: A multicenter clinical trial. *J. Am. Anim. Hosp. Assoc.* **2000**, *36*, 431–438. [CrossRef]
175. Goldenberg-Cohen, N.; Dadon-Bar-El, S.; Hasanreisoglu, M.; Avraham-Lubin, B.C.R.; Dratviman-Storobinsky, O.; Cohen, Y.; Weinberger, D. Possible neuroprotective effect of brimonidine in a mouse model of ischaemic optic neuropathy. *Clin. Exp. Ophthalmol.* **2009**, *37*, 718–729. [CrossRef]
176. Acheampong, A.A.; Small, D.; Baumgarten, V.; Welty, D.; Tang-Liu, D. Formulation effects on ocular absorption of brimonidine in rabbit eyes. *J. Ocul. Pharmacol. Ther.* **2002**, *18*, 325–337. [CrossRef]
177. Gelatt, K.N.; MacKay, E.O. Effect of single and multiple doses of 0.2% brimonidine tartrate in the glaucomatous Beagle. *Vet. Ophthalmol.* **2002**, *5*, 253–262. [CrossRef]
178. Burke, J.; Schwartz, M. Preclinical evaluation of brimonidine. *Surv. Ophthalmol.* **1996**, *41*, S9–S18. [CrossRef]
179. Schnichels, S.; Hurst, J.; de Vries, J.W.; Ullah, S.; Frößl, K.; Gruszka, A.; Löscher, M.; Bartz-Schmidt, K.-U.; Spitzer, M.S.; Herrmann, A. Improved Treatment Options for Glaucoma with Brimonidine-Loaded Lipid DNA Nanoparticles. *ACS Appl. Mater. Interfaces* **2021**, *13*, 9445–9456. [CrossRef]
180. Tamhane, M.; Luu, K.T.; Attar, M. Ocular pharmacokinetics of brimonidine drug delivery system in monkeys and translational modeling for selection of dose and frequency in clinical trials. *J. Pharmacol. Exp. Ther.* **2021**, *378*, 207–214. [CrossRef]
181. Toris, C.B.; Gleason, M.L.; Camras, C.B.; Yablonski, M.E. Effects of brimonidine on aqueous humor dynamics in human eyes. *Arch. Ophthalmol.* **1995**, *113*, 1514–1517. [CrossRef] [PubMed]
182. Liu, Y.; Wang, Y.; Lv, H.; Jiang, X.; Zhang, M.; Li, X. α-adrenergic agonist brimonidine control of experimentally induced myopia in guinea pigs: A pilot study. *Mol. Vis.* **2017**, *23*, 785–798. [PubMed]
183. Morrison, J.C.; Nylander, K.B.; Lauer, A.K.; Cepurna, W.O.; Johnson, E. Glaucoma drops control intraocular pressure and protect optic nerves in a rat model of glaucoma. *Investig. Ophthalmol. Vis. Sci.* **1998**, *39*, 526–531.
184. Gabelt, B.T.; Robinson, J.C.; Hubbard, W.C.; Peterson, C.M.; Debink, N.; Wadhwa, A.; Kaufman, P.L. Apraclonidine and brimonidine effects on anterior ocular and cardiovascular physiology in normal and sympathectomized monkeys. *Exp. Eye Res.* **1994**, *59*, 633–644. [CrossRef] [PubMed]
185. Toris, C.B.; Tafoya, M.E.; Camras, C.B.; Yablonski, M.E. Effects of apraclonidine on aqueous humor dynamics in human eyes. *Ophthalmology* **1995**, *102*, 456–461. [CrossRef]
186. Orgül, S.; Bacon, D.R.; Van Buskirk, E.M.; Cioffi, G.A. Optic nerve vasomotor effects of topical apraclonidine hydrochloride. *Br. J. Ophthalmol.* **1996**, *80*, 82–84. [CrossRef]
187. Miller, P.E.; Nelson, M.J.; Rhaesa, S.L. Effects of topical administration of 0.5% apraclonidine on intraocular pressure, pupil size, and heart rate in clinically normal dogs. *Am. J. Vet. Res.* **1996**, *57*, 79–82.
188. Miller, P.E.; Rhaesa, S.L. Effects of topical administration of 0.5% apraclonidine on intraocular pressure, pupil size, and heart rate in clinically normal cats. *Am. J. Vet. Res.* **1996**, *57*, 83–86.
189. Li, T.; Wang, Y.; Chen, J.; Gao, X.; Pan, S.; Su, Y.; Zhou, X. Co-delivery of brinzolamide and miRNA-124 by biodegradable nanoparticles as a strategy for glaucoma therapy. *Drug Deliv.* **2020**, *27*, 410–421. [CrossRef]
190. Desantis, L. Preclinical overview of brinzolamide1. *Surv. Ophthalmol.* **2000**, *44*, S119–S129. [CrossRef]
191. Li, N.; Shi, H.-M.; Cong, L.; Lu, Z.-Z.; Ye, W.; Zhang, Y.-Y. Outflow facility efficacy of five drugs in enucleated porcine eyes by a method of constant-pressure perfusion. *Int. J. Clin. Exp. Med.* **2015**, *8*, 7184–7191. [PubMed]

192. Di, Y.; Luo, X.-M.; Qiao, T.; Lu, N. Intraocular pressure with rebound tonometry and effects of topical intraocular pressure reducing medications in guinea pigs. *Int. J. Ophthalmol.* **2017**, *10*, 186–190. [CrossRef] [PubMed]
193. Toris, C.B.; Zhan, G.-L.; McLaughlin, M.A. Effects of brinzolamide on aqueous humor dynamics in monkeys and rabbits. *J. Ocul. Pharmacol. Ther.* **2003**, *19*, 397–404. [CrossRef] [PubMed]
194. Cvetkovic, R.S.; Perry, C.M. Brinzolamide: A review of its use in the management of primary open-angle glaucoma and ocular hypertension. *Drugs Aging* **2003**, *20*, 919–947. [CrossRef] [PubMed]
195. Ingram, C.J.; Brubaker, R.F. Effect of brinzolamide and dorzolamide on aqueous humor flow in human eyes. *Am. J. Ophthalmol.* **1999**, *128*, 292–296. [CrossRef]
196. Chandra, S.; Muir, E.R.; Deo, K.; Kiel, J.W.; Duong, T.Q. Effects of dorzolamide on retinal and choroidal blood flow in the DBA/2J mouse model of glaucoma. *Investig. Ophthalmol. Vis. Sci.* **2016**, *57*, 826–831. [CrossRef]
197. Pitha, I.; Kimball, E.C.; Oglesby, E.N.; Pease, M.E.; Fu, J.; Schaub, J.; Kim, Y.-C.; Hu, Q.; Hanes, J.; Quigley, H.A. Sustained Dorzolamide Release Prevents Axonal and Retinal Ganglion Cell Loss in a Rat Model of IOP-Glaucoma. *Transl. Vis. Sci. Technol.* **2018**, *7*, 13. [CrossRef]
198. Percicot, C.L.; Schnell, C.R.; Debon, C.; Hariton, C. Continuous intraocular pressure measurement by telemetry in alpha-chymotrypsin-induced glaucoma model in the rabbit: Effects of timolol, dorzolamide, and epinephrine. *J. Pharmacol. Toxicol. Methods* **1996**, *36*, 223–228. [CrossRef]
199. Stefánsson, E.; Jensen, P.K.; Eysteinsson, T.; Bang, K.; Kiilgaard, J.F.; Dollerup, J.; Scherfig, E.; la Cour, M. Optic Nerve Oxygen Tension in Pigs and the Effect of Carbonic Anhydrase Inhibitors. *Investig. Ophthalmol. Vis. Sci.* **1999**, *40*, 2756–2761.
200. Dietrich, U.M.; Chandler, M.J.; Cooper, T.; Vidyashankar, A.; Chen, G. Effects of topical 2% dorzolamide hydrochloride alone and in combination with 0.5% timolol maleate on intraocular pressure in normal feline eyes. *Vet. Ophthalmol.* **2007**, *10*, 95–100. [CrossRef]
201. Gelatt, K.N.; MacKay, E.O. Changes in intraocular pressure associated with topical dorzolamide and oral methazolamide in glaucomatous dogs. *Vet. Ophthalmol.* **2001**, *4*, 61–67. [CrossRef] [PubMed]
202. Wang, R.F.; Serle, J.B.; Gagliuso, D.J.; Podos, S.M. Comparison of the ocular hypotensive effect of brimonidine, dorzolamide, latanoprost, or artificial tears added to timolol in glaucomatous monkey eyes. *J. Glaucoma* **2000**, *9*, 458–462. [CrossRef]
203. Larsson, L.I.; Alm, A. Aqueous humor flow in human eyes treated with dorzolamide and different doses of acetazolamide. *Arch. Ophthalmol.* **1998**, *116*, 19–24. [CrossRef] [PubMed]
204. Avila, M.Y.; Stone, R.A.; Civan, M.M. Knockout of A3 Adenosine Receptors Reduces Mouse Intraocular Pressure. *Investig. Ophthalmol. Vis. Sci.* **2002**, *43*, 3021–3026.
205. Findl, O.; Hansen, R.M.; Fulton, A.B. The effects of acetazolamide on the electroretinographic responses in rats. *Investig. Ophthalmol. Vis. Sci.* **1995**, *36*, 1019–1026.
206. Kaur, I.P.; Singh, M.; Kanwar, M. Formulation and evaluation of ophthalmic preparations of acetazolamide. *Int. J. Pharm.* **2000**, *199*, 119–127. [CrossRef]
207. Maren, T.H. Ion secretion into the posterior aqueous humor of dogs and monkeys. *Exp. Eye Res.* **1977**, *25*, 245–247. [CrossRef]
208. Macri, F.J.; Dixon, R.L.; Rall, D.P. Aqueous humor turnover rates in the cat. I. Effect of acetazolamide. *Investig. Ophthalmol.* **1965**, *4*, 927–934.
209. Fridriksdóttir, H.; Loftsson, T.; Stefánsson, E. Formulation and testing of methazolamide cyclodextrin eye drop solutions. *J. Control. Release* **1997**, *44*, 95–99. [CrossRef]
210. Guđmundsdóttir, E.; Stefánsson, E.; Bjarnadóttir, G.; Sigurjónsdóttir, J.F.; Guđmundsdóttir, G.; Masson, M.; Loftsson, T. Methazolamide 1% in Cyclodextrin Solution Lowers IOP in Human Ocular Hypertension. *Investig. Ophthalmol. Vis. Sci.* **2000**, *41*, 3552–3554.
211. Li, G.; Mukherjee, D.; Navarro, I.; Ashpole, N.E.; Sherwood, J.M.; Chang, J.; Overby, D.R.; Yuan, F.; Gonzalez, P.; Kopczynski, C.C.; et al. Visualization of conventional outflow tissue responses to netarsudil in living mouse eyes. *Eur. J. Pharmacol.* **2016**, *787*, 20–31. [CrossRef] [PubMed]
212. Ren, R.; Li, G.; Le, T.D.; Kopczynski, C.; Stamer, W.D.; Gong, H. Netarsudil increases outflow facility in human eyes through multiple mechanisms. *Investig. Ophthalmol. Vis. Sci.* **2016**, *57*, 6197–6209. [CrossRef] [PubMed]
213. Leary, K.A.; Lin, K.-T.; Steibel, J.P.; Harman, C.D.; Komáromy, A.M. Safety and efficacy of topically administered netarsudil (Rhopressa^{TM}) in normal and glaucomatous dogs with ADAMTS10-open-angle glaucoma (ADAMTS10-OAG). *Vet. Ophthalmol.* **2021**, *24*, 75–86. [CrossRef] [PubMed]
214. Kitaoka, Y.; Sase, K.; Tsukahara, C.; Fujita, N.; Arizono, I.; Kogo, J.; Tokuda, N.; Takagi, H. Axonal Protection by Netarsudil, a ROCK Inhibitor, Is Linked to an AMPK-Autophagy Pathway in TNF-Induced Optic Nerve Degeneration. *Investig. Ophthalmol. Vis. Sci.* **2022**, *63*, 4. [CrossRef] [PubMed]
215. Lin, C.-W.; Sherman, B.; Moore, L.A.; Laethem, C.L.; Lu, D.-W.; Pattabiraman, P.P.; Rao, P.V.; deLong, M.A.; Kopczynski, C.C. Discovery and preclinical development of netarsudil, a novel ocular hypotensive agent for the treatment of glaucoma. *J. Ocul. Pharmacol. Ther.* **2018**, *34*, 40–51. [CrossRef]
216. Isobe, T.; Kasai, T.; Kawai, H. Ocular penetration and pharmacokinetics of ripasudil following topical administration to rabbits. *J. Ocul. Pharmacol. Ther.* **2016**, *32*, 405–414. [CrossRef]
217. Kamiya, T.; Omae, T.; Nakabayashi, S.; Takahashi, K.; Tanner, A.; Yoshida, A. Effect of Rho Kinase Inhibitor Ripasudil (K-115) on Isolated Porcine Retinal Arterioles. *J. Ocul. Pharmacol. Ther.* **2021**, *37*, 104–111. [CrossRef]

218. Nakabayashi, S.; Kawai, M.; Yoshioka, T.; Song, Y.-S.; Tani, T.; Yoshida, A.; Nagaoka, T. Effect of intravitreal Rho kinase inhibitor ripasudil (K-115) on feline retinal microcirculation. *Exp. Eye Res.* **2015**, *139*, 132–135. [CrossRef]
219. Nishijima, E.; Namekata, K.; Kimura, A.; Guo, X.; Harada, C.; Noro, T.; Nakano, T.; Harada, T. Topical ripasudil stimulates neuroprotection and axon regeneration in adult mice following optic nerve injury. *Sci. Rep.* **2020**, *10*, 15709. [CrossRef]
220. Wada, Y.; Higashide, T.; Nagata, A.; Sugiyama, K. Effects of ripasudil, a rho kinase inhibitor, on blood flow in the optic nerve head of normal rats. *Graefe's Arch. Clin. Exp. Ophthalmol.* **2019**, *257*, 303–311. [CrossRef]
221. Inoue, T.; Tanihara, H. Ripasudil hydrochloride hydrate: Targeting Rho kinase in the treatment of glaucoma. *Expert Opin. Pharmacother.* **2017**, *18*, 1669–1673. [CrossRef] [PubMed]
222. Yamamoto, K.; Maruyama, K.; Himori, N.; Omodaka, K.; Yokoyama, Y.; Shiga, Y.; Morin, R.; Nakazawa, T. The novel Rho kinase (ROCK) inhibitor K-115: A new candidate drug for neuroprotective treatment in glaucoma. *Investig. Ophthalmol. Vis. Sci.* **2014**, *55*, 7126–7136. [CrossRef] [PubMed]
223. Song, H.; Gao, D. Fasudil, a Rho-associated protein kinase inhibitor, attenuates retinal ischemia and reperfusion injury in rats. *Int. J. Mol. Med.* **2011**, *28*, 193–198. [CrossRef]
224. Khallaf, A.M.; El-Moslemany, R.M.; Ahmed, M.F.; Morsi, M.H.; Khalafallah, N.M. Exploring a Novel Fasudil-Phospholipid Complex Formulated as Liposomal Thermosensitive in situ Gel for Glaucoma. *Int. J. Nanomed.* **2022**, *17*, 163–181. [CrossRef] [PubMed]
225. Ichikawa, M.; Yoshida, J.; Saito, K.; Sagawa, H.; Tokita, Y.; Watanabe, M. Differential effects of two ROCK inhibitors, Fasudil and Y-27632, on optic nerve regeneration in adult cats. *Brain Res.* **2008**, *1201*, 23–33. [CrossRef]
226. Pakravan, M.; Beni, A.N.; Ghahari, E.; Varshochian, R.; Yazdani, S.; Esfandiari, H.; Ahmadieh, H. The Ocular Hypotensive Efficacy of Topical Fasudil, a Rho-Associated Protein Kinase Inhibitor, in Patients with End-Stage Glaucoma. *Am. J. Ther.* **2016**, *24*, e676–e680. [CrossRef]
227. Da, B.; Cao, Y.; Wei, H.; Chen, Z.; Shui, Y.; Li, Z. Antagonistic effects of tranilast on proliferation and collagen synthesis induced by TGF-beta2 in cultured human trabecular meshwork cells. *J. Huazhong Univ. Sci. Technol. Med. Sci.* **2004**, *24*, 490–496. [CrossRef]
228. Cao, Y.; Hu, Y.; Li, J.; Shui, Y.; Da, B.; Wei, H. Effect of Tranilast on Collagen Synthesis and TGF–Beta2 Expression of Cultured Human Lamina Cribrosa Astrocytes. *Investig. Ophthalmol. Vis. Sci.* **2006**, *47*, 1544.
229. Spitzer, M.S.; Sat, M.; Schramm, C.; Schnichels, S.; Schultheiss, M.; Yoeruek, E.; Dzhelebov, D.; Szurman, P. Biocompatibility and antifibrotic effect of UV-cross-linked hyaluronate as a release-system for tranilast after trabeculectomy in a rabbit model—A pilot study. *Curr. Eye Res.* **2012**, *37*, 463–470. [CrossRef]
230. Pfeiffer, N.; Voykov, B.; Renieri, G.; Bell, K.; Richter, P.; Weigel, M.; Thieme, H.; Wilhelm, B.; Lorenz, K.; Feindor, M.; et al. First-in-human phase I study of ISTH0036, an antisense oligonucleotide selectively targeting transforming growth factor beta 2 (TGF-β2), in subjects with open-angle glaucoma undergoing glaucoma filtration surgery. *PLoS ONE* **2017**, *12*, e0188899. [CrossRef]
231. Hasenbach, K.; Van Bergen, T.; Vandewalle, E.; De Groef, L.; Van Hove, I.; Moons, L.; Stalmans, I.; Fettes, P.; Leo, E.; Wosikowski, K.; et al. Potent and selective antisense oligonucleotides targeting the transforming growth factor beta (TGF-β) isoforms in advanced glaucoma: A preclinical evaluation. *MAIO* **2016**, *1*, 20–28. [CrossRef]
232. Nakamura, H.; Siddiqui, S.S.; Shen, X.; Malik, A.B.; Pulido, J.S.; Kumar, N.M.; Yue, B.Y.J.T. RNA interference targeting transforming growth factor-beta type II receptor suppresses ocular inflammation and fibrosis. *Mol. Vis.* **2004**, *10*, 703–711. [PubMed]
233. Mead, A.L.; Wong, T.T.L.; Cordeiro, M.F.; Anderson, I.K.; Khaw, P.T. Evaluation of Anti-TGF-β2 Antibody as a New Postoperative Anti-scarring Agent in Glaucoma Surgery. *Investig. Ophthalmol. Vis. Sci.* **2003**, *44*, 3394. [CrossRef]
234. CAT-152 0102 Trabeculectomy Study Group; Khaw, P.; Grehn, F.; Holló, G.; Overton, B.; Wilson, R.; Vogel, R.; Smith, Z. A phase III study of subconjunctival human anti-transforming growth factor beta(2) monoclonal antibody (CAT-152) to prevent scarring after first-time trabeculectomy. *Ophthalmology* **2007**, *114*, 1822–1830. [CrossRef] [PubMed]
235. Shan, S.-W.; Do, C.-W.; Lam, T.C.; Li, H.-L.; Stamer, W.D.; To, C.-H. Thrombospondin-1 mediates Rho-kinase inhibitor-induced increase in outflow-facility. *J. Cell. Physiol.* **2021**, *236*, 8226–8238. [CrossRef]
236. Chen, W.-S.; Cao, Z.; Krishnan, C.; Panjwani, N. Verteporfin without light stimulation inhibits YAP activation in trabecular meshwork cells: Implications for glaucoma treatment. *Biochem. Biophys. Res. Commun.* **2015**, *466*, 221–225. [CrossRef]
237. Matsubara, A.; Nakazawa, T.; Husain, D.; Iliaki, E.; Connolly, E.; Michaud, N.A.; Gragoudas, E.S.; Miller, J.W. Investigating the effect of ciliary body photodynamic therapy in a glaucoma mouse model. *Investig. Ophthalmol. Vis. Sci.* **2006**, *47*, 2498–2507. [CrossRef]
238. Parodi, M.B.; Iacono, P. Photodynamic therapy with verteporfin for anterior segment neovascularizations in neovascular glaucoma. *Am. J. Ophthalmol.* **2004**, *138*, 157–158. [CrossRef]
239. Ko, M.-L.; Chen, C.-F.; Peng, P.-H.; Peng, Y.-H. Simvastatin upregulates Bcl-2 expression and protects retinal neurons from early ischemia/reperfusion injury in the rat retina. *Exp. Eye Res.* **2011**, *93*, 580–585. [CrossRef]
240. Krempler, K.; Schmeer, C.W.; Isenmann, S.; Witte, O.W.; Löwel, S. Simvastatin improves retinal ganglion cell survival and spatial vision after acute retinal ischemia/reperfusion in mice. *Investig. Ophthalmol. Vis. Sci.* **2011**, *52*, 2606–2618. [CrossRef]
241. Nagaoka, T.; Takahashi, A.; Sato, E.; Izumi, N.; Hein, T.W.; Kuo, L.; Yoshida, A. Effect of systemic administration of simvastatin on retinal circulation. *Arch. Ophthalmol.* **2006**, *124*, 665–670. [CrossRef] [PubMed]
242. Nagaoka, T.; Hein, T.W.; Yoshida, A.; Kuo, L. Simvastatin elicits dilation of isolated porcine retinal arterioles: Role of nitric oxide and mevalonate-rho kinase pathways. *Investig. Ophthalmol. Vis. Sci.* **2007**, *48*, 825–832. [CrossRef] [PubMed]

243. Kim, M.-L.; Sung, K.R.; Shin, J.A.; Young Yoon, J.; Jang, J. Statins reduce TGF-beta2-modulation of the extracellular matrix in cultured astrocytes of the human optic nerve head. *Exp. Eye Res.* **2017**, *164*, 55–63. [CrossRef]
244. Kim, M.; Shin, J.; Sung, K. Statins regulate MMP-2 and MMP-9 secretion and activation in human ONH astrocytes. *Investig. Ophthalmol. Vis. Sci.* **2018**, *59*, 6145.
245. Villarreal, G.; Chatterjee, A.; Oh, S.S.; Oh, D.-J.; Rhee, D.J. Pharmacological regulation of SPARC by lovastatin in human trabecular meshwork cells. *Investig. Ophthalmol. Vis. Sci.* **2014**, *55*, 1657–1665. [CrossRef]
246. Park, J.-H.; Yoo, C.; Kim, Y.Y. Effect of Lovastatin on Wound-Healing Modulation After Glaucoma Filtration Surgery in a Rabbit Model. *Investig. Ophthalmol. Vis. Sci.* **2016**, *57*, 1871–1877. [CrossRef]
247. Song, X.-Y.; Chen, Y.-Y.; Liu, W.-T.; Cong, L.; Zhang, J.-L.; Zhang, Y.; Zhang, Y.-Y. Atorvastatin reduces IOP in ocular hypertension in vivo and suppresses ECM in trabecular meshwork perhaps via FGD4. *Int. J. Mol. Med.* **2022**, *49*, 76. [CrossRef]
248. Kim, M.-L.; Sung, K.R.; Kwon, J.; Choi, G.W.; Shin, J.A. Neuroprotective effect of statins in a rat model of chronic ocular hypertension. *Int. J. Mol. Sci.* **2021**, *22*, 12500. [CrossRef]
249. Cong, L.; Fu, S.; Zhang, J.; Zhao, J.; Zhang, Y. Effects of atorvastatin on porcine aqueous humour outflow and trabecular meshwork cells. *Exp. Ther. Med.* **2018**, *15*, 210–216. [CrossRef]
250. Agarwal, R.; Krasilnikova, A.; Mohamed, S.N.L. Topical losartan reduces IOP by altering TM morphology in rats with steroid-induced ocular hypertension. *Indian J. Physiol.* **2018**, *62*, 238–248.
251. Shah, G.B.; Sharma, S.; Mehta, A.A.; Goyal, R.K. Oculohypotensive effect of angiotensin-converting enzyme inhibitors in acute and chronic models of glaucoma. *J. Cardiovasc. Pharmacol.* **2000**, *36*, 169–175. [CrossRef] [PubMed]
252. Costagliola, C.; Verolino, M.; De Rosa, M.L.; Iaccarino, G.; Ciancaglini, M.; Mastropasqua, L. Effect of oral losartan potassium administration on intraocular pressure in normotensive and glaucomatous human subjects. *Exp. Eye Res.* **2000**, *71*, 167–171. [CrossRef] [PubMed]
253. Sawaguchi, S.; Yue, B.Y.; Yeh, P.; Tso, M.O. Effects of intracameral injection of chondroitinase ABC in vivo. *Arch. Ophthalmol.* **1992**, *110*, 110–117. [CrossRef] [PubMed]
254. Murienne, B.J.; Chen, M.L.; Quigley, H.A.; Nguyen, T.D. The contribution of glycosaminoglycans to the mechanical behaviour of the posterior human sclera. *J. R. Soc. Interface* **2016**, *13*, 20160367. [CrossRef]
255. Kirihara, T.; Shimazaki, A.; Nakamura, M.; Miyawaki, N. Ocular hypotensive efficacy of Src-family tyrosine kinase inhibitors via different cellular actions from Rock inhibitors. *Exp. Eye Res.* **2014**, *119*, 97–105. [CrossRef]
256. Belmadani, S.; Bernal, J.; Wei, C.-C.; Pallero, M.A.; Dell'italia, L.; Murphy-Ullrich, J.E.; Berecek, K.H. A thrombospondin-1 antagonist of transforming growth factor-beta activation blocks cardiomyopathy in rats with diabetes and elevated angiotensin II. *Am. J. Pathol.* **2007**, *171*, 777–789. [CrossRef]
257. Lu, A.; Miao, M.; Schoeb, T.R.; Agarwal, A.; Murphy-Ullrich, J.E. Blockade of TSP1-dependent TGF-β activity reduces renal injury and proteinuria in a murine model of diabetic nephropathy. *Am. J. Pathol.* **2011**, *178*, 2573–2586. [CrossRef]
258. Leask, A. Breathe, breathe in the air: The anti-CCN2 antibody pamrevlumab (FG-3019) completes a successful phase II clinical trial for idiopathic pulmonary fibrosis. *J. Cell Commun. Signal.* **2019**, *13*, 441–442. [CrossRef]
259. Wang, J.; Harris, A.; Prendes, M.A.; Alshawa, L.; Gross, J.C.; Wentz, S.M.; Rao, A.B.; Kim, N.J.; Synder, A.; Siesky, B. Targeting Transforming Growth Factor-β Signaling in Primary Open-Angle Glaucoma. *J. Glaucoma* **2017**, *26*, 390–395. [CrossRef]
260. Webber, H.C.; Bermudez, J.Y.; Sethi, A.; Clark, A.F.; Mao, W. Crosstalk between TGFβ and Wnt signaling pathways in the human trabecular meshwork. *Exp. Eye Res.* **2016**, *148*, 97–102. [CrossRef]
261. Wordinger, R.J.; Sharma, T.; Clark, A.F. The role of TGF-β2 and bone morphogenetic proteins in the trabecular meshwork and glaucoma. *J. Ocul. Pharmacol. Ther.* **2014**, *30*, 154–162. [CrossRef] [PubMed]
262. Tanihara, H.; Inoue, T.; Yamamoto, T.; Kuwayama, Y.; Abe, H.; Suganami, H.; Araie, M.; K-115 Clinical Study Group. Intra-ocular pressure-lowering effects of a Rho kinase inhibitor, ripasudil (K-115), over 24 hours in primary open-angle glaucoma and ocular hypertension: A randomized, open-label, crossover study. *Acta Ophthalmol.* **2015**, *93*, e254–e260. [CrossRef]
263. Tanihara, H.; Inoue, T.; Yamamoto, T.; Kuwayama, Y.; Abe, H.; Araie, M.; K-115 Clinical Study Group. Phase 2 randomized clinical study of a Rho kinase inhibitor, K-115, in primary open-angle glaucoma and ocular hypertension. *Am. J. Ophthalmol.* **2013**, *156*, 731–736. [CrossRef] [PubMed]
264. Sato, S.; Hirooka, K.; Nitta, E.; Ukegawa, K.; Tsujikawa, A. Additive intraocular pressure lowering effects of the rho kinase inhibitor, ripasudil in glaucoma patients not able to obtain adequate control after other maximal tolerated medical therapy. *Adv. Ther.* **2016**, *33*, 1628–1634. [CrossRef]
265. Pokrovskaya, O.; Wallace, D.; O'Brien, C. The emerging role of statins in glaucoma pathological mechanisms and therapeutics. *Open J. Ophthalmol.* **2014**, *4*, 124–138. [CrossRef]
266. McCann, P.; Hogg, R.E.; Fallis, R.; Azuara-Blanco, A. The Effect of Statins on Intraocular Pressure and on the Incidence and Progression of Glaucoma: A Systematic Review and Meta-Analysis. *Investig. Ophthalmol. Vis. Sci.* **2016**, *57*, 2729–2748. [CrossRef]
267. Yuan, Y.; Xiong, R.; Wu, Y.; Ha, J.; Wang, W.; Han, X.; He, M. Associations of statin use with the onset and progression of open-angle glaucoma: A systematic review and meta-analysis. *EClinicalMedicine* **2022**, *46*, 101364. [CrossRef]
268. McGwin, G.; McNeal, S.; Owsley, C.; Girkin, C.; Epstein, D.; Lee, P.P. Statins and other cholesterol-lowering medications and the presence of glaucoma. *Arch. Ophthalmol.* **2004**, *122*, 822–826. [CrossRef]
269. Weinreb, R.N. Enhancement of scleral macromolecular permeability with prostaglandins. *Trans. Am. Ophthalmol. Soc.* **2001**, *99*, 319–343.

International Journal of *Molecular Sciences*

MDPI

Review

The Role of miR-29 Family in TGF-β Driven Fibrosis in Glaucomatous Optic Neuropathy

Aoife Smyth [1,*,†], Breedge Callaghan [2,†], Colin E. Willoughby [2] and Colm O'Brien [1]

1 UCD Clinical Research Centre, Mater Misericordiae University Hospital, D07 R2WY Dublin, Ireland
2 Genomic Medicine, Biomedical Sciences Research Institute, Ulster University, Coleraine BT52 1SA, UK
* Correspondence: aoife.smyth@ucdconnect.ie
† These authors contributed equally to this work.

Abstract: Primary open angle glaucoma (POAG), a chronic optic neuropathy, remains the leading cause of irreversible blindness worldwide. It is driven in part by the pro-fibrotic cytokine transforming growth factor beta (TGF-β) and leads to extracellular matrix remodelling at the lamina cribrosa of the optic nerve head. Despite an array of medical and surgical treatments targeting the only known modifiable risk factor, raised intraocular pressure, many patients still progress and develop significant visual field loss and eventual blindness. The search for alternative treatment strategies targeting the underlying fibrotic transformation in the optic nerve head and trabecular meshwork in glaucoma is ongoing. MicroRNAs are small non-coding RNAs known to regulate post-transcriptional gene expression. Extensive research has been undertaken to uncover the complex role of miRNAs in gene expression and miRNA dysregulation in fibrotic disease. MiR-29 is a family of miRNAs which are strongly anti-fibrotic in their effects on the TGF-β signalling pathway and the regulation of extracellular matrix production and deposition. In this review, we discuss the anti-fibrotic effects of miR-29 and the role of miR-29 in ocular pathology and in the development of glaucomatous optic neuropathy. A better understanding of the role of miR-29 in POAG may aid in developing diagnostic and therapeutic strategies in glaucoma.

Keywords: glaucoma; glaucomatous optic neuropathy; fibrosis; miR-29; extracellular matrix

Citation: Smyth, A.; Callaghan, B.; Willoughby, C.E.; O'Brien, C. The Role of miR-29 Family in TGF-β Driven Fibrosis in Glaucomatous Optic Neuropathy. *Int. J. Mol. Sci.* **2022**, *23*, 10216. https://doi.org/10.3390/ijms231810216

Academic Editors: Neil R. Miller and Rongkung Tsai

Received: 7 August 2022
Accepted: 2 September 2022
Published: 6 September 2022

1. Introduction

Glaucoma is the leading cause of irreversible blindness worldwide, affecting over 60 million people, a number which is predicted to rise to 118.8 million by 2040 [1]. Glaucoma refers to a group of clinical conditions rather than to an individual disorder. In general, these conditions are related by the presence of a progressive optic neuropathy. The most common form of glaucoma, primary open angle glaucoma (POAG) is characterised by raised intraocular pressure (IOP), loss of retinal ganglion cell (RGC) axons, and excavation of the optic nerve head (ONH), leading to characteristic peripheral visual field loss [2]. The key site of damage at the ONH in glaucoma is the lamina cribrosa (LC), which consists of a series of porous connective tissue plates, allowing the passage of RGC axons to exit the eye whilst maintaining structural support to the ONH. Surrounding these laminar plates are the LC cells and ONH astrocytes, which produce essential growth factors and the extracellular matrix (ECM) [3]. The laminar plates consisting of ECM components, including collagen and elastin, are subject to fibrotic remodelling, including excess deposition of elastin and collagen fibres [4,5]. Increased IOP is believed to lead to mechanical strain on the LC, disruption of these porous pathways, and resultant damage to the RGC axons, which are seen in glaucomatous injury [6].

The primary and only known modifiable risk factor in POAG is raised intra-ocular pressure (IOP). IOP is maintained by a balance between the rate of production of aqueous humour from the ciliary body and the rate of drainage of aqueous via the trabecular meshwork (TM) and the uveoscleral pathway. Resistance to outflow occurs primarily at the juxtacanalicular connective tissue due to ECM remodelling leading to raised IOP [7]. IOP-lowering treatment reduces the risk of glaucoma development and progression. Several multi-centre studies have shown that reducing IOP is neuro-protective and can delay structural and functional damage to the optic nerve axons [8]. In the Ocular Hypertension Treatment Study (OHTS), treatment reduced the risk of developing glaucoma from 9.5% to 4.4% [9]. In the Early Manifest Glaucoma Trial (EMGT) a 25% reduction in IOP resulted in less frequent and later progression compared to untreated patients [10]. However, despite adequate reduction in IOP with medical or surgical intervention, many patients still progress and develop significant visual field loss. The cumulative risk of unilateral blindness due to glaucoma is estimated to be 26.5% after 10 years and 38.1% at 20 years, while bilateral blindness has been found to occur in 5.5% of patients after 10 years and 13.5% after 20 years [11]. This suggests that the nature of POAG is multi-factorial, involving complex molecular networks and aberrant growth factor signalling working synergistically to result in the glaucomatous changes that are observed in the ONH [12]. Multiple research groups have identified transforming growth factor beta (TGF-β) as one of the major fibrotic players in glaucoma [13].

2. TGF-β Drives Fibrosis in Glaucoma

TGF-β is a multifunctional cytokine known to play a major role on the molecular pathways that modulate ECM in glaucomatous eyes [14,15]. The TGF-β family consists of the TGF-β1, TGF-β2, and TGF-β3 isoforms and regulates proliferation, differentiation, ECM remodelling, epithelial-mesenchymal transition (EMT), tumour progression, and apoptosis [13]. TGF-β signalling occurs via canonical (Smad dependent) and non-canonical (non-Smad dependent) pathways. The specific cellular effects of TGF-β are dependent of the isoform concentration and target tissue. Normal regulation of TGF-β is required for maintenance of tissue homeostasis; however, aberrant overexpression has been implicated in several ocular, fibrotic, and neuro-degenerative diseases. TGF-β plays a central role in fibrosis and wound healing as it induces the differentiation of fibroblasts to highly contractile myofibroblasts characterized by the enhanced expression of ECM proteins [16].

Strong evidence extrapolated from ex vivo and in vitro studies demonstrates a link between TGF-β and ocular hypertension. Raised IOP has been associated with the TGF-β-induced fibrotic response in the eye. Cultured human and animal anterior ocular models have shown that TGF-β can directly increase IOP, while animal models mimicking glaucoma suggest that elevated IOP induces physical changes at the ONH, resulting in the compression of the optic nerve, blockage of axoplasmic flow, and retinal ganglion cell death [17–22]. The LC site is considered a significant location of optic nerve fibre damage in glaucoma as LC cells are similar to myofibroblasts, which are known to be responsible for fibrotic disease development elsewhere in the human body [23] Profibrotic changes elicited by TGF-β within the ONH have been implicated in POAG and pseudoexfoliation glaucoma (PXFG) and include altered turnover of ECM components, formation of cross-linked actin networks (CLANS), upregulation of alpha smooth muscle actin (αSMA), and actin stress fibre formation [4,11–13,19–24].

TGF-β1 is among 183 genes upregulated in POAG LC cells compared to normal controls [22]. In eyes with POAG, over 10-fold immunoreactivity for TGF-β2 has been observed in the region of the ONH. Specifically, in the glaucomatous ONH, there is a massive increase in the levels of TGF-β2 which is mainly localized to reactive astrocytes that line the vitreous surface and occupy the prelaminar region, the compressed cribriform plates, and the nerve bundles in the lamina cribrosa [25]. In addition, exogenous treatment with TGF-β1 induces expression of ECM genes in the LC and the TM [26]. As a central mediator of myofibroblast trans-differentiation and fibrosis, TGF-β is a promising therapeutic target for glaucoma. However, clinical implementation of global TGF-β antagonism deserves cautious consideration since TGF-β exerts important immunomodulatory and tumour-suppressive effects. The complete inhibition of TGF-β as a therapeutic strategy may prove counter effective as it has multiple effects on different cells within the same organ. This highlights the need for a more targeted therapeutic strategy that can regulate the TGF-β signalling pathway at several different levels.

3. MicroRNAs

MicroRNAs (miRNAs) are small endogenous non-coding RNAs approximately 19–25 nucleotides in length and are located in the exons or introns of coding genes [27]. They are important negative regulators of post-transcriptional gene expression, with reports suggesting that over 60% of protein-coding genes in humans are regulated by miRNAs [28]. MiRNAs bind to partially complementary sequences within the 3′ untranslated region of target mRNAs and either induce nonsense mediated decay or translational repression. They were initially discovered in the nematode *Caenorhabditis elegans* in 1993 [29,30], and since then over 2500 miRNAs have been identified in the human genome [31].

Most miRNAs are transcribed by RNA polymerase II from long primary transcripts known as pri-miRNAs [32]. Only pri-miRNAs which contain the suitable stem length, a large flexible terminal loop of about 10 base pairs (bp) and the ability to produce 5′ and 3′ single-stranded RNA overhangs will be efficiently processed and mature to functional miRNAs. Pri-miRNA is cropped into the hairpin loop precursor molecule (pre-miRNAs), approximately 70 nucleotides in length, in the nucleus by nuclear RNase III Drosha [33]. This liberated hairpin structure, referred to as pre-miRNA, is transported from the nucleus to the cytoplasm via the transport receptor exportin 5 [34], where it is processed into ~22-nucleotide-long double-stranded mature miRNAs by Dicer RNAse III enzyme [35]. Pre-miRNAs often contain the sequences for multiple mature miRNAs. One strand of mature miRNA is degraded, while the other then integrates into an RNA-induced silencing complex (RISC) via loading onto the Argonaut proteins [36] (Figure 1). The uncapitalized prefix "mir-" refers to the precursor form, whereas "miR-" refers to the mature form. The suffix -3p or -3q is used to denote which end of the pre-miRNA the mature miRNA originates from.

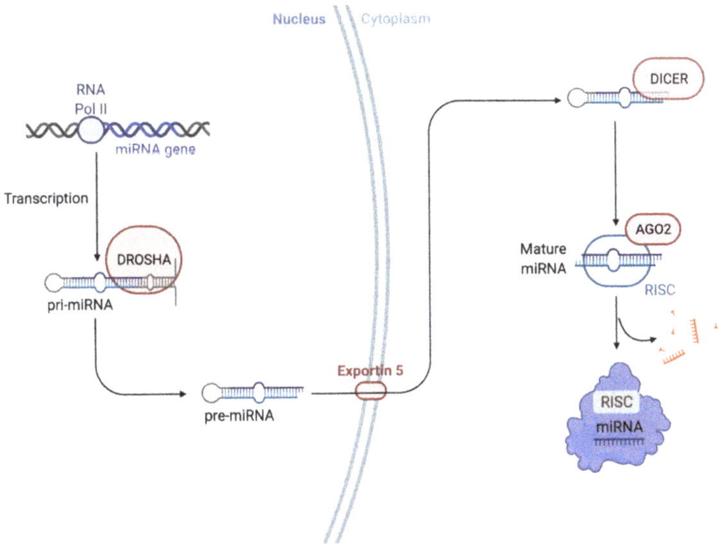

Figure 1. MiRNA biogenesis. miRNA genes are transcribed by RNA polymerase II into pri-miRNA, which are cleaved into pre-miRNA by nuclear RNase III Drosha. Pre-miRNA is transported to the cytoplasm by Exportin 5, where it is then processed into mature double-stranded miRNA by Dicer a RNase III enzyme. Finally, either strand of the mature miRNA duplex is loaded onto the Argonaut (AGO) protein to form the miRNA induced silencing complex (RISC).

Although some miRNAs function as a switch by repressing a single target, the majority exert their effects as modest alterations on several targets through imperfect binding which cumulatively can alter cellular phenotypes [37]. Gene regulation mediated by miRNAs occurs via two main mechanisms. Firstly, via translational repression of target mRNA by miRNAs blocking initiation of translation and/or elongation [38,39]. Secondly, miRNAs can bind to mRNAs, promoting RNA degradation through accelerated deadenylation and decapping [40,41].

MiRNAs play critical roles in multiple physiological and pathological processes. Due to their unique expression patterns and their ability to target numerous transcripts often in the same biological process, miRNAs can potentially regulate the expression of many genes in a tissue- or cell-specific manner. They operate in complex networks in which one mRNA can be regulated by multiple miRs and one miR can regulate multiple genes targets [42]. An entire signalling pathway can be regulated by miRNAs in physiological and disease processes. The dysregulation of miRNAs in disease states can be used to develop biomarkers [43] and provide insight into the underlying pathophysiological basis of the disease [44]. Abnormally expressed miRNAs have been identified in cancer, fibrosis, Alzheimer's, and cardiovascular disease [45–48]. In POAG, many miRNAs have been detected in patient-derived samples [49] and play a role in the TM [50], retina [51], and ONH [52].

4. MicroRNAs That Regulate TGF-β Signalling

By targeting up- or downstream signalling molecules in the TGF-β signalling pathways, miRNAs can promote or inhibit the development of fibrosis. MiRNA-based manipulation of the TGF-β signalling pathway is a new approach to target fibrosis [53] and numerous studies have been published detailing the reciprocal crosstalk between miRNAs and TGF-β [54–57]. Both in-silico and experimental validation analysis has shown that miRNAs can influence TGF-β signalling at several transcriptional and post-transcriptional levels. Nearly all the TGF-β members involved in the canonical signalling pathway have been shown to be influenced by miRNAs. Reports have also demonstrated the regulation of non-canonical TGF-β/PI3K/AKT signalling pathways by miRNAs, supporting their potential role in the diagnostic and therapeutic management of fibrotic diseases [54]. Interestingly, TGF-β signalling itself can enhance the maturation of miRNAs by binding to a component of the Drosha complex (p68) and initiating a bidirectional functional loop [57–59].

TGF-β induced fibrosis related miRNAs has been studied more extensively in other tissues, such as the lung, liver, kidney, heart, and skin [60,61]. In cardiac fibrosis, miR-92a regulates the inhibitory Smad7, promoting the fibrotic process while miR-26a has been shown to directly target Smad1 [62]. The miR-200 family targets TGF-βR1 and SMAD2; therefore, downregulation of the miR-200 family results in increased EMT [59]. In the kidney, miR-29 can inhibit disintegrin metalloproteases (ADAMs) involved in TGF-β signalling, reducing collagen expression and the subsequent development of renal fibrosis [63]. In the eye, many miRNAs have been found to be abundantly expressed and play important roles in ocular physiology and pathology. These include miR-200 [64] miR-184 [65] miR-29 family [66] and miR-21 [67]. Expression profiling of miRNAs in the anterior segment of healthy donors including cornea, TM, and ciliary body samples reported 378 miRs collectively expressed [68].

5. MiR-29 Family

The microRNA-29 (miR-29) family, which this review will discuss in more detail, includes miR-29a, miR-29b-1, miR-29b-2, and miR-29c. MiR-29b-1 and miR-29b-2 have identical mature sequences and are therefore collectively known as miR-29b. MiR-29a and -29b-1 are encoded on chromosome 7q32.3, while the miR-29b-2 and -29c cluster are found on chromosome 1q32.2 (Figure 2). All four members have a common seed sequence in nucleotides 2 to 8 and largely regulate a similar group of target mRNAs [69]. Mir-29, like other miRNAs, is transcribed by RNA polymerase II [70]. MiR-29a and -29b-1 are transcribed as a primary transcript unit [71].

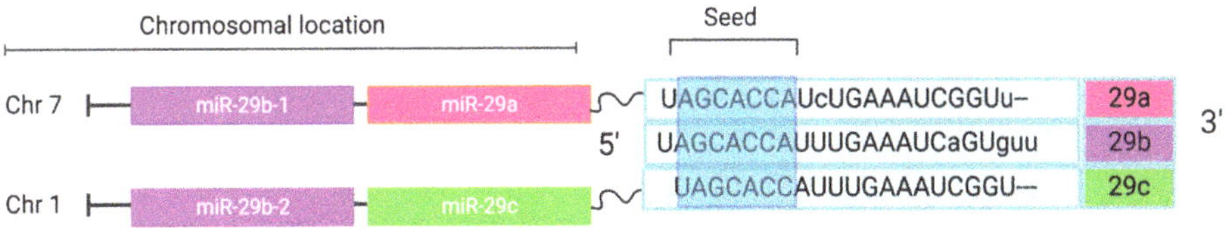

Figure 2. Schematic representation of the miR-29 family members: miR-29a, -29b, and -29c. The family is transcribed from two chromosomal positions forming a bi-cistronic transcriptional unit; both miR-29a and miR-29b1 are found on chr7, while miR-29b2 and miR-29c are located on chr1. miR-29 family members have identical seed sequences (darker blue box) along with similar mature miRNA sequences.

MIR-29 expression is regulated at both a transcriptional and post transcriptional level. Multiple transcriptional factor binding sites on miR-29 have been identified, including a Smad3 binding site in miR-29b-2 [72], a myc binding site in both the miR-29b-1/a and -29-2/c clusters [73] and three NF-kB binding sites in miR-29-1/a region [74]. Similarly, post transcriptional regulation of miR-29 has been reported in anaplastic large cell lymphoma, where t(6;7)(p25.3;q32.3) spontaneous translocation was associated with upregulation of miR-29 on 7q32.3 [75].

Although each miR-29 family member shares the common 7-nt seed sequence, unique sequence features have been reported. One notable difference is that miR- 29b, unlike -29a or c, has a distinct hexanucleotide terminal motif required for nuclear localization [76]. In exogenous delivery of miR-29b, mutations in this region impair localization to the nucleus [77]. Deletion of this hexanucleotide motif led to higher cytoplasmic localization of miR-29b and enhanced effects with downregulation of its target, knowledge of which may be beneficial in enhancing miR-29b therapeutic effects [78]. MiR-29a is mainly localized to the cytoplasm and has a distinct cytosine residue at position 10 [77]. Deep sequencing analysis found -29c to be enriched to a greater extent in the nucleus than the cytoplasm [79]. Alternatively, miR-29b and -29c contain a tri-uracil sequence at position 9–11, responsible for rapid decay. Replacement with the cytosine residue in -29a leads to greater stability [80].

The miR-29 family have been implicated in many cellular functions, including apoptosis [81,82], proliferation, and differentiation [83], and play an essential role in development and normal physiology. MiR-29 knockout (KO) mice demonstrate developmental defects and growth retardation [84]. Downregulation of miR-29 has also been linked to the development of many cancers, including lung [85], colon [86], liver [87], and acute myeloid leukaemia [88]. Tumour suppressor effects of miR-29b were demonstrated in xenograft leukaemia models and exogenous delivery of miR-29b induced apoptosis of tumour cells and dramatic reduction in tumorigenicity [88,89]. In contradiction to this, other reports propose that miR-29 is an oncogene in gastric and pancreatic cancers [73], strengthening the argument that the biological function of miRNAs is cell-type- and organ-specific.

6. MiR-29 in Fibrosis

The miR-29 family are key players in fibrotic activity in multiple organs including the heart, lungs and kidney. Each family member targets many different genes encoding proteins essential for both the physiological and pathological formation of ECM including collagen, laminin, fibrillin, and elastin [90,91]. The miR-29 family is unique in that in targets 20 collagen mRNA species, with no other reported miRNA targeting more than 11 collagen transcripts, proposing it is a "master regulator" of fibrosis or the "master fibromiRNA" [46,92].

MiR-29a has been found to be a negative regulator of TAB1, a gene responsible for the regulation of inflammation. An increase in TAB1 leads to elevated expression of tissue inhibitor of matrix metalloproteinase-1 (TIMP-1), a widespread inhibitor of MMPs, demonstrating its role in fibrosis [93]. Interestingly, the expression levels of miR-29 differ with organ-specific cell types. MiR-29 levels were 100 times higher in hepatic stellate cells (HSCs) than hepatocytes [94] Similarly, higher levels were reported in cardiac fibroblasts than in myocytes [95]. Both studies demonstrate high expression levels in cell types that play a role in the regulation of ECM.

The suppression of miR-29 is strongly linked to the pro-fibrotic TGF-β. By binding to TGF-β receptors, TGF-β1 phosphorylates Smad2 and Smad3 leading to nuclear translocation and regulation of the expression of approximately 60 target ECM genes [63]. MiR-29 is a known downstream target in the TGF-β/Smad pathway [96], and Smad3 signalling results in downregulation of miR-29 [97].

The antifibrotic role of miR-29 has been extensively investigated in pulmonary fibrosis [93]. In both bleomycin-induced fibrotic lung disease and idiopathic pulmonary fibrosis, miR-29 family member levels were significantly reduced [96,98]. MiR29 expression levels are inversely correlated with the severity of pulmonary fibrosis [92]. TGF-β stimulation reduced miR-29a-c levels further and upregulated collagen I, III and fibronectin in the fibrotic lung. This downregulation of miR-29 was prevented in Smad3 knockout mice, indicating regulation of miR-29 via the Smad3 signalling pathway. Similarly, knockdown of miR-29 in human foetal lung fibroblasts correlated with an increase in profibrotic genes including ADAM12 and ADAMTS9 [99]. In IMR90 cells, TGF-β1 induced COL1a1 expression was blocked by miR-29 mimics for each family member. The overexpression of miR-29 using specific mimics for miR-29a, b and c family members demonstrated a disruption to PI3K/AKT phosphorylation and resulted in atypical collagen expression, suggesting targeting of the PI3k-Akt pathway [100]. In a model of liver fibrosis, all three members of the miR-29 family were downregulated [101]. MiR-29b is also reduced in HSCs, a primary producer of collagen in the liver. Transfection of HSCs with miR-29b significantly attenuated the expression of Col1a1 and Col1a2 [102]. MiR-29b has been reported to be the most effective suppressor of type 1 collagen in HSCs among several miRNA whose expression levels were under the control of TGF-β1 [100]. In addition, over expression of miR-29b in rat HSCs inhibited lysyl oxidase and heat shock protein 47, two essential proteins in ECM maturation [103].

The anti-fibrotic reports of miR-29 are also evident in cardiac pathophysiology. MiR-29c expression was decreased in a model of cardiac hypertrophy in mice [104]. Following acute myocardial infarction in mice, all mir-29 family member levels were downregulated in cardiac tissue adjacent to the infarct compared to remotely isolated tissue from the same donor [92]. In congestive heart failure, miR-29 expression was reduced in atrial fibroblasts with an associated increase in ECM target genes including fibrillin and COL1A1 and COL3A1 [105]. In contrast to its protective antifibrotic effects in myocardial cells, one report states miR-29a and miR-29c overexpression promoted apoptosis, whereas downregulation protected against myocardial ischaemia–reperfusion injury [106]. The pro-apoptotic effects of miR-29 have been reported in several cell type [107–109]. MiR-29 has been shown to activate p53 via p85α and CDC42 and therefore promote apoptosis [108,109]. However, under mild stress conditions, p53 can function as an antioxidant and promote cell survival [110]. Thus, the pro-apoptotic effects of miR-29 through p53 signalling may be dependent on the specific cell type and stress level.

The TGF-β/Smad signalling pathway is a well-known regulator of renal fibrosis. In renal tubular epithelial cells, TGF-β1 negatively regulates miR-29b expression via Smad3. Induction of renal fibrosis by unilateral ureteric obstruction in mice induced a significant reduction in miR-29a,b, and c [63]. As reported in pulmonary fibrosis, expression of miR-29 was significantly upregulated in Smad3 knockout mice, with subsequent inhibition of renal fibrosis [72]. In diabetic nephropathy, miR-29b was downregulated in mesangial cells via TGF-β/Smad mechanisms [111]. Loss of miR-29b led to progression of microalbuminuria and renal fibrosis. In systemic sclerosis (SS), a multisystem fibrotic disorder, miR-29a was strongly downregulated compared to healthy controls. TGF-β, PDGF-B, and IL-4 also reduced miR-29a levels in controls similar to levels seen in SS fibroblasts [112,113]. In keloid vs. healthy fibroblasts, miR-29a–c levels were significantly reduced—miR-29b expression in particular. In keloid fibroblasts transfected with pre-miR-29a, type I and III collagen mRNA and protein levels were decreased [114].

It is clear that miR-29 plays a crucial role in fibrosis in many organs via regulation of multiple signalling pathways in addition to direct inhibition of ECM proteins. Novel research on miR-29 as a therapeutic strategy in fibrosis is ongoing. Exogenous miR-29b gene delivery following bleomycin administration in normal lung tissue prevented the development of pulmonary fibrosis [96]. In diabetic nephropathy, ultrasound assisted gene therapy restored miR-29b expression levels thus attenuating fibrotic changes [111]. Multiple studies have shown that the level of fibrotic transformation in varying pathological processes can be regulated by targeting the TGF-β driven downregulation of the miR-29 family in specific tissues [113–115].

7. MiR-29 Family in Eye Disease

The majority of research on miR-29 in ocular pathology focuses on its role in glaucoma. However, it has also been reported in several anterior [66] and posterior segment conditions [116]. In Fuchs endothelial corneal dystrophy (FECD), a common condition resulting in disruption of the corneal endothelium [28], the differential expression of 87 significant miRNAs was analysed. The miR-29 family was the most significantly downregulated in the endothelial tissue from FECD patients. Transcriptional overexpression of the miR-29 target genes, COL1A1 and COL4A1, was noted in the same samples. Interestingly, given its role in miR-29 downregulation, TGFβ-1 has been reported to be upregulated in FECD samples [117]. In another study, treatment of corneal endothelial cells in FECD with miR-29b led to a significant drop in expression levels of ECM genes, including COL1A1, COL4A1, and LAMC1 [118]. In a guinea pig model of myopia, miR-29a,b, and c expression was increased in the sclera and the expression levels of Col1a1 was reduced [119]. The differential expression of the miR-29 family was also investigated in diabetic retinopathy models [115] and these studies proposed that miR-29 may play a protective role in the regulation of retinal pigment epithelium (RPE) apoptosis induced by hyperglycaemia [120].

8. MiR-29 Family in Glaucoma

Given the well-reported role of miR-29 in ECM production and fibrotic transformation in various tissues, it is not surprising that research on miR-29 in ocular pathology focuses mainly on its role in the development of fibrosis at the TM and ONH in POAG. MiR-29a, 29b, and 29c are expressed in TM cells [121] and lamina cribrosa cells [52]. In aqueous humour samples from healthy and glaucomatous human donors, miR-29a, b, and c were detected and are among the most prevalent miRNAs isolated from glaucomatous samples [122,123]. In array studies, miR-29b was downregulated in Tenon's ocular fibroblasts (TF) stimulated with TGF-β1. TGF-β2 also reduced miR-29b expression in both normal and glaucomatous TF cells in vitro [124]. Overexpressing miR-29b in TF cells also inhibited the expression of COL1a1, SP1, and PI3Kp85a, supporting the role of miR-29b in the regulation of PI3K signalling in fibrosis and subsequent collagen production [125]. In vivo, miR-29 was found to be downregulated in the retina of a CNS-injury-induced model of glaucoma [126]. Contradictory to other reports, Liu et al. demonstrated reduced miR-29b expression in the retinal tissues of glaucoma rats vs. control [127]. In addition, they suggested that miR-29b may induce apoptosis in human TM cells and silencing of miR-29 protected HTM cells against oxidative injury via ERK pathway.

ECM remodelling of the LC is a key process in the development of glaucomatous optic neuropathy. There is limited published research on miR-29 specifically at the lamina. However, an important paper by Lopez et al. found that miR-29a and miR-29c expression levels were downregulated in glaucomatous LC cells compared to age-matched controls. They also found miR-29b was downregulated in glaucoma samples. However, this was not statistically significant [52]. Interestingly, treatment of LC cells with TGF-β2 resulted in an additional reduction in miR-29c expression. LC cells were subsequently transfected with miR-29c, which resulted in the downregulation of type I and IV collagen, suggesting that TGF-β2 and miR-29 regulate ECM synthesis in the LC cell [52]. Restoration of miR-29 expression levels at the ONH may aid in the regulation of TGF-β-induced ECM overproduction.

Induction of oxidative stress in cultured human TM cells resulted in the downregulation of miR-29b and increased expression of ECM genes [128]. Transfection of these cells with a miR-29b mimic resulted in reduced expression of an array of collagen genes (COL1A1, COL1A2, COL4A1, COL5A1, COL5A2, COL3A1) and ADAM12, a profibrotic gene which was also identified as a direct target of miR-29b. This suggests that miR-29b may be able to prevent excess ECM deposition in TM and modulate changes in IOP due to outflow restriction [128]. Further research from Luna et al. demonstrated that TGF-β2, but not TGF-β1, downregulated all three members of the miR-29 family in TM cells [67]. However, Villarreal et al. found that TM cells treated with TGF-β2 induced miR-29a expression and miR-29b suppression [121]. Additionally, in TGF-β2-treated TM cells, upregulation of miR-29 reduced the expression of previously upregulated ECM proteins. SMAD3 modulates miR-29b expression via the TGF-β signalling pathway under both basal and TGF-β2 conditions in the cultured TM cells [121].

The canonical Wnt signalling pathway is also crucial in the regulation of ECM expression and aqueous outflow [129]. Lithium chloride (LiCl) stimulation, a known activator of β-catenin, upregulated miR-29b levels, but no significant change was observed in miR-29a or c expression in primary TM cells [129]. These studies suggest that miR-29b expression is modulated by a variety of factors, including LiCl, TGF-β, and oxidative stress, and that miR-29b plays a central role in ECM synthesis. MiR-29b is regulated by the TGF-β signalling pathway and the canonical Wnt signalling pathway, both essential ECM pathways. Evidence of cross-inhibition between the TGF-β/SMAD and canonical Wnt pathways in the TM has been reported [130]. Interestingly, miR-29a was also shown to be upregulated in TM cells following mechanical stretch [131]. The crosstalk between different signalling pathways plays a role in ocular fibrosis associated with glaucoma.

Although targeting fibrotic transformation at the TM is beneficial for aqueous outflow and IOP modulation, targeting fibrosis of the LC may crucially alter the common endpoint of glaucoma, irreversible ONH damage. Despite the limited amount of research published on miR-29 at the ONH in glaucoma, available evidence demonstrates the importance of miR-29 in TGF-β-induced fibrosis at the ONH in POAG. TGF-β2 expression levels are elevated in LC cells isolated from glaucoma patients compared to age-matched controls [22]. Our research group has previously demonstrated that the LC cells are sensitive to mechanical stress/strain, and in response they upregulate the expression of ECM genes and TGF-β [26]. Upregulation of TGF-β and ECM genes leads to increased collagen deposition and the disorganization of collagen and elastin fibres, resulting in destruction of the normal porous pathways of LC and RGC axon degeneration [4,5]. Previously, we have shown that TGF-β upregulated collagen expression at the LC [26]. As demonstrated by Lopez et al., induction of ECM proteins by TGF-β2 is attenuated by miR-29c, indicating miR-29c may also regulate TGF-β2 signalling. Together, these results support the concept that miR-29 can influence the TGF-β2 signalling pathway in ECM synthesis in LC cells [54]. Further research is required to expand on the role of miR-29 in the development of glaucomatous optic neuropathy. Investigating whether TGF-β inhibits the transcription of miR-29 or affects the processing of this microRNA would be a beneficial next step.

There is increasing evidence of the role of miR-29 in the development of fibrosis in POAG. Future research on the development of miRNA therapies to control ECM production may offer a novel disease-modifying therapeutic approach in POAG. Multiple papers investigate the possibility of restoring downregulated miR-29 levels either through transfection with mimics or the use of viral vectors. Subconjunctival injection of lentivirus-mediated miR-29b following glaucoma filtration surgery in rabbits found reduced collagen 1a1 expression and fibroblast numbers at post-operative day 28, resulting in lower IOP and sustained bleb function compared to controls [132]. Interestingly, it was noted that overexpression of miR-29b provided protection to subconjunctival tissue against collagen production and fibrosis, suggesting it may play a role in attenuating bleb scarring following glaucoma filtration surgery [124]. In a study examining corneal and retinal fibrosis, an oligonucleotide mimic of miR-29b, MRG-201, was administered topically to both a rat cornea post-alkali burn and via intravitreal injection to a rabbit model of proliferative vitreoretinopathy. MRG-201 was found to reduce collagen expression and inhibit corneal and retinal fibrosis [133].

9. Conclusions

Understanding the role of miRNAs in health and disease in the eye may prove central to dissecting the physiological and pathophysiological mechanisms impacting glaucoma. The ability of miRNA manipulations to alter gene expression in vitro and in vivo has raised the possibility of miRNA-based therapeutics [112,133]. Several miRNA therapeutics are undergoing evaluation in preclinical and clinical studies, including miRNAs which target fibrotic responses in the lung, liver, heart, and kidney [133–136]. There are several methods of manipulating miRNA expression, including miR mimics, anti-miRs, target site blockers, and miRNA sponges [133]. The anterior segment and TM offer many advantages for miRNA-based therapies, including accessibility and non-invasive observation of the phenotypic effects of therapy in vivo. Several potential delivery options are feasible [136,137]. Several challenges must be overcome, and understanding the miRNA–mRNA interactome is critical to development miRNA therapeutics for fibrosis in the LC and TM.

Funding: AS and COB have received no financial support for this study. BC and CEW were funded by Fight for Sight (UK) and Glaucoma (UK).

Institutional Review Board Statement: Not applicable.

Informed Consent Statement: Not applicable.

Data Availability Statement: Not applicable.

Conflicts of Interest: The authors declare no conflict of interest.

References

1. Tham, Y.C.; Li, X.; Wong, T.Y.; Quigley, H.A.; Aung, T.; Cheng, C.Y. Global prevalence of glaucoma and projections of glaucoma burden through 2040: A systematic review and meta-analysis. *Ophthalmology* **2014**, *121*, 2081–2090. [CrossRef]
2. Myers, J.S.; Fudemberg, S.J.; Lee, D. Evolution of optic nerve photography for glaucoma screening: A review. *Clin. Exp. Ophthalmol.* **2017**, *46*, 169–176. [CrossRef]
3. Kim, T.-W.; Kagemann, L.; Girard, M.J.A.; Strouthidis, N.G.; Sung, K.R.; Leung, C.K.; Schuman, J.S.; Wollstein, G. Imaging of the Lamina Cribrosa in Glaucoma: Perspectives of Pathogenesis and Clinical Applications. *Curr. Eye Res.* **2013**, *38*, 903–909. [CrossRef]
4. Pena, J.D.; Netland, P.A.; Vidal, I.; Dorr, D.A.; Rasky, A.; Hernandez, M. Elastosis of the Lamina Cribrosa in Glaucomatous Optic Neuropathy. *Exp. Eye Res.* **1998**, *67*, 517–524. [CrossRef]
5. Hernandez, M.R.; Andrzejewska, W.M.; Neufeld, A.H. Changes in the Extracellular Matrix of the Human Optic Nerve Head in Primary Open-Angle Glaucoma. *Am. J. Ophthalmol.* **1990**, *109*, 180–188. [CrossRef]
6. Downs, J.C.; Girkin, C.A. Lamina cribrosa in glaucoma. *Curr. Opin. Ophthalmol.* **2017**, *28*, 113. [CrossRef]
7. Quigley, H.A.; Hohman, R.M.; Addicks, E.M.; Massof, R.W.; Green, W.R. Morphologic Changes in the Lamina Cribrosa Correlated with Neural Loss in Open-Angle Glaucoma. *Am. J. Ophthalmol.* **1983**, *95*, 673–691. [CrossRef]
8. Kass, M.A.; Heuer, D.K.; Higginbotham, E.J.; Johnson, C.A.; Keltner, J.L.; Miller, J.P.; Parrish, R.K.; Wilson, M.R.; Gordon, M.O.; Ocular Hypertension Treatment Study Group. The Ocular Hypertension Treatment Study: A randomized trial determines that top-ical ocular hypotensive medication delays or prevents the onset of primary open-angle glaucoma. *Arch. Ophthalmol.* **2002**, *120*, 701–713. [CrossRef]
9. Wormald, R.; Virgili, G.; Azuara-Blanco, A. Systematic reviews and randomised controlled trials on open angle glaucoma. *Eye* **2019**, *34*, 161–167. [CrossRef]
10. Heijl, A.; Leske, M.C.; Bengtsson, B.; Hyman, L.; Bengtsson, B.; Hussein, M.; Early Manifest Glaucoma Trial Group. Reduction of intraocular pressure and glaucoma progression: Results from the Early Manifest Glaucoma Trial. *Arch. Ophthalmol.* **2002**, *120*, 1268–1279. [CrossRef]

11. Peters, D.; Bengtsson, B.; Heijl, A. Lifetime Risk of Blindness in Open-Angle Glaucoma. *Am. J. Ophthalmol.* **2013**, *156*, 724–730. [CrossRef]
12. Wang, H.W.; Sun, P.; Chen, Y.; Jiang, L.P.; Wu, H.P.; Zhang, W.; Gao, F. Research progress on human genes involved in the patho-genesis of glaucoma. *Mol. Med. Rep.* **2018**, *18*, 656–674.
13. Weiss, A.; Attisano, L. The TGFbeta superfamily signaling pathway. *Wiley Interdiscip. Rev. Dev. Biol.* **2013**, *2*, 47–63. [CrossRef]
14. Prendes, M.A.; Harris, A.; Wirostko, B.M.; Gerber, A.L.; Siesky, B. The role of transforming growth factor β in glaucoma and the therapeutic implications. *Br. J. Ophthalmol.* **2013**, *97*, 680–686. [CrossRef]
15. Wordinger, R.J.; Sharma, T.; Clark, A.F. The Role of TGF-β2 and Bone Morphogenetic Proteins in the Trabecular Meshwork and Glaucoma. *J. Ocul. Pharmacol. Ther.* **2014**, *30*, 154–162. [CrossRef]
16. Fuchshofer, R.; Tamm, E.R. The role of TGF-β in the pathogenesis of primary open-angle glaucoma. *Cell Tissue Res.* **2011**, *347*, 279–290. [CrossRef]
17. Fleenor, D.L.; Shepard, A.R.; Hellberg, P.E.; Jacobson, N.; Pang, I.H.; Clark, A.F. TGFβ2-induced changes in human trabecular mesh-work: Implications for intraocular pressure. *Investig. Ophthalmol. Vis. Sci.* **2006**, *47*, 226–234. [CrossRef]
18. Bhattacharya, S.K.; Gabelt, B.T.; Ruiz, J.; Picciani, R.; Kaufman, P.L. Cochlin Expression in Anterior Segment Organ Culture Models after TGFβ2 Treatment. *Investig. Ophthalmol. Vis. Sci.* **2009**, *50*, 551–559. [CrossRef]
19. Birke, M.T.; Birke, K.; Lütjen-Drecoll, E.; Schlötzer-Schrehardt, U.; Hammer, C.M. Cytokine-Dependent ELAM-1 Induction and Concomitant Intraocular Pressure Regulation in Porcine Anterior Eye Perfusion Culture. *Investig. Ophthalmol. Vis. Sci.* **2011**, *52*, 468–475. [CrossRef]
20. Rocha-Sousa, A.; Rodrigues-Araújo, J.; Gouveia, P.; Barbosa-Breda, J.; Azevedo-Pinto, S.; Pereira-Silva, P.; Leite-Moreira, A. New Therapeutic Targets for Intraocular Pressure Lowering. *ISRN Ophthalmol.* **2013**, *2013*, 261386. [CrossRef]
21. Angayarkanni, N.; Coral, K.; Bharathi Devi, S.R.; Saijyothi, A.V. The Biochemistry of the Eye. In *Pharmacology of Ocular Thera-Peutics*; Adis: Cham, Switzerland, 2016; pp. 83–157.
22. Kirwan, R.P.; Wordinger, R.J.; Clark, A.F.; O'Brien, C.J. Differential global and extra-cellular matrix focused gene expression pat-terns between normal and glaucomatous human lamina cribrosa cells. *Mol. Vis.* **2009**, *15*, 76. [PubMed]
23. Liu, B.; McNally, S.; Kilpatrick, J.I.; Jarvis, S.P.; O'Brien, C.J. Aging and ocular tissue stiffness in glaucoma. *Surv. Ophthalmol.* **2018**, *63*, 56–74. [CrossRef] [PubMed]
24. Wallace, D.M.; Pokrovskaya, O.; O'Brien, C.J. The Function of Matricellular Proteins in the Lamina Cribrosa and Trabecular Meshwork in Glaucoma. *J. Ocul. Pharmacol. Ther.* **2015**, *31*, 386–395. [CrossRef] [PubMed]
25. Fuchshofer, R. The pathogenic role of transforming growth factor-β2 in glaucomatous damage to the optic nerve head. *Exp. Eye Res.* **2011**, *93*, 165–169. [CrossRef] [PubMed]
26. Kirwan, R.P.; Leonard, M.O.; Murphy, M.; Clark, A.F.; O'Brien, C.J. Transforming growth factor-β-regulated gene transcription and protein expression in human GFAP-negative lamina cribrosa cells. *Glia* **2005**, *52*, 309–324. [CrossRef]
27. Rodriguez, A.; Griffiths-Jones, S.; Ashurst, J.L.; Bradley, A. Identification of Mammalian microRNA Host Genes and Transcription Units. *Genome Res.* **2004**, *14*, 1902–1910. [CrossRef]
28. Friedman, R.C.; Farh, K.K.-H.; Burge, C.B.; Bartel, D.P. Most mammalian mRNAs are conserved targets of microRNAs. *Genome Res.* **2009**, *19*, 92–105. [CrossRef]
29. Lee, R.C.; Feinbaum, R.L.; Ambros, V. The *C. elegans* heterochronic gene lin-4 encodes small RNAs with antisense complemen-tarity to lin-14. *Cell* **1993**, *75*, 843–854. [CrossRef]
30. Wightman, B.; Ha, I. Wightman, Ha, Ruvkun-1993-Cell-Posttranscriptional regulation of the heterochronic gene lin-14 by lin-4 mediates temporal pattern. PDF. *Cell* **1993**, *75*, 855–862. [CrossRef]
31. Bentwich, I.; Avniel, A.; Karov, Y.; Aharonov, R.; Gilad, S.; Barad, O.; Barzilai, A.; Einat, P.; Einav, U.; Meiri, E.; et al. Identification of hundreds of conserved and nonconserved human microRNAs. *Nat. Genet.* **2005**, *37*, 766–770. [CrossRef]
32. Lee, Y.; Kim, M.; Han, J.; Yeom, K.-H.; Lee, S.; Baek, S.H.; Kim, V.N. MicroRNA genes are transcribed by RNA polymerase II. *EMBO J.* **2004**, *23*, 4051–4060. [CrossRef] [PubMed]
33. Lee, Y.; Ahn, C.; Han, J.; Choi, H.; Kim, J.; Yim, J.; Lee, J.; Provost, P.; Rådmark, O.; Kim, S.; et al. The nuclear RNase III drosha initiates microRNA processing. *Nature* **2003**, *425*, 415–419. [CrossRef] [PubMed]
34. Lund, E.; Güttinger, S.; Calado, A.; Dahlberg, J.E.; Kutay, U. Nuclear Export of MicroRNA Precursors. *Science* **2004**, *303*, 95–98. [CrossRef]
35. Ketting, R.F.; Fischer, S.E.; Bernstein, E.; Sijen, T.; Hannon, G.J.; Plasterk, R.H. Dicer functions in RNA interference and in synthesis of small RNA involved in developmental timing in *C. elegans*. *Genes Dev.* **2001**, *15*, 2654–2659. [CrossRef]
36. Pratt, A.J.; MacRae, I.J. The RNA-induced Silencing Complex: A Versatile Gene-silencing Machine. *J. Biol. Chem.* **2009**, *284*, 17897–17901. [CrossRef]
37. Baek, D.; Villén, J.; Shin, C.; Camargo, F.D.; Gygi, S.P.; Bartel, D.P. The impact of microRNAs on protein output. *Nature* **2008**, *455*, 64–71. [CrossRef] [PubMed]
38. Pillai, R.S.; Bhattacharyya, S.N.; Artus, C.G.; Zoller, T.; Cougot, N.; Basyuk, E.; Bertrand, E.; Filipowicz, W. Inhibition of Translational Initiation by Let-7 MicroRNA in Human Cells. *Science* **2005**, *309*, 1573–1576. [CrossRef]
39. Nottrott, S.; Simard, M.; Richter, J.D. Human let-7a miRNA blocks protein production on actively translating polyribosomes. *Nat. Struct. Mol. Biol.* **2006**, *13*, 1108–1114. [CrossRef]

40. Huntzinger, E.; Izaurralde, E. Gene silencing by microRNAs: Contributions of translational repression and mRNA decay. *Nat. Rev. Genet.* **2011**, *12*, 99–110. [CrossRef]
41. Ipsaro, J.J.; Joshua-Tor, L. From guide to target: Molecular insights into eukaryotic RNA-interference machinery. *Nat. Struct. Mol. Biol.* **2015**, *22*, 20–28. [CrossRef]
42. Esquela-Kerscher, A.; Slack, F.J. Oncomirs—microRNAs with a role in cancer. *Nat. Rev. Cancer* **2006**, *6*, 259–269. [CrossRef] [PubMed]
43. Wang, J.; Chen, J.; Sen, S. MicroRNA as Biomarkers and Diagnostics. *J. Cell. Physiol.* **2015**, *231*, 25–30. [CrossRef] [PubMed]
44. Ardekani, A.M.; Naeini, M.M. The role of microRNAs in human diseases. *Avicenna J. Med. Biotechnol.* **2010**, *2*, 161. [PubMed]
45. Peng, Y.; Croce, C.M. The role of MicroRNAs in human cancer. *Signal Transduct. Target. Ther.* **2016**, *1*, 15004. [CrossRef] [PubMed]
46. O'Reilly, S. MicroRNAs in fibrosis: Opportunities and challenges. *Arthritis Res. Ther.* **2016**, *18*, 11. [CrossRef]
47. Swarbrick, S.; Wragg, N.; Ghosh, S.; Stolzing, A. Systematic Review of miRNA as Biomarkers in Alzheimer's Disease. *Mol. Neurobiol.* **2019**, *56*, 6156–6167. [CrossRef]
48. Colpaert, R.M.; Calore, M. MicroRNAs in Cardiac Diseases. *Cells* **2019**, *8*, 737. [CrossRef]
49. Lobo, J.; Gillis, A.J.M.; van den Berg, A.; Dorssers, L.C.J.; Belge, G.; Dieckmann, K.-P.; Roest, H.P.; Van Der Laan, L.J.W.; Gietema, J.; Hamilton, R.J.; et al. Identification and Validation Model for Informative Liquid Biopsy-Based microRNA Biomarkers: Insights from Germ Cell Tumor in Vitro, in Vivo and Patient-Derived Data. *Cells* **2019**, *8*, 1637. [CrossRef]
50. Callaghan, B.; Lester, K.; Lane, B.; Fan, X.; Goljanek-Whysall, K.; Simpson, D.A.; Sheridan, C.; Willoughby, C.E. Genome-wide tran-scriptome profiling of human trabecular meshwork cells treated with TGF-β2. *Sci. Rep.* **2022**, *12*, 9564.
51. Seong, H.; Cho, H.K.; Kee, C.; Song, D.H.; Cho, M.C.; Kang, S.S. Profiles of microRNA in aqueous humor of normal tension glauco-ma patients using RNA sequencing. *Sci. Rep.* **2021**, *11*, 19024.
52. Lopez, N.; Rangan, R.; Clark, A.; Tovar-Vidales, T. Mirna Expression in Glaucomatous and TGFβ2 Treated Lamina Cribrosa Cells. *Int. J. Mol. Sci.* **2021**, *22*, 6178. [CrossRef] [PubMed]
53. Kang, H. Role of MicroRNAs in TGF-β Signaling Pathway-Mediated Pulmonary Fibrosis. *Int. J. Mol. Sci.* **2017**, *18*, 2527. [CrossRef] [PubMed]
54. Suzuki, H.I. MicroRNA control of TGF-β signaling. *Int. J. Mol. Sci.* **2018**, *19*, 1901. [CrossRef] [PubMed]
55. Luo, K. Signaling Cross Talk between TGF-β/Smad and Other Signaling Pathways. *Cold Spring Harb. Perspect. Biol.* **2016**, *9*, a022137. [CrossRef]
56. Meng, X.-M.; Nikolic-Paterson, D.J.; Lan, H.Y. TGF-β: The master regulator of fibrosis. *Nat. Rev. Nephrol.* **2016**, *12*, 325–338. [CrossRef]
57. Yang, C.; Zheng, S.-D.; Wu, H.-J.; Chen, S.-J. Regulatory Mechanisms of the Molecular Pathways in Fibrosis Induced by MicroRNAs. *Chin. Med. J.* **2016**, *129*, 2365–2372. [CrossRef]
58. Davis-Dusenbery, B.; Hilyard, A.C.; Lagna, G.; Hata, A. SMAD proteins control DROSHA-mediated microRNA maturation. *Nature* **2008**, *454*, 56–61. [CrossRef]
59. Butz, H.; Rácz, K.; Hunyady, L.; Patócs, A. Crosstalk between TGF-β signaling and the microRNA machinery. *Trends Pharmacol. Sci.* **2012**, *33*, 382–393. [CrossRef]
60. Liu, X.; Hu, H.; Yin, J.Q. Therapeutic strategies against TGF-β signaling pathway in hepatic fibrosis. *Liver Int.* **2005**, *26*, 8–22. [CrossRef]
61. Cutroneo, K.R. TGF-β–induced fibrosis and SMAD signaling: Oligo decoys as natural therapeutics for inhibition of tissue fibrosis and scarring. *Wound Repair Regen.* **2007**, *15*, S54–S60. [CrossRef]
62. Zhang, B.; Zhou, M.; Li, C.; Zhou, J.; Li, H.; Zhu, D.; Wang, Z.; Chen, A.; Zhao, Q. MicroRNA-92a inhibition attenuates hypox-ia/reoxygenation-induced myocardiocyte apoptosis by targeting Smad7. *PLoS ONE* **2014**, *9*, e100298.
63. Ramdas, V.; McBride, M.; Denby, L.; Baker, A.H. Canonical transforming growth factor-β signaling regulates disintegrin metal-loprotease expression in experimental renal fibrosis via miR-29. *Am. J. Pathol.* **2013**, *183*, 1885–1896. [CrossRef]
64. Xue, L.; Xiong, C.; Li, J.; Ren, Y.; Zhang, L.; Jiao, K.; Chen, C.; Ding, P. miR-200-3p suppresses cell proliferation and reduces apoptosis in diabetic retinopathy via blocking the TGF-β2/Smad pathway. *Biosci. Rep.* **2020**, *40*, 11. [CrossRef] [PubMed]
65. Luo, Y.; Liu, S.; Yao, K. Transcriptome-wide Investigation of mRNA/circRNA in miR-184 and Its r.57c > u Mutant Type Treatment of Human Lens Epithelial Cells. *Mol. Ther.-Nucleic Acids* **2017**, *7*, 71–80. [CrossRef] [PubMed]
66. Luna, C.; Li, G.; Qiu, J.; Epstein, D.L.; Gonzalez, P. Cross-talk between miR-29 and Transforming Growth Factor-Betas in Trabecular Meshwork Cells. *Investig. Ophthalmol. Vis. Sci.* **2011**, *52*, 3567–3572. [CrossRef]
67. Tan, C.; Song, M.; Stamer, W.D.; Qiao, Y.; Chen, X.; Sun, X.; Lei, Y.; Chen, J. miR-21-5p: A viable therapeutic strategy for regulating intraocular pressure. *Exp. Eye Res.* **2020**, *200*, 108197. [CrossRef]
68. Drewry, M.; Helwa, I.; Allingham, R.R.; Hauser, M.A.; Liu, Y. miRNA Profile in Three Different Normal Human Ocular Tissues by miRNA-Seq. *Investig. Ophthalmol. Vis. Sci.* **2016**, *57*, 3731–3739. [CrossRef]
69. Kwon, J.J.; Factora, T.D.; Dey, S.; Kota, J. A Systematic Review of miR-29 in Cancer. *Mol. Ther.-Oncolytics* **2018**, *12*, 173–194. [CrossRef] [PubMed]
70. Michlewski, G.; Cáceres, J.F. Post-transcriptional control of miRNA biogenesis. *RNA* **2018**, *25*, 1–16. [CrossRef]
71. Kriegel, A.J.; Liu, Y.; Fang, Y.; Ding, X.; Liang, M. The miR-29 family: Genomics, cell biology, and relevance to renal and cardio-vascular injury. *Physiol. Genom.* **2012**, *44*, 237–244. [CrossRef]

72. Qin, W.; Chung, A.C.; Huang, X.R.; Meng, X.-M.; Hui, D.; Yu, C.-M.; Sung, J.J.Y.; Lan, H.Y. TGF-β/Smad3 Signaling Promotes Renal Fibrosis by Inhibiting miR-29. *J. Am. Soc. Nephrol.* **2011**, *22*, 1462–1474. [CrossRef] [PubMed]
73. Chang, T.C.; Yu, D.; Lee, Y.S.; Wentzel, E.A.; Arking, D.E.; West, K.M.; Dang, C.V.; Thomas-Tikhonenko, A.; Mendell, J.T. Widespread mi-croRNA repression by Myc contributes to tumorigenesis. *Nat. Genet.* **2008**, *40*, 43–50. [CrossRef] [PubMed]
74. Mott, J.L.; Kurita, S.; Cazanave, S.C.; Bronk, S.F.; Werneburg, N.W.; Fernandez-Zapico, M.E. Transcriptional suppression of mir-29b-1/mir-29a promoter by c-Myc, hedgehog, and NF-kappaB. *J. Cell. Biochem.* **2010**, *110*, 1155–1164. [CrossRef] [PubMed]
75. Feldman, A.L.; Dogan, A.; Smith, D.I.; Law, M.E.; Ansell, S.M.; Johnson, S.H.; Porcher, J.C.; Özsan, N.; Wieben, E.D.; Eckloff, B.W.; et al. Discovery of recurrent t (6; 7)(p25. 3; q32. 3) translocations in ALK-negative anaplastic large cell lymphomas by mas-sively parallel genomic sequencing. *Blood J. Am. Soc. Hematol.* **2011**, *117*, 915–919.
76. Liu, Y.; Taylor, N.E.; Lu, L.; Usa, K.; Cowley, A.W., Jr.; Ferreri, N.R.; Yeo, N.C.; Liang, M. Renal medullary microRNAs in Dahl salt-sensitive rats: miR-29b regulates several collagens and related genes. *Hypertension* **2010**, *55*, 974–982. [CrossRef]
77. Hwang, H.-W.; Wentzel, E.A.; Mendell, J.T. A Hexanucleotide Element Directs MicroRNA Nuclear Import. *Science* **2007**, *315*, 97–100. [CrossRef]
78. Jagannathan, S.; Vad, N.; Vallabhapurapu, S.; Anderson, K.C.; Driscoll, J. MiR-29b replacement inhibits proteasomes and disrupts aggresome+autophagosome formation to enhance the antimyeloma benefit of bortezomib. *Leukemia* **2014**, *29*, 727–738. [CrossRef]
79. Liao, J.-Y.; Ma, L.-M.; Guo, Y.-H.; Zhang, Y.-C.; Zhou, H.; Shao, P.; Chen, Y.-Q.; Qu, L.-H. Deep Sequencing of Human Nuclear and Cytoplasmic Small RNAs Reveals an Unexpectedly Complex Subcellular Distribution of miRNAs and tRNA 3′ Trailers. *PLoS ONE* **2010**, *5*, e10563. [CrossRef]
80. Zhang, Z.; Zou, J.; Wang, G.-K.; Zhang, J.-T.; Huang, S.; Qin, Y.-W.; Jing, Q. Uracils at nucleotide position 9–11 are required for the rapid turnover of miR-29 family. *Nucleic Acids Res.* **2011**, *39*, 4387–4395. [CrossRef]
81. Kole, A.J.; Swahari, V.; Hammond, S.M.; Deshmukh, M. miR-29b is activated during neuronal maturation and targets BH3-only genes to restrict apoptosis. *Genes Dev.* **2011**, *25*, 125–130. [CrossRef]
82. Wei, W.; He, H.-B.; Zhang, W.-Y.; Zhang, H.-X.; Bai, J.-B.; Liu, H.-Z.; Cao, J.-H.; Chang, K.-C.; Li, X.-Y.; Zhao, S.-H. miR-29 targets Akt3 to reduce proliferation and facilitate differentiation of myoblasts in skeletal muscle development. *Cell Death Dis.* **2013**, *4*, e668. [CrossRef] [PubMed]
83. Zhu, K.; Liu, L.; Zhang, J.; Wang, Y.; Liang, H.; Fan, G.; Jiang, Z.; Zhang, C.-Y.; Chen, X.; Zhou, G. MiR-29b suppresses the proliferation and migration of osteosarcoma cells by targeting CDK6. *Protein Cell* **2016**, *7*, 434–444. [CrossRef] [PubMed]
84. Cushing, L.; Costinean, S.; Xu, W.; Jiang, Z.; Madden, L.; Kuang, P.; Huang, J.; Weisman, A.; Hata, A.; Croce, C.M.; et al. Disruption of miR-29 Leads to Aberrant Differentiation of Smooth Muscle Cells Selectively Associated with Distal Lung Vasculature. *PLoS Genet.* **2015**, *11*, e1005238. [CrossRef] [PubMed]
85. Yanaihara, N.; Caplen, N.J.; Bowman, E.; Seike, M.; Kumamoto, K.; Yi, M.; Stephens, R.M.; Okamoto, A.; Yokota, J.; Tanaka, T.; et al. Unique microRNA molecular profiles in lung cancer diagnosis and prognosis. *Cancer Cell* **2006**, *9*, 189–198. [CrossRef] [PubMed]
86. Cummins, J.M.; He, Y.; Leary, R.J.; Pagliarini, R.; Diaz, L.A., Jr.; Sjoblom, T.; Barad, O.; Bentwich, Z.; Szafranska, A.E.; Labourier, E.; et al. The colorectal microRNAome. *Proc. Natl. Acad. Sci. USA* **2006**, *103*, 3687–3692. [CrossRef] [PubMed]
87. Xiong, Y.; Fang, J.H.; Yun, J.P.; Yang, J.; Zhang, Y.; Jia, W.H.; Zhuang, S.M. Effects of MicroRNA-29 on apoptosis, tumorigenicity, and prognosis of hepatocellular carcinoma. *Hepatology* **2010**, *51*, 836–845. [CrossRef] [PubMed]
88. Garzon, R.; Heaphy, C.E.; Havelange, V.; Fabbri, M.; Volinia, S.; Tsao, T.; Zanesi, N.; Kornblau, S.M.; Marcucci, G.; Calin, G.A.; et al. MicroRNA 29b functions in acute myeloid leukemia. *Blood J. Am. Soc. Hematol.* **2009**, *114*, 5331–5341. [CrossRef]
89. Gebeshuber, C.A.; Zatloukal, K.; Martinez, J. miR-29a suppresses tristetraprolin, which is a regulator of epithelial polarity and metastasis. *EMBO Rep.* **2009**, *10*, 400–405. [CrossRef]
90. Li, Z.; Hassan, M.Q.; Jafferji, M.; Aqeilan, R.I.; Garzon, R.; Croce, C.M.; Van Wijnen, A.J.; Stein, J.L.; Stein, G.S.; Lian, J.B. Biological functions of miR-29b contribute to positive regulation of osteoblast differentiation. *J. Biol. Chem.* **2009**, *284*, 15676–15684. [CrossRef]
91. Sengupta, S.; den Boon, J.A.; Chen, I.H.; Newton, M.A.; Stanhope, S.A.; Cheng, Y.J.; Chen, C.J.; Hildesheim, A.; Sugden, B.; Ahlquist, P. Mi-croRNA 29c is down-regulated in nasopharyngeal carcinomas, up-regulating mRNAs encoding extracellular matrix pro-teins. *Proc. Natl. Acad. Sci. USA* **2008**, *105*, 5874–5878. [CrossRef]
92. Cushing, L.; Kuang, P.; Lü, J. The role of miR-29 in pulmonary fibrosis. *Biochem. Cell Biol.* **2015**, *93*, 109–118. [CrossRef] [PubMed]
93. Ciechomska, M.; O'Reilly, S.; Suwara, M.; Bogunia-Kubik, K.; van Laar, J.M. MiR-29a reduces TIMP-1 production by dermal fibro-blasts via targeting TGF-β activated kinase 1 binding protein 1, implications for systemic sclerosis. *PLoS ONE* **2014**, *9*, e115596. [CrossRef] [PubMed]
94. Roderburg, C.; Urban, G.-W.; Bettermann, K.; Vucur, M.; Zimmermann, H.W.; Schmidt, S.; Janssen, J.; Koppe, C.; Knolle, P.; Castoldi, M.; et al. Micro-RNA profiling reveals a role for miR-29 in human and murine liver fibrosis. *Hepatology* **2011**, *53*, 209–218. [CrossRef] [PubMed]
95. Van Rooij, E.; Sutherland, L.B.; Thatcher, J.E.; DiMaio, J.M.; Naseem, R.H.; Marshall, W.S.; Hill, J.A.; Olson, E.N. Dysregulation of mi-croRNAs after myocardial infarction reveals a role of miR-29 in cardiac fibrosis. *Proc. Natl. Acad. Sci. USA* **2008**, *105*, 13027–13032. [CrossRef] [PubMed]
96. Xiao, J.; Meng, X.-M.; Huang, X.R.; Chung, A.C.; Feng, Y.-L.; Hui, D.; Yu, C.-M.; Sung, J.J.Y.; Lan, H.Y. miR-29 Inhibits Bleomycin-induced Pulmonary Fibrosis in Mice. *Mol. Ther.* **2012**, *20*, 1251–1260. [CrossRef] [PubMed]

97. Zhou, L.; Wang, L.; Lu, L.; Jiang, P.; Sun, H.; Wang, H. Inhibition of miR-29 by TGF-beta-Smad3 signaling through dual mecha-nisms promotes transdifferentiation of mouse myoblasts into myofibroblasts. *PLoS ONE* **2012**, *7*, e33766.
98. Pandit, K.; Kaminski, N. MicroRNAs in Idiopathic Pulmonary Fibrosis. *Transl. Res.* **2017**, 179–202. [CrossRef]
99. Cushing, L.; Kuang, P.P.; Qian, J.; Shao, F.; Wu, J.; Little, F.; Thannickal, V.J.; Cardoso, W.V.; Lü, J. miR-29 Is a Major Regulator of Genes Associated with Pulmonary Fibrosis. *Am. J. Respir. Cell Mol. Biol.* **2011**, *45*, 287–294. [CrossRef] [PubMed]
100. Yang, T.; Liang, Y.; Lin, Q.; Liu, J.; Luo, F.; Li, X.; Zhou, H.; Zhuang, S.; Zhang, H. MiR-29 mediates TGFβ1-induced extracellular matrix synthesis through activation of PI3K-AKT pathway in human lung fibroblasts. *J. Cell. Biochem.* **2012**, *114*, 1336–1342. [CrossRef] [PubMed]
101. Sekiya, Y.; Ogawa, T.; Yoshizato, K.; Ikeda, K.; Kawada, N. Suppression of hepatic stellate cell activation by microRNA-29b. *Biochem. Biophys. Res. Commun.* **2011**, *412*, 74–79. [CrossRef]
102. Ogawa, T.; Iizuka, M.; Sekiya, Y.; Yoshizato, K.; Ikeda, K.; Kawada, N. Suppression of type I collagen production by mi-croRNA-29b in cultured human stellate cells. *Biochem. Biophys. Res. Commun.* **2010**, *391*, 316–321. [CrossRef] [PubMed]
103. Zhang, Y.; Ghazwani, M.; Li, J.; Sun, M.; Stolz, D.B.; He, F.; Fan, J.; Xie, W.; Li, S. MiR-29b inhibits collagen maturation in hepatic stel-late cells through down-regulating the expression of HSP47 and lysyl oxidase. *Biochem. Biophys. Res. Com-Munications* **2014**, *446*, 940–944. [CrossRef] [PubMed]
104. Van Rooij, E.; Sutherland, L.B.; Liu, N.; Williams, A.H.; McAnally, J.; Gerard, R.D.; Richardson, J.A.; Olson, E.N. A signature pattern of stress-responsive microRNAs that can evoke cardiac hypertrophy and heart failure. *Proc. Natl. Acad. Sci. USA* **2006**, *103*, 18255–18260. [CrossRef]
105. Dawson, K.; Wakili, R.; Ördög, B.; Clauss, S.; Chen, Y.; Iwasaki, Y.; Voigt, N.; Qi, X.Y.; Sinner, M.F.; Dobrev, D.; et al. MicroRNA29: A mechanistic contributor and potential biomarker in atrial fibrillation. *Circulation* **2013**, *127*, 1466–1475. [CrossRef] [PubMed]
106. Ye, Y.; Hu, Z.; Lin, Y.; Zhang, C.; Perez-Polo, J.R. Downregulation of microRNA-29 by antisense inhibitors and a PPAR-γ agonist protects against myocardial ischaemia–reperfusion injury. *Cardiovasc. Res.* **2010**, *87*, 535–544. [CrossRef] [PubMed]
107. Mott, J.L.; Kobayashi, S.; Bronk, S.F.; Gores, G.J. mir-29 regulates Mcl-1 protein expression and apoptosis. *Oncogene* **2007**, *26*, 6133–6140. [CrossRef]
108. Park, S.-Y.; Lee, J.H.; Ha, M.; Nam, J.-W.; Kim, V.N. miR-29 miRNAs activate p53 by targeting p85α and CDC42. *Nat. Struct. Mol. Biol.* **2008**, *16*, 23–29. [CrossRef]
109. Wang, Y.; Lee, C.G. MicroRNA and cancer–focus on apoptosis. *J. Cell. Mol. Med.* **2009**, *13*, 12–23. [CrossRef]
110. Sablina, A.A.; Budanov, A.V.; Ilyinskaya, G.V.; Agapova, L.S.; Kravchenko, J.E.; Chumakov, P. The antioxidant function of the p53 tumor suppressor. *Nat. Med.* **2005**, *11*, 1306–1313. [CrossRef]
111. Chen, H.Y.; Zhong, X.; Huang, X.R.; Meng, X.-M.; You, Y.; Chung, A.C.; Lan, H.Y. MicroRNA-29b Inhibits Diabetic Nephropathy in db/db Mice. *Mol. Ther.* **2014**, *22*, 842–853. [CrossRef]
112. Maurer, B.; Stanczyk, J.; Jüngel, A.; Akhmetshina, A.; Trenkmann, M.; Brock, M.; Kowal-Bielecka, O.; Gay, R.E.; Michel, B.A.; Distler, J.H.W.; et al. MicroRNA-29, a key regulator of collagen expression in systemic sclerosis. *Arthritis Rheumatol.* **2010**, *62*, 1733–1743. [CrossRef] [PubMed]
113. Zhu, H.; Li, Y.; Qu, S.; Luo, H.; Zhou, Y.; Wang, Y.; Zhao, H.; You, Y.; Xiao, X.; Zuo, X. MicroRNA Expression Abnormalities in Limited Cutaneous Scleroderma and Diffuse Cutaneous Scleroderma. *J. Clin. Immunol.* **2012**, *32*, 514–522. [CrossRef] [PubMed]
114. Zhang, G.-Y.; Wu, L.-C.; Liao, T.; Chen, G.-C.; Chen, Y.-H.; Zhao, Y.-X.; Chen, S.-Y.; Wang, A.-Y.; Lin, K.; Lin, D.-M.; et al. A novel regulatory function for miR-29a in keloid fibrogenesis. *Clin. Exp. Dermatol.* **2015**, *41*, 341–345. [CrossRef] [PubMed]
115. Gong, Q.; Su, G. Roles of miRNAs and long noncoding RNAs in the progression of diabetic retinopathy. *Biosci. Rep.* **2017**, *37*, BSR20171157. [CrossRef] [PubMed]
116. Fuller-Carter, P.I.; Carter, K.W.; Anderson, D.; Harvey, A.R.; Giles, K.M.; Rodger, J. Integrated analyses of zebrafish miRNA and mRNA expression profiles identify miR-29b and miR-223 as potential regulators of optic nerve regeneration. *BMC Genom.* **2015**, *16*, 591. [CrossRef]
117. Weller, J.M.; Zenkel, M.; Schlötzer-Schrehardt, U.; Bachmann, B.O.; Tourtas, T.; Kruse, F.E. Extracellular Matrix Alterations in Late-Onset Fuchs' Corneal Dystrophy. *Investig. Ophthalmol. Vis. Sci.* **2014**, *55*, 3700–3708. [CrossRef]
118. Toyono, T.; Usui, T.; Villarreal, G., Jr.; Kallay, L.; Matthaei, M.; Vianna, L.M.; Zhu, A.Y.; Kuroda, M.; Amano, S.; Jun, A.S. MicroRNA-29b over-expression decreases extracellular matrix mRNA and protein production in human corneal endothelial cells. *Cornea* **2016**, *35*, 1466. [CrossRef]
119. Wang, M.; Yang, Z.K.; Liu, H.; Li, R.Q.; Liu, Y.; Zhong, W.J. Genipin inhibits the scleral expression of miR-29 and MMP2 and pro-motes COL1A1 expression in myopic eyes of guinea pigs. *Graefe's Arch. Clin. Exp. Ophthalmol.* **2020**, *258*, 1031–1038. [CrossRef]
120. Lin, X.; Zhou, X.; Liu, D.; Yun, L.; Zhang, L.; Chen, X.; Chai, Q.; Li, L. MicroRNA-29 regulates high-glucose-induced apoptosis in hu-man retinal pigment epithelial cells through PTEN. *Vitr. Cell. Dev. Biol.-Anim.* **2016**, *52*, 419–426. [CrossRef]
121. Villarreal, G.; Oh, D.J.; Kang, M.H.; Rhee, D.J. Coordinated regulation of extracellular matrix synthesis by the microRNA-29 family in the trabecular meshwork. *Investig. Ophthalmol. Vis. Sci.* **2011**, *52*, 3391–3397. [CrossRef]
122. Dunmire, J.J.; Lagouros, E.; Bouhenni, R.A.; Jones, M.; Edward, D.P. MicroRNA in aqueous humor from patients with cataract. *Exp. Eye Res.* **2013**, *108*, 68–71. [CrossRef] [PubMed]

123. Wecker, T.; Hoffmeier, K.; Plötner, A.; Grüning, B.; Horres, R.; Backofen, R.; Reinhard, T.; Schlunck, G. MicroRNA Profiling in Aqueous Humor of Individual Human Eyes by Next-Generation Sequencing. *Investig. Ophthalmol. Vis. Sci.* **2016**, *57*, 1706–1713. [CrossRef] [PubMed]
124. Ran, W.; Zhu, D.; Feng, Q. TGF-β2 stimulates Tenon's capsule fibroblast proliferation in patients with glaucoma via suppres-sion of miR-29b expression regulated by Nrf2. *Int. J. Clin. Exp. Pathol.* **2015**, *8*, 4799. [PubMed]
125. Li, N.; Cui, J.; Duan, X.; Chen, H.; Fan, F. Suppression of Type I Collagen Expression by miR-29b via PI3K, Akt, and Sp1 Pathway in Human Tenon's Fibroblasts. *Investig. Ophthalmol. Vis. Sci.* **2012**, *53*, 1670–1678. [CrossRef] [PubMed]
126. Jayaram, H.; Cepurna, W.O.; Johnson, E.C.; Morrison, J.C. MicroRNA Expression in the Glaucomatous Retina. *Investig. Ophthalmol. Vis. Sci.* **2015**, *56*, 7971–7982. [CrossRef]
127. Liu, H.; Xiu, Y.; Zhang, Q.; Xu, Y.; Wan, Q.; Tao, L. Silencing microRNA-29b-3p expression protects human trabecular meshwork cells against oxidative injury via upregulation of RNF138 to activate the ERK pathway. *Int. J. Mol. Med.* **2021**, *47*, 101. [CrossRef]
128. Luna, C.; Li, G.; Qiu, J.; Epstein, D.L.; Gonzalez, P. Role of miR-29b on the regulation of the extracellular matrix in human trabec-ular meshwork cells under chronic oxidative stress. *Mol. Vis.* **2009**, *15*, 2488.
129. Villarreal, G.; Chatterjee, A.; Oh, S.S.; Oh, D.J.; Kang, M.H.; Rhee, D.J. Canonical wnt signaling regulates extracellular matrix expres-sion in the trabecular meshwork. *Investig. Ophthalmol. Vis. Sci.* **2014**, *55*, 7433–7440. [CrossRef]
130. Webber, H.C.; Bermudez, J.Y.; Sethi, A.; Clark, A.F.; Mao, W. Crosstalk between TGFβ and Wnt signaling pathways in the human trabecular meshwork. *Exp. Eye Res.* **2016**, *148*, 97–102. [CrossRef]
131. Youngblood, H.; Cai, J.; Drewry, M.D.; Helwa, I.; Hu, E.; Liu, S.; Yu, H.; Mu, H.; Hu, Y.; Perkumas, K.; et al. Expression of mRNAs, miRNAs, and lncRNAs in Human Trabecular Meshwork Cells Upon Mechanical Stretch. *Investig. Ophthalmol. Vis. Sci.* **2020**, *61*, 2. [CrossRef]
132. Yu, J.; Luo, H.; Li, N.; Duan, X. Suppression of Type I Collagen Expression by miR-29b Via PI3K, Akt, and Sp1 Pathway, Part II: An in Vivo Investigation. *Investig. Ophthalmol. Vis. Sci.* **2015**, *56*, 6019. [CrossRef] [PubMed]
133. Gallant-Behm, C.L.; Propp, S.; Jackson, A. Inhibition of ocular fibrosis with a miR-29b mimic. *Investig. Ophthalmol. Vis. Sci.* **2018**, *59*, 5316.
134. Wahid, F.; Shehzad, A.; Khan, T.; Kim, Y.Y. MicroRNAs: Synthesis, mechanism, function, and recent clinical trials. *Biochim. Et Biophys. Acta Mol. Cell Res.* **2010**, *1803*, 1231–1243. [CrossRef]
135. Baumann, V.; Winkler, J. miRNA-based therapies: Strategies and delivery platforms for oligonucleotide and non-oligonucleotide agents. *Future Med. Chem.* **2014**, *6*, 1967–1984. [CrossRef]
136. Berber, P.; Grassmann, F.; Kiel, C.; Weber, B.H.F. An Eye on Age-Related Macular Degeneration: The Role of MicroRNAs in Disease Pathology. *Mol. Diagn. Ther.* **2016**, *21*, 31–43. [CrossRef] [PubMed]
137. Li, H.; Ye, Z.; Li, Z. Identification of the potential biological target molecules related to primary open-angle glaucoma. *BMC Ophthalmol.* **2022**, *22*, 188. [CrossRef]

International Journal of
Molecular Sciences

MDPI

Review

Neuromyelitis Optica Spectrum Disorder: From Basic Research to Clinical Perspectives

Tzu-Lun Huang [1,2,*], Jia-Kang Wang [1,2,3,4,5], Pei-Yao Chang [1,2], Yung-Ray Hsu [1,2], Cheng-Hung Lin [2,6], Kung-Hung Lin [7] and Rong-Kung Tsai [8,9,*]

1 Department of Ophthalmology, Far Eastern Memorial Hospital, Banqiao Dist., New Taipei City 220, Taiwan; jiakangw2158@gmail.com (J.-K.W.); peiyao@seed.net.tw (P.-Y.C.); scherzoray@gmail.com (Y.-R.H.)
2 Department of Electrical Engineering, Yuan Ze University, Chung-Li, Taoyuan 320, Taiwan; chlin@saturn.yzu.edu.tw
3 Department of Medicine, National Yang-Ming University, Taipei City 112, Taiwan
4 Department of Medicine, National Taiwan University, Taipei City 106, Taiwan
5 Department of Healthcare Administration and Department of Nursing, Oriental Institute of Technology, New Taipei City 220, Taiwan
6 Biomedical Engineering Research Center, Yuan Ze University, Taoyuan 320, Taiwan
7 Department of Neurology, Taiwan Adventist Hospital, Taipei City 105, Taiwan; kksao.lin@gmail.com
8 Institute of Eye Research, Hualien Tzu Chi Hospital, Buddhist Tzu Chi Medical Foundation, Tzu Chi University, 707 Sec. 3 Chung-Yung Road, Hualien 970, Taiwan
9 Institute of Medical Sciences, Tzu Chi University, Hualien 970, Taiwan
* Correspondence: huang.tzulum@gmail.com (T.-L.H.); rktsai@tzuchi.com.tw (R.-K.T.); Tel.: +886-3-8561825 (ext. 2112) (R.-K.T.); Fax: +886-3-8577161 (R.-K.T.)

Abstract: Neuromyelitis optica spectrum disorder (NMOSD) is an inflammatory disease of the central nervous system characterized by relapses and autoimmunity caused by antibodies against the astrocyte water channel protein aquaporin-4. Over the past decade, there have been significant advances in the biologic knowledge of NMOSD, which resulted in the IDENTIFICATION of variable disease phenotypes, biomarkers, and complex inflammatory cascades involved in disease pathogenesis. Ongoing clinical trials are looking at new treatments targeting NMOSD relapses. This review aims to provide an update on recent studies regarding issues related to NMOSD, including the pathophysiology of the disease, the potential use of serum and cerebrospinal fluid cytokines as disease biomarkers, the clinical utilization of ocular coherence tomography, and the comparison of different animal models of NMOSD.

Keywords: neuromyelitis optica spectrum disease; aquaporin-4; myelin oligodendrocyte glycoprotein; ocular coherence tomography; complement; microcystic macular degeneration; Müller cell; astrocyte; oligodendrocyte; microglia

Citation: Huang, T.-L.; Wang, J.-K.; Chang, P.-Y.; Hsu, Y.-R.; Lin, C.-H.; Lin, K.-H.; Tsai, R.-K. Neuromyelitis Optica Spectrum Disorder: From Basic Research to Clinical Perspectives. *Int. J. Mol. Sci.* **2022**, *23*, 7908. https://doi.org/10.3390/ijms23147908

Academic Editor: Zsuzsanna Helyes

Received: 8 June 2022
Accepted: 15 July 2022
Published: 18 July 2022

1. Introduction

Neuromyelitis optica spectrum disorder (NMOSD) is a common cause of optic neuritis (ON) in Taiwan. In 2015, the prevalence of NMOSD was 1.47/100,000, and the age-standardized annual incidence rate was 0.61/100,000 person-years [1]. The reported prevalence of NMOSD in different racial groups is approximately 1/100,000 in White individuals, 3.5/100,000 in Asians, and 10/100,000 in Black individuals [2]. The differential diagnosis of NMOSD and multiple sclerosis (MS) was challenging until the discovery of neuromyelitis optica (NMO) autoantibodies by Lennon et al. [3,4]. In most cases, NMOSD is caused by pathogenic NMO immunoglobulin G (IgG) autoantibodies that bind to the aquaporin-4 (AQP4) target antigen, a water channel expressed on the end-feet membranes of astrocytes along the blood–brain barrier (BBB) and in Müller cells distributed on the fovea centralis in the retina [4–9]. The pathology most often occurs in the periventricular zone, involving astrocyte plasma membrane domains facing the pia and vessels, whereas the least-affected site in the central nervous system (CNS) is the area postrema in the dorsal medulla [10,11].

Currently, the clinical diagnosis of NMOSD is mainly based on the detection of serum NMO-IgG (AQP4-IgG) antibodies and the presence of core symptoms included in the diagnostic criteria developed by the International Panel for NMO Diagnosis in 2015 (Table 1) [10,12,13]. The revised criteria that replaced the previous 2006 criteria for NMO diagnosis resulted in a significant increase in the diagnostic sensitivity of NMOSD by 76% (62% in the AQP4-IgG-positive group and 14% in the seronegative group) [14]. For AQP4-IgG-positive patients, at least one of six sites within the CNS, including the spinal cord, optic nerves, area postrema, diencephalon, brainstem, and cerebrum, must be attacked. In seronegative patients, at least two core sites have to be affected and additional magnetic resonance imaging (MRI) criteria fulfilled [13]. The rate of seropositivity for myelin oligodendrocyte glycoprotein (MOG-IgG) antibodies in AQP4-IgG-seronegative patients with NMOSD was reported to reach up to 41.6% [15].

Table 1. NMOSD diagnostic criteria for adult patients.

Diagnostic criteria for NMOSD with AQP4 IgG

1. At least one core clinical characteristic
2. Positive test for AQP-IgG using an available detection method (CBA recommended)
3. Exclusion of alternative diagnoses

Diagnostic criteria for NMOSD without AQP4-IgG or NMOSD with unknown AQP4-IgG status

1. At least two core clinical characteristics occurring as a result of one or more clinical attacks and meeting all the following requirements:
    a. At least one core clinical characteristic must be optic neuritis, acute myelitis with longitudinal extensive neuritis, acute myelitis with LETM, or area postrema syndrome
    b. Dissemination in space (two or more different core clinical characteristics)
    c. Fulfillment of additional MRI criteria *
2. Negative tests of AQP4-IgG using an available detection method, or testing unavailable
3. Exclusion of alternative diagnoses

Core clinical characteristics

1. Optic neuritis
2. Acute myelitis
3. Area postrema syndrome: episode of otherwise unexplained hiccups or nausea and vomiting
4. Acute brainstem syndrome
5. Symptomatic narcolepsy or acute diencephalic clinical syndrome with NMOSD-typical diencephalic MRI lesions
6. Symptomatic cerebral syndrome with NMOSD-typical brain lesions

Modified IPND 2015 NMOSD Criteria [13].

*** Additional MRI criteria**

1. Acute optic neuritis: requires brain MRI showing normal findings or only nonspecific white matter lesions, or optic nerve MRI with T2-hyperintense lesion or T1-weighted gadolinium-enhancing lesion extending >1/2 optic nerve length or involving optic chiasm.
2. Acute myelitis: requires associated intramedullary MRI lesion extending ≥3 contiguous segments (LETM) OR ≥3 contiguous segments of focal spinal cord atrophy.
3. Area postrema syndrome: requires associated dorsal medulla/area postrema lesions.
4. Acute brainstem syndrome: requires associated periependymal brainstem lesions.

Abbreviations: NMOSD = neuromyelitis optica spectrum disorders; AQP4 = aquaporin-4; LETM = longitudinal extensive transverse myelitis; CBA = cell-based assay.

From the perspective of clinical application, biological biomarkers may be important for predicting the future risk of relapse and disease prognosis [10,16]. AQP4-IgG antibody titers seem to be linked to clinical presentation and immune response, with higher titers associated with worse visual function and more extensive cerebral involvement on MRI [16]. On the other hand, AQP4-IgG antibodies might represent a byproduct resulting from complex immunoinflammatory processes in NMOSD, with no significant variations in antibody titers between different disease stages [17]. Beyond autoantibodies, the clinical presentation and demographic features may be more reliable in terms of prognosis prediction [18]. Age was reported to be predictive of the involvement site, and ON seems to be the most common inflammatory lesion in NMOSD patients younger than 30 years [19].

AQP4-IgG-seropositive NMOSD indicates the entity of astrocytopathy, and MOG-IgG is a protein expressed by oligodendrocytes on the most superficial surface of myelin sheaths, which results in oligodendropathy [20–22]. MOG antibody-associated disease (MOGAD) exhibits different clinical features from those of AQP4-IgG-seropositive NMOSD [23–25]. The phenotype difference between AQP4-IgG- and MOG-IgG-positive ON can be assessed by the length of the optic nerve involvement and preferable involvement site on MRI, the morphology of the optic disc, laterality, and the pattern of the ganglion cell–inner plexiform layer (GC-IPL) on optical coherence tomography (OCT) [24,26]. MRI image characteristics add evidence to the differential diagnosis of ON. AQP4-ON preferentially presents with a longer, more unilateral, more posterior portion of the optic nerve with T1 gadolinium enhancement [13,27,28]. In contrast, MOG-ON usually presents with a longer, more bilateral and more anterior portion of the optic nerve accompanied by intraorbital optic nerve swelling and perineural T1 gadolinium enhancement [29].

Sex difference is low due to the higher proportion of males in the MOGAD group compared with that in the AQP4-IgG group. For MOGAD, 41% (7/17 case) to 44% (4/9 case) of female cases were noted [24,30]. MOG-ON may present at multiple ages and shows no sex bias, but the female/male ratio is 7.2:1.0 in the AQP4-ON group [26,29,31]. Moreover, only 9% of MOG-IgG-positive cases have a concurrent autoimmune disorder, and 80% of MOGAD cases will relapse but have a better clinical prognosis [32,33].

Although most neuronal damage occurs during the first episode, the treatment of a relapse episode in patients with NMOSD is essential for preserving as much of the neuron reservoir as possible. Most patients with NMOSD achieve good functional improvement after corticosteroid treatment and add-on plasmapheresis in the acute stage. However, clinical relapse occurs in most cases, resulting in cumulative neurologic damage. The new strategies may provide additional options for patients who are refractory to current maintenance therapies including treatments interfering with eosinophilic function, monoclonal antibodies that target neutrophil elastase, complement activation, interleukin IL-6 receptor (IL-6R) signaling, and plasma cells producing AQP4, and MOG-IgG antibodies [34–40]. Recently, three monoclonal antibody therapies approved by the Food and Drug Administration for the treatment of NMOSD demonstrated safety and efficacy in reducing the risk of relapse during remission; these are eculizumab (inhibitor of complement protein C5), inebilizumab (humanized monoclonal antibody against CD19 B cell protein), and satralizumab (humanized recombinant monoclonal antibody targeting IL-6R).

2. The Pathogenesis of NMOSD

AQP4 contributes to the stabilization of extracellular osmolality during neuronal activity. Moreover, it maintains glutamate homeostasis and energy balance as well as buffers the metabolic load in the BBB [5,41]. The pathological features of NMOSD include activated complement with extensive vasculocentric immune complex deposition, the loss of AQP4 expression in astrocytes, neutrophil/macrophage/microglial infiltration and eosinophil degranulation, myelin loss, and thickened hyalinization blood [4,5,42–45].The two major AQP4 isoforms, M1 and M23, exhibit locational and maturational differences in the ratio of M1 to M23 proteins along the astrocytic membrane, which possibly determines the pathogenicity and a different anatomical distribution in the CNS and at different stages of CNS maturation in pediatric and adult patients [46–49]. The proportion of the largest AQP4 aggregate is the highest in the optic nerve followed by the spinal cord; this is relevant to why NMO selectively targets the CNS tissue and spares non-CNS AQP4-expressing tissues [50]. The M1 protein is completely internalized, but M23 resists internalization and activates the complement more efficiently than M1 when bound by the antigen [46,51]. The relative components of AQP4 isoforms are tissue-specific, with an approximate 3:1 ratio of AQP4-M23 to AQP4-M1 in rat brain [52]. Formation of supramolecular structures, called orthogonal arrays of particles (OAPs), by AQP4 is essential in NMOSD pathogenesis and enhances complement-dependent cytotoxicity (CDC) by the pathogenic AQP4-IgG [53]. It remains unclear if the OAP composition varies in pediatric and adult patients or whether OAP differences may cause different phenotypes [54].

Müller cells and neuronal axons are the main targets in an experimental model of NMO [55]. After intravitreal injection of AQP4-IgG antibodies, complement activation and immunoglobulin deposition was found in Müller cells and caused a retinal pathology [56]. AQP4 is also coexpressed with the Kir4.1 potassium channel subunit in cells, and the electrogenic bicarbonate transporter contributes to changes in the extracellular space, involved in buffering K+ [8]. In clinical practice, Müller cell dysfunction was shown to significantly reduce the b-wave amplitude in the scotopic electroretinogram of AQP4-IgG-positive patients compared with normal controls [57]. However, the results were inconclusive regarding a relationship between the b-wave amplitude and the volume of the outer retinal segment on OCT as well as disease severity, assessed on the basis of the Expanded Disability Status Scale (EDSS) or visual acuity [57].

3. Cytotoxicity Pathway

Complement-dependent cytotoxicity (CDC), complement-dependent cellular cytotoxicity (CDCC), and antibody-dependent cellular cytotoxicity (ADCC) are responsible for astrocyte injury in NMOSD [58,59]. ADCC seems to play a main role in facilitating macrophage and natural killer (NK) cell activation after binding to the CH3 region of IgG antibodies via the effector cells' Fc receptors in the outer zone of developing lesions (penumbra) [59–61]. In CDC, antibody binding to a target antigen triggers the classic complement pathway and results in the formation of the membrane attack complex (MAC). In CDCC, another protein, C3b, is expressed during the complement cascade activation and interacts with NK cells and macrophages to facilitate cell lysis [62].

Peripheral autoimmune dysregulation starts after the modulation of peripheral T cells. Pathogenic autoreactive T cells (Th17 cells) and IL-6 disrupt BBB tight junctions, resulting in CNS inflammation due to the effect of numerous chemokines and cytokines (Figure 1) [63–65]. IL-6 is a proinflammatory cytokine that amplifies inflammation, increases the survival of plasmablasts capable of producing AQP4-IgG antibodies, supports the differentiation of B cells to plasma cells, and induces BBB injury [66,67]. Because B cells and autoantibodies were found to be disease beginners in experimental autoimmune encephalomyelitis (EAE), inebilizumab is instructive for modeling the therapeutic effects with enhanced ADCC against CD19-positive B cells, as confirmed in MS and NMOSD [68,69].

The activation of the complement cascade in patients with NMOSD was reported to increase membrane permeability and promote the influx of serum AQP4-IgG antibodies, which further amplified the inflammatory reaction at the BBB of the CNS [70]. Basic research demonstrated that AQP4 antibodies trigger the complement system and lead to MAC formation via the CDC pathway, which results in astrocyte damage and secondary neuronal injury [71,72]. C1q-targeted monoclonal antibodies were demonstrated to effectively inhibit AQP4-IgG-mediated CDC, which interfered with MAC, and also IgG-mediated CDCC, which influenced the formation of the Cb3–Cb3R complex on macrophage and NK cells in an in vivo study [73]. Eculizumab is a humanized monoclonal antibody that inhibits terminal C5 complement protein cleavage into the C5a (inducing proinflammatory activity) and C5b fragments (inducing the MAC formation) [74–76]. Serum C4 levels were found to be lower in patients with AQP4-IgG-positive NMOSD in clinical remission than in those with MOGAD and MS as well as in healthy controls [77]. Immune features and the cytokine profile in the cerebrospinal fluid (CSF) significantly vary in patients with MS, AQP4-positive NMOSD, and MOGAD, suggesting that these are different autoimmune demyelinating diseases [78,79]. The role of complement in MOGAD has not been fully elucidated so far. It is possible that MOG-IgG could cause reversible myelin damage without complement activation [80]. On the other hand, a subset of human MOG-IgG antibodies was shown to induce complement-dependent pathogenic effects in a murine animal model [81]. Increased levels of proteins indicating classic and alternative complement activation were observed in patients with MOGAD compared with the control groups. Therefore, complement activation could be a potential therapeutic target in patients with MOGAD [82].

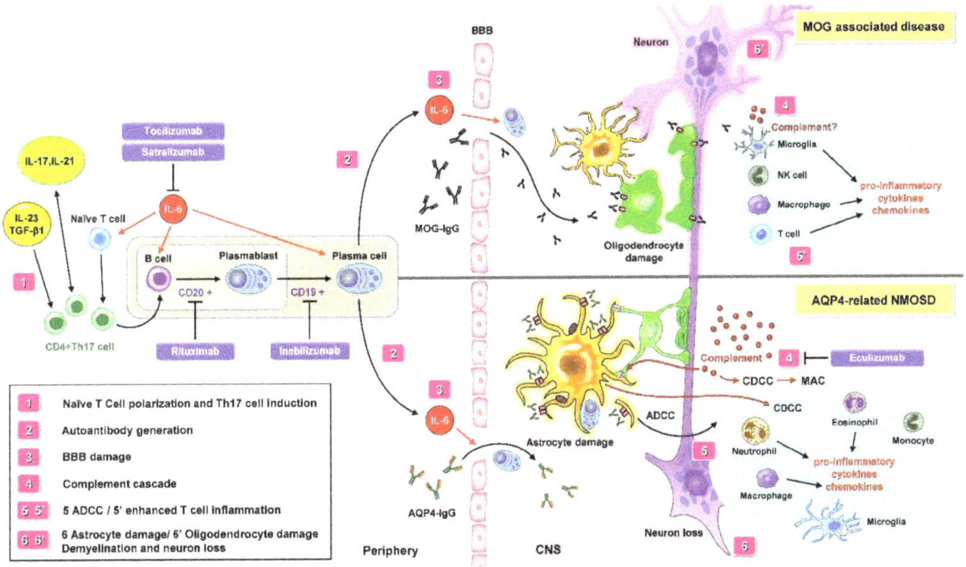

Figure 1. The pathological mechanism of NMOSD may involve peripheral autoimmune dysregulation. Interleukin 6 (IL-6) is a key factor in AQP4-related NMOSD pathophysiology. A similar role of IL-6 is also reported in MOG-associated disease (MOGAD). Besides IL-6, Th17 cells differentiation may be induced by IL-17, IL-21, IL-23, and TGF-β1. It is thought that an impaired innate immune system may promote naive T cell transformation into Th 17 cell and stimulate B cell differentiation to plasmablasts, then to plasma cells producing AQP4-IgG or MOG-IgG autoantibody. A leaky BBB contributes to the migration of AQP4-IgG from the periphery into the CNS. AQP4-IgG bind to AQP4 and activate the complement cascade (CDC and CDCC) and ADCC. Cytokine and chemokine production leads to the recruitment of macrophages, eosinophils, neutrophils, and monocytes to the inflammation site. After microglia and macrophage infiltration, astrocytes and oligodendrocyte are damaged, which leads to advanced axonal degeneration and neuronal death. AQP4-IgG-seropositivity in NMOSD indicates the entity of astrocytopathy, and MOG-IgG results in oligodendropathy, named MOGAD. Current maintenance therapies include interfering with complement activation (Eculizumab), IL-6 R signaling (Tocilizumab and Satralizumab), and plasma cells producing AQP-4 and MOG IgG Abs (Rituximab and Inebilizumab). Abbreviations: NMOSD = neuromyelitis optica spectrum disorders; BBB = blood–brain barrier; CDC = complement-dependent cytotoxicity; CDCC = complement-dependent cellular cytotoxicity; ADCC = antibody-dependent cellular cytotoxicity; MOG = myelin oligodendrocyte glycoprotein; AQP-4 = aquaporin-4; IL-6 = interleukin 6; IL-17 = interleukin 17; Th17 cell = T helper 17 cell; TGF-β1 = transforming growth factor beta 1; IL-6 R = IL-6 receptor.

The new evidence on NMOSD pathophysiology highlights promising treatment modalities as well as clinical studies [83]. Restoring immune tolerance might provide an interesting treatment strategy in the future [84]. Some success was achieved by using autologous hematopoietic stem cell transplantation [85], peptide-loaded tolerogenic dendritic cells [86], DNA vaccine encoding myelin basic protein, [87], autoreactive T cell vaccination, and regulatory T cells [88,89]. Further alternative targets for NMOSD treatments are the blood–brain barrier, [90], the complement cascade [91], and B cells [92].

4. Genetic Susceptibility to NMOSD

Despite important breakthroughs in the understanding of AQP4 and MOG antibodies and their involvement in NMOSD, the genetic factors underlying the disease pathogenesis have not been fully understood. More recently, genome-wide single-nucleotide polymorphism arrays have shown some susceptibility loci for NMOSD [93]. It is predominantly a sporadic disorder, although familial NMOSD occurs in 3% of the cases [93,94]. Human leukocyte antigen (HLA) haplotypes were reported to be highly correlated with NMOSD. HLA is located on chromosome 6, and the main variations are observed in DQA1, DQB1, DRB1, and DPB1 [95–97]. Whole-genome sequence studies that have been conducted in Europeans since 2009 identified a C4A deletion and a fourfold reduction of C4a levels as the most likely functional drivers of an increased risk for AQP4-IgG production. Furthermore, HLA-DQA1*102, HLA-DQA1*501, HLA-DQB1*0201, and HLA-DRB1*03 alleles were significantly associated with NMOSD [96,98]. In Japan, Ogawa et al. found that HLA-DQA1*05:03 was significantly associated with NMOSD, whereas Watanabe et al. reported that HLA-DRB1*08:02 and HLA-DPB1*05:01 were associated with susceptibility to NMOSD and that HLA-DRB1*09:01 was protective against NMOSD [99–101]. In addition, distinct genetic and infectious profiles in Japanese patients with NMOSD demonstrated that the HLA-DRB1*1602 and HLA-DPB1*0501 alleles as well as infection with *Helicobacter pylori* and *Chlamydia pneumonia* were associated with higher susceptibility to AQP4-IgG-seropositive NMOSD [102]. Future studies should evaluate response to treatment as well as genetic and cytokine profiles in association with distinct genetic backgrounds in patients with NMOSD.

In summary, the potential molecular mechanisms underlying AQP4-seropositive NMOSD may be related to proteins encoded by the novel genes involved in complement activation, antigen presentation, antibody-dependent cytotoxicity, and immune regulation [103].

5. Potential Biomarkers in NMOSD

5.1. Surrogate Serum Biomarkers

Evidence shows that AQP-4 IgG antibodies are not strongly associated with clinical indices, such as the EDSS, risk of relapse, or visual prognosis in NMOSD [17]. On the other hand, there are data suggesting that the activation of complements, cytokines, and chemokines contributes to the complex pathogenesis of the disorder [104,105]. Naive T-helper cells differentiate into a new lineage called Th17 and have the capacity to produce large amounts of IL-17, a cytokine linked to autoimmune diseases [67,106]. IL-6 signaling involving Th17 cells and Th17-associated cytokines may play a crucial role in the pathogenesis of NMOSD (Figure 1) [66,107–110]. Apart from IL-17, Th17-cell differentiation may be induced by IL-6, IL-23, and transforming growth factor β1 [111,112]. Granulocyte macrophage colony-stimulating factor acts as a proinflammatory cytokine and could critically be involved in the formation of Th17 cells and the activation of macrophages and dendritic cells involving the secretion IL-23 and IL-6 [113]. Patients with NMOSD were shown to have higher levels of IL-6, IL-17, and IL-21 in both CSF and serum, as well as higher levels of IL-1, IL-8, IL-13, and granulocyte colony-stimulating factor in the CSF than those with MS [66,107]. The IL-6 levels in CSF correlate with neural damage biomarkers in NMOSD, and increased plasma IL-6 levels correlate with the EDSS [114]. As for the pathological mechanisms, IL6 signaling is thought to contribute in multiple ways, as shown in Figure 1. Two monoclonal antibodies, satralizumab and tocilizumab, activate the same mechanism, in that they both target IL-6 receptor- (IL-6R) and IL-6-associated immune cascades, leading to T-cell activation, IgG secretion, BBB damage, activation of the complement cascade, and enhancement of macrophage and microglia activity [84,109,115,116]. In a novel in vitro BBB model, the proposed role of IL-6 on the BBB was confirmed [117]. AQP4-IgG induced IL-6 release from astrocytes, then the BBB was impaired by IL-6 signaling in endothelial cells, and reversal of the BBB impairment was enhanced by anti-IL-6 receptor (IL-6R) antibodies [110,118,119].

Complex processes involving activated microglia ultimately promote the pathological course of NMOSD, and that suggests that microglia may serve as a therapeutic target in NMO [120]. Briefly, complement C3a secreted from activated astrocytes may induce the secretion of complement C1q and inflammatory cytokines by microglia, facilitating injury to microglia, astrocytes, oligodendrocytes, and neurons in an autocrine or paracrine manner [121].

Serum biomarkers including glial fibrillary acidic protein (GFAP) and neurofilament light chain (NfL) may help guide the design of effective therapies for the management of disease [22,26,122–124]. In a subgroup analysis, the CSF levels of IL-6, NfL, and GFAP were higher in AQP4-IgG-positive cases and might be used as indicators of disease activity, relapse risk, and therapy efficacy [124–126]. Factors involving the tight junctions seem to be other candidates for key biomarkers. Epidermal growth factor may be involved in the disruption of the BBB by downregulating claudin-5 in NMOSD, and women were shown to exhibit higher urinary levels of this factors, which might explain their greater susceptibility to NMOSD [127]. Interferon-γ reduces BBB integrity in cultured brain endothelial cells through Rho kinase-mediated cytoskeletal contraction, causing junction irregularity and cell–cell disconnections leading to deformity in adherence and tight junction proteins [128,129]. Serum vascular endothelial growth factor, myeloid progenitor inhibitory factor 1, and neuron–glia-related cell-adhesion molecule were positively associated with AQP4-IgG titers; thus, they could be potential biomarkers of NMOSD [127]. A study on plasma chemokine levels in NMOSD during remission confirmed that IL-1β and tumor necrosis factor α stimulate eosinophilic chemoattraction, suggesting that the elevated secretion of monocyte chemotactic protein (C–C motif chemokine ligand 13, CCL13) and eotaxins (CCL11 and CCL26) may be a critical step in eosinophil recruitment during remission [130].

5.2. OCT Biomarker

The international CROCTINO program uses OCT as a standardized method to assess the clinical course and pathophysiology of NMOSD as well as to monitor therapeutic efficacy [131,132]. OCT was shown to provide unique insights into the identification of foveal pitting in NMOSD likely due to the loss of Müller cells [133].

6. Optic Nerve Structure in NMOSD

The use of OCT to discriminate the microstructures of the retinal nerve fiber layer and GC-IPL has been debated in recent studies on NMOSD and MS. Moreover, while current therapies were demonstrated to improve the visual function after acute treatment, structural improvement remains an unmet need. GC-IPL thickness associated with visual ability in NMOSD-ON eyes leads to more severe retinal thinning and visual impairment than that found in MS [134]. A cross-sectional collaborative retrospective study reported that the average GC-IPL loss was 22.7 µm after the first ON attack, and the average loss after a recurrent episode was 3.5 µm, with noticeable subclinical GC-IPL loss in non-optic neuritis (NON) eyes [132]. NMOSD-NON eyes exhibited reduced thickness in the GC-IPL but not in the pRNFL compared with normal eyes, and relative changes in the parvocellular layer of NMOSD-NON eyes were not fully confirmed in recent studies [132,134,135]. Due to the presence of numerous confounding factors when determining the thickness of the anterior visual pathway, parafoveal segmentation on OCT may enable a more sensitive detection of neuronal loss and reflect a neurodegenerative reaction of retinal ganglion cells (RGC) and Müller cell damage in NMOSD [136,137]. Contrarily, pRNFL in the papillomacular bundle exhibited a reduction in MS-NON due to parvocellular axons being more vulnerable to energy depletion in MS studies [138–140]. GC-IPL damage on OCT spatial relationship and papillomacular bundle loss in neurodegenerative disease such as mitochondriopathy or neuroinflammmatory disease require further research to elucidate the damage in the megacellular and parvocellular layers in the lateral genicular nucleus [139,141]. There were no significant differences in the annual changes in mGC-IPL, pRNFL, total macular volume, and disc cup ratio in the NMOSD-ON eyes when comparing patients treated with different immunosuppressive therapies [142].

7. Macular Structure in NMOSD

The foveal structure on OCT has been discussed as a potential biomarker of NMOSD. The foveal structure, including foveal pit shape, depth or total macular volume (mm^3), or central foveal thickness, may be an early diagnostic marker of NMOSD [136,143,144]. This hypothesis is supported by data from animal studies, which showed Müller cell death after intravitreal injection of AQP4 antibodies and revealed a lysosomal degradation mechanism for AQP4 loss on Müller cells [145].

In the parafoveal region, which is rich in astrocytes and AQP4-expressing Müller cells, a positive association between attack-independent neural loss and visual function was observed [57]. Microcystic macular degeneration (MMD) may contribute to loss in both high- and low-contrast visual testing after an NMOSD-ON episode [136,137]. The inner nuclear layer (INL) and outer retinal layer were thicker in the NMOSD-ON eyes compared with NMOSD-NON and control healthy eyes, due to the presence of MMD in the episode of ON [134,137,146]. MMD is predominantly localized in the INL, but also extends to the outer nuclear layer [136]. Interestingly, a previous study demonstrated that the INL thickness was negatively correlated with the GC-IPL content in NMOSD [147].

To date, there have been no cross-sectional and longitudinal studies to elucidate whether MMD is a temporary change or secondary to optic neuropathy. Although the pathophysiologic mechanism of MMD in NMO is complex, degeneration is believed to be caused by the disruption of the blood–retinal barrier and the transition of microglial cells to phagocytose apoptotic RGCs [148]. Another possibility is vitreomacular traction, but fluorescein angiography is needed to confirm the cause–effect relationship [149]. MMD exhibited no progression over a 20-month follow-up, and the risk of MMD was observed in 4.7% of patients with MS and in 13.3–26% of patients with NMOSD [136,137,150]. MMD is not a specific sign of NMOSD, and the exclusion of other secondary insults, such as uveitis, diabetes, or Fingolimod exposure, is required [150,151]. In hereditary optic neuropathy, MMD may be associated with vitreomacular traction or the epiphenomenon of optic atrophy, unrelated to inflammation or retrograde transsynaptic degeneration [152]. In advanced glaucomatous optic atrophy, MMD in the superior and nasal macular quadrants was also documented on OCT [147]. Furthermore, the INL cyst secondary to retinitis pigmentosa was not an uncommon sign [153,154].

To summarize, INL cystoid lesions are a nonspecific indicator of degenerative optic neuropathy or retinopathy, and MMD could be linked to Müller cell pathology in NMOSD [155–157]. However, further research is required to prove this hypothesis.

8. OCT Angiography in NMOSD

Subclinical vascular changes in the parafoveal retina might occur during an ON attack and could be associated with astrocyte damage with increased levels of sNfL/sGFAP [158]. Patients with NMOSD exhibited an enlargement of the foveal avascular zone independent of an ON attack [158]. This could be explained by damage of the blood–retinal barrier resulting from Müller cell loss, leading to the enlargement of the foveal avascular zone on OCT angiography in patients with NMOSD but not in those with MS [137,144,158,159]. A strong correlation between the deep vascular complex and visual acuity was reported, and decreased microvascular density in the superficial and deep vascular complex was significantly correlated with the frequency of NMO-ON attacks [160]. OCT angiography with a measurable analysis offers a new possibilities in the study of microvascular impairment in NMOSD and may become an objective clinical tool for patient monitoring.

9. Animal Models of Neuromyelitis Optica

The available animal models of NMO are largely based on a passive transfer of AQP4-IgG antibodies or AQP4-sensitized T cells to rodents and are often combined with proinflammatory maneuvers (coinfusion of proinflammatory factors or additional needle trauma) [60,161–163]. The models exhibit T cell and B cell activation, macrophage/microglial infiltration, eosinophil aggregation, immune complex deposition, loss of AQP4 and GFAP expression, and astrocyte/axonal injury [42,45,60,162] (Table 2). There are currently two main methods for generating animal models of NMO: one is NMO-IgG immunization in the EAE model [162–166], and the other is coinjection of the NMO-IgG/human complement into the target, which can be a route of intraventricular, intra-spinal cord, perichiasmal, or transoptic nerve sheath [42,92,161,167–170].

Table 2. Animal models of NMO-optic neuritis without experimental autoimmune encephalomyelitis.

Reference	Animal	Model System	Significance
Matsumoto et al., 2014 [169]	Adult Lewis rats	NMO patients' sera were applied on the optic nerve after desheathing	7 days after treatment: lost expression of both AQP4 and GFAP on IHC, leading to regional astrocytic degeneration and inflammatory cell invasion, which resulted in secondary loss of RGCs and their axons
Asavapanumas et al., 2014 [42]	8- to 10-week-old, weight-matched AQP4+/+ and AQP4−/− mice in CD1 genetic background	Passive transfer of NMO-IgG and complement by continuous 3-day intracranial infusion near the optic chiasm	Loss of AQP4 and GFAP immunoreactivity, granulocyte and macrophage infiltration, deposition of activated complement, and demyelination and axonal loss
Asavapanumas et al., 2014 [161]	Adult Lewis rats	A single intracerebral needle insertion, without pre-existing inflammation or infusion of proinflammatory factors	At 5 days, there was marked loss of AQP4, GFAP, and myelin. Granulocyte and macrophage infiltration, complement deposition, BBB disruption, microglial activation, and neuron death. The penumbra was associated with a complement-independent mechanism (antibody-dependent cellular cytotoxicity).
Saadoun et al., 2010 [92]	8- to 10-week-old, wild-type and AQP4-null mice on a CD1 genetic background	Intracerebral coinjection of Ig G from NMO patients with human complement	Within 12 h of injection, striking loss of AQP4, glial cell edema, demyelination, and axonal loss, but little intraparenchymal inflammation. At 7 days, there was extensive inflammatory cell infiltration, perivascular deposition of activated complement, extensive demyelination and loss of astrocytes, and neuronal cell death.

Abbreviations: NMO = neuromyelitis optica; AQP4 = aquaporin-4; IHC = immunohistochemistry; RGCs = retinal ganglion cells; GFAP = glial fibrillary acidic protein; BBB = blood–brain barrier.

10. Animal Model of NMO

Passive immunization by intraperitoneal injection of AQP4-specific T cells in EAE rats allows EAE to develop faster via specific targeting of the astrocytes and the entry of pathogenic AQP4 antibodies to produce NMO-like lesions in the CNS after 10 to 14 days from the injection [171]. The extent and location of inflammation and demyelination mainly vary according to the specific antigen introduced and rodent species and strain [170]. Lewis rats can produce high titers of antibodies against specific epitopes of human AQP4 [172]. However, Saadoun et al. recently demonstrated that the coinjection of NMO-IgG with human complement could produce NMO-like lesions in naive mice without EAE [92]. Asavapanumas et al. reported that a single intracerebral or intraperitoneal injection of NMO-IgG antibodies after intracerebral needle stab injury without the administration of complement or proinflammatory cytokines was able to produce a mouse model of NMO [60,161]. Evidence suggests that the coadministration of the complement is required for developing a complete NMO lesion but is not needed for the development of the penumbra, which emphasizes the pathogenic role of macrophage/microglia involving ADCC in NMO [59,60].

Studies demonstrated that a passive transfer by intravenous or intraperitoneal injection of the AQP4 antibodies from seropositive NMO patients was insufficient to cause NMO-like lesions in rodents, as the low levels of antibodies could not penetrate into the CNS [163,173]. When applying patient sera without any filtration modification, it is likely that coexisting human complements may play a synergic role in the development of strong neuroinflammation [169,174,175]. Optic nerve susceptibility in NMO might also arise from the abundant AQP4 expression along the optic nerve compared with the brain [65]. Aside from the optic nerve, AQP4 is also highly expressed in astrocyte-like Müller cells in the inner retina and the ciliary epithelium [7]. A study using intravitreal AQP4-IgG passive transfer resulted in a complement-independent retinal pathology that reduced AQP4 expression and increased GFAP levels by 5 days [145]. We summarize the rodent models regarding ON without existence of EAE in Table 2. The passive cotransfer of NMO-IgG antibodies and complement via a continuous 3-day infusion near the optic chiasm in mice seemed to be sufficient to develop NMO-ON [42]. However, continuous infusion with precise needle placement is technically challenging and might cause additional irreversible damage. On the other hand, retrobulbar infusion, intravitreal injection, or a single intracranial injection may result in a limited or transient pathology [42]. We believe that local retrobulbar injection of NMO-IgG-positive serum is difficult to perform, as this approach easily causes optic nerve unpredictable traumas. However, Matsumoto et al. injected human NMO-IgG-positive serum directly into the space of the optic nerve sheath after desheathing, which led to infiltration of inflammatory cells into the optic nerve and regional astrocyte loss with progressive loss of RGCs and demyelination at day 14 [169].

11. Limitations of the Animal Models of NMO

Although each model was shown to have features of human NMO-like lesions, multiple factors may limit direct comparisons between animal and human data. First, in human NMOSD, AQP4-IgG antibodies are produced continuously, then astrocyte loss is associated with loss of myelin. Second, astrocytes and RGCs in the human CNS and eye are more complex than in rodents [176,177]. Third, the coinjection of AQP4-IgG antibodies and complement can activate the complement system in rats but not in mice and may lead to underestimation of the complement inhibitory function. Finally, EAE models in rats are Th1-cell-mediated, whereas AQP4-specific T cells in NMO reportedly show a preferential involvement of Th17/Th2 lymphocytes including IL-6- and Th17-polarizing cytokine interactions [65,108,178].

Animal models may enable us to understand the early pathogenetic mechanisms in the immune cascade of nerve inflammation and develop potential drug therapies; however, they partially recapitulate the pathological features of human NMO in animal model as the complement system and humoral/cytotoxic immunity vary between different species [170,172,179].

12. Conclusions

NMOSD is a complex multifactorial neuroinflammatory disease; extensive research is ongoing on the pathogenesis, genetic background, serum biomarkers, OCT segmentation. Novel drugs targeting the complement cascade system, IL-6R, and B cells are being studied. Restoring the blood–brain barrier and enhancing immune tolerance by using stem cell transplantation, dendritic cells, vaccine and regulatory T cells might provide potential therapeutic strategies in the future. Animal models may help gain a better understanding of the detailed immune mechanisms involved and could lead to the development of potential future treatments, for example, based on the inhibition of AQP4 antibody formation that could prevent the activation of inflammatory cells and offer neuroprotection.

Author Contributions: T.-L.H., writing—original draft preparation; J.-K.W., resources; P.-Y.C., resources; Y.-R.H., investigation; C.-H.L., funding acquisition; K.-H.L., resources; R.-K.T., supervision. All authors have read and agreed to the published version of the manuscript.

Funding: Grant: Ministry of Science and Technology Taiwan (MOST 110-2221E155013).

Institutional Review Board Statement: Not applicable.

Informed Consent Statement: Not applicable.

Data Availability Statement: Not applicable.

Conflicts of Interest: The authors declare no conflict of interest.

References

1. Fang, C.W.; Wang, H.P.; Chen, H.M.; Lin, J.W.; Lin, W.S. Epidemiology and Comorbidities of Adult Multiple Sclerosis and Neuromyelitis Optica in Taiwan, 2001–2015. *Mult. Scler. Relat. Disord.* **2020**, *45*, 102425. [CrossRef]
2. Hor, J.Y.; Asgari, N.; Nakashima, I.; Broadley, S.A.; Leite, M.I.; Kissani, N.; Jacob, A.; Marignier, R.; Weinshenker, B.G.; Paul, F.; et al. Epidemiology of Neuromyelitis Optica Spectrum Disorder and Its Prevalence and Incidence Worldwide. *Front. Neurol.* **2020**, *11*, 501. [CrossRef] [PubMed]
3. Jarius, S.; Wildemann, B. The Case of the Marquis De Causan (1804): An Early Account of Visual Loss Associated with Spinal Cord Inflammation. *J. Neurol.* **2012**, *259*, 1354–1357. [CrossRef] [PubMed]
4. Lennon, V.A.; Wingerchuk, D.M.; Kryzer, T.J.; Pittock, S.J.; Lucchinetti, C.F.; Fujihara, K.; Nakashima, I.; Weinshenker, B.G. A Serum Autoantibody Marker of Neuromyelitis Optica: Distinction from Multiple Sclerosis. *Lancet* **2004**, *364*, 2106–2112. [CrossRef]
5. Roemer, S.F.; Parisi, J.E.; Lennon, V.A.; Benarroch, E.E.; Lassmann, H.; Bruck, W.; Mandler, R.N.; Weinshenker, B.G.; Pittock, S.J.; Wingerchuk, D.M.; et al. Pattern-Specific Loss of Aquaporin-4 Immunoreactivity Distinguishes Neuromyelitis Optica from Multiple Sclerosis. *Brain* **2007**, *130*, 1194–1205. [CrossRef] [PubMed]
6. Lennon, V.A.; Kryzer, T.J.; Pittock, S.J.; Verkman, A.S.; Hinson, S.R. Igg Marker of Optic-Spinal Multiple Sclerosis Binds to the Aquaporin-4 Water Channel. *J. Exp. Med.* **2005**, *202*, 473–477. [CrossRef] [PubMed]
7. Hamann, S.; Zeuthen, T.; La Cour, M.; Nagelhus, E.A.; Ottersen, O.P.; Agre, P.; Nielsen, S. Aquaporins in Complex Tissues: Distribution of Aquaporins 1–5 in Human and Rat Eye. *Am. J. Physiol.* **1998**, *274*, C1332–C1345. [CrossRef] [PubMed]
8. Nagelhus, E.A.; Mathiisen, T.M.; Ottersen, O.P. Aquaporin-4 in the Central Nervous System: Cellular and Subcellular Distribution and Coexpression with Kir4.1. *Neuroscience* **2004**, *129*, 905–913. [CrossRef]
9. Nagelhus, E.A.; Veruki, M.L.; Torp, R.; Haug, F.M.; Laake, J.H.; Nielsen, S.; Agre, P.; Ottersen, O.P. Aquaporin-4 Water Channel Protein in the Rat Retina and Optic Nerve: Polarized Expression in Muller Cells and Fibrous Astrocytes. *J. Neurosci.* **1998**, *18*, 2506–2519. [CrossRef]
10. Whittam, D.; Wilson, M.; Hamid, S.; Keir, G.; Bhojak, M.; Jacob, A. What's New in Neuromyelitis Optica? A Short Review for the Clinical Neurologist. *J. Neurol.* **2017**, *264*, 2330–2344. [CrossRef]
11. Nielsen, S.; Nagelhus, E.A.; Amiry-Moghaddam, M.; Bourque, C.; Agre, P.; Ottersen, O.P. Specialized Membrane Domains for Water Transport in Glial Cells: High-Resolution Immunogold Cytochemistry of Aquaporin-4 in Rat Brain. *J. Neurosci.* **1997**, *17*, 171–180. [CrossRef]
12. Trebst, C.; Jarius, S.; Berthele, A.; Paul, F.; Schippling, S.; Wildemann, B., Borisow, N.; Kleiter, I.; Aktas, O.; Kumpfel, T.; et al. Update on the Diagnosis and Treatment of Neuromyelitis Optica: Recommendations of the Neuromyelitis Optica Study Group (Nemos). *J. Neurol.* **2014**, *261*, 1–16. [CrossRef]
13. Wingerchuk, D.M.; Banwell, B.; Bennett, J.L.; Cabre, P.; Carroll, W.; Chitnis, T.; De Seze, J.; Fujihara, K.; Greenberg, B.; Jacob, A.; et al. International Consensus Diagnostic Criteria for Neuromyelitis Optica Spectrum Disorders. *Neurology* **2015**, *85*, 177–189. [CrossRef]
14. Hamid, S.H.; Elsone, L.; Mutch, K.; Solomon, T.; Jacob, A. The Impact of 2015 Neuromyelitis Optica Spectrum Disorders Criteria on Diagnostic Rates. *Mult. Scler.* **2017**, *23*, 228–233. [CrossRef]
15. Li, X.; Zhang, C.; Jia, D.; Fan, M.; Li, T.; Tian, D.C.; Liu, Y.; Shi, F.D. The Occurrence of Myelin Oligodendrocyte Glycoprotein Antibodies in Aquaporin-4-Antibody Seronegative Neuromyelitis Optica Spectrum Disorder: A Systematic Review and Meta-Analysis. *Mult. Scler. Relat. Disord.* **2021**, *53*, 103030. [CrossRef]
16. Takahashi, T.; Fujihara, K.; Nakashima, I.; Misu, T.; Miyazawa, I.; Nakamura, M.; Watanabe, S.; Shiga, Y.; Kanaoka, C.; Fujimori, J.; et al. Anti-Aquaporin-4 Antibody Is Involved in the Pathogenesis of Nmo: A Study on Antibody Titre. *Brain* **2007**, *130*, 1235–1243. [CrossRef]
17. Schmetzer, O.; Lakin, E.; Roediger, B.; Duchow, A.; Asseyer, S.; Paul, F.; Siebert, N. Anti-Aquaporin 4 Igg Is Not Associated with Any Clinical Disease Characteristics in Neuromyelitis Optica Spectrum Disorder. *Front. Neurol.* **2021**, *12*, 635419. [CrossRef]
18. Rotstein, D.; Kim, S.H.; Hacohen, Y.; Levy, M. Editorial: Epidemiology of Atypical Demyelinating Diseases. *Front. Neurol.* **2021**, *12*, 662353. [CrossRef]
19. Palace, J.; Lin, D.Y.; Zeng, D.; Majed, M.; Elsone, L.; Hamid, S.; Messina, S.; Misu, T.; Sagen, J.; Whittam, D.; et al. Outcome Prediction Models in Aqp4-Igg Positive Neuromyelitis Optica Spectrum Disorders. *Brain* **2019**, *142*, 1310–1323. [CrossRef]
20. Kitley, J.; Woodhall, M.; Waters, P.; Leite, M.I.; Devenney, E.; Craig, J.; Palace, J.; Vincent, A. Myelin-Oligodendrocyte Glycoprotein Antibodies in Adults with a Neuromyelitis Optica Phenotype. *Neurology* **2012**, *79*, 1273–1277. [CrossRef]

21. Probstel, A.K.; Dornmair, K.; Bittner, R.; Sperl, P.; Jenne, D.; Magalhaes, S.; Villalobos, A.; Breithaupt, C.; Weissert, R.; Jacob, U.; et al. Antibodies to Mog Are Transient in Childhood Acute Disseminated Encephalomyelitis. *Neurology* **2011**, *77*, 580–588. [CrossRef]
22. Kaneko, K.; Sato, D.K.; Nakashima, I.; Nishiyama, S.; Tanaka, S.; Marignier, R.; Hyun, J.W.; Oliveira, L.M.; Reindl, M.; Seifert-Held, T.; et al. Myelin Injury without Astrocytopathy in Neuroinflammatory Disorders with Mog Antibodies. *J. Neurol. Neurosurg. Psychiatry* **2016**, *87*, 1257–1259. [CrossRef] [PubMed]
23. Kim, H.; Lee, E.J.; Kim, S.; Choi, L.K.; Kim, K.; Kim, H.W.; Kim, K.K.; Lim, Y.M. Serum Biomarkers in Myelin Oligodendrocyte Glycoprotein Antibody-Associated Disease. *Neurol. Neuroimmunol. Neuroinflamm.* **2020**, *7*, e708. [CrossRef] [PubMed]
24. Tanaka, S.; Hashimoto, B.; Izaki, S.; Oji, S.; Fukaura, H.; Nomura, K. Clinical and Immunological Differences between Mog Associated Disease and Anti Aqp4 Antibody-Positive Neuromyelitis Optica Spectrum Disorders: Blood-Brain Barrier Breakdown and Peripheral Plasmablasts. *Mult. Scler. Relat. Disord.* **2020**, *41*, 102005. [CrossRef] [PubMed]
25. Fujihara, K.; Cook, L.J. Neuromyelitis Optica Spectrum Disorders and Myelin Oligodendrocyte Glycoprotein Antibody-Associated Disease: Current Topics. *Curr. Opin. Neurol.* **2020**, *33*, 300–308. [CrossRef]
26. De Lott, L.B.; Bennett, J.L.; Costello, F. The Changing Landscape of Optic Neuritis: A Narrative Review. *J. Neurol.* **2022**, *269*, 111–124. [CrossRef]
27. Khanna, S.; Sharma, A.; Huecker, J.; Gordon, M.; Naismith, R.T.; Van Stavern, G.P. Magnetic Resonance Imaging of Optic Neuritis in Patients with Neuromyelitis Optica Versus Multiple Sclerosis. *J. Neuroophthalmol.* **2012**, *32*, 216–220. [CrossRef]
28. Storoni, M.; Davagnanam, I.; Radon, M.; Siddiqui, A.; Plant, G.T. Distinguishing Optic Neuritis in Neuromyelitis Optica Spectrum Disease from Multiple Sclerosis: A Novel Magnetic Resonance Imaging Scoring System. *J. Neuroophthalmol.* **2013**, *33*, 123–127. [CrossRef]
29. Chen, J.J.; Flanagan, E.P.; Jitprapaikulsan, J.; Lopez-Chiriboga, A.S.S.; Fryer, J.P.; Leavitt, J.A.; Weinshenker, B.G.; Mckeon, A.; Tillema, J.M.; Lennon, V.A.; et al. Myelin Oligodendrocyte Glycoprotein Antibody-Positive Optic Neuritis: Clinical Characteristics, Radiologic Clues, and Outcome. *Am. J. Ophthalmol.* **2018**, *195*, 8–15. [CrossRef]
30. Kitley, J.; Waters, P.; Woodhall, M.; Leite, M.I.; Murchison, A.; George, J.; Küker, W.; Chandratre, S.; Vincent, A.; Palace, J. Neuromyelitis Optica Spectrum Disorders with Aquaporin-4 and Myelin-Oligodendrocyte Glycoprotein Antibodies: A Comparative Study. *JAMA Neurol.* **2014**, *71*, 276–283. [CrossRef]
31. Sato, D.K.; Callegaro, D.; Lana-Peixoto, M.A.; Waters, P.J.; De Haidar Jorge, F.M.; Takahashi, T.; Nakashima, I.; Apostolos-Pereira, S.L.; Talim, N.; Simm, R.F.; et al. Distinction between Mog Antibody-Positive and Aqp4 Antibody-Positive Nmo Spectrum Disorders. *Neurology* **2014**, *82*, 474–481. [CrossRef]
32. Jarius, S.; Ruprecht, K.; Kleiter, I.; Borisow, N.; Asgari, N.; Pitarokoili, K.; Pache, F.; Stich, O.; Beume, L.A.; Hummert, M.W.; et al. Mog-Igg in Nmo and Related Disorders: A Multicenter Study of 50 Patients. Part 2: Epidemiology, Clinical Presentation, Radiological and Laboratory Features, Treatment Responses, and Long-Term Outcome. *J. Neuroinflamm.* **2016**, *13*, 280. [CrossRef]
33. Jiao, Y.; Fryer, J.P.; Lennon, V.A.; Jenkins, S.M.; Quek, A.M.; Smith, C.Y.; Mckeon, A.; Costanzi, C.; Iorio, R.; Weinshenker, B.G.; et al. Updated Estimate of Aqp4-Igg Serostatus and Disability Outcome in Neuromyelitis Optica. *Neurology* **2013**, *81*, 1197–1204. [CrossRef]
34. Selmaj, K.; Selmaj, I. Novel Emerging Treatments for Nmosd. *Neurol. Neurochir. Pol.* **2019**, *53*, 317–326. [CrossRef]
35. Traboulsee, A.; Greenberg, B.M.; Bennett, J.L.; Szczechowski, L.; Fox, E.; Shkrobot, S.; Yamamura, T.; Terada, Y.; Kawata, Y.; Wright, P.; et al. Safety and Efficacy of Satralizumab Monotherapy in Neuromyelitis Optica Spectrum Disorder: A Randomised, Double-Blind, Multicentre, Placebo-Controlled Phase 3 Trial. *Lancet Neurol.* **2020**, *19*, 402–412. [CrossRef]
36. Cree, B.a.C.; Bennett, J.L.; Kim, H.J.; Weinshenker, B.G.; Pittock, S.J.; Wingerchuk, D.M.; Fujihara, K.; Paul, F.; Cutter, G.R.; Marignier, R.; et al. Inebilizumab for the Treatment of Neuromyelitis Optica Spectrum Disorder (N-Momentum): A Double-Blind, Randomised Placebo-Controlled Phase 2/3 Trial. *Lancet* **2019**, *394*, 1352–1363. [CrossRef]
37. Wingerchuk, D.M.; Zhang, I.; Kielhorn, A.; Royston, M.; Levy, M.; Fujihara, K.; Nakashima, I.; Tanvir, I.; Paul, F.; Pittock, S.J. Network Meta-Analysis of Food and Drug Administration-Approved Treatment Options for Adults with Aquaporin-4 Immunoglobulin G-Positive Neuromyelitis Optica Spectrum Disorder. *Neurol. Ther.* **2022**, *11*, 123–135. [CrossRef]
38. Pittock, S.J.; Lennon, V.A.; Mckeon, A.; Mandrekar, J.; Weinshenker, B.G.; Lucchinetti, C.F.; O'toole, O.; Wingerchuk, D.M. Eculizumab in Aqp4-Igg-Positive Relapsing Neuromyelitis Optica Spectrum Disorders: An Open-Label Pilot Study. *Lancet Neurol.* **2013**, *12*, 554–562. [CrossRef]
39. Katz Sand, I.; Fabian, M.T.; Telford, R.; Kraus, T.A.; Chehade, M.; Masilamani, M.; Moran, T.; Farrell, C.; Ebel, S.; Cook, L.J.; et al. Open-Label, Add-on Trial of Cetirizine for Neuromyelitis Optica. *Neurol. Neuroimmunol. Neuroinflamm.* **2018**, *5*, e441. [CrossRef]
40. Herges, K.; De Jong, B.A.; Kolkowitz, I.; Dunn, C.; Mandelbaum, G.; Ko, R.M.; Maini, A.; Han, M.H.; Killestein, J.; Polman, C.; et al. Protective Effect of an Elastase Inhibitor in a Neuromyelitis Optica-Like Disease Driven by a Peptide of Myelin Oligodendroglial Glycoprotein. *Mult. Scler.* **2012**, *18*, 398–408. [CrossRef]
41. Ransom, B.; Behar, T.; Nedergaard, M. New Roles for Astrocytes (Stars at Last). *Trends Neurosci.* **2003**, *26*, 520–522. [CrossRef]
42. Asavapanumas, N.; Ratelade, J.; Papadopoulos, M.C.; Bennett, J.L.; Levin, M.H.; Verkman, A.S. Experimental Mouse Model of Optic Neuritis with Inflammatory Demyelination Produced by Passive Transfer of Neuromyelitis Optica-Immunoglobulin G. *J. Neuroinflamm.* **2014**, *11*, 16. [CrossRef]

43. Bennett, J.L.; De Seze, J.; Lana-Peixoto, M.; Palace, J.; Waldman, A.; Schippling, S.; Tenembaum, S.; Banwell, B.; Greenberg, B.; Levy, M.; et al. Neuromyelitis Optica and Multiple Sclerosis: Seeing Differences through Optical Coherence Tomography. *Mult. Scler.* **2015**, *21*, 678–688. [CrossRef]
44. Lucchinetti, C.F.; Mandler, R.N.; Mcgavern, D.; Bruck, W.; Gleich, G.; Ransohoff, R.M.; Trebst, C.; Weinshenker, B.; Wingerchuk, D.; Parisi, J.E.; et al. A Role for Humoral Mechanisms in the Pathogenesis of Devic's Neuromyelitis Optica. *Brain* **2002**, *125*, 1450–1461. [CrossRef] [PubMed]
45. Lucchinetti, C.F.; Guo, Y.; Popescu, B.F.G.; Fujihara, K.; Itoyama, Y.; Misu, T. The Pathology of an Autoimmune Astrocytopathy: Lessons Learned from Neuromyelitis Optica. *Brain Pathol.* **2014**, *24*, 83–97. [CrossRef] [PubMed]
46. Hinson, S.R.; Romero, M.F.; Popescu, B.F.; Lucchinetti, C.F.; Fryer, J.P.; Wolburg, H.; Fallier-Becker, P.; Noell, S.; Lennon, V.A. Molecular Outcomes of Neuromyelitis Optica (Nmo)-Igg Binding to Aquaporin-4 in Astrocytes. *Proc. Natl. Acad. Sci. USA* **2012**, *109*, 1245–1250. [CrossRef] [PubMed]
47. Crane, J.M.; Tajima, M.; Verkman, A.S. Live-Cell Imaging of Aquaporin-4 Diffusion and Interactions in Orthogonal Arrays of Particles. *Neuroscience* **2010**, *168*, 892–902. [CrossRef] [PubMed]
48. Abe, Y.; Yasui, M. Aquaporin-4 in Neuromyelitis Optica Spectrum Disorders: A Target of Autoimmunity in the Central Nervous System. *Biomolecules* **2022**, *12*, 591. [CrossRef]
49. Mckeon, A.; Lennon, V.A.; Lotze, T.; Tenenbaum, S.; Ness, J.M.; Rensel, M.; Kuntz, N.L.; Fryer, J.P.; Homburger, H.; Hunter, J.; et al. Cns Aquaporin-4 Autoimmunity in Children. *Neurology* **2008**, *71*, 93–100. [CrossRef]
50. Matiello, M.; Schaefer-Klein, J.; Sun, D.; Weinshenker, B.G. Aquaporin 4 Expression and Tissue Susceptibility to Neuromyelitis Optica. *JAMA Neurol.* **2013**, *70*, 1118–1125. [CrossRef]
51. Crane, J.M.; Van Hoek, A.N.; Skach, W.R.; Verkman, A.S. Aquaporin-4 Dynamics in Orthogonal Arrays in Live Cells Visualized by Quantum Dot Single Particle Tracking. *Mol. Biol. Cell* **2008**, *19*, 3369–3378. [CrossRef]
52. Neely, J.D.; Christensen, B.M.; Nielsen, S.; Agre, P. Heterotetrameric Composition of Aquaporin-4 Water Channels. *Biochemistry* **1999**, *38*, 11156–11163. [CrossRef]
53. Phuan, P.W.; Ratelade, J.; Rossi, A.; Tradtrantip, L.; Verkman, A.S. Complement-Dependent Cytotoxicity in Neuromyelitis Optica Requires Aquaporin-4 Protein Assembly in Orthogonal Arrays. *J. Biol. Chem.* **2012**, *287*, 13829–13839. [CrossRef]
54. Li, J.; Bazzi, S.A.; Schmitz, F.; Tanno, H.; Mcdaniel, J.R.; Lee, C.-H.; Joshi, C.; Kim, J.E.; Monson, N.; Greenberg, B.M.; et al. Molecular Level Characterization of Circulating Aquaporin-4 Antibodies in Neuromyelitis Optica Spectrum Disorder. *Neurol. Neuroimmunol. Neuroinflamm.* **2021**, *8*, e1034. [CrossRef]
55. Zeka, B.; Lassmann, H.; Bradl, M. Muller Cells and Retinal Axons Can Be Primary Targets in Experimental Neuromyelitis Optica Spectrum Disorder. *Clin. Exp. Neuroimmunol.* **2017**, *8*, 3–7. [CrossRef]
56. Wingerchuk, D.M. Neuromyelitis Optica: Potential Roles for Intravenous Immunoglobulin. *J. Clin. Immunol.* **2013**, *33* (Suppl. 1), S33–S37. [CrossRef]
57. You, Y.; Zhu, L.; Zhang, T.; Shen, T.; Fontes, A.; Yiannikas, C.; Parratt, J.; Barton, J.; Schulz, A.; Gupta, V.; et al. Evidence of Müller Glial Dysfunction in Patients with Aquaporin-4 Immunoglobulin G-Positive Neuromyelitis Optica Spectrum Disorder. *Ophthalmology* **2019**, *126*, 801–810. [CrossRef]
58. Ratelade, J.; Asavapanumas, N.; Ritchie, A.M.; Wemlinger, S.; Bennett, J.L.; Verkman, A.S. Involvement of Antibody-Dependent Cell-Mediated Cytotoxicity in Inflammatory Demyelination in a Mouse Model of Neuromyelitis Optica. *Acta Neuropathol.* **2013**, *126*, 699–709. [CrossRef]
59. Duan, T.; Smith, A.J.; Verkman, A.S. Complement-Independent Bystander Injury in Aqp4-Igg Seropositive Neuromyelitis Optica Produced by Antibody-Dependent Cellular Cytotoxicity. *Acta Neuropathol. Commun.* **2019**, *7*, 112. [CrossRef]
60. Asavapanumas, N.; Ratelade, J.; Verkman, A.S. Unique Neuromyelitis Optica Pathology Produced in Naive Rats by Intracerebral Administration of Nmo-Igg. *Acta Neuropathol.* **2014**, *127*, 539–551. [CrossRef]
61. Seidel, U.J.; Schlegel, P.; Lang, P. Natural Killer Cell Mediated Antibody-Dependent Cellular Cytotoxicity in Tumor Immunotherapy with Therapeutic Antibodies. *Front. Immunol.* **2013**, *4*, 76. [CrossRef]
62. Imai, K.; Takaoka, A. Comparing Antibody and Small-Molecule Therapies for Cancer. *Nat. Rev. Cancer* **2006**, *6*, 714–727. [CrossRef]
63. Huppert, J.; Closhen, D.; Croxford, A.; White, R.; Kulig, P.; Pietrowski, E.; Bechmann, I.; Becher, B.; Luhmann, H.J.; Waisman, A.; et al. Cellular Mechanisms of Il-17-Induced Blood-Brain Barrier Disruption. *FASEB J.* **2010**, *24*, 1023–1034. [CrossRef]
64. Carlson, T.; Kroenke, M.; Rao, P.; Lane, T.E.; Segal, B. The Th17–Elr+ Cxc Chemokine Pathway Is Essential for the Development of Central Nervous System Autoimmune Disease. *J. Exp. Med.* **2008**, *205*, 811–823. [CrossRef] [PubMed]
65. Varrin-Doyer, M.; Spencer, C.M.; Schulze-Topphoff, U.; Nelson, P.A.; Stroud, R.M.; Cree, B.A.C.; Zamvil, S.S. Aquaporin 4-Specific T Cells in Neuromyelitis Optica Exhibit a Th17 Bias and Recognize Clostridium Abc Transporter. *Ann. Neurol.* **2012**, *72*, 53–64. [CrossRef] [PubMed]
66. Uzawa, A.; Mori, M.; Arai, K.; Sato, Y.; Hayakawa, S.; Masuda, S.; Taniguchi, J.; Kuwabara, S. Cytokine and Chemokine Profiles in Neuromyelitis Optica: Significance of Interleukin-6. *Mult. Scler. J.* **2010**, *16*, 1443–1452. [CrossRef] [PubMed]
67. Passos, G.R.D.; Sato, D.K.; Becker, J.; Fujihara, K. Th17 Cells Pathways in Multiple Sclerosis and Neuromyelitis Optica Spectrum Disorders: Pathophysiological and Therapeutic Implications. *Mediat. Inflamm.* **2016**, *2016*, 5314541. [CrossRef] [PubMed]
68. Chen, D.; Gallagher, S.; Monson, N.L.; Herbst, R.; Wang, Y. Inebilizumab, a B Cell-Depleting Anti-Cd19 Antibody for the Treatment of Autoimmune Neurological Diseases: Insights from Preclinical Studies. *J. Clin. Med.* **2016**, *5*, 107. [CrossRef]

69. Challa, D.K.; Bussmeyer, U.; Khan, T.; Montoyo, H.P.; Bansal, P.; Ober, R.J.; Ward, E.S. Autoantibody Depletion Ameliorates Disease in Murine Experimental Autoimmune Encephalomyelitis. *mAbs* **2013**, *5*, 655–659. [CrossRef]
70. Hinson, S.R.; Pittock, S.J.; Lucchinetti, C.F.; Roemer, S.F.; Fryer, J.P.; Kryzer, T.J.; Lennon, V.A. Pathogenic Potential of Igg Binding to Water Channel Extracellular Domain in Neuromyelitis Optica. *Neurology* **2007**, *69*, 2221–2231. [CrossRef]
71. Yao, X.; Verkman, A.S. Complement Regulator Cd59 Prevents Peripheral Organ Injury in Rats Made Seropositive for Neuromyelitis Optica Immunoglobulin G. *Acta Neuropathol. Commun.* **2017**, *5*, 57. [CrossRef]
72. Soltys, J.; Liu, Y.; Ritchie, A.; Wemlinger, S.; Schaller, K.; Schumann, H.; Owens, G.P.; Bennett, J.L. Membrane Assembly of Aquaporin-4 Autoantibodies Regulates Classical Complement Activation in Neuromyelitis Optica. *J. Clin. Investig.* **2019**, *129*, 2000–2013. [CrossRef]
73. Phuan, P.W.; Zhang, H.; Asavapanumas, N.; Leviten, M.; Rosenthal, A.; Tradtrantip, L.; Verkman, A.S. C1q-Targeted Monoclonal Antibody Prevents Complement-Dependent Cytotoxicity and Neuropathology in In Vitro and Mouse Models of Neuromyelitis Optica. *Acta Neuropathol.* **2013**, *125*, 829–840. [CrossRef]
74. Brachet, G.; Bourquard, T.; Gallay, N.; Reiter, E.; Gouilleux-Gruart, V.; Poupon, A.; Watier, H. Eculizumab Epitope on Complement C5: Progress towards a Better Understanding of the Mechanism of Action. *Mol. Immunol.* **2016**, *77*, 126–131. [CrossRef]
75. Hillmen, P.; Young, N.S.; Schubert, J.; Brodsky, R.A.; Socie, G.; Muus, P.; Roth, A.; Szer, J.; Elebute, M.O.; Nakamura, R.; et al. The Complement Inhibitor Eculizumab in Paroxysmal Nocturnal Hemoglobinuria. *N. Engl. J. Med.* **2006**, *355*, 1233–1243. [CrossRef]
76. Merle, N.S.; Noe, R.; Halbwachs-Mecarelli, L.; Fremeaux-Bacchi, V.; Roumenina, L.T. Complement System Part II: Role in Immunity. *Front. Immunol.* **2015**, *6*, 257. [CrossRef]
77. Pache, F.; Ringelstein, M.; Aktas, O.; Kleiter, I.; Jarius, S.; Siebert, N.; Bellmann-Strobl, J.; Paul, F.; Ruprecht, K. C3 and C4 Complement Levels in Aqp4-Igg-Positive Nmosd and in Mogad. *J. Neuroimmunol.* **2021**, *360*, 577699. [CrossRef]
78. Takai, Y.; Misu, T.; Kaneko, K.; Chihara, N.; Narikawa, K.; Tsuchida, S.; Nishida, H.; Komori, T.; Seki, M.; Komatsu, T.; et al. Myelin Oligodendrocyte Glycoprotein Antibody-Associated Disease: An Immunopathological Study. *Brain* **2020**, *143*, 1431–1446. [CrossRef]
79. Kaneko, K.; Sato, D.K.; Nakashima, I.; Ogawa, R.; Akaishi, T.; Takai, Y.; Nishiyama, S.; Takahashi, T.; Misu, T.; Kuroda, H.; et al. Csf Cytokine Profile in Mog-Igg+ Neurological Disease Is Similar to Aqp4-Igg+ Nmosd but Distinct from Ms: A Cross-Sectional Study and Potential Therapeutic Implications. *J. Neurol. Neurosurg. Psychiatry* **2018**, *89*, 927–936. [CrossRef]
80. Saadoun, S.; Waters, P.; Owens, G.P.; Bennett, J.L.; Vincent, A.; Papadopoulos, M.C. Neuromyelitis Optica Mog-Igg Causes Reversible Lesions in Mouse Brain. *Acta Neuropathol. Commun.* **2014**, *2*, 35. [CrossRef]
81. Peschl, P.; Schanda, K.; Zeka, B.; Given, K.; Bohm, D.; Ruprecht, K.; Saiz, A.; Lutterotti, A.; Rostasy, K.; Hoftberger, R.; et al. Human Antibodies against the Myelin Oligodendrocyte Glycoprotein Can Cause Complement-Dependent Demyelination. *J. Neuroinflamm.* **2017**, *14*, 208. [CrossRef]
82. Keller, C.W.; Lopez, J.A.; Wendel, E.M.; Ramanathan, S.; Gross, C.C.; Klotz, L.; Reindl, M.; Dale, R.C.; Wiendl, H.; Rostásy, K.; et al. Complement Activation Is a Prominent Feature of Mogad. *Ann. Neurol.* **2021**, *90*, 976–982. [CrossRef]
83. Carnero Contentti, E.; Correale, J. Neuromyelitis Optica Spectrum Disorders: From Pathophysiology to Therapeutic Strategies. *J. Neuroinflamm.* **2021**, *18*, 208. [CrossRef]
84. Papadopoulos, M.C.; Bennett, J.L.; Verkman, A.S. Treatment of Neuromyelitis Optica: State-of-the-Art and Emerging Therapies. *Nat. Rev. Neurol.* **2014**, *10*, 493–506. [CrossRef]
85. Zhang, P.; Liu, B. Effect of Autologous Hematopoietic Stem Cell Transplantation on Multiple Sclerosis and Neuromyelitis Optica Spectrum Disorder: A Prisma-Compliant Meta-Analysis. *Bone Marrow Transplant.* **2020**, *55*, 1928–1934. [CrossRef]
86. Zubizarreta, I.; Flórez-Grau, G.; Vila, G.; Cabezón, R.; España, C.; Andorra, M.; Saiz, A.; Llufriu, S.; Sepulveda, M.; Sola-Valls, N.; et al. Immune Tolerance in Multiple Sclerosis and Neuromyelitis Optica with Peptide-Loaded Tolerogenic Dendritic Cells in a Phase 1b Trial. *Proc. Natl. Acad. Sci. USA* **2019**, *116*, 8463–8470. [CrossRef]
87. Garren, H.; Robinson, W.H.; Krasulová, E.; Havrdová, E.; Nadj, C.; Selmaj, K.; Losy, J.; Nadj, I.; Radue, E.W.; Kidd, B.A.; et al. Phase 2 Trial of a DNA Vaccine Encoding Myelin Basic Protein for Multiple Sclerosis. *Ann. Neurol.* **2008**, *63*, 611–620. [CrossRef]
88. Bar-Or, A.; Steinman, L.; Behne, J.M.; Benitez-Ribas, D.; Chin, P.S.; Clare-Salzler, M.; Healey, D.; Kim, J.I.; Kranz, D.M.; Lutterotti, A.; et al. Restoring Immune Tolerance in Neuromyelitis Optica: Part II. *Neurol. Neuroimmunol. Neuroinflamm.* **2016**, *3*, e277. [CrossRef]
89. Steinman, L.; Bar-Or, A.; Behne, J.M.; Benitez-Ribas, D.; Chin, P.S.; Clare-Salzler, M.; Healey, D.; Kim, J.I.; Kranz, D.M.; Lutterotti, A.; et al. Restoring Immune Tolerance in Neuromyelitis Optica: Part I. *Neurol. Neuroimmunol. Neuroinflamm.* **2016**, *3*, e276. [CrossRef]
90. Shimizu, F.; Nishihara, H.; Kanda, T. Blood-Brain Barrier Dysfunction in Immuno-Mediated Neurological Diseases. *Immunol. Med.* **2018**, *41*, 120–128. [CrossRef]
91. Asavapanumas, N.; Tradtrantip, L.; Verkman, A.S. Targeting the Complement System in Neuromyelitis Optica Spectrum Disorder. *Expert Opin. Biol. Ther.* **2021**, *21*, 1073–1086. [CrossRef] [PubMed]
92. Saadoun, S.; Waters, P.; Bell, B.A.; Vincent, A.; Verkman, A.S.; Papadopoulos, M.C. Intra-Cerebral Injection of Neuromyelitis Optica Immunoglobulin G and Human Complement Produces Neuromyelitis Optica Lesions in Mice. *Brain* **2010**, *133*, 349–361. [CrossRef] [PubMed]
93. Ghafouri-Fard, S.; Azimi, T.; Taheri, M. A Comprehensive Review on the Role of Genetic Factors in Neuromyelitis Optica Spectrum Disorder. *Front. Immunol.* **2021**, *12*, 737673. [CrossRef] [PubMed]

94. Matiello, M.; Kim, H.J.; Kim, W.; Brum, D.G.; Barreira, A.A.; Kingsbury, D.J.; Plant, G.T.; Adoni, T.; Weinshenker, B.G. Familial Neuromyelitis Optica. *Neurology* **2010**, *75*, 310–315. [CrossRef] [PubMed]
95. Zhong, X.; Chen, C.; Sun, X.; Wang, J.; Li, R.; Chang, Y.; Fan, P.; Wang, Y.; Wu, Y.; Peng, L.; et al. Whole-Exome Sequencing Reveals the Major Genetic Factors Contributing to Neuromyelitis Optica Spectrum Disorder in Chinese Patients with Aquaporin 4-Igg Seropositivity. *Eur. J. Neurol.* **2021**, *28*, 2294–2304. [CrossRef] [PubMed]
96. Zéphir, H.; Fajardy, I.; Outteryck, O.; Blanc, F.; Roger, N.; Fleury, M.; Rudolf, G.; Marignier, R.; Vukusic, S.; Confavreux, C.; et al. Is Neuromyelitis Optica Associated with Human Leukocyte Antigen? *Mult. Scler.* **2009**, *15*, 571–579. [CrossRef] [PubMed]
97. Matsushita, T.; Masaki, K.; Isobe, N.; Sato, S.; Yamamoto, K.; Nakamura, Y.; Watanabe, M.; Suenaga, T.; Kira, J.I. Genetic Factors for Susceptibility to and Manifestations of Neuromyelitis Optica. *Ann. Clin. Transl. Neurol.* **2020**, *7*, 2082–2093. [CrossRef]
98. Estrada, K.; Whelan, C.W.; Zhao, F.; Bronson, P.; Handsaker, R.E.; Sun, C.; Carulli, J.P.; Harris, T.; Ransohoff, R.M.; Mccarroll, S.A.; et al. A Whole-Genome Sequence Study Identifies Genetic Risk Factors for Neuromyelitis Optica. *Nat. Commun.* **2018**, *9*, 1929. [CrossRef]
99. Ogawa, K.; Okuno, T.; Hosomichi, K.; Hosokawa, A.; Hirata, J.; Suzuki, K.; Sakaue, S.; Kinoshita, M.; Asano, Y.; Miyamoto, K.; et al. Next-Generation Sequencing Identifies Contribution of Both Class I and Ii Hla Genes on Susceptibility of Multiple Sclerosis in Japanese. *J. Neuroinflamm.* **2019**, *16*, 162. [CrossRef]
100. Beppu, S.; Kinoshita, M.; Wilamowski, J.; Suenaga, T.; Yasumizu, Y.; Ogawa, K.; Ishikura, T.; Tada, S.; Koda, T.; Murata, H.; et al. High Cell Surface Expression and Peptide Binding Affinity of Hla-Dqa1*05:03, a Susceptible Allele of Neuromyelitis Optica Spectrum Disorders (Nmosd). *Sci. Rep.* **2022**, *12*, 106. [CrossRef]
101. Watanabe, M.; Nakamura, Y.; Sato, S.; Niino, M.; Fukaura, H.; Tanaka, M.; Ochi, H.; Kanda, T.; Takeshita, Y.; Yokota, T.; et al. Hla Genotype-Clinical Phenotype Correlations in Multiple Sclerosis and Neuromyelitis Optica Spectrum Disorders Based on Japan Ms/Nmosd Biobank Data. *Sci. Rep.* **2021**, *11*, 607. [CrossRef]
102. Yoshimura, S.; Isobe, N.; Matsushita, T.; Yonekawa, T.; Masaki, K.; Sato, S.; Kawano, Y.; Kira, J. Distinct Genetic and Infectious Profiles in Japanese Neuromyelitis Optica Patients According to Anti-Aquaporin 4 Antibody Status. *J. Neurol. Neurosurg. Psychiatry* **2013**, *84*, 29–34. [CrossRef]
103. Li, T.; Li, H.; Li, Y.; Dong, S.A.; Yi, M.; Zhang, Q.X.; Feng, B.; Yang, L.; Shi, F.D.; Yang, C.S. Multi-Level Analyses of Genome-Wide Association Study to Reveal Significant Risk Genes and Pathways in Neuromyelitis Optica Spectrum Disorder. *Front. Genet.* **2021**, *12*, 690537. [CrossRef]
104. Uzawa, A.; Mori, M.; Kuwabara, S. Cytokines and Chemokines in Neuromyelitis Optica: Pathogenetic and Therapeutic Implications. *Brain Pathol.* **2014**, *24*, 67–73. [CrossRef]
105. Rocca, M.A.; Cacciaguerra, L.; Filippi, M. Moving Beyond Anti-Aquaporin-4 Antibodies: Emerging Biomarkers in the Spectrum of Neuromyelitis Optica. *Expert Rev. Neurother.* **2020**, *20*, 601–618. [CrossRef]
106. Park, H.; Li, Z.; Yang, X.O.; Chang, S.H.; Nurieva, R.; Wang, Y.-H.; Wang, Y.; Hood, L.; Zhu, Z.; Tian, Q.; et al. A Distinct Lineage of Cd4 T Cells Regulates Tissue Inflammation by Producing Interleukin 17. *Nat. Immunol.* **2005**, *6*, 1133–1141. [CrossRef]
107. Hou, M.M.; Li, Y.F.; He, L.L.; Li, X.Q.; Zhang, Y.; Zhang, S.X.; Li, X.Y. Proportions of Th17 Cells and Th17-Related Cytokines in Neuromyelitis Optica Spectrum Disorders Patients: A Meta-Analysis. *Int. Immunopharmacol.* **2019**, *75*, 105793. [CrossRef]
108. Maciak, K.; Pietrasik, S.; Dziedzic, A.; Redlicka, J.; Saluk-Bijak, J.; Bijak, M.; Włodarczyk, T.; Miller, E. Th17-Related Cytokines as Potential Discriminatory Markers between Neuromyelitis Optica (Devic's Disease) and Multiple Sclerosis—A Review. *Int. J. Mol. Sci.* **2021**, *22*, 8946. [CrossRef]
109. Fujihara, K.; Bennett, J.L.; De Seze, J.; Haramura, M.; Kleiter, I.; Weinshenker, B.G.; Kang, D.; Mughal, T.; Yamamura, T. Interleukin-6 in Neuromyelitis Optica Spectrum Disorder Pathophysiology. *Neurol. Neuroimmunol. Neuroinflamm.* **2020**, *7*, e841. [CrossRef]
110. Takeshita, Y.; Fujikawa, S.; Serizawa, K.; Fujisawa, M.; Matsuo, K.; Nemoto, J.; Shimizu, F.; Sano, Y.; Tomizawa-Shinohara, H.; Miyake, S.; et al. New Bbb Model Reveals That Il-6 Blockade Suppressed the Bbb Disorder, Preventing Onset of Nmosd. *Neurol. Neuroimmunol. Neuroinflamm.* **2021**, *8*, e1076. [CrossRef]
111. Langrish, C.L.; Chen, Y.; Blumenschein, W.M.; Mattson, J.; Basham, B.; Sedgwick, J.D.; Mcclanahan, T.; Kastelein, R.A.; Cua, D.J. Il-23 Drives a Pathogenic T Cell Population That Induces Autoimmune Inflammation. *J. Exp. Med.* **2005**, *201*, 233–240. [CrossRef]
112. Korn, T.; Bettelli, E.; Oukka, M.; Kuchroo, V.K. Il-17 and Th17 Cells. *Annu. Rev. Immunol.* **2009**, *27*, 485–517. [CrossRef]
113. El-Behi, M.; Ciric, B.; Dai, H.; Yan, Y.; Cullimore, M.; Safavi, F.; Zhang, G.-X.; Dittel, B.N.; Rostami, A. The Encephalitogenicity of Th17 Cells Is Dependent on Il-1- and Il-23-Induced Production of the Cytokine Gm-Csf. *Nat. Immunol.* **2011**, *12*, 568–575. [CrossRef] [PubMed]
114. Monteiro, C.; Fernandes, G.; Kasahara, T.M.; Barros, P.O.; Dias, A.S.O.; Araujo, A.; Ornelas, A.M.M.; Aguiar, R.S.; Alvarenga, R.; Bento, C.a.M. The Expansion of Circulating Il-6 and Il-17-Secreting Follicular Helper T Cells Is Associated with Neurological Disabilities in Neuromyelitis Optica Spectrum Disorders. *J. Neuroimmunol.* **2019**, *330*, 12–18. [CrossRef] [PubMed]
115. Uchida, T.; Mori, M.; Uzawa, A.; Masuda, H.; Muto, M.; Ohtani, R.; Kuwabara, S. Increased Cerebrospinal Fluid Metalloproteinase-2 and Interleukin-6 Are Associated with Albumin Quotient in Neuromyelitis Optica: Their Possible Role on Blood-Brain Barrier Disruption. *Mult. Scler.* **2017**, *23*, 1072–1084. [CrossRef] [PubMed]
116. Kimura, A.; Naka, T.; Kishimoto, T. Il-6-Dependent and -Independent Pathways in the Development of Interleukin 17-Producing T Helper Cells. *Proc. Natl. Acad. Sci. USA* **2007**, *104*, 12099–12104. [CrossRef]

117. Takeshita, Y.; Obermeier, B.; Cotleur, A.C.; Spampinato, S.F.; Shimizu, F.; Yamamoto, E.; Sano, Y.; Kryzer, T.J.; Lennon, V.A.; Kanda, T.; et al. Effects of Neuromyelitis Optica-Igg at the Blood-Brain Barrier in Vitro. *Neurol. Neuroimmunol. Neuroinflamm.* **2017**, *4*, e311. [CrossRef]
118. Uzawa, A.; Mori, M.; Kuwabara, S. Role of Interleukin-6 in the Pathogenesis of Neuromyelitis Optica. *Clin. Exp. Neuroimmunol.* **2013**, *4*, 167–172. [CrossRef]
119. Kaplin, A.I.; Deshpande, D.M.; Scott, E.; Krishnan, C.; Carmen, J.S.; Shats, I.; Martinez, T.; Drummond, J.; Dike, S.; Pletnikov, M.; et al. Il-6 Induces Regionally Selective Spinal Cord Injury in Patients with the Neuroinflammatory Disorder Transverse Myelitis. *J. Clin. Investig.* **2005**, *115*, 2731–2741. [CrossRef]
120. Moinfar, Z.; Zamvil, S.S. Microglia Complement Astrocytes in Neuromyelitis Optica. *J. Clin. Investig.* **2020**, *130*, 3961–3964. [CrossRef]
121. Li, W.; Liu, J.; Tan, W.; Zhou, Y. The Role and Mechanisms of Microglia in Neuromyelitis Optica Spectrum Disorders. *Int. J. Med. Sci.* **2021**, *18*, 3059–3065. [CrossRef]
122. Takano, R.; Misu, T.; Takahashi, T.; Sato, S.; Fujihara, K.; Itoyama, Y. Astrocytic Damage Is Far More Severe Than Demyelination in Nmo: A Clinical Csf Biomarker Study. *Neurology* **2010**, *75*, 208–216. [CrossRef]
123. Wang, J.; Cui, C.; Lu, Y.; Chang, Y.; Wang, Y.; Li, R.; Shan, Y.; Sun, X.; Long, Y.; Wang, H.; et al. Therapeutic Response and Possible Biomarkers in Acute Attacks of Neuromyelitis Optica Spectrum Disorders: A Prospective Observational Study. *Front. Immunol.* **2021**, *12*, 720907. [CrossRef]
124. Watanabe, M.; Nakamura, Y.; Michalak, Z.; Isobe, N.; Barro, C.; Leppert, D.; Matsushita, T.; Hayashi, F.; Yamasaki, R.; Kuhle, J.; et al. Serum Gfap and Neurofilament Light as Biomarkers of Disease Activity and Disability in Nmosd. *Neurology* **2019**, *93*, e1299–e1311. [CrossRef]
125. Aktas, O.; Smith, M.A.; Rees, W.A.; Bennett, J.L.; She, D.; Katz, E.; Cree, B.a.C.; N-MOmentum Scientific Group and the N-MOmentum Study Investigators. Serum Glial Fibrillary Acidic Protein: A Neuromyelitis Optica Spectrum Disorder Biomarker. *Ann. Neurol.* **2021**, *89*, 895–910. [CrossRef]
126. Schindler, P.; Grittner, U.; Oechtering, J.; Leppert, D.; Siebert, N.; Duchow, A.S.; Oertel, F.C.; Asseyer, S.; Kuchling, J.; Zimmermann, H.G.; et al. Serum Gfap and Nfl as Disease Severity and Prognostic Biomarkers in Patients with Aquaporin-4 Antibody-Positive Neuromyelitis Optica Spectrum Disorder. *J. Neuroinflamm.* **2021**, *18*, 105. [CrossRef]
127. Fu, C.C.; Gao, C.; Zhang, H.H.; Mao, Y.Q.; Lu, J.Q.; Petritis, B.; Huang, A.S.; Yang, X.G.; Long, Y.M.; Huang, R.P. Serum Molecular Biomarkers in Neuromyelitis Optica and Multiple Sclerosis. *Mult. Scler. Relat. Disord.* **2022**, *59*, 103527. [CrossRef]
128. Sonar, S.A.; Shaikh, S.; Joshi, N.; Atre, A.N.; Lal, G. Ifn-Gamma Promotes Transendothelial Migration of $Cd4^+$ T Cells across the Blood-Brain Barrier. *Immunol. Cell Biol.* **2017**, *95*, 843–853. [CrossRef]
129. Bonney, S.; Seitz, S.; Ryan, C.A.; Jones, K.L.; Clarke, P.; Tyler, K.L.; Siegenthaler, J.A. Gamma Interferon Alters Junctional Integrity Via Rho Kinase, Resulting in Blood-Brain Barrier Leakage in Experimental Viral Encephalitis. *mBio* **2019**, *10*, e01675-19. [CrossRef]
130. Tong, Y.; Yang, T.; Wang, J.; Zhao, T.; Wang, L.; Kang, Y.; Cheng, C.; Fan, Y. Elevated Plasma Chemokines for Eosinophils in Neuromyelitis Optica Spectrum Disorders during Remission. *Front. Neurol.* **2018**, *9*, 44. [CrossRef]
131. Specovius, S.; Zimmermann, H.G.; Oertel, F.C.; Chien, C.; Bereuter, C.; Cook, L.J.; Lana Peixoto, M.A.; Fontenelle, M.A.; Kim, H.J.; Hyun, J.W.; et al. Cohort Profile: A Collaborative Multicentre Study of Retinal Optical Coherence Tomography in 539 Patients with Neuromyelitis Optica Spectrum Disorders (Croctino). *BMJ Open* **2020**, *10*, e035397. [CrossRef]
132. Oertel, F.C.; Specovius, S.; Zimmermann, H.G.; Chien, C.; Motamedi, S.; Bereuter, C.; Cook, L.; Lana Peixoto, M.A.; Fontanelle, M.A.; Kim, H.J.; et al. Retinal Optical Coherence Tomography in Neuromyelitis Optica. *Neurol. Neuroimmunol. Neuroinflamm.* **2021**, *8*, e1068. [CrossRef]
133. Graves, J.S.; Oertel, F.C.; Van Der Walt, A.; Collorone, S.; Sotirchos, E.S.; Pihl-Jensen, G.; Albrecht, P.; Yeh, E.A.; Saidha, S.; Frederiksen, J.; et al. Leveraging Visual Outcome Measures to Advance Therapy Development in Neuroimmunologic Disorders. *Neurol. Neuroimmunol. Neuroinflamm.* **2022**, *9*, e1126. [CrossRef]
134. Schneider, E.; Zimmermann, H.; Oberwahrenbrock, T.; Kaufhold, F.; Kadas, E.M.; Petzold, A.; Bilger, F.; Borisow, N.; Jarius, S.; Wildemann, B.; et al. Optical Coherence Tomography Reveals Distinct Patterns of Retinal Damage in Neuromyelitis Optica and Multiple Sclerosis. *PLoS ONE* **2013**, *8*, e66151. [CrossRef] [PubMed]
135. Wingerchuk, D.M.; Pittock, S.J.; Lucchinetti, C.F.; Lennon, V.A.; Weinshenker, B.G. A Secondary Progressive Clinical Course Is Uncommon in Neuromyelitis Optica. *Neurology* **2007**, *68*, 603–605. [CrossRef] [PubMed]
136. Sotirchos, E.S.; Saidha, S.; Byraiah, G.; Mealy, M.A.; Ibrahim, M.A.; Sepah, Y.J.; Newsome, S.D.; Ratchford, J.N.; Frohman, E.M.; Balcer, L.J.; et al. In Vivo Identification of Morphologic Retinal Abnormalities in Neuromyelitis Optica. *Neurology* **2013**, *80*, 1406–1414. [CrossRef] [PubMed]
137. Oertel, F.C.; Kuchling, J.; Zimmermann, H.; Chien, C.; Schmidt, F.; Knier, B.; Bellmann-Strobl, J.; Korn, T.; Scheel, M.; Klistorner, A.; et al. Microstructural Visual System Changes in Aqp4-Antibody–Seropositive Nmosd. *Neurol. Neuroimmunol. Neuroinflamm.* **2017**, *4*, e334. [CrossRef] [PubMed]
138. Van Horssen, J.; Witte, M.E.; Ciccarelli, O. The Role of Mitochondria in Axonal Degeneration and Tissue Repair in Ms. *Mult. Scler.* **2012**, *18*, 1058–1067. [CrossRef]
139. Evangelou, N.; Konz, D.; Esiri, M.M.; Smith, S.; Palace, J.; Matthews, P.M. Size-Selective Neuronal Changes in the Anterior Optic Pathways Suggest a Differential Susceptibility to Injury in Multiple Sclerosis. *Brain* **2001**, *124*, 1813–1820. [CrossRef]

140. Al-Nosairy, K.O.; Horbrügger, M.; Schippling, S.; Wagner, M.; Haghikia, A.; Pawlitzki, M.; Hoffmann, M.B. Structure–Function Relationship of Retinal Ganglion Cells in Multiple Sclerosis. *Int. J. Mol. Sci.* **2021**, *22*, 3419. [CrossRef]
141. La Morgia, C.; Di Vito, L.; Carelli, V.; Carbonelli, M. Patterns of Retinal Ganglion Cell Damage in Neurodegenerative Disorders: Parvocellular vs Magnocellular Degeneration in Optical Coherence Tomography Studies. *Front. Neurol.* **2017**, *8*, 710. [CrossRef]
142. Zeng, P.; Du, C.; Zhang, R.; Jia, D.; Jiang, F.; Fan, M.; Zhang, C. Optical Coherence Tomography Reveals Longitudinal Changes in Retinal Damage under Different Treatments for Neuromyelitis Optica Spectrum Disorder. *Front. Neurol.* **2021**, *12*, 669567. [CrossRef]
143. Jeong, I.H.; Kim, H.J.; Kim, N.H.; Jeong, K.S.; Park, C.Y. Subclinical Primary Retinal Pathology in Neuromyelitis Optica Spectrum Disorder. *J. Neurol.* **2016**, *263*, 1343–1348. [CrossRef]
144. Roca-Fernandez, A.; Oertel, F.C.; Yeo, T.; Motamedi, S.; Probert, F.; Craner, M.J.; Sastre-Garriga, J.; Zimmermann, H.G.; Asseyer, S.; Kuchling, J.; et al. Foveal Changes in Aquaporin-4 Antibody Seropositive Neuromyelitis Optica Spectrum Disorder Are Independent of Optic Neuritis and Not Overtly Progressive. *Eur. J. Neurol.* **2021**, *28*, 2280–2293. [CrossRef]
145. Felix, C.M.; Levin, M.H.; Verkman, A.S. Complement-Independent Retinal Pathology Produced by Intravitreal Injection of Neuromyelitis Optica Immunoglobulin G. *J. Neuroinflamm.* **2016**, *13*, 275. [CrossRef]
146. Chen, X.; Kuehlewein, L.; Pineles, S.L.; Tandon, A.K.; Bose, S.X.; Klufas, M.A.; Sadda, S.R.; Sarraf, D. En Face Optical Coherence Tomography of Macular Microcysts Due to Optic Neuropathy from Neuromyelitis Optica. *Retin Cases Brief Rep.* **2015**, *9*, 302–306. [CrossRef]
147. Wolff, B.; Basdekidou, C.; Vasseur, V.; Mauget-Faysse, M.; Sahel, J.A.; Vignal, C. Retinal Inner Nuclear Layer Microcystic Changes in Optic Nerve Atrophy: A Novel Spectral-Domain Oct Finding. *Retina* **2013**, *33*, 2133–2138. [CrossRef]
148. Zhang, S.; Wang, H.; Lu, Q.; Qing, G.; Wang, N.; Wang, Y.; Li, S.; Yang, D.; Yan, F. Detection of Early Neuron Degeneration and Accompanying Glial Responses in the Visual Pathway in a Rat Model of Acute Intraocular Hypertension. *Brain Res.* **2009**, *1303*, 131–143. [CrossRef]
149. Mirza, R.G.; Johnson, M.W.; Jampol, L.M. Optical Coherence Tomography Use in Evaluation of the Vitreoretinal Interface: A Review. *Surv. Ophthalmol.* **2007**, *52*, 397–421. [CrossRef]
150. Gelfand, J.M.; Nolan, R.; Schwartz, D.M.; Graves, J.; Green, A.J. Microcystic Macular Oedema in Multiple Sclerosis Is Associated with Disease Severity. *Brain* **2012**, *135*, 1786–1793. [CrossRef]
151. Kappos, L.; Radue, E.W.; O'connor, P.; Polman, C.; Hohlfeld, R.; Calabresi, P.; Selmaj, K.; Agoropoulou, C.; Leyk, M.; Zhang-Auberson, L.; et al. A Placebo-Controlled Trial of Oral Fingolimod in Relapsing Multiple Sclerosis. *N. Engl. J. Med.* **2010**, *362*, 387–401. [CrossRef]
152. Barboni, P.; Carelli, V.; Savini, G.; Carbonelli, M.; La Morgia, C.; Sadun, A.A. Microcystic Macular Degeneration from Optic Neuropathy: Not Inflammatory, Not Trans-Synaptic Degeneration. *Brain* **2013**, *136*, e239. [CrossRef]
153. Strong, S.A.; Hirji, N.; Quartilho, A.; Kalitzeos, A.; Michaelides, M. Retrospective Cohort Study Exploring Whether an Association Exists between Spatial Distribution of Cystoid Spaces in Cystoid Macular Oedema Secondary to Retinitis Pigmentosa and Response to Treatment with Carbonic Anhydrase Inhibitors. *Br. J. Ophthalmol.* **2019**, *103*, 233–237. [CrossRef]
154. Hajali, M.; Fishman, G.A.; Anderson, R.J. The Prevalence of Cystoid Macular Oedema in Retinitis Pigmentosa Patients Determined by Optical Coherence Tomography. *Br. J. Ophthalmol.* **2008**, *92*, 1065. [CrossRef]
155. Abegg, M.; Zinkernagel, M.; Wolf, S. Microcystic Macular Degeneration from Optic Neuropathy. *Brain* **2012**, *135*, e225. [CrossRef]
156. Balk, L.J.; Killestein, J.; Polman, C.H.; Uitdehaag, B.M.; Petzold, A. Microcystic Macular Oedema Confirmed, but Not Specific for Multiple Sclerosis. *Brain* **2012**, *135*, e226. [CrossRef]
157. Agte, S.; Junek, S.; Matthias, S.; Ulbricht, E.; Erdmann, I.; Wurm, A.; Schild, D.; Käs, J.A.; Reichenbach, A. Müller Glial Cell-Provided Cellular Light Guidance through the Vital Guinea-Pig Retina. *Biophys. J.* **2011**, *101*, 2611–2619. [CrossRef]
158. Aly, L.; Strauß, E.M.; Feucht, N.; Weiß, I.; Berthele, A.; Mitsdoerffer, M.; Haass, C.; Hemmer, B.; Maier, M.; Korn, T.; et al. Optical Coherence Tomography Angiography Indicates Subclinical Retinal Disease in Neuromyelitis Optica Spectrum Disorders. *Mult. Scler.* **2021**, *28*, 522–531. [CrossRef] [PubMed]
159. Lin, T.-Y.; Chien, C.; Lu, A.; Paul, F.; Zimmermann, H.G. Retinal Optical Coherence Tomography and Magnetic Resonance Imaging in Neuromyelitis Optica Spectrum Disorders and Mog-Antibody Associated Disorders: An Updated Review. *Expert Rev. Neurother.* **2021**, *21*, 1101–1123. [CrossRef] [PubMed]
160. Kwapong, W.R.; Peng, C.; He, Z.; Zhuang, X.; Shen, M.; Lu, F. Altered Macular Microvasculature in Neuromyelitis Optica Spectrum Disorders. *Am. J. Ophthalmol.* **2018**, *192*, 47–55. [CrossRef] [PubMed]
161. Asavapanumas, N.; Verkman, A.S. Neuromyelitis Optica Pathology in Rats following Intraperitoneal Injection of Nmo-Igg and Intracerebral Needle Injury. *Acta Neuropathol. Commun.* **2014**, *2*, 48. [CrossRef]
162. Kinoshita, M.; Nakatsuji, Y.; Kimura, T.; Moriya, M.; Takata, K.; Okuno, T.; Kumanogoh, A.; Kajiyama, K.; Yoshikawa, H.; Sakoda, S. Neuromyelitis Optica: Passive Transfer to Rats by Human Immunoglobulin. *Biochem. Biophys. Res. Commun.* **2009**, *386*, 623–627. [CrossRef]
163. Kurosawa, K.; Misu, T.; Takai, Y.; Sato, D.K.; Takahashi, T.; Abe, Y.; Iwanari, H.; Ogawa, R.; Nakashima, I.; Fujihara, K.; et al. Severely Exacerbated Neuromyelitis Optica Rat Model with Extensive Astrocytopathy by High Affinity Anti-Aquaporin-4 Monoclonal Antibody. *Acta Neuropathol. Commun.* **2015**, *3*, 82. [CrossRef]
164. Bennett, J.L.; Lam, C.; Kalluri, S.R.; Saikali, P.; Bautista, K.; Dupree, C.; Glogowska, M.; Case, D.; Antel, J.P.; Owens, G.P.; et al. Intrathecal Pathogenic Anti-Aquaporin-4 Antibodies in Early Neuromyelitis Optica. *Ann. Neurol.* **2009**, *66*, 617–629. [CrossRef]

165. Bradl, M.; Lassmann, H. Experimental Models of Neuromyelitis Optica. *Brain Pathol.* **2014**, *24*, 74–82. [CrossRef]
166. Bradl, M.; Misu, T.; Takahashi, T.; Watanabe, M.; Mader, S.; Reindl, M.; Adzemovic, M.; Bauer, J.; Berger, T.; Fujihara, K.; et al. Neuromyelitis Optica: Pathogenicity of Patient Immunoglobulin in Vivo. *Ann. Neurol.* **2009**, *66*, 630–643. [CrossRef]
167. Geis, C.; Ritter, C.; Ruschil, C.; Weishaupt, A.; Grunewald, B.; Stoll, G.; Holmoy, T.; Misu, T.; Fujihara, K.; Hemmer, B.; et al. The Intrinsic Pathogenic Role of Autoantibodies to Aquaporin 4 Mediating Spinal Cord Disease in a Rat Passive-Transfer Model. *Exp. Neurol.* **2015**, *265*, 8–21. [CrossRef]
168. Zhang, H.; Verkman, A.S. Longitudinally Extensive Nmo Spinal Cord Pathology Produced by Passive Transfer of Nmo-Igg in Mice Lacking Complement Inhibitor Cd59. *J. Autoimmun.* **2014**, *53*, 67–77. [CrossRef]
169. Matsumoto, Y.; Kanamori, A.; Nakamura, M.; Takahashi, T.; Nakashima, I.; Negi, A. Sera from Patients with Seropositive Neuromyelitis Optica Spectral Disorders Caused the Degeneration of Rodent Optic Nerve. *Exp. Eye Res.* **2014**, *119*, 61–69. [CrossRef]
170. Redler, Y.; Levy, M. Rodent Models of Optic Neuritis. *Front. Neurol.* **2020**, *11*, 580951. [CrossRef]
171. Pohl, M.; Fischer, M.-T.; Mader, S.; Schanda, K.; Kitic, M.; Sharma, R.; Wimmer, I.; Misu, T.; Fujihara, K.; Reindl, M.; et al. Pathogenic T Cell Responses against Aquaporin 4. *Acta Neuropathol.* **2011**, *122*, 21–34. [CrossRef]
172. Jones, M.V.; Collongues, N.; De Seze, J.; Kinoshita, M.; Nakatsuji, Y.; Levy, M. Review of Animal Models of Neuromyelitis Optica. *Mult. Scler. Relat. Disord.* **2012**, *1*, 174–179. [CrossRef]
173. Ratelade, J.; Bennett, J.L.; Verkman, A.S. Intravenous Neuromyelitis Optica Autoantibody in Mice Targets Aquaporin-4 in Peripheral Organs and Area Postrema. *PLoS ONE* **2011**, *6*, e27412. [CrossRef]
174. Hinson, S.R.; Roemer, S.F.; Lucchinetti, C.F.; Fryer, J.P.; Kryzer, T.J.; Chamberlain, J.L.; Howe, C.L.; Pittock, S.J.; Lennon, V.A. Aquaporin-4-Binding Autoantibodies in Patients with Neuromyelitis Optica Impair Glutamate Transport by Down-Regulating Eaat2. *J. Exp. Med.* **2008**, *205*, 2473–2481. [CrossRef] [PubMed]
175. Waters, P.; Jarius, S.; Littleton, E.; Leite, M.I.; Jacob, S.; Gray, B.; Geraldes, R.; Vale, T.; Jacob, A.; Palace, J.; et al. Aquaporin-4 Antibodies in Neuromyelitis Optica and Longitudinally Extensive Transverse Myelitis. *Arch Neurol.* **2008**, *65*, 913–919. [CrossRef] [PubMed]
176. Oberheim, N.A.; Wang, X.; Goldman, S.; Nedergaard, M. Astrocytic Complexity Distinguishes the Human Brain. *Trends Neurosci.* **2006**, *29*, 547–553. [CrossRef] [PubMed]
177. Sanes, J.R.; Masland, R.H. The Types of Retinal Ganglion Cells: Current Status and Implications for Neuronal Classification. *Annu. Rev. Neurosci.* **2015**, *38*, 221–246. [CrossRef] [PubMed]
178. Traub, J.; Hausser-Kinzel, S.; Weber, M.S. Differential Effects of Ms Therapeutics on B Cells-Implications for Their Use and Failure in Aqp4-Positive Nmosd Patients. *Int. J. Mol. Sci.* **2020**, *21*, 5021. [CrossRef]
179. Bergman, I.; Basse, P.H.; Barmada, M.A.; Griffin, J.A.; Cheung, N.K. Comparison of in Vitro Antibody-Targeted Cytotoxicity Using Mouse, Rat and Human Effectors. *Cancer Immunol. Immunother.* **2000**, *49*, 259–266. [CrossRef]

International Journal of
Molecular Sciences

MDPI

Review

Erythropoietin in Optic Neuropathies: Current Future Strategies for Optic Nerve Protection and Repair

Yi-Fen Lai [1], Ting-Yi Lin [1], Pin-Kuan Ho [2], Yi-Hao Chen [1], Yu-Chuan Huang [3,4,*] and Da-Wen Lu [1,*]

1 Department of Ophthalmology, Tri-Service General Hospital, National Defense Medical Center, Taipei 11490, Taiwan; iris92929@gmail.com (Y.-F.L.); pa735210@gmail.com (T.-Y.L.); doc30879@mail.ndmctsgh.edu.tw (Y.-H.C.)
2 School of Dentistry, National Defense Medical Center, Taipei 11490, Taiwan; james.sonicho@gmail.com
3 School of Pharmacy, National Defense Medical Center, Taipei 11490, Taiwan
4 Department of Research and Development, National Defense Medical Center, Taipei 11490, Taiwan
* Correspondence: yuh@mail.ndmctsgh.edu.tw (Y.-C.H.); ludawen@yahoo.com (D.-W.L.); Tel.: +886-2-87923100 (Y.-C.H.); +886-2-87927163 (D.-W.L.)

Abstract: Erythropoietin (EPO) is known as a hormone for erythropoiesis in response to anemia and hypoxia. However, the effect of EPO is not only limited to hematopoietic tissue. Several studies have highlighted the neuroprotective function of EPO in extra-hematopoietic tissues, especially the retina. EPO could interact with its heterodimer receptor (EPOR/βcR) to exert its anti-apoptosis, anti-inflammation and anti-oxidation effects in preventing retinal ganglion cells death through different intracellular signaling pathways. In this review, we summarized the available pre-clinical studies of EPO in treating glaucomatous optic neuropathy, optic neuritis, non-arteritic anterior ischemic optic neuropathy and traumatic optic neuropathy. In addition, we explore the future strategies of EPO for optic nerve protection and repair, including advances in EPO derivates, and EPO deliveries. These strategies will lead to a new chapter in the treatment of optic neuropathy.

Keywords: erythropoietin; neuroprotection; retinal ganglion cell; optic neuropathy; optic nerve protection

Citation: Lai, Y.-F.; Lin, T.-Y.; Ho, P.-K.; Chen, Y.-H.; Huang, Y.-C.; Lu, D.-W. Erythropoietin in Optic Neuropathies: Current Future Strategies for Optic Nerve Protection and Repair. *Int. J. Mol. Sci.* **2022**, *23*, 7143. https://doi.org/10.3390/ijms23137143

Academic Editor: Katalin Prokai-Tatrai

Received: 11 May 2022
Accepted: 24 June 2022
Published: 27 June 2022

1. Introduction

Erythropoietin (EPO) is a hormone that can stimulate erythropoiesis [1]. Its expression is regulated by hypoxia-inducible factors (HIF), a transduction factor sensitive to anemia and hypoxia [2]. EPO is produced by interstitial cells in the adult kidney [3]. It is secreted into the plasma and stimulates hematopoietic stem cell differentiation into red blood cells; however, the effect of EPO is not limited to erythroid tissues. EPO and EPO receptors (EPOR) have autocrine and paracrine functions in extra-hematopoietic tissues such as the endothelium, the heart, and the central nervous system, including the retina [4–7]. The role of EPO in paracrine signaling in the retina, which occurs inside the blood-retinal barrier, suggests its physiological roles other than erythropoiesis.

An abundance of EPO and EPOR has been demonstrated in the retina of humans [8]. EPO, the product of ganglion cells and retinal pigment epithelium cells is capable of targeting EPOR on photoreceptor cells, bipolar cells and amacrine cells [9]. A study indicated that EPOR upregulation is important for neuroprotection in retinal ischemic preconditioning [10]. Another study supported that exogenous EPO could protect neuron from damage in a model of transient global retinal ischemia [11]. In our previous studies, we found that EPO could protect cultured adult rat retinal ganglion cells (RGCs) against N-methyl-d-aspartate (NMDA) toxicity, tumor necrosis factor-alpha (TNF-α) toxicity and trophic factor withdrawal (TFW) [12]. Our in vivo study also found that intravitreal injection of EPO could attenuate NMDA-mediated excitotoxic retinal damage [13]. Except for the studies mentioned, many researchers have stated that EPO possesses antiapoptosis [14], antioxidative [15] and anti-inflammatory [16] properties. These properties are factors to why EPO is characterized to have neuroprotective effect in an organism's retina. Understanding the features of EPO might result in the development of beneficial optic neuropathy treatments, including new delivery systems and derivatives with prolonged drug action of tissue protection and without erythropoietic side effects. Therefore, we summarize the available studies involving the neuroprotective effects of EPO in optic neuropathies and propose future strategies involving EPO in optic nerve repair and protection.

2. EPOR: Different Isoforms with Pleiotropic Functions

The structure of EPOR consists of a cytoplasmic domain with 235 amino acids, a single transmembrane domain with 23 amino acids, and an extracellular domain with 225 amino acids [17]. There are two subdomains, D1 and D2, in the extracellular domain, both of which are necessary for EPO binding [17]. Different isoforms of EPOR have been identified and characterized to have pleiotropic functions:

2.1. The Homodimer Isoform: $EPOR_2$

The homodimer isoform is present in erythroblasts [17]. During hematopoiesis, EPO binds to its receptor and results in homodimerization of EPOR (Figure 1) [18]. Following binding, Janus kinase-2 (JAK-2) activates several secondary signal molecules [17,19], such as STAT5 [20], MAPK, and PI3-K/Akt [21]. The activation of these molecules contributes to the differentiation and maturation of erythroid progenitor cells [22].

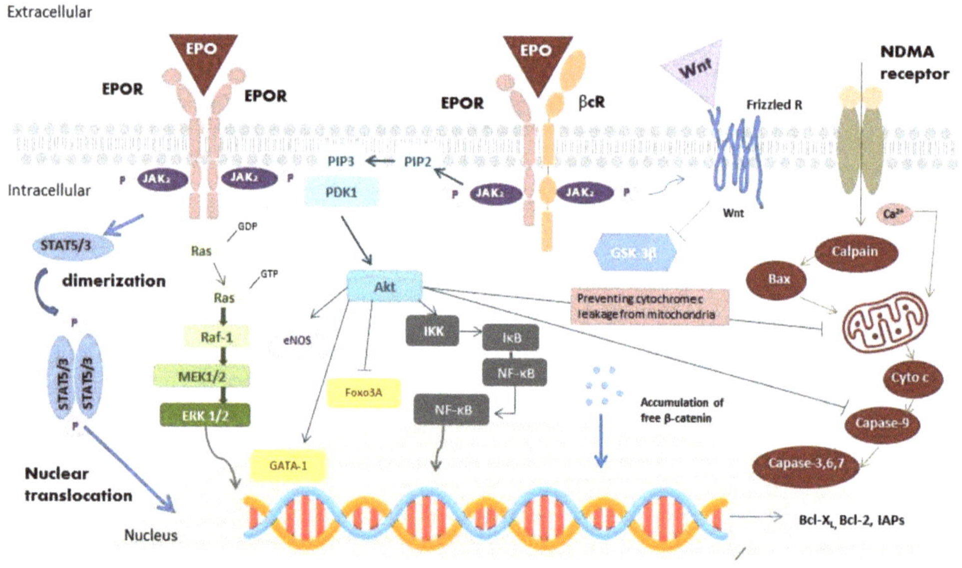

Figure 1. Binding of EPO to EPOR induces JAK-2 phosphorylation, dimerization, and subsequently activate STAT5/3, Ras/Raf/MEK/ERK, PI3-K/Akt, and NF-κB pathways. JAK-2 phosphorylates STAT5 or STAT3, leading to the dimerization of STAT5 (STAT3). STAT5 (STAT3) and the last signaling molecule in the MAPK pathway translocate into the nucleus and upregulate the expression of antiapoptotic Bcl-2 and Bcl-xL. Activation of PI3-k/Akt pathway increases endothelial nitric oxide synthase (eNOS) protein expression and NO production, which could increase blood flow and attenuate regional injury. PI3-k/Akt pathway also phosphorylates transcription factor GATA-1 and

Foxo3 A, which enhance the expression of antiapoptosis proteins. Activation of the IKK complex by Akt phosphorylates IκB, resulting in its ubiquitination, and degradation, and in the releases of bound NF-κB. Free NF-κB translocates into the nucleus and exerts its antiapoptosis activity through the expression of inhibitors of apoptotic proteins (IAPs). Furthermore, binding of EPO to EPOR/βcR activates Wnt signaling, which inhibits GSK-3β phosphorylation and allow β-catenin to stabilize and accumulate in the cytoplasm in a non-phosphorylated form. Free β-catenin translocates into the nucleus and trigger transcription of Wnt-target gene responsible for cell antiapoptosis and the development of nervous system. Activation of NMDA receptors allows the influx of Ca^{2+}, which induces excitotoxicity via initiation of the μ-calpain/Bax/cytochrome c/caspase-9 pathway. The caspases result in DNA fragmentation and lead to cell apoptosis. Activation of PI3-K/Akt pathway could also inhibit caspase activity by preventing cytochrome c leakage from mitochondria, thus inhibiting DNA degradation.

2.2. Heterodimer Isoform: EPOR/βcR

In addition to the homodimerization, there are other types of EPO receptors, which involve affinities 8–16 times weaker [23,24]. A study confirmed the receptor was a heterodimer consisting of EPOR and the β common receptor (βcR), a subunit of granulocyte-macrophage colony stimulating factor, interleukin 5, and interleukin 3 [25]. Since the EpoR/βcR heterodimer has the properties against tissue injury and inflammation, some authors named it as the "tissue-protective receptor" or "innate repair receptor" [26]. Recent data found the presence of this heterodimer complex in the RGCs, inner nuclear layer and photoreceptors [27]. In experimental studies, EPO binding to the EPOR/βcR heterodimer could reduce light-induced photoreceptor cell death [27]. Additionally, EPO binding to the EPOR/βcR heterodimer could activate Wingless (Wnt) signaling (Figure 1) [28], which could regulate cells survival, and differentiation. Wnt signaling is an important pathway responsible for the development of different ocular structure [29]. This heterodimer receptor contributes to the majority of the protective effects of EPO, which potentially underlines a vast quantity of therapeutic approaches.

2.3. Extracellular Soluble Isoform: sEPOR

The extracellular soluble isoform of EPOR (sEPOR), which lacks the transmembrane and cytoplasmic domains, is found in human plasma [30]. During hypoxia, in contrast to the expression of the full-length form increased through HIF transduction, the expression of the sEPOR is downregulated. In many studies, sEPOR is viewed as an endogenous antagonist of EPO, which blocks the neuroprotective effects of EPO. This form interacts with EPO without further activation of any downstream pathways. Moreover, its binding with EPO restricts the interaction of EPO with other receptor isoforms, resulting in a lower availability and bioactivity of EPO [10,31].

3. Effects of EPO

3.1. Angiogenic Effects

The transcription factor, HIF, has a vital role in hematopoiesis. In normoxic conditions, prolyl hydroxylase domain proteins (PHDs) hydroxylate all HIF-α subunit. After binding to von Hippel–Lindau tumor suppressor protein (VHL), hydroxylated HIF-α is then ubiquitinated. The ubiquitination of hydroxylated HIFs results in its degradation by the proteasome. In hypoxic conditions, the action of PHDs is inhibited. The stabilized HIF-α thus binds to HIF-β and translocates into the nucleus to regulate erythropoiesis via regulation of the expression of the EPO gene, vascular endothelial growth factor (VEGF) [32], as well as genes coding for proteins involved in iron metabolism [33], which are important for tissue oxygenation. After translation of EPO, the EPO is secreted into the circulation to reach hematopoietic cells. EPO binds with EPOR on erythroid cells, which triggers homodimerization of EPOR and activates the EPOR-associated JAK-2 by autophosphorylation (Figure 1) [17]. The active kinase JAK-2 results in the phosphorylation of tyrosine residues on the cytoplasmic portion of the EPOR [17]. The phospho-tyrosine residues recruit various proteins, which subsequently activate a series of pathways, including JAK-2/STAT5 (STAT3), PI3-K/Akt, and MAPK pathway [20,21]. JAK-2 phosphorylates STAT5 or STAT3, once it binds to the cytoplasmic portion of EPOR. STAT5 (STAT3) homodimerizes and translocates into the nucleus as a gene transcription factor. Activating the JAK-2/STAT5 (STAT3) pathway also leads to the upregulation of the antiapoptotic B-cell lymphoma-extra-large (Bcl-X_L) protein, therefore protecting proerythroblasts from apoptosis [34]. After the activation of Ras by adaptor proteins, initiation of RAF/mitogen-activated protein kinase (MEK)/extracellular signal-regulated kinase (ERK) pathway would occur. RAF-1 protein kinase phosphorylates MEK, which subsequently phosphorylates MAPK/ERK1/2 [35]. The last molecules in the cascades translocate into the nucleus and activate various gene transcription factors for erythropoiesis regulation. PI3-K/Akt pathway is one of the main activating signaling pathways. PI3-K could lead to the phosphorylation of Akt, which could activate other proteins involved in erythropoiesis regulation. Akt phosphorylates the transcription factor GATA binding protein-1 (GATA-1), which is an important transcription factor for the anti-apoptotic Bcl-X_L expression and erythroid-specific genes. Phosphorylation of GATA-1 could enhance GATA-1 activity in erythroid cell [36]. The forkhead box O3A (Foxo3A), another Akt targeted transcription factor, has proapoptotic functions; in contrast, phosphorylation of Foxo3A inhibits its transcriptional activity [37]. Figure 1 illustrates the intracellular signaling pathway of EPO. Dysfunction in these signaling pathway leads to abnormal erythropoiesis by disrupting cells proliferation and apoptosis.

3.2. Antiapoptotic Effects

Binding of EPO to EPOR results in JAK2 phosphorylation and initiates STAT5 (STAT3), MAPK, PI3-K/Akt and nuclear factor kappa-light-chain-enhancer (NF-κB) downstream pathways, which execute the antiapoptotic effect of EPO (Figure 1) [38]. The last molecules in the STAT5 (STAT3) and MAPK pathways could translocate into the nucleus and activate the apoptotic regulators of Bcl-2 family, antiapoptotic Bcl-2 and Bcl-X_L, to inhibit apoptosis [39]. Activation of PI3-K/Akt pathway also prevents cell apoptosis. Cell death signaling can be initiated by caspases or mitochondrial membrane depolarization. When the mitochondria membrane is depolarized, cytochrome c would be released into the cytoplasm and form the apoptosome complex with apoptotic protease activating factor-1 (Apaf-1) [40]. Pro-caspase-9 is activated by the apoptosome, which initiates downstream caspase activation. The activated caspases would cause DNA fragmentation and lead to cell apoptosis [40]. Activation of PI3-K/Akt pathway could inhibit caspase activity by preventing cytochrome c leakage from the mitochondria [41]. IκB kinase (IKK), another Akt target, is also associated with cell survival. In resting cells, NF-κB is held by the IκB. Activation of the IKK complex phosphorylates IκB, resulting in its ubiquitination and degradation, and in the releases of bound NF-κB. NF-κB exerts its protective effects through the increase in inhibitors of apoptotic protein (IAPs) [42], blocking of caspase activity [42], suppression of TNF-α related apoptosis [42], direct enhancing activation of Bcl-X_L, and removal of cellular reactive oxygen species (ROS) [43].

In addition, Wnt signaling was proven to inhibit cancer therapy-mediated apoptosis and exhibit its oncogenic properties through the antiapoptosis effect [44]. Binding of EPO to EPOR/βcR heterodimer, present in RGCs and ocular stem cells, also activates Wnt signaling (Figure 1). Wnt binds to the Frizzled transmembrane receptors, which inhibits β-catenin phosphorylated by glycogen synthase kinase (GSK)-3β [45]. Free β-catenin accumulates and thus translocate into the nucleus. The binding of β-catenin to T-cell factor (Tcf) regulates cells survivability [44].

3.3. Anti-Inflammatory Effects

In inflammatory conditions, EPO was detected at the borders of the injury sites. Hence, the potential anti-inflammatory effect of EPO has also been investigated. EPO was found to decrease pro-inflammatory cytokine production, including intercellular adhesion molecule-1 (ICAM-1) [46], interleukin-6 (IL-6) [47], and TNF-α [48,49]. EPO also increased the production of the anti-inflammatory cytokine IL-10 [48]. Additionally, EPO could increase endothelial nitric oxide synthase (eNOS) protein expression (Figure 1) [50], which increase nitric oxide production. Nitric oxide could increase blood flow, and attenuate regional injury [51]. As regards the innate immune system, EPO could facilitate phagocytosis in macrophages [52], mediate dendritic cell maturation and immunomodulation [53], and reduce inflammation caused by mast cells [54]. In previous literature, these effects were thought to be mediated by the inhibition of pro-inflammatory cytokines. However, recent studies have confirmed the existence of EPORs on human T and B lymphocytes, suggesting that EPO could potentially have a direct impact on the immune cells [55]. In the adaptive immune system, EPO could directly promote the proliferation of regulatory T cells, but inhibit the proliferation of conventional T cells without inducing apoptosis [56]. These anti-inflammatory effects of EPO have been observed in several experimental studies of kidney transplant, colitis and encephalomyelitis [56–58]. Thus, EPO is thought to be an important hormone that facilitates immune homeostasis.

3.4. Antioxidant Effects

EPO has the ability to attenuate oxidative stress, allowing it to be categorized as a cytoprotective agent [59,60]. EPO could induce heme oxygenase-1 expression via PI3K/Akt pathway [61], which could provide a cytoprotective effect in astrocytes [62]. EPO also increases the level of glutathione peroxidase, a potent antioxidant protein, which can decrease the toxic activity of ROS [63]. Apart from direct antioxidative effects of EPO, indirect antioxidative effects have been reported. For example, the increase in the number of red blood cells resulting from EPO activity results in an increase in total level of antioxidative enzymes. [64]. EPO could also indirectly inhibit iron-dependent oxidative injury by depleting iron, a major catalyst for free radial reaction [65].

4. Current Strategy of EPO for Optic Nerve Protection and Repair

Encouraging results of EPO from basic research support the possibility of integrating its therapeutic effects in glaucomatous optic neuropathy, optic neuritis, non-arteritic anterior ischemic optic neuropathy (NAION), and traumatic optic neuropathy (TON). We summarize the available studies in the literature on the use of erythropoietin in these optic neuropathies (listed in Table 1).

Glaucomatous optic neuropathy, a neurodegenerative disease, is characterized by progressive loss of RGCs. Elevated intraocular pressure (IOP) is considered the most important risk factor of glaucomatous optic neuropathy. However, some patients experienced continued RGCs loss despite good intraocular pressure control, suggesting the presence of other complicated mechanisms stimulating RGC death. Multifactorial mechanisms have been postulated for glaucomatous optic neuropathy, including vascular insufficiency, inflammation [66,67], excitotoxicity [68] and neurotrophic factor withdrawal [69]. Due to the complex pathogenesis of glaucoma, EPO was developed to prevent the IOP-independent RGCs loss. Several studies have reported that the EPO level in the aqueous humor increased in patients with glaucoma [70]. The cause of the elevated aqueous EPO in glaucomatous eyes might be related to the ischemia, hypoxia, or elevated ROS caused by glaucomatous damage [71]. The increase in EPO is identified as a compensatory response due to the presence of glutamate, nitric oxide and the free radicals after the glaucomatous damage [72].

Previous studies have reported glutamate and NMDA excitotoxicity as the probable mechanism of glaucoma. This involves the opening of ion channels which allows the entry of extracellular Ca^{2+} into neurons. Ca^{2+} acts as second messenger to activate downstream signaling pathways leading to RGCs apoptosis [73]. TNF-α and TNF-α receptor 1 signaling could also induce RGC hyper-excitability by upregulating Na^{+} channels, which contribute to RGCs apoptosis in glaucoma [74]. In our previous study, we cultured RGCs from adult rats in a medium containing neurotrophic factors [12]. Cytotoxicity was induced by NMDA, TFW, and TNF-α. EPO was found to provide neuroprotection to cultured adult rat RGCs against NMDA-, TFW-, and TNF-α -induced toxicity. The efficacy of EPO is similar with memantine (an NMDA receptor antagonist), glial cell-derived neurotrophic factor (GDNF), and Z-IETD-FMK (a caspase-8 inhibitor). Additionally, inhibiting STAT5, MAPK/ERK and PI3K/Akt signal impaired the protective effects of EPO [12]. We subsequently investigated the effect of EPO in vivo study [13]. Wistar rats were randomly assigned to different groups treated with intravitreal NMDA and EPO. We found that EPO had dose-dependent neuroprotective effect against NDMA-mediated neurotoxicity. Through histological findings, EPO was also found to reverse the NMDA-induced damage to bipolar cell axon terminals in the inner plexiform layer. We also observed that in the excitotoxic signaling pathway of NDMA-induced toxicity, μ-calpain is activated first, followed by Bax, and then caspase-9 (Figure 1). EPO could protect RGCs by downregulating the activity of μ-calpain, Bax as well as caspase-9 [13].

Apart from our previous research results, EPO was also found to be neuroprotective via systemic, intravitreal, subconjunctival and retrobulbar administration in rat model of glaucoma. The DBA/2J mice, which spontaneously develop glaucomatous loss of RGC and are used to mimic human hereditary glaucoma, were intraperitoneally injected with EPO. Treatment with EPO could promote RGC survival without affecting IOP [75]. Subconjunctival injection of EPO in a rat model of glaucoma demonstrated increase in electroretinography wave amplitudes and retinal thickness [76]. Retrobulbar injection of EPO could preserve RGCs in rats with acute elevated IOP [77]. A single intravitreal injection of EPO could provide protective effects on RGC viability in rat model of glaucoma [78]. Based on the aforementioned studies, EPO is found to have neuroprotective effects regardless of the EPO administration methods. However, the discussion of EPO in the treatment of glaucoma is limited to animal studies. In humans, there are only a few observational studies investigating the correlation between EPO and glaucoma, especially neovascular glaucoma [79–81]. To date, human studies using EPO for the treatment of glaucoma are still lacking. Future studies could focus the application of EPO in patients with primary open-angle glaucoma to see if EPO exhibits the same neuroprotective effects in animal experiments.

Optic neuritis is another high occurring disease among the world population. For optic neuritis, methylprednisolone is the standard treatment in clinical practices. Although steroid treatment could accelerate visual acuity recovery, recent study demonstrates that steroids could not influence the visual outcome or atrophy of the optic nerve [82]. An animal study even demonstrated that methylprednisolone could increase RGCs degeneration by inhibiting the neurotrophin pathway [83]. Since EPO has shown multiple neurotrophin-like properties in various neuronal disorders, the efficacy of EPO is evaluated as an add-on therapy to methylprednisolone in autoimmune optic neuritis by investigators. In an experimental autoimmune encephalomyelitis (EAE) rat model, intraperitoneal injection of EPO (5000 U/kg) significantly increased the survivability and functionality of RGCs in rats afflicted with myelin oligodendrocyte glycoprotein (MOG)-induced optic neuritis [84]. In the model of MOG-EAE, Sättler et al. concluded that the PI3-K/Akt pathway plays an important role in RGCs survivability under systemic treatment with EPO [84]. Establishment of potentially relevant intracellular conduction pathways might make the application of EPO more feasible in MOG-EAE. Human studies have been performed, but the results were not conclusive. A comparatives study in humans demonstrated no difference in visual acuity, visual field and contrast sensitivity between the intravenous EPO (20,000 IU/day) accompanied with methylprednisolone group, and the methylprednisolone only group [85]. A comparative study reported intravenous EPO (33,000 IU/day) as an add-on therapy to methylprednisolone improved median deviation of perimetry in acute optic neuritis [86], but post-intervention retinal nerve fiber layer (RNFL) thickness demonstrated no significant difference from the methylprednisolone only group [86]. One double-blinded randomized control study demonstrated decreased structural and functional impairments in EPO add-on group [87]. Retinal nerve fiber thinning was less apparent, and visual evoked potential latencies were shorter in the EPO add-on group than in the control group. One randomized, placebo-controlled, double blind, phase 3 study compared patients receiving intravenous EPO (33,000 IU/day) plus methylprednisolone to patients receiving placebo plus methylprednisolone [88]. Mean RNFL thickness atrophy and mean low contrast letter acuity scores showed no difference between these two groups [88]. Most of the studies failed to demonstrate EPO to be a structurally and functionally neuroprotective agent as an add-on therapy in optic neuritis. The reason might be that most of these studies chose longer disease-treatment duration (0–10 days), and did not stratify the severity of optic neuritis. The application of EPO on the injured tissues might lack receptors activity since severe inflammation might decrease tissue bioavailability for drugs to interact. Additionally, all studies administrated EPO systemically in a short duration (3 days). The efficacy of EPO might therefore be limited. Future studies into this matter could classify the severity of optic neuritis, administer EPO more closely to disease onset and extend the treatment duration to see the therapeutic effects of EPO.

Table 1. Summary of clinical studies that evaluate the effect of erythropoietin on optic neuropathies.

Authors	Year	Study Design	Number of Eyes/Patients (Animals)	Intervention	Main Outcomes
Glaucoma (Animal Studies)					
Cheng et al. [13]	2020	Randomized intervention study	125 Wistar rats	Randomly assigned into five groups: (1) Control (2) Intravitreal NMDA80 (3) Intravitreal NMDA80 + 10 ng EPO (4) Intravitreal NMDA80 + 50 ng EPO (5) Intravitreal NMDA80 + 250 ng EPO	EPO protects RGCs and bipolar cell axon terminals in IPL by downregulating apoptotic factors to attenuate NMDA-mediated excitotoxic retinal damage.
Zhong et al. [75]	2007	Intervention study	91 C57BL/6J mice and 294 DBA/2J mice	Assigned into 5 groups: (1) Control (2) Intraperitoneal Memantine (70 mg/kg/wk) (3) Intraperitoneal EPO (3000 IU/Kg/wk) (4) Intraperitoneal EPO (6000 IU/Kg/wk) (5) Intraperitoneal EPO (12,000 U/Kg/wk)	EPO's effects were similar to those of memantine, a known neuroprotective agent. EPO promoted RGCs survival in DBA/2J glaucomatous mice without affecting IOP.
Resende et al. [76]	2018	Comparative study	26 Wistar Hannover albino rats with unilateral glaucoma induced by coagulation of 3 episcleral veins in the right eye Case (right eye): 13 eyes Control (left eye): 13 eyes	Subconjunctival injection of 1000 IU EPO versus placebo	EPO improved both scoptopic and photopic amplitude. Retinal thickness is thicker in EPO group.
Zhong et al. [77]	2008	Intervention study	75 rats with unilateral glaucoma induced by saline infused into anterior chamber. The IOP was raised to 70 mm Hg for a duration of up to 60 min.	Assigned into 5 groups: (1) Unoperated control (2) Operated control (3) Acute elevated IOP group (4) Acute elevated IOP + retrobulbar EPO (1000 U/100 μL) (5) Acute elevated IOP + vehicle solution retrobulbar injection (i.e., EPO diluted in a vehicle solution)	EPO with a retrobulbar administration could protect RGCs from acute elevated IOP.
Tsai et al. [78]	2005	Intervention study	29 Sprague Dawley rats with EVC glaucoma model	Assigned into 4 groups: (1) Unoperated control (2) Episcleral vessel cautery (3) EVC + intravitreal normal saline (4) EVC + intravitreal EPO(200 ng/5 μL)	RGC counts were significantly decreased in both the EVC and EVC+ intravitreal normal saline groups but not significantly decreased in the EVC-EPO treated retinas.

Table 1. *Cont.*

Authors	Year	Study Design	Number of Eyes/Patients (Animals)	Intervention	Main Outcomes
Optic Neuritis (Human Studies)					
Sanjari et al. [85]	2019	Nonrandomized comparative case–control study	62 patients with isolated retrobulbar optic neuritis (onset <10 days) Cases: 35 patients Control: 27 patients	Intravenous EPO 20,000 IU/day for 3 days + intravenous methylprednisolone versus intravenous methylprednisolone	No difference was observed between the two groups in BCVA, contrast sensitivity, MD of visual field, and pace of recovery of visual acuity at 120-day follow-up.
Shayegannejad et al. [86]	2015	Nonrandomized comparative case–control study	30 patients with acute optic neuritis with unknown origin or demyelinative origin (onset < 4 days) Cases: 15 patients Control: 15 patients	Intravenous EPO 33,000 IU/day for 3 days + intravenous methylprednisolone versus intravenous methylprednisolone	The amount of MD improvement was significantly higher in EPO-treated group. No difference was observed between the two groups in post-intervention PSD, amount of PSD improvement, post-intervention RNFL, and RNFL loss at 6-month follow up.
Sühs et al. [87]	2012	Randomized double-blind clinical trial	37 patients with unilateral optic neuritis (onset < 10 days) Case: 20 patients Control: 17 patients	Intravenous EPO 33,000 IU/day for 3 days + methylprednisolone versus intravenous methylprednisolone	EPO group had less RNFL thinning, shorter VEP latencies, and smaller decrease in retrobulbar diameter of optic nerve. No difference was observed between the two groups in recovery of visual acuity and visual field perception at 16-week follow-up.
Lagrèze et al. [88]	2021	Randomized double-blind clinical trial	103 patients with unilateral optic neuritis (onset < 10 days) Case: 52 patients Control: 51 patients	Intravenous EPO 33,000 IU/day for 3 days + methylprednisolone versus intravenous methylprednisolone	No difference was observed between the two groups in post-intervention RNFL thickness, low contrast visual acuity at 26-week follow up. One patient in EPO group developed a venous sinus thrombosis, which was treated with anticoagulants and resolved without sequelae.
Non-Arteritic Anterior Ischemic Optic Neuropathy(Human Studies)					
Modarres et al. [89]	2011	Case series	31 patients with NAION (onset ≤ 1 month)	Intravitreal injection of EPO (2000 IU/0.2 mL).	EPO improved visual acuity and MD at 3-month follow up. The effect of EPO began to wear off after 3 months. The improvement in BCVA from baseline persisted at 6-month follow-up.
Pakravan et al. [90]	2017	Nonrandomized comparative case series	113 patients with NAION (onset < 14 days) I.V. Steroid + EPO: 40 patients I.V. Steroid: 43 patients Observation: 30 patients	Assigned into 3 groups: (1) Intravenous EPO 10,000 IU BID for 3 days + intravenous methylprednisolone (2) Intravenous methylprednisolone (3) Observation	No significant differences were observed among the three groups in visual acuity, peripapillary RNFL thickness, and visual field at 6-month follow-up.
Nikkhan et al. [91]	2020	Randomized clinical trial	99 patients with NAION (onset ≤ 5 days) EPO: 34 patients Oral steroid: 33 patients Placebo: 32 patients	Assigned into 3 groups: (1) Intravenous EPO 10,000 IU BID for 3 days (2) Oral prednisolone (3) Placebo	More patients in the EPO group gained at least 3 lines of BCVA. Patients in EPO group preserved more peripapillary RNFL. No significant differences in visual acuity and MD of visual field among the three groups at 6-month follow-up.
Traumatic Optic Neuropathy(Human Studies)					
Kashkouli et al. [92]	2011	Nonrandomized comparative case–control study	15 patients with iTON (onset < 3 weeks) EPO: 7 patients Observation: 8 patients	Intravenous injection of EPO (10,000 IU/day) for 3 days	BCVA was significantly higher in the EPO group at last follow up (mean follow up time: EPO group: 7.0 months, observation group: 5.8 months)

Table 1. *Cont.*

Authors	Year	Study Design	Number of Eyes/Patients (Animals)	Intervention	Main Outcomes
Enterzari et al. [93]	2014	Case series	18 patients with iTON (onset < 2 weeks)	Intravenous injection of EPO (20,000 IU/day) for 3 days	EPO improve BCVA at 3-month follow-up.
Kashkouli et al. [94]	2017	Clinical trial	100 patients with TON (onset < 3 weeks) EPO: 69 patients Steroid: 15 patients Observation: 16 patients	Assigned into 3 groups: (1) Intravenous EPO (10,000 or 20,000 IU/day) for 3 days (2) Intravenous methylprednisolone (3) Observation	All three groups showed a significant improvement of BCVA. Differences between groups were not statistically significant. Color vision was significantly improved in the EPO group at 3-month follow-up.
Rashad et al. [95]	2018	Case series	Recent iTON (<3 month): 7 eyes Old iTON (3–36 months): 7 eyes	Intravitreal injection of EPO (2000 IU/0.2 mL)	Both groups have improvement in BCVA, visual evoked response amplitude, and latency at 6-month follow-up.

NMDA: N-Methyl-D-aspartic acid; EPO: erythropoietin; RGC: retinal ganglion cell; IOP: intraocular pressure; EVC: episcleral vessel cautery; BCVA: best-corrected visual acuity; MD: mean deviation; PSD: pattern standard deviation; RNFL: retinal nerve fiber layer; VEP: visual evoked potentials; NAION: non-arteritic anterior ischemic optic neuropathy; TON: traumatic optic neuropathy.

Non-arteritic anterior ischemic optic neuropathy is thought to result from vascular insufficiency. Patients with hypertension or obstructive sleep apnea have higher risk of developing NAION since the disease could result in hypoperfusion of the optic nerve. The hypoperfusion causes ischemia and swelling of the axons, thus increasing the pressure on the nervous tissues confined within the tight borders of the posterior scleral outlet. The axon swelling results in further ischemia and neuron swelling. The vicious cycle leads to severe ganglion cells damage. Due to the evidence showing neuroprotection effect of EPO, investigators also determined the efficacy of EPO in NAION. Modarres et al. conducted a prospective interventional case series by intravitreally injecting EPO (2000 IU/0.2 mL) into thirty-one patients within 1 month of the NAION onset [89]. Within the first month, 61.2% of patients had shown improvement in visual acuity, after 3 months, the protective effect of EPO began to wear off. Nevertheless, the visual acuity remained significantly better than baseline after a 6-month follow up [89]. Pakravan et al. performed another prospective comparative case series in 113 patients diagnosed as recent onset NAION (less than 14 days) [90]. Patients were categorized into three groups: intravenous methylprednisolone with intravenous EPO (10,000 IU twice a day for 3 days), intravenous methylprednisolone, and control group. Among the three experimental groups, there were no statistically significant differences in best-corrected visual acuity (BCVA), mean deviation, and peripapillary RNFL thickness after a 6-month follow up. The same research group later performed a randomized clinical trial to compare the effect of systemic EPO (10,000 IU twice a day for 3 days) versus oral steroids (75 mg daily tapered off within 6 weeks) versus placebo [91]. A total of 99 patients diagnosed as acute-onset (<5 days) NAION were included. The EPO-treated group did not improve visual acuity and mean deviation of visual field when compared to the oral steroid-treated group and placebo group. However, more patients (55%) in the EPO group gained at least three lines of BCVA. Patients in EPO group preserved more peripapillary RNFL [91]. Among the aforementioned studies, the case series by Modarres et al. reported that EPO was beneficial in NAION, but its limitation was the lack of a comparison group. The subsequent interventional comparative study by Pakravan et al. failed to demonstrate the benefits of EPO in NAION. They were debated involving the concomitant use of systemic steroid and EPO because high-dose steroid has shown to inhibit pro-inflammatory cytokines and neurotrophic factors. The postulated systemic steroid might blunt EPO's neuroprotective effects. Limitations of the study include the lack of randomized study design and the broad inclusion window (14 days), so the neuroprotective effect of EPO might not be demonstrated. The research team subsequently improved the limitations of their study by publishing a randomized study and narrowing the inclusion window (5 days), which proved that EPO did have some structural and functional benefits although EPO group did not have significantly better visual acuity than that in the steroid and placebo groups at the end of the tracking. Since existing studies shows intravenous EPO appears to have limitations in the treatment of NAION, future studies should be directed toward a larger randomized study to replicate the benefit of intravitreal EPO in NAION in Modarres's study.

For **traumatic optic neuropathy**, indirect TON is the more common type. The shearing force could lead to small vessel and neuron axon injury around the optic nerve by inducing ischemia, inflammation, and oxidative stress, all of which result in ganglion cell death. Currently, the common treatments are observation, corticosteroids and optic canal decompression. However, none of these managements are proven to be effective. Since EPO has shown to be neuroprotective, EPO might play a role in treating indirect TON. Intravenous EPO was first commenced in patients with indirect TON by Kashkouli et al. in 2011 [92]. Indirect TON patients with intravenous EPO (10,000 IU in 3 days) were compared to indirect TON patients without treatment. They found that the EPO-treated group has higher BCVA than that in the observation group. They advocated intravenous EPO may be a new effective and safe treatment in patients with indirect TON [92]. The efficacy of EPO in indirect TON was re-tested by Enterzari et al. in 2014. In the case series, EPO was also shown to improve the mean BCVA [93]. In 2017, Kashkouli et al. performed a phase 3, multicenter study. They enrolled TON patients with trauma-treatment duration less than 3 weeks [94]. The mean BCVA was compared among the three groups, including the EPO group, the methylprednisolone group and the observational group. The dosage of EPO was given according to patient's age, where 10,000 units EPO per day were infused into patients under 13 years of age and 20,000 units EPO per day were infused into patients above 13 years of age for 3 consecutive days. The EPO-treated group has better color vision than other groups. All three groups demonstrated improvement of BCVA. Although a better final vision was seen in the EPO group, but the results were insignificant between the groups [94]. They also reported late treatment (>3 days) and initial BCVA of no light perception as poor prognosis factors, but then another study takes a different view. Another study by Rashad et al. investigated the efficacy of intravitreal EPO in treating recent (<3 months trauma-treatment duration) and old (3–36 months) TON in 2018 [95]. They reported intravitreal injection of EPO (2000 IU/0.2 mL) improved BCVA, visual evoked response amplitude and latency in either recent and old indirect TON [95]. All of the above studies reported EPO could improve BCVA in TON patients either in the case series or in a larger clinical trial. Although EPO seems to bring promising experiment results, these studies still lack randomized study designs. The results need to be interpreted with care. The American Academy of Ophthalmology presented a report exploring the efficacy of surgery, steroids, EPO and other drugs for TON; however, they were also unable to reach a conclusion due to lack of level I evidence [96]. Notably, Rashad's study reported that intravitreal EPO could improve vision in old TON patients. The conclusion is highly anticipated since there has been no effective treatment for old TON patients. Future studies should prioritize a large, randomized study, while investigating the efficacy of intravitreal EPO in recent or old TON patients.

5. Advances in EPO Derivatives

For more than a decade, the use of EPO to treat hematopoietic anemia in chronic kidney disease has played an integral role in clinical practice. On non-hematopoietic cells, high-dose systemic EPO administration is required to promote tissue repair and neuroprotection due to the low affinity toward heterodimeric EPOR/βcR [23]. However, high doses of EPO have the potential to trigger undesirable side effects such as polycythemia and thromboembolic events. The development of EPO derivatives with a higher affinity toward the heterodimeric EPOR/βcR would further improve medical protocols by eliminating undesirable and detrimental effects. In addition, the availability of EPO derivatives could potentially lower the costs of EPO treatment and provide new series of treatment options to counteract different neurodegenerative diseases. Recently, newly modified EPO possesses improved characteristics as an erythropoiesis-stimulating agent (ESA), including diminished side effects, extended half-life, and reduced clearance rate during circulation.

Epoetin alfa (Epogen), a type of ESA medicine, has been the standard of care for patients with kidney disease and cancer-related anemia. **Epoetin alfa-epbx** (RetacritTM) shares the same amino acid sequence and similar carbohydrate composition as epoetin alfa (EpogenTM). In 2018, the protein was approved by the FDA, making it the first biosimilar EPO molecules approved in the USA [97]. **Darbepoetin alfa** (DA, Aranesp), an alternative agent of Epoetin alfa and a hyperglycosylated EPO analog, is a novel ESA with two additional N-glycosylation sites accompanied by 22 sialic acid moieties. In the attempt to extend the molecule's half-life by three-fold longer than EPO in vivo, glycoengineering was conducted to increase the structure's resistance to degradation. Darbepoetin alfa was approved for treating anemia resulting from renal diseases and cancer chemotherapy. The treatment protocol only requires a once-per-week visit and is accompanied by lower clinical costs [98,99]. **C.E.R.A.** (continuous erythropoietin receptor activator), a third-generation ESA, is an EPO (~34 kDa) integrated with methoxypolyethylene glycol (PEG, 30 kDa). Compared with other EPO derivatives, C.E.R.A. has a unique pharmacological profile with the longest half-life and slowest clearance rate. These unique pharmacological properties exist because of methoxypolyethylene glycol (PEG) integration into EPO. Notably, EPO pegylation (the process of connecting a hydrophilic polymer to EPO) significantly prolongs the duration of EPO action, and enhances proteolytic resistance in cell-free plasma [100].

Two types of modified EPO molecules with no affinity towards canonical EPOR have been developed, each of which possesses tissue protective effects by binding onto heterodimeric EPOR/βcR. The two enzymatically desialyated EPO are asialoerythropoietin (asialoEpo) and carbamylated EPO (cEpo), with each having neuron and oligodendrocyte protection capabilities without erythropoietic functions. **Asialerythropoietin** (asialoEPO) was evaluated to be a safe drug for clinical treatments. However, asialoEPO's half-life (t1/2~1.14 min) is much shorter than that of EPO (t1/2~5.6 h). The short half-life gives asialoEPO insufficient persistence time to stimulate hematopoiesis. Based on the above concept, researchers found that chemical modification of the EPO binding sites could abolish erythropoiesis function but retain the tissue-protective effect. **Carbamylated EPO (cEpo),** a chemically modified derivative of EPO's lysine residues, was found to act through the heterodimeric EPOR/βcR rather than classical $EPOR_2$ primarily because of the modified structure of cEpo. The study has confirmed that cEpo possesses neuron anti-apoptotic effects similar to EPO but instead does not induce neovascularization [101]. Investigators emphasized the future pharmacological role of cEpo as a non-hematopoietic neuroprotective agent. In recent years, the neuroprotective effects of cEpo makes it a rising candidate for prospective drugs [102].

Helix B of EPO, exposed to aqueous medium away from the binding sites of EPO and EPOR2, is important for the recognition of heterodimer EPOR/βcR. Based on the finding, investigators developed an eleven-amino acid linear peptide, mimicking the structure of the external surface of the helix B peptide and named it as ARA290 or Cibinetide or **helix B surface peptide (HBSP)**. As predicted, HSBP were not erythropoieitic but has properties in protecting against neuronal injury. McVicar et al. demonstrated that HBSP is sufficient in activating tissue-protective pathways without altering hematocrit or exacerbating neovascularization [103]. Although it has clear advantages, the 2 min plasma half-life of HBSP limits its application in vivo. Based on the amino acid sequence of HBSP, Zhang et al. designed and synthesized **thioether-cyclized helix B peptide (CHBP)** to increase structure integrity, prevent proteolytic degradation, and improve tissue-protective potency [98,104]. More recently, Cho et al. further designed a next-generation modified helix C peptide (**ML1-h3**) capable of improving neuroprotective effects against oxidative stress. This innovation would promote EPOR-mediated cell survival and proliferation in vitro and in vivo. This process signifies a brighter prospective for clinical applications and promotes the value of developing EPO derivatives for clinical use [105].

6. Advances in EPO Delivery

6.1. Protein-Based Ocular Delivery

Many EPO studies involve frequent injections of ophthalmic proteins via invasive procedures, which might result in a variety of adverse effects and increase the probability of irreversible damage to the patient's eye. Topical sustain released formulations are non-invasive drugs, that effectively reaches the posterior segment of the eye. According to Silva et al., mucoadhesive polymers such as chitosan and hyaluronic acid can improve the ocular bioavailability of drugs with the support of nanoparticulate delivery systems [106]. The formulation was found to be non-cytotoxic toward ARPE-19 and HaCa T cell lines. CS/HA6-rhEPO may be a promising topical formulation after enhancing its bioavailability through different ocular barriers. For the intraocular route of administration, De Julius et al. developed two polymer microparticles, poly (propylene sulfide) (PPS) and poly (lactic-co-glycolic acid) (PLGA), to prolong His-tagged rhEPO-R76E (42kDa) release [107]. The rhEPO-R76E was loaded into the polymeric microparticles to prolong in vivo release for at least 28 days to resolve the issue involving short half-life of the rhEPO-R76E (t1/2~13 min). PPS-based microparticles platform is especially promising because it is degradable by ROS. The delivery system provides extended neuroprotection and inherent antioxidant benefits, which reinforces its ability in ocular delivery of EPO.

6.2. Gene-Based Ocular Delivery

Under the gene delivery approaches, EPO has significant therapeutic potential in neurodegenerative diseases due to its neuroprotective effects. However, recombinant EPO is limited in clinical treatment of glaucoma patients due to its short half-life. As regards this issue, Bond et al. constructed a viral gene delivery system for EPO-R76E [108]. Treatment with recombinant adeno-associated virus (rAAV) provides sustainable, long-term delivery of EPO-R76E without a critical rise in hematocrit [108,109]. AAV-mediated long-term EPO expression is achievable in animal models with the primary functions of promoting red blood cells proliferation and neuroprotection.

Another challenge in applying gene therapy in humans is the improvement of drug selectivity. For systemically secreted hormone, such as EPO, it is vital to use an inducible genetic delivery system to avoid excess expression and side effects. However, precise expression control is highly desirable when maintaining steady-state red blood cell counts within a narrow therapeutic window. Hines-Beard et al. packaged EPOR76E into a recombinant adeno-associated viral vector under the control of the tetracycline inducible promoter [110]. In the retina, tetracycline-controlled expression of green fluoresce protein (GFP) in retinal pigmented epithelium and photoreceptor cells becomes apparent in rats following subretinal injections of rAAV-2/2 vector. The outer nuclear layer in the eyes was approximately 8 μm thicker in mice that received doxycycline water as compared to the control groups.

The morpholino-regulated hammerhead ribozyme was selected as another inducible genetic delivery system by Zhong et al. [111]. One of the designed ribozymes enabled regulation of AAV-delivered transgenes, allowing dose-dependent and more than 200 folds of protein to be expressed. The induction rate of morpholino becomes functional when interacting within EPO-encoding switchable AAV vectors. By controlling the dose of morpholino, EPO levels can be maintained for several weeks after a single injection while preventing hematocrit level fluctuations.

6.3. Surface Receptor-Targeted Ocular Delivery

Through surface receptor-targeted delivery results, most suggest that the tissue-protective effect of EPO and injury response are mediated by the EPOR/βcR heterodimer and not by the EPOR homodimer [112]. In addition to some well-known derivatives of EPO with better affinity for the EPOR/βcR heterodimer, such as asialoEPO, cEpo and HBSP (see above), traptamers of transmembrane domain (TMD) proteins of EPOR/βcR are also an option. He et al. constructed ELI-3 traptamer that specifically targets the TMD of human EPOR and triggers cooperative JAK/STAT signaling for proliferation and tissue protection [113]. Moreover, ELI-3 fails to induce erythroid differentiation from primary human hematopoietic progenitor cells. This traptamer-mediated delivery strategy not only provides selective receptor binding but also enhances binding affinity, and facilitates better EPO delivery efficiency.

6.4. Cell-Based Ocular Delivery

Mesenchymal stem cell (MSC) therapy is potential in treating optic neuropathies. MSCs have demonstrated to possess neuroprotective effects in numerous neurodegenerative diseases while maintaining retinal morphology [114,115]. They could also regulate inflammatory responses [116] and increase the secretion of neurotrophic factors [117]. Furthermore, they could transdifferentiate into retinal progenitor cells [118]. Johnson et al. intravitreally transplanted MSCs in a rat model of glaucoma and found an increased in axon survivability and decreased in axon loss of RGCs [119]. However, successful stem cell transplantation depends on the survivability of MSCs in a pathological environment. This can be addressed using EPO, which could enhance the engraftment of MSCs [120]. MSCs could be the vector of EPO because these cells could cross the brain-retinal barrier and localize into the inflamed sites [121]. The phenomenon emphasizes a mutualistic relationship between MSCs and EPO. Hence, some investigators attempt to evaluate the efficacy of EPO-expressing MSC in treating retinal degenerative diseases. Ding et al. transduced MSCs with lentiviral particles encoding EPO. They found that co-treatment with EPO and MSCs instead of only with MSC could attenuate human retinal neuron apoptosis by restoring the mitochondrial membrane potential and protect human retinal neurons from glutamate neurotoxicity [122]. The ability for EPO to synchronize with MSCs may become beneficial in producing medical protocols involving the treatment of patients with glaucomatous optic neuropathy. Given their endogenous long-term therapeutic effects, MSCs-based therapy could be the future direction in optic nerve repair.

7. Conclusions

EPO plays a vital role from the time of eye development to the many protective actions in optic neuropathies. EPO binding to heterodimeric EPOR/βcR initiates intracellular pathways, including JAK-2/STAT5 (STAT3), PI3-k/Akt, MAPK, NF-κB and Wnt signaling, which contributes to its anti-apoptosis, anti-inflammation, anti-oxidative effects. The above effects have brought promising neuroprotective results in several pre-clinical studies of glaucomatous optic neuropathy, optic neuritis, NAION and TON. However, the practical application of EPO is still limited by its hematopoietic side effects due to the lower affinity toward EPOR/βcR heterodimer. For this purpose, investigators developed EPO derivatives with extended half-life in plasma, decreased clearance rate and higher affinity toward EPOR/βcR heterodimer. These strategies enhance the tissue protection and reduce erythropoiesis. In addition, creating new EPO delivery systems is also a hurdle required to address. The development of topical drugs, microsphere, specific traptamer toward transmembrane domain of EPOR/βcR heterodimer, promoter-regulated gene therapy and even more appealing candidate, EPO-modified MSC therapy are promising therapeutic strategies in the future, which would bring endogenous long-term therapeutic effect in current noncurable optic degenerative diseases. We foresee that more clinical trials will be conducted to address on the safety and efficacy of these new strategies. Incorporating these therapeutic approaches with a better-controlled regulation could potentially magnify the beneficial effect of EPO for optic neuropathies in the future.

Author Contributions: Conceptualization, Y.-C.H. and D.-W.L.; software, Y.-F.L.; validation, P.-K.H., Y.-C.H. and D.-W.L.; resources, Y.-H.C. and D.-W.L.; writing—original draft preparation, Y.-F.L.; writing—review and editing, T.-Y.L. and P.-K.H.; visualization, Y.-F.L.; supervision, Y.-C.H. and D.-W.L.; funding acquisition, Y.-C.H. and D.-W.L. All authors have read and agreed to the published version of the manuscript.

Funding: This work was supported by grants from Tri-Service General Hospital (TSGH-E-111239) and the Ministry of National Defense-Medical Affairs Bureau (MND-MAB-D-111137).

Informed Consent Statement: Patient consent was waived because this is a review article.

Data Availability Statement: Not applicable.

Conflicts of Interest: The authors declare no conflict of interest.

References

1. Annese, T.; Tamma, R.; Ruggieri, S.; Ribatti, D. Erythropoietin in tumor angiogenesis. *Exp. Cell Res.* **2019**, *374*, 266–273. [CrossRef] [PubMed]
2. Tirpe, A.A.; Gulei, D.; Ciortea, S.M.; Crivii, C.; Berindan-Neagoe, I. Hypoxia: Overview on hypoxia-mediated mechanisms with a focus on the role of HIF genes. *Int. J. Mol. Sci.* **2019**, *20*, 6140. [CrossRef] [PubMed]
3. Yasuoka, Y.; Fukuyama, T.; Izumi, Y.; Nakayama, Y.; Inoue, H.; Yanagita, K.; Oshima, T.; Yamazaki, T.; Uematsu, T.; Kobayashi, N.; et al. Erythropoietin production by the kidney and the liver in response to severe hypoxia evaluated by Western blotting with deglycosylation. *Physiol. Rep.* **2020**, *8*, e14485. [CrossRef] [PubMed]
4. Kimáková, P.; Solár, P.; Solárová, Z.; Komel, R.; Debeljak, N. Erythropoietin and its angiogenic activity. *Int. J. Mol. Sci.* **2017**, *18*, 1519. [CrossRef] [PubMed]
5. Ostrowski, D.; Heinrich, R. Alternative erythropoietin receptors in the nervous system. *J. Clin. Med.* **2018**, *7*, 24. [CrossRef]
6. Klopsch, C.; Skorska, A.; Ludwig, M.; Lemcke, H.; Maass, G.; Gaebel, R.; Beyer, M.; Lux, C.; Toelk, A.; Müller, K.; et al. Intramyocardial angiogenetic stem cells and epicardial erythropoietin save the acute ischemic heart. *Dis. Models Mech.* **2018**, *11*, dmm033282. [CrossRef]
7. Bretz, C.A.; Ramshekar, A.; Kunz, E.; Wang, H.; Hartnett, M.E. Signaling through the erythropoietin receptor affects angiogenesis in retinovascular disease. *Investig. Ophthalmol. Vis. Sci.* **2020**, *61*, 23. [CrossRef]
8. Samson, F.P.; He, W.; Sripathi, S.R.; Patrick, A.T.; Madu, J.; Chung, H.; Frost, M.C.; Jee, D.; Gutsaeva, D.R.; Jahng, W.J. Dual switch mechanism of erythropoietin as an antiapoptotic and pro-angiogenic determinant in the retina. *ACS Omega* **2020**, *5*, 21113–21126. [CrossRef]
9. García-Ramírez, M.; Hernández, C.; Simó, R. Expression of erythropoietin and its receptor in the human retina: A comparative study of diabetic and nondiabetic subjects. *Diabetes Care* **2008**, *31*, 1189–1194. [CrossRef]
10. Dreixler, J.C.; Hagevik, S.; Hemmert, J.W.; Shaikh, A.R.; Rosenbaum, D.M.; Roth, S. Involvement of erythropoietin in retinal ischemic preconditioning. *Anesthesiology* **2009**, *110*, 774–780. [CrossRef]
11. Junk, A.K.; Mammis, A.; Savitz, S.I.; Singh, M.; Roth, S.; Malhotra, S.; Rosenbaum, P.S.; Cerami, A.; Brines, M.; Rosenbaum, D.M. Erythropoietin administration protects retinal neurons from acute ischemia-reperfusion injury. *Proc. Natl. Acad. Sci. USA* **2002**, *99*, 10659–10664. [CrossRef]
12. Chang, Z.Y.; Yeh, M.K.; Chiang, C.H.; Chen, Y.H.; Lu, D.W. Erythropoietin protects adult retinal ganglion cells against NMDA-, trophic factor withdrawal-, and TNF-α-induced damage. *PLoS ONE* **2013**, *8*, e55291. [CrossRef] [PubMed]
13. Cheng, W.S.; Lin, I.H.; Feng, K.M.; Chang, Z.Y.; Huang, Y.C.; Lu, D.W. Neuroprotective effects of exogenous erythropoietin in Wistar rats by downregulating apoptotic factors to attenuate N-methyl-D-aspartate-mediated retinal ganglion cells death. *PLoS ONE* **2020**, *15*, e0223208. [CrossRef] [PubMed]
14. Si, W.; Wang, J.; Li, M.; Qu, H.; Gu, R.; Liu, R.; Wang, L.; Li, S.; Hu, X. Erythropoietin protects neurons from apoptosis via activating PI3K/AKT and inhibiting Erk1/2 signaling pathway. *3 Biotech* **2019**, *9*, 131. [CrossRef] [PubMed]
15. Pathipati, P.; Ferriero, D.M. The differential effects of erythropoietin exposure to oxidative stress on microglia and astrocytes in vitro. *Dev. Neurosci.* **2017**, *39*, 310–322. [CrossRef] [PubMed]
16. Zhou, Z.W.; Li, F.; Zheng, Z.T.; Li, Y.D.; Chen, T.H.; Gao, W.W.; Chen, J.L.; Zhang, J.N. Erythropoietin regulates immune/inflammatory reaction and improves neurological function outcomes in traumatic brain injury. *Brain Behav.* **2017**, *7*, e00827. [CrossRef]
17. Constantinescu, S.N.; Ghaffari, S.; Lodish, H.F. The erythropoietin receptor: Structure, activation and intracellular signal transduction. *Trends Endocrinol. Metab. TEM* **1999**, *10*, 18–23. [CrossRef]
18. Watowich, S.S.; Hilton, D.J.; Lodish, H.F. Activation and inhibition of erythropoietin receptor function: Role of receptor dimerization. *Mol. Cell. Biol.* **1994**, *14*, 3535–3549. [CrossRef]
19. Kim, A.R.; Ulirsch, J.C.; Wilmes, S.; Unal, E.; Moraga, I.; Karakukcu, M.; Yuan, D.; Kazerounian, S.; Abdulhay, N.J.; King, D.S.; et al. Functional selectivity in cytokine signaling revealed through a pathogenic EPO mutation. *Cell* **2017**, *168*, 1053–1064. [CrossRef]
20. Tóthová, Z.; Tomc, J.; Debeljak, N.; Solár, P. STAT5 as a key protein of erythropoietin signalization. *Int. J. Mol. Sci.* **2021**, *22*, 7109. [CrossRef]
21. Tóthová, Z.; Šemeláková, M.; Solárová, Z.; Tomc, J.; Debeljak, N.; Solár, P. The role of PI3K/AKT and MAPK signaling pathways in erythropoietin signalization. *Int. J. Mol. Sci.* **2021**, *22*, 7682. [CrossRef] [PubMed]
22. Sanghera, K.P.; Mathalone, N.; Baigi, R.; Panov, E.; Wang, D.; Zhao, X.; Hsu, H.; Wang, H.; Tropepe, V.; Ward, M.; et al. The PI3K/Akt/mTOR pathway mediates retinal progenitor cell survival under hypoxic and superoxide stress. *Mol. Cell. Neurosci.* **2011**, *47*, 145–153. [CrossRef] [PubMed]

23. Masuda, S.; Nagao, M.; Takahata, K.; Konishi, Y.; Gallyas, F., Jr.; Tabira, T.; Sasaki, R. Functional erythropoietin receptor of the cells with neural characteristics. Comparison with receptor properties of erythroid cells. *J. Biol. Chem.* **1993**, *268*, 11208–11216. [CrossRef]
24. Kebschull, L.; Theilmann, L.F.C.; Mohr, A.; Uennigmann, W.; Stoeppeler, S.; Heitplatz, B.; Spiegel, H.U.; Bahde, R.; Palmes, D.M.; Becker, F. $EPOR_2/\beta cR_2$-independendent effects of low-dose epoetin-α in porcine liver transplantation. *Biosci. Rep.* **2017**, *37*, BSR20171007. [CrossRef]
25. Jubinsky, P.T.; Krijanovski, O.I.; Nathan, D.G.; Tavernier, J.; Sieff, C.A. The beta chain of the interleukin-3 receptor functionally associates with the erythropoietin receptor. *Blood* **1997**, *90*, 1867–1873. [CrossRef]
26. Peng, B.; Kong, G.; Yang, C.; Ming, Y. Erythropoietin and its derivatives: From tissue protection to immune regulation. *Cell Death Dis.* **2020**, *11*, 79. [CrossRef]
27. Colella, P.; Iodice, C.; Di Vicino, U.; Annunziata, I.; Surace, E.M.; Auricchio, A. Non-erythropoietic erythropoietin derivatives protect from light-induced and genetic photoreceptor degeneration. *Hum. Mol. Genet.* **2011**, *20*, 2251–2262. [CrossRef]
28. Wang, Z.; Liu, C.H.; Huang, S.; Chen, J. Wnt signaling in vascular eye diseases. *Prog. Retin. Eye Res.* **2019**, *70*, 110–133. [CrossRef]
29. Wagstaff, P.E.; Heredero Berzal, A.; Boon, C.J.F.; Quinn, P.M.J.; Ten Asbroek, A.; Bergen, A.A. The role of small molecules and their effect on the molecular mechanisms of early retinal organoid development. *Int. J. Mol. Sci.* **2021**, *22*, 7081. [CrossRef]
30. Vizcardo-Galindo, G.; León-Velarde, F.; Villafuerte, F.C. High-altitude hypoxia decreases plasma erythropoietin soluble receptor concentration in lowlanders. *High Alt. Med. Biol.* **2020**, *21*, 92–98. [CrossRef]
31. Khankin, E.V.; Mutter, W.P.; Tamez, H.; Yuan, H.T.; Karumanchi, S.A.; Thadhani, R. Soluble erythropoietin receptor contributes to erythropoietin resistance in end-stage renal disease. *PLoS ONE* **2010**, *5*, e9246. [CrossRef] [PubMed]
32. Zhang, D.; Lv, F.L.; Wang, G.H. Effects of HIF-1α on diabetic retinopathy angiogenesis and VEGF expression. *Eur. Rev. Med. Pharmacol. Sci.* **2018**, *22*, 5071–5076. [CrossRef]
33. Ogawa, C.; Tsuchiya, K.; Tomosugi, N.; Maeda, K. A hypoxia-inducible factor stabilizer improves hematopoiesis and iron metabolism early after administration to treat anemia in hemodialysis patients. *Int. J. Mol. Sci.* **2020**, *21*, 7153. [CrossRef] [PubMed]
34. Socolovsky, M.; Nam, H.; Fleming, M.D.; Haase, V.H.; Brugnara, C.; Lodish, H.F. Ineffective erythropoiesis in Stat5a(−/−)5b(−/−) mice due to decreased survival of early erythroblasts. *Blood* **2001**, *98*, 3261–3273. [CrossRef] [PubMed]
35. Tu, P.S.; Lin, E.C.; Chen, H.W.; Chen, S.W.; Lin, T.A.; Gau, J.P.; Chang, Y.I. The extracellular signal-regulated kinase 1/2 modulates the intracellular localization of DNA methyltransferase 3A to regulate erythrocytic differentiation. *Am. J. Transl. Res.* **2020**, *12*, 1016–1030.
36. Dai, T.Y.; Lan, J.J.; Gao, R.L.; Zhao, Y.N.; Yu, X.L.; Liang, S.X.; Liu, W.B.; Sun, X. Panaxdiol saponins component promotes hematopoiesis by regulating GATA transcription factors of intracellular signaling pathway in mouse bone marrow. *Ann. Transl. Med.* **2022**, *10*, 38. [CrossRef]
37. Das, T.P.; Suman, S.; Alatassi, H.; Ankem, M.K.; Damodaran, C. Inhibition of AKT promotes FOXO3a-dependent apoptosis in prostate cancer. *Cell Death Dis.* **2016**, *7*, e2111. [CrossRef]
38. Digicaylioglu, M.; Lipton, S.A. Erythropoietin-mediated neuroprotection involves cross-talk between Jak2 and NF-kappaB signalling cascades. *Nature* **2001**, *412*, 641–647. [CrossRef]
39. Shen, J.; Wu, Y.; Xu, J.Y.; Zhang, J.; Sinclair, S.H.; Yanoff, M.; Xu, G.; Li, W.; Xu, G.T. ERK- and Akt-dependent neuroprotection by erythropoietin (EPO) against glyoxal-AGEs via modulation of Bcl-xL, Bax, and BAD. *Investig. Ophthalmol. Vis. Sci.* **2010**, *51*, 35–46. [CrossRef] [PubMed]
40. Chong, Z.Z.; Kang, J.Q.; Maiese, K. Apaf-1, Bcl-xL, cytochrome c, and caspase-9 form the critical elements for cerebral vascular protection by erythropoietin. *J. Cereb. Blood Flow Metab. Off. J. Int. Soc. Cereb. Blood Flow Metab.* **2003**, *23*, 320–330. [CrossRef] [PubMed]
41. Wang, Z.Y.; Shen, L.J.; Tu, L.; Hu, D.N.; Liu, G.Y.; Zhou, Z.L.; Lin, Y.; Chen, L.H.; Qu, J. Erythropoietin protects retinal pigment epithelial cells from oxidative damage. *Free Radic. Biol. Med.* **2009**, *46*, 1032–1041. [CrossRef] [PubMed]
42. Wang, C.Y.; Mayo, M.W.; Korneluk, R.G.; Goeddel, D.V.; Baldwin, A.S., Jr. NF-kappaB antiapoptosis: Induction of TRAF1 and TRAF2 and c-IAP1 and c-IAP2 to suppress caspase-8 activation. *Science* **1998**, *281*, 1680–1683. [CrossRef] [PubMed]
43. Chen, C.; Edelstein, L.C.; Gélinas, C. The Rel/NF-kappaB family directly activates expression of the apoptosis inhibitor Bcl-x(L). *Mol. Cell. Biol.* **2000**, *20*, 2687–2695. [CrossRef] [PubMed]
44. Chen, S.; Guttridge, D.C.; You, Z.; Zhang, Z.; Fribley, A.; Mayo, M.W.; Kitajewski, J.; Wang, C.Y. Wnt-1 signaling inhibits apoptosis by activating beta-catenin/T cell factor-mediated transcription. *J. Cell Biol.* **2001**, *152*, 87–96. [CrossRef]
45. Duda, P.; Akula, S.M.; Abrams, S.L.; Steelman, L.S.; Martelli, A.M.; Cocco, L.; Ratti, S.; Candido, S.; Libra, M.; Montalto, G.; et al. Targeting GSK3 and associated signaling pathways involved in cancer. *Cells* **2020**, *9*, 1110. [CrossRef]
46. Kwak, J.; Kim, J.H.; Jang, H.N.; Jung, M.H.; Cho, H.S.; Chang, S.H.; Kim, H.J. Erythropoietin ameliorates ischemia/reperfusion-induced acute kidney injury via inflammasome suppression in mice. *Int. J. Mol. Sci.* **2020**, *21*, 3453. [CrossRef]
47. Gong, Q.; Zeng, J.; Zhang, X.; Huang, Y.; Chen, C.; Quan, J.; Ling, J. Effect of erythropoietin on angiogenic potential of dental pulp cells. *Exp. Ther. Med.* **2021**, *22*, 1079. [CrossRef]
48. Lin, X.; Ma, X.; Cui, X.; Zhang, R.; Pan, H.; Gao, W. Effects of erythropoietin on lung injury induced by cardiopulmonary bypass after cardiac surgery. *Med. Sci. Monit. Int. Med. J. Exp. Clin. Res.* **2020**, *26*, e920039. [CrossRef]

49. Cui, J.; Zhang, F.; Cao, W.; Wang, Y.; Liu, J.; Liu, X.; Chen, T.; Li, L.; Tian, J.; Yu, B. Erythropoietin alleviates hyperglycaemia-associated inflammation by regulating macrophage polarization via the JAK2/STAT3 signalling pathway. *Mol. Immunol.* **2018**, *101*, 221–228. [CrossRef]
50. Elshiekh, M.; Kadkhodaee, M.; Seifi, B.; Ranjbaran, M.; Askari, H. Up-regulation of nitric oxide synthases by erythropoietin alone or in conjunction with ischemic preconditioning in ischemia reperfusion injury of rat kidneys. *Gen. Physiol. Biophys.* **2017**, *36*, 281–288. [CrossRef]
51. Cruz Navarro, J.; Pillai, S.; Ponce, L.L.; Van, M.; Goodman, J.C.; Robertson, C.S. Endothelial nitric oxide synthase mediates the cerebrovascular effects of erythropoietin in traumatic brain injury. *Front. Immunol.* **2014**, *5*, 494. [CrossRef] [PubMed]
52. Govindappa, P.K.; Elfar, J.C. Erythropoietin promotes M2 macrophage phagocytosis of Schwann cells in peripheral nerve injury. *Cell Death Dis.* **2022**, *13*, 245. [CrossRef] [PubMed]
53. Einwächter, H.; Heiseke, A.; Schlitzer, A.; Gasteiger, G.; Adler, H.; Voehringer, D.; Manz, M.G.; Ruzsics, Z.; Dölken, L.; Koszinowski, U.H.; et al. The innate immune response to infection induces erythropoietin-dependent replenishment of the dendritic cell compartment. *Front. Immunol.* **2020**, *11*, 1627. [CrossRef] [PubMed]
54. Korkmaz, T.; Kahramansoy, N.; Kilicgun, A.; Firat, T. The effect of erythropoietin to pulmonary injury and mast cells secondary to acute pancreatitis. *BMC Res. Notes* **2014**, *7*, 267. [CrossRef]
55. Cantarelli, C.; Angeletti, A.; Cravedi, P. Erythropoietin, a multifaceted protein with innate and adaptive immune modulatory activity. *Am. J. Transpl. Off. J. Am. Soc. Transpl. Am. Soc. Transpl. Sur.* **2019**, *19*, 2407–2414. [CrossRef]
56. Purroy, C.; Fairchild, R.L.; Tanaka, T.; Baldwin, W.M., 3rd; Manrique, J.; Madsen, J.C.; Colvin, R.B.; Alessandrini, A.; Blazar, B.R.; Fribourg, M.; et al. Erythropoietin receptor-mediated molecular crosstalk promotes T cell immunoregulation and transplant survival. *J. Am. Soc. Nephrol. JASN* **2017**, *28*, 2377–2392. [CrossRef]
57. Arıkan, T.; Akcan, A.; Dönder, Y.; Yılmaz, Z.; Sözüer, E.; Öz, B.; Baykan, M.; Gök, M.; Poyrazoğlu, B. Effects of erythropoietin on bacterial translocation in a rat model of experimental colitis. *Turk. J. Surg.* **2019**, *35*, 202–209. [CrossRef]
58. Moransard, M.; Bednar, M.; Frei, K.; Gassmann, M.; Ogunshola, O.O. Erythropoietin reduces experimental autoimmune encephalomyelitis severity via neuroprotective mechanisms. *J. Neuroinflamm.* **2017**, *14*, 202. [CrossRef]
59. Shokrzadeh, M.; Etebari, M.; Ghassemi-Barghi, N. An engineered non-erythropoietic erythropoietin-derived peptide, ARA290, attenuates doxorubicin induced genotoxicity and oxidative stress. *Toxicol. Vitr. Int. J. Publ. Assoc. BIBRA* **2020**, *66*, 104864. [CrossRef]
60. Dang, J.Z.; Tu, Y.F.; Wang, J.; Yang, Y.J. Carbamylated erythropoietin alleviates kidney damage in diabetic rats by suppressing oxidative stress. *Curr. Med. Sci.* **2021**, *41*, 513–521. [CrossRef]
61. Salinas, M.; Wang, J.; Rosa de Sagarra, M.; Martín, D.; Rojo, A.I.; Martin-Perez, J.; Ortiz de Montellano, P.R.; Cuadrado, A. Protein kinase Akt/PKB phosphorylates heme oxygenase-1 in vitro and in vivo. *FEBS Lett.* **2004**, *578*, 90–94. [CrossRef] [PubMed]
62. Diaz, Z.; Assaraf, M.I.; Miller, W.H., Jr.; Schipper, H.M. Astroglial cytoprotection by erythropoietin pre-conditioning: Implications for ischemic and degenerative CNS disorders. *J. Neurochem.* **2005**, *93*, 392–402. [CrossRef] [PubMed]
63. Thompson, A.M.; Farmer, K.; Rowe, E.M.; Hayley, S. Erythropoietin modulates striatal antioxidant signalling to reduce neurodegeneration in a toxicant model of Parkinson's disease. *Mol. Cell. Neurosci.* **2020**, *109*, 103554. [CrossRef] [PubMed]
64. Glass, G.A.; Gershon, D. Decreased enzymic protection and increased sensitivity to oxidative damage in erythrocytes as a function of cell and donor aging. *Biochem. J.* **1984**, *218*, 531–537. [CrossRef]
65. Bany-Mohammed, F.M.; Slivka, S.; Hallman, M. Recombinant human erythropoietin: Possible role as an antioxidant in premature rabbits. *Pediatr. Res.* **1996**, *40*, 381–387. [CrossRef]
66. Pulukool, S.K.; Bhagavatham, S.K.S.; Kannan, V.; Sukumar, P.; Dandamudi, R.B.; Ghaisas, S.; Kunchala, H.; Saieesh, D.; Naik, A.A.; Pargaonkar, A.; et al. Elevated dimethylarginine, ATP, cytokines, metabolic remodeling involving tryptophan metabolism and potential microglial inflammation characterize primary open angle glaucoma. *Sci. Rep.* **2021**, *11*, 9766. [CrossRef]
67. Krishnan, A.; Kocab, A.J.; Zacks, D.N.; Marshak-Rothstein, A.; Gregory-Ksander, M. A small peptide antagonist of the Fas receptor inhibits neuroinflammation and prevents axon degeneration and retinal ganglion cell death in an inducible mouse model of glaucoma. *J. Neuroinflamm.* **2019**, *16*, 184. [CrossRef]
68. Li, Q.; Jin, R.; Zhang, S.; Sun, X.; Wu, J. Group II metabotropic glutamate receptor agonist promotes retinal ganglion cell survival by reducing neuronal excitotoxicity in a rat chronic ocular hypertension model. *Neuropharmacology* **2020**, *170*, 108016. [CrossRef]
69. Cha, Y.W.; Kim, S.T. Serum and aqueous humor levels of brain-derived neurotrophic factor in patients with primary open-angle glaucoma and normal-tension glaucoma. *Int. Ophthalmol.* **2021**, *41*, 3869–3875. [CrossRef]
70. Mokbel, T.H.; Ghanem, A.A.; Kishk, H.; Arafa, L.F.; El-Baiomy, A.A. Erythropoietin and soluble CD44 levels in patients with primary open-angle glaucoma. *Clin. Exp. Ophthalmol.* **2010**, *38*, 560–565. [CrossRef]
71. Arjamaa, O.; Nikinmaa, M. Oxygen-dependent diseases in the retina: Role of hypoxia-inducible factors. *Exp. Eye Res.* **2006**, *83*, 473–483. [CrossRef] [PubMed]
72. Kawakami, M.; Sekiguchi, M.; Sato, K.; Kozaki, S.; Takahashi, M. Erythropoietin receptor-mediated inhibition of exocytotic glutamate release confers neuroprotection during chemical ischemia. *J. Biol. Chem.* **2001**, *276*, 39469–39475. [CrossRef]
73. Chader, G.J. Advances in glaucoma treatment and management: Neurotrophic agents. *Investig. Opthalmol. Vis. Sci.* **2012**, *53*, 2501–2505. [CrossRef] [PubMed]

74. Cheng, S.; Wang, H.N.; Xu, L.J.; Li, F.; Miao, Y.; Lei, B.; Sun, X.; Wang, Z. Soluble tumor necrosis factor-alpha-induced hyperexcitability contributes to retinal ganglion cell apoptosis by enhancing Nav1.6 in experimental glaucoma. *J. Neuroinflamm.* **2021**, *18*, 182. [CrossRef] [PubMed]
75. Zhong, L.; Bradley, J.; Schubert, W.; Ahmed, E.; Adamis, A.P.; Shima, D.T.; Robinson, G.S.; Ng, Y.S. Erythropoietin promotes survival of retinal ganglion cells in DBA/2J glaucoma mice. *Investig. Opthalmol. Vis. Sci.* **2007**, *48*, 1212–1218. [CrossRef]
76. Resende, A.P.; Rosolen, S.G.; Nunes, T.; São Braz, B.; Delgado, E. Functional and structural effects of erythropoietin subconjunctival administration in glaucomatous animals. *Biomed. Hub* **2018**, *3*, 488970. [CrossRef] [PubMed]
77. Zhong, Y.S.; Liu, X.H.; Cheng, Y.; Min, Y.J. Erythropoietin with retrobulbar administration protects retinal ganglion cells from acute elevated intraocular pressure in rats. *J. Ocul. Pharmacol. Ther. Off. J. Assoc. Ocul. Pharmacol. Ther.* **2008**, *24*, 453–459. [CrossRef]
78. Tsai, J.C.; Wu, L.; Worgul, B.; Forbes, M.; Cao, J. Intravitreal administration of erythropoietin and preservation of retinal ganglion cells in an experimental rat model of glaucoma. *Curr. Eye Res.* **2005**, *30*, 1025–1031. [CrossRef]
79. Zhou, M.; Chen, S.; Wang, W.; Huang, W.; Cheng, B.; Ding, X.; Zhang, X. Levels of erythropoietin and vascular endothelial growth factor in surgery-required advanced neovascular glaucoma eyes before and after intravitreal injection of bevacizumab. *Investig. Opthalmol. Vis. Sci.* **2013**, *54*, 3874–3879. [CrossRef]
80. Sun, Y.; Zhao, H.; Shen, Y.; Guan, W. Comparison of erythropoietin, semaphorins 3A and pigment epithelium derived factor levels in serum and aqueous humor of patients with neovascular glaucoma and cataract. *J. Coll. Phys. Surg. Pak. JCPSP* **2019**, *29*, 900–901. [CrossRef]
81. Watanabe, D.; Suzuma, K.; Matsui, S.; Kurimoto, M.; Kiryu, J.; Kita, M.; Suzuma, I.; Ohashi, H.; Ojima, T.; Murakami, T.; et al. Erythropoietin as a retinal angiogenic factor in proliferative diabetic retinopathy. *N. Engl. J. Med.* **2005**, *353*, 782–792. [CrossRef]
82. Mackay, D.D. Should patients with optic neuritis be treated with steroids? *Curr. Opin. Ophthalmol.* **2015**, *26*, 439–444. [CrossRef] [PubMed]
83. Diem, R.; Hobom, M.; Maier, K.; Weissert, R.; Storch, M.K.; Meyer, R.; Bähr, M. Methylprednisolone increases neuronal apoptosis during autoimmune CNS inflammation by inhibition of an endogenous neuroprotective pathway. *J. Neurosci. Off. J. Soc. Neurosci.* **2003**, *23*, 6993–7000. [CrossRef]
84. Sättler, M.B.; Merkler, D.; Maier, K.; Stadelmann, C.; Ehrenreich, H.; Bähr, M.; Diem, R. Neuroprotective effects and intracellular signaling pathways of erythropoietin in a rat model of multiple sclerosis. *Cell Death Differ.* **2004**, *11* (Suppl. 2), S181–S192. [CrossRef] [PubMed]
85. Soltan Sanjari, M.; Pakdel, F.; Moosavi, F.; Pirmarzdashti, N.; Nojomi, M.; Haghighi, A.; Hashemi, M.; Bahmani Kashkouli, M. Visual outcomes of adding erythropoietin to methylprednisolone for treatment of retrobulbar optic neuritis. *J. Ophthalmic Vis. Res.* **2019**, *14*, 299–305. [CrossRef]
86. Shayegannejad, V.; Shahzamani, S.; Dehghani, A.; Dast Borhan, Z.; Rahimi, M.; Mirmohammadsadeghi, A. A double-blind, placebo-controlled trial of adding erythropoietin to intravenous methylprednisolone for the treatment of unilateral acute optic neuritis of unknown or demyelinative origin. *Graefe's Archive Clin. Exp. Ophthalmol.* **2015**, *253*, 797–801. [CrossRef]
87. Sühs, K.W.; Hein, K.; Sättler, M.B.; Görlitz, A.; Ciupka, C.; Scholz, K.; Käsmann-Kellner, B.; Papanagiotou, P.; Schäffler, N.; Restemeyer, C.; et al. A randomized, double-blind, phase 2 study of erythropoietin in optic neuritis. *Ann. Neurol.* **2012**, *72*, 199–210. [CrossRef]
88. Lagrèze, W.A.; Küchlin, S.; Ihorst, G.; Grotejohann, B.; Beisse, F.; Volkmann, M.; Heinrich, S.P.; Albrecht, P.; Ungewiss, J.; Wörner, M.; et al. Safety and efficacy of erythropoietin for the treatment of patients with optic neuritis (TONE): A randomised, double-blind, multicentre, placebo-controlled study. *Lancet Neurol.* **2021**, *20*, 991–1000. [CrossRef]
89. Modarres, M.; Falavarjani, K.G.; Nazari, H.; Sanjari, M.S.; Aghamohammadi, F.; Homaii, M.; Samiy, N. Intravitreal erythropoietin injection for the treatment of non-arteritic anterior ischaemic optic neuropathy. *Br. J. Ophthalmol.* **2011**, *95*, 992–995. [CrossRef]
90. Pakravan, M.; Esfandiari, H.; Hassanpour, K.; Razavi, S.; Pakravan, P. The effect of combined systemic erythropoietin and steroid on non-arteritic anterior ischemic optic neuropathy: A prospective study. *Curr. Eye Res.* **2017**, *42*, 1079–1084. [CrossRef]
91. Nikkhah, H.; Golalipour, M.; Doozandeh, A.; Pakravan, M.; Yaseri, M.; Esfandiari, H. The effect of systemic erythropoietin and oral prednisolone on recent-onset non-arteritic anterior ischemic optic neuropathy: A randomized clinical trial. *Graefe's Archive Clin. Exp. Ophthalmol.* **2020**, *258*, 2291–2297. [CrossRef] [PubMed]
92. Kashkouli, M.B.; Pakdel, F.; Sanjari, M.S.; Haghighi, A.; Nojomi, M.; Homaee, M.H.; Heirati, A. Erythropoietin: A novel treatment for traumatic optic neuropathy-a pilot study. *Graefe's Archive Clin. Exp. Ophthalmol.* **2011**, *249*, 731–736. [CrossRef] [PubMed]
93. Entezari, M.; Esmaeili, M.; Yaseri, M. A pilot study of the effect of intravenous erythropoetin on improvement of visual function in patients with recent indirect traumatic optic neuropathy. *Graefe's Archive Clin. Exp. Ophthalmol.* **2014**, *252*, 1309–1313. [CrossRef]
94. Kashkouli, M.B.; Yousefi, S.; Nojomi, M.; Sanjari, M.S.; Pakdel, F.; Entezari, M.; Etezad-Razavi, M.; Razeghinejad, M.R.; Esmaeli, M.; Shafiee, M.; et al. Traumatic optic neuropathy treatment trial (TONTT): Open label, phase 3, multicenter, semi-experimental trial. *Graefe's Archive Clin. Exp. Ophthalmol.* **2018**, *256*, 209–218. [CrossRef] [PubMed]
95. Rashad, M.A.; Abdel Latif, A.A.M.; Mostafa, H.A.; Fawzy, S.M.; Abdel Latif, M.A.M. Visual-evoked-response-supported outcome of intravitreal erythropoietin in management of indirect traumatic optic neuropathy. *J. Ophthalmol.* **2018**, *2018*, 2750632. [CrossRef]
96. Wladis, E.J.; Aakalu, V.K.; Sobel, R.K.; McCulley, T.J.; Foster, J.A.; Tao, J.P.; Freitag, S.K.; Yen, M.T. Interventions for indirect traumatic optic neuropathy: A report by the American academy of ophthalmology. *Ophthalmology* **2021**, *128*, 928–937. [CrossRef] [PubMed]

97. Anand, S.; Al-Mondhiry, J.; Fischer, K.; Glaspy, J. Epoetin alfa-epbx: A new entrant into a crowded market. a historical review of the role of erythropoietin stimulating agents and the development of the first epoetin biosimilar in the United States. *Expert Rev. Clin. Pharmacol.* **2021**, *14*, 1–8. [CrossRef]
98. Lee, D.E.; Son, W.; Ha, B.J.; Oh, M.S.; Yoo, O.J. The prolonged half-lives of new erythropoietin derivatives via peptide addition. *Biochem. Biophys. Res. Commun.* **2006**, *339*, 380–385. [CrossRef]
99. Powell, J.; Gurk-Turner, C. Darbepoetin alfa (Aranesp). *Bayl. Univ. Med. Cent. Proc.* **2002**, *15*, 332–335. [CrossRef]
100. Aizawa, K.; Kawasaki, R.; Tashiro, Y.; Hirata, M.; Endo, K.; Shimonaka, Y. Epoetin beta pegol, but not recombinant erythropoietin, retains its hematopoietic effect in vivo in the presence of the sialic acid-metabolizing enzyme sialidase. *Int. J. Hematol.* **2016**, *104*, 182–189. [CrossRef]
101. Liu, X.; Zhu, B.; Zou, H.; Hu, D.; Gu, Q.; Liu, K.; Xu, X. Carbamylated erythropoietin mediates retinal neuroprotection in streptozotocin-induced early-stage diabetic rats. *Graefe's Archive Clin. Exp. Ophthalmol.* **2015**, *253*, 1263–1272. [CrossRef] [PubMed]
102. Chen, J.; Yang, Z.; Zhang, X. Carbamylated erythropoietin: A prospective drug candidate for neuroprotection. *Biochem. Insights* **2015**, *8*, 25–29. [CrossRef] [PubMed]
103. McVicar, C.M.; Hamilton, R.; Colhoun, L.M.; Gardiner, T.A.; Brines, M.; Cerami, A.; Stitt, A.W. Intervention with an erythropoietin-derived peptide protects against neuroglial and vascular degeneration during diabetic retinopathy. *Diabetes* **2011**, *60*, 2995–3005. [CrossRef] [PubMed]
104. Zhang, C.; Yang, C.; Zhu, T. From erythropoietin to its peptide derivatives: Smaller but stronger. *Curr. Protein Pept. Sci.* **2017**, *18*, 1191–1194. [CrossRef] [PubMed]
105. Cho, B.; Yoo, S.J.; Kim, S.Y.; Lee, C.H.; Lee, Y.I.; Lee, S.R.; Moon, C. Second-generation non-hematopoietic erythropoietin-derived peptide for neuroprotection. *Redox Biol.* **2022**, *49*, 102223. [CrossRef]
106. Silva, B.; Marto, J.; Braz, B.S.; Delgado, E.; Almeida, A.J.; Gonçalves, L. New nanoparticles for topical ocular delivery of erythropoietin. *Int. J. Pharm.* **2020**, *576*, 119020. [CrossRef]
107. DeJulius, C.R.; Bernardo-Colón, A.; Naguib, S.; Backstrom, J.R.; Kavanaugh, T.; Gupta, M.K.; Duvall, C.L.; Rex, T.S. Microsphere antioxidant and sustained erythropoietin-R76E release functions cooperate to reduce traumatic optic neuropathy. *J. Control. Release Off. J. Control. Release Soc.* **2021**, *329*, 762–773. [CrossRef]
108. Bond, W.S.; Hines-Beard, J.; GoldenMerry, Y.L.; Davis, M.; Farooque, A.; Sappington, R.M.; Calkins, D.J.; Rex, T.S. Virus-mediated EpoR76E therapy slows optic nerve axonopathy in experimental glaucoma. *Mol. Ther. J. Am. Soc. Gene Ther.* **2016**, *24*, 230–239. [CrossRef]
109. Tao, Y.; Zhu, Q.; Wang, L.; Zha, X.; Teng, D.; Xu, L. Adeno-associated virus (AAV)-mediated neuroprotective effects on the degenerative retina: The therapeutic potential of erythropoietin. *Fundam. Clin. Pharmacol.* **2020**, *34*, 131–147. [CrossRef]
110. Hines-Beard, J.; Desai, S.; Haag, R.; Esumi, N.; D'Surney, L.; Parker, S.; Richardson, C.; Rex, T.S. Identification of a therapeutic dose of continuously delivered erythropoietin in the eye using an inducible promoter system. *Curr. Gene Ther.* **2013**, *13*, 275–281. [CrossRef]
111. Zhong, G.; Wang, H.; He, W.; Li, Y.; Mou, H.; Tickner, Z.J.; Tran, M.H.; Ou, T.; Yin, Y.; Diao, H.; et al. A reversible RNA on-switch that controls gene expression of AAV-delivered therapeutics in vivo. *Nat. Biotechnol.* **2020**, *38*, 169–175. [CrossRef] [PubMed]
112. Bohr, S.; Patel, S.J.; Vasko, R.; Shen, K.; Iracheta-Vellve, A.; Lee, J.; Bale, S.S.; Chakraborty, N.; Brines, M.; Cerami, A.; et al. Modulation of cellular stress response via the erythropoietin/CD131 heteroreceptor complex in mouse mesenchymal-derived cells. *J. Mol. Med.* **2015**, *93*, 199–210. [CrossRef] [PubMed]
113. He, L.; Cohen, E.B.; Edwards, A.P.B.; Xavier-Ferrucio, J.; Bugge, K.; Federman, R.S.; Absher, D.; Myers, R.M.; Kragelund, B.B.; Krause, D.S.; et al. Transmembrane protein aptamer induces cooperative signaling by the EPO receptor and the cytokine receptor β-common subunit. *iScience* **2019**, *17*, 167–181. [CrossRef]
114. Liu, W.; Rong, Y.; Wang, J.; Zhou, Z.; Ge, X.; Ji, C.; Jiang, D.; Gong, F.; Li, L.; Chen, J.; et al. Exosome-shuttled miR-216a-5p from hypoxic preconditioned mesenchymal stem cells repair traumatic spinal cord injury by shifting microglial M1/M2 polarization. *J. Neuroinflamm.* **2020**, *17*, 47. [CrossRef] [PubMed]
115. Kim, J.; Lee, Y.; Lee, S.; Kim, K.; Song, M.; Lee, J. Mesenchymal stem cell therapy and alzheimer's disease: Current status and future perspectives. *J. Alzheimer's Dis. JAD* **2020**, *77*, 1–14. [CrossRef]
116. Luque-Campos, N.; Contreras-López, R.A.; Jose Paredes-Martínez, M.; Torres, M.J.; Bahraoui, S.; Wei, M.; Espinoza, F.; Djouad, F.; Elizondo-Vega, R.J.; Luz-Crawford, P. Mesenchymal stem cells improve rheumatoid arthritis progression by controlling memory T cell response. *Front. Immunol.* **2019**, *10*, 798. [CrossRef] [PubMed]
117. Jiang, Y.; Gao, H.; Yuan, H.; Xu, H.; Tian, M.; Du, G.; Xie, W. Amelioration of postoperative cognitive dysfunction in mice by mesenchymal stem cell-conditioned medium treatments is associated with reduced inflammation, oxidative stress and increased BDNF expression in brain tissues. *Neurosci. Lett.* **2019**, *709*, 134372. [CrossRef]
118. Hu, Y.; Liang, J.; Cui, H.; Wang, X.; Rong, H.; Shao, B.; Cui, H. Wharton's jelly mesenchymal stem cells differentiate into retinal progenitor cells. *Neural Regen. Res.* **2013**, *8*, 1783–1792. [CrossRef]
119. Johnson, T.V.; Bull, N.D.; Hunt, D.P.; Marina, N.; Tomarev, S.I.; Martin, K.R. Neuroprotective effects of intravitreal mesenchymal stem cell transplantation in experimental glaucoma. *Investig. Opthalmol. Vis. Sci.* **2010**, *51*, 2051–2059. [CrossRef]
120. Daga, A.; Muraglia, A.; Quarto, R.; Cancedda, R.; Corte, G. Enhanced engraftment of EPO-transduced human bone marrow stromal cells transplanted in a 3D matrix in non-conditioned NOD/SCID mice. *Gene Ther.* **2002**, *9*, 915–921. [CrossRef]

121. Omoto, M.; Katikireddy, K.R.; Rezazadeh, A.; Dohlman, T.H.; Chauhan, S.K. Mesenchymal stem cells home to inflamed ocular surface and suppress allosensitization in corneal transplantation. *Investig. Opthalmol. Vis. Sci.* **2014**, *55*, 6631–6638. [CrossRef] [PubMed]
122. Shirley Ding, S.L.; Kumar, S.; Ali Khan, M.S.; Ling Mok, P. Human mesenchymal stem cells expressing erythropoietin enhance survivability of retinal neurons against oxidative stress: An in vitro study. *Front. Cell. Neurosci.* **2018**, *12*, 190. [CrossRef] [PubMed]

International Journal of
Molecular Sciences

MDPI

Article

Neuroprotection and Neuroregeneration Strategies Using the rNAION Model: Theory, Histology, Problems, Results and Analytical Approaches

Steven L. Bernstein [1,2,*], Yan Guo [1], Zara Mehrabian [1] and Neil R. Miller [3]

1 Department of Ophthalmology and Visual Sciences, University of Maryland at Baltimore School of Medicine, 10 S. Pine St., Baltimore, MD 21201, USA
2 Department of Anatomy and Neurobiology, University of Maryland at Baltimore School of Medicine, 10 S. Pine St., Baltimore, MD 21201, USA
3 Wilmer Eye Institute, Johns Hopkins University School of Medicine, 600 N. Wolfe St., Baltimore, MD 21205, USA
* Correspondence: sbernstein@som.umaryland.edu; Tel.: +1-410-706-3712

Abstract: Nonarteritic anterior ischemic optic neuropathy (NAION) is the most common cause of sudden optic nerve (ON)-related vision loss in humans. Study of this disease has been limited by the lack of available tissue and difficulties in evaluating both treatments and the window of effectiveness after symptom onset. The rodent nonarteritic anterior ischemic optic neuropathy model (rNAION) closely resembles clinical NAION in its pathophysiological changes and physiological responses. The rNAION model enables analysis of the specific responses to sudden ischemic axonopathy and effectiveness of potential treatments. However, there are anatomic and genetic differences between human and rodent ON, and the inducing factors for the disease and the model are different. These variables can result in marked differences in lesion development between the two species, as well as in the possible responses to various treatments. These caveats are discussed in the current article, as well as some of the species-associated differences that may be related to ischemic lesion severity and responses.

Keywords: nonarteritic anterior ischemic optic neuropathy; retinal ganglion cells; optic nerve; neuroprotection; rodents; gene expression; models

Citation: Bernstein, S.L.; Guo, Y.; Mehrabian, Z.; Miller, N.R. Neuroprotection and Neuroregeneration Strategies Using the rNAION Model: Theory, Histology, Problems, Results and Analytical Approaches. *Int. J. Mol. Sci.* **2022**, *23*, 15604. https://doi.org/10.3390/ijms232415604

Academic Editor: Stephanie C. Joachim

Received: 28 September 2022
Accepted: 23 November 2022
Published: 9 December 2022

1. Introduction

Nonarteritic anterior ischemic optic neuropathy (NAION) is an ischemic lesion in the anterior portion of the optic nerve, which results in sudden vision loss, visible edema of the optic nerve head (the optic disc), and ultimately retinal ganglion cell (RGC) neuron death and loss of RGC axons by Wallerian degeneration (progressive axon degeneration in both directions from the site of the lesion). Most clinical NAION cases are believed to be due to a post-ischemic compartment syndrome associated with vascular (capillary) dysregulation at the site of the initial lesion [1]. However, a number of associated factors potentially contribute to this disease, and the relative degree of severity of each case. These include the size of the optic nerve as it enters the eye (morphology), vascular dysregulation due to underlying systemic disorders such as hypertension and diabetes, familial genetics and mitochondrial mutations, and possible other spontaneous pathologic processes. These include such things as microemboli to the optic nerve head, elevated central venous pressure, and differential cerebrospinal fluid pressure gradients [2–4]. Importantly, no currently available drug has been shown to be consistently effective in reducing the damage or in ameliorating the visual debilitation that occurs in NAION. One reason for this lack of progress in clinical treatment is a dearth of knowledge of the pathophysiological mechanisms responsible for permanent visual loss after NAION. Another reason is the variable time from onset of

NAION symptoms to clinical recognition and possible treatment. Finally, it is clear that some patients have some degree of optic disc swelling, for an unknown amount of time, before clinical symptoms develop. Thus, we largely lack an understanding of the processes and time window opportunities that may be available for different treatment approaches. The rodent NAION (rNAION) and primate NAION (pNAION) models are now available for intensive analysis of pathophysiological mechanisms associated with clinical NAION, evaluation of potential treatments, and to identify the time windows of opportunity for treating this disorder [5–7].

The rNAION Model: Histology and Comparison with Human Disease

The optic nerve head (ONH) has a vasculature far more complex than the distal optic nerve, with circulatory contributions from the retina, choroid and optic nerve-pial vessels. Thus there are possibilities for dysregulation from multiple components (see Figure 1).

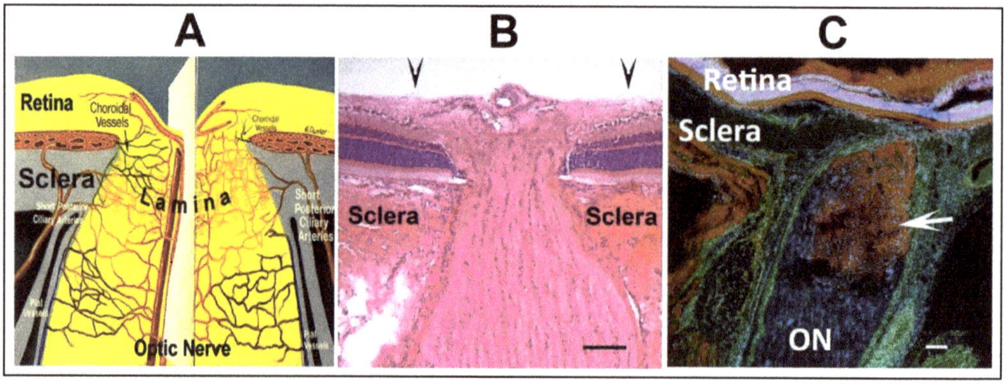

Figure 1. Overview of the ONH and contributory vascular components, and limitations of vascular leakage in rNAION. (**A**). Schematic of the vascular supply of the primate ONH, The ONH is partially bounded by the thick scleral wall, which resists lateral expansion. The fenestrated lamina within the ONH enables transit of the RGC axons. ONH circulation is a plexus formed with contributions from intraretinal, choroidal, optic nerve intraneural and pial circulations, as well as direct contribution from the short posterior ciliary arteries (SPCAs) in primates. (**B**). H&E-stained cross-section of the rat ONH. The unmyelinated portion of the ONH is bounded by the sclera, and smaller in diameter than the myelinated distal ON. The arrowheads above the figure indicate 500 μm boundary. (**C**). Limits of ONH vascular leakage following rNAION induction (arrow) 1d post-induction in the rNAION model. Immunohistochemistry using labeled 3 kDa (red-Dextran) and 55 kDa (green-FITC/BSA) probes. Serum leaks from decompensated capillaries in the ONH in a focal manner, with distal ON vasculature unimpaired. Scale bar: 100 μm in (**B**,**C**).

The ONH is bounded within the thick-walled sclera and in primates, the individual axon bundles are enclosed between collagenous columns. Thus there is little room for compensatory tissue expansion in the setting of edema. This problem is compounded in individuals with only a small opening in the sclera where the optic nerve emerges to form the optic nerve (the 'disk-at-risk') [3].

In prototypical human NAION, vascular dysregulation anywhere in the optic nerve head can result in some degree of interstitial (extravascular) or intracellular edema. This causes expansion of the fascicles containing the ON axons until resistance is met by either the tissue surrounding the fascicles or the optic nerve sheath. At that point, extracellular pressure increases by hydraulic action until the resistance is sufficient to close off capillary circulation, resulting in a compartment syndrome with tissue ischemia. Human ON axons are thickly fasciculated: that is, individual groups of axons (fascicles) are separated by relatively dense collagenous partitions within the nerve. Thus, compartment syndromes can occur in only a portion of the human ON, affecting individual fascicles.

The farther away in evolution an animal model is from humans, the more retinal and optic nerve dissimilarities may occur that can confound both the interpretations of pathology and possible treatments. Thus, animal models of NAION are just that: Models that are representative of various components of the disease and potentially useful for analysis of disease mechanisms and treatments, but that must always be considered with a number of caveats, including reliance on individual pathways to a greater or lesser degree. Although rats and humans share ~99% of their overall genes [8], different species can express individual genes that may be relevant to a specific neuroprotective mechanism at different levels. For example, L-type calcium channel blockers are highly effective neuroprotectants in models of rodent central nervous system (CNS) ischemia [9] but relatively ineffective in humans [10]. This may be partly because rats express L-type calcium channels in ON tissue at levels ~5-fold higher than in humans or other old world primates [11], suggesting that rats rely on these channels to a greater degree than primates.

The initial NAION model was defined in rats and called rodent anterior ischemic optic neuropathy (rAION) or rodent NAION (rNAION). Both terms are used in the literature. The intraocular optic disk diameter in the rat examined through a plano-convex contact lens is 500 μm (Figure 1B, arrows), but narrows within the sclera to ~250 μm (Figure 1B). A 500 μm laser spot thus irradiates both the optic nerve and the peripapillary retina and its supporting vessels. While the collagen sheaths in the human ON surrounding the axon fascicles are quite dense, the sheaths surrounding rodent ON axons are extremely thin. The laser/rose Bengal-induced vascular decompensation causes focal serum leakage in the ONH (Figure 1C), resulting in intraneural edema limited by the sclera and ON sheath (Figure 1C). This gross expansion is easily seen in vivo using spectral-domain optical coherence tomography (SD-OCT), where it can be measured at the anterior portion of the ON, including its intraretinal portion (compare Figure 2F, control rat ONH, with Figure 2H; post-induction). ONH capillaries are likely compromised by a rise in overall intraneural pressure, rather than from compromise of individual fascicles. Axon loss in rNAION thus is likely a function of the total size of the nerve, rather than associated with individual regions, as occurs in humans and in the nonhuman primate (NHP) NAION model (pNAION) [7,12]. The laser spot must be precisely focused; if laser irradiation extends over the surrounding peripapillary retina, this can result in decompensation of retinal vasculature, causing both ON and retinal ischemia. Including animals with mixed ischemic lesions in the evaluation of rNAION can confound individual analyses and confuse subsequent treatment approaches. In particular, as retinal responses to neuroprotective agents can be vastly different than those of the ON, it can be difficult to separate treatment responses to the retinal ischemic and optic nerve head-axon ischemic components. A ganzfeld electroretinogram can be used to distinguish animals with mixed lesions from those with pure ON ischemia.

Mice ONs have fewer axons than rat ONs (mice: ~50,000 vs. rat: ~100,000), and a correspondingly smaller ONH, which means that a 300μm laser spot size at 50 mW is required for mouse induction, rather than the 500 μm spot used for rats. The same 50 mW of radiant power is distributed over a smaller area (mouse ON circumference is only 36% the size of the rat ON). There is, therefore, correspondingly more power per unit area, and a potential for greater capillary decompensation. Additionally, ON ischemic induction that results in large percentages (>75%) of RGC loss can be associated with amacrine retinal neuron loss [13]. This suggests that conditions required to generate severe ONH edema also can induce a state of overlapping retinal ischemia. Following mouse rNAION induction, great care is needed to identify animals with pure ON ischemic lesions, so that animals with mixed retinal and ON ischemia can be eliminated from further analyses.

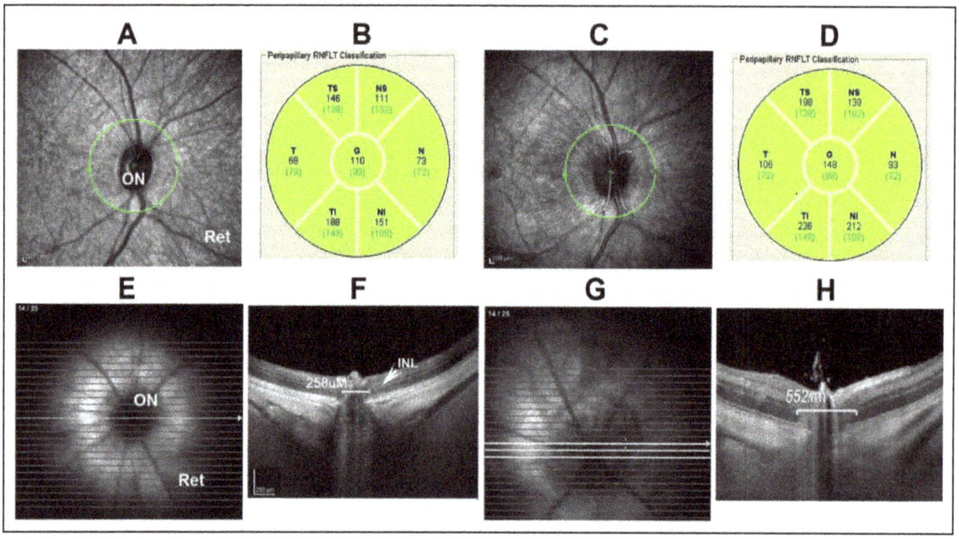

Figure 2. Comparison of OCT appearance of the ON in two NAION (pNAION and rNAION) models: (**A**). OCT image of uninduced NHP. (**B**). Quantification of peripapillary nerve fiber layer (RGC axonal layer) thickness in uninduced NHP. The global nerve fiber layer thickness (**G**) is 110 μm, with quantification of individual regions. (**C**). OCT image of 2d post-induced NHP ONH. There is edema of the ONH, with striae extending out into the superior retina. (**D**). Quantification of the RGC axon layer. There is increased thickness of the global peripapillary nerve fiber layer, indicating ONH edema. (**E**). OCT *en face* view of uninduced rat ON. The ONH is dark, and relatively small in diameter. (**F**). Cross section enabled by planoconcave contact lens. The width of the ONH at mid-diameter, as measured by the distance in microns between the boundary of inner nuclear layer (INL) on either side of the nerve, is 258 μm. (**G**). OCT *en face* view of rNAION 2d post-induced ON. The nerve head is pale and enlarged. (**H**). ONH cross sectional view after rNAION induction. The ONH diameter (in brackets) has expanded to 552 μm; compare with panel F, indicating ONH edema.

Some of the advantages of the rNAION model, then, are balanced by the differences from human NAION as well as pNAION in ON morphology. Identifying additional species whose ONH and ON structure more closely resemble that of primates may help reduce some of the drawbacks associated with the rodent model, but the rNAION model, with its ease of induction, the relative inexpense of the animals and of animal upkeep, and the availability of complete genomic information for both rats and mice make this model an invaluable tool to use in ischemic optic neuropathy research.

2. Results

2.1. Analytical Approaches and Correlation

Although the initiating events that result in ONH edema may be different between the human disease and its animal models, the pathophysiological changes that ultimately result in axon ischemia are likely similar. In both clinical disease and in the nonhuman primate and rodent models, vascular decompensation and leakage results in ONH edema within a tightly restricted space. The edema in turn causes capillary compression and compromise, causing a compartment syndrome that generates axon ischemia. Axon ischemia results in subsequent localized loss of axon transport and electrical conductivity, followed by inflammation, RGC axon collapse and, eventually, isolated RGC loss.

Acute ONH edema is present in human NAION [3], and also in the rodent and primate models [7,14]. This edema can be quantified by optical coherence tomography (OCT) in clinical NAION [15], pNAION [12], and rNAION, [14,16]. The primate retina and ONH can be evaluated using a standard OCT device such as a Heidelberg spectral domain-optical coherence tomograph (SD-OCT), and the ONH changes associated with pNAION are similar to those of clinical NAION (Figure 2A–D). However, the small size of the rodent eye requires additional optical adjustment, depending on whether or not a rodent-specialized imaging device such as a bio-optigen OCT is used. We initially developed a simple plano-concave contact lens for use in rats and mice that is now commercially available (Micro-R and Micro-M; Cantor and Nissel, UK) and that can be used with standard OCT devices such as the Heidelberg spectral domain-OCT in combination with a high-plus (28-diopter) correcting lens. The use of the plano-convex lens enables both a cross-sectional and *en face* view of the rodent retina (Figure 2E–H).

2.2. ONH Vascular Leakage in the rNAION Model

Following rNAION induction, ONH vascular leakage is demonstrable within 5 h. We performed post-induction leakage analysis using indocyanine green (ICGA) and fluorescein angiography (IVFA) (Figure 3). ICG signal at the ONH was found to be more robust than fluorescein, likely because ICG is >95% protein bound, limiting diffusion [16]. We used a 5 h post-rNAION ICGA to determine if the relative degree of early leakage is useful as a biomarker for later rNAION severity (Figure 3I–G leakage). While all induced eyes showed some degree of ICG-leakage signal, the degree of early leakage by either method was not sufficiently robust to predict the ultimate level of rNAION severity, as measured by RGC loss at 30 days [16]. Animals with strong early signals can ultimately have little neuronal loss, whereas animals with less intense leakage could yield significant loss of RGCs (Figure 3). These findings may be associated with a number of factors, including ON sheath resistance, and the relative size of each animal's ON. Thus, very early biomarkers (<1d) of rNAION lesion severity remain to be identified.

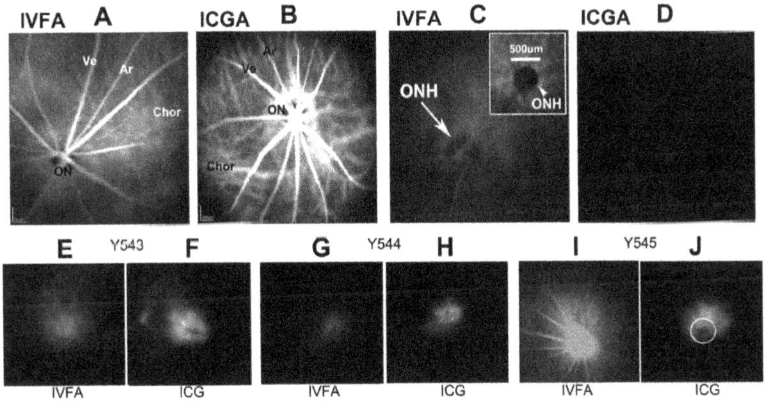

Figure 3. Markers of ONH vascular leakage in rNAION. (**A**,**B**). Baseline retinal fundus photos taken 30 s post-intravenous dye injection in a naïve (uninduced) animal of A. Fluorescein (IVFA). The intraretinal veins (Ve) and arteries (Ar) are visible, but the optic nerve circulation is muted due to the presence of melanin pigment, which blocks visible light. (**B**). Indocyanine green (ICGA). ICG fluorescence is visualized via infrared light, which passes through melanin. The choroidal circulation below the retinal pigment epithelium is clearly visible, as is the enhanced circulation around the ON. (**C**). fluorescein dye fluorescence 5 min post-injection. The ONH is barely visible. (**D**). ICG fluorescence 5 min post-injection. No leakage is visible. (**E**–**J**): fluorescein and ICG image pairs of the same eyes in three animals (Y543, Y544, Y545) taken 5 h post-rNAION induction. There are significant differences in the amount of post-injection fluorescence revealed by the two dye types. In general, the ICG dye signal is more stable, due to its nearly 100% binding to serum proteins and reduced diffusion. The ICG patterns are indicative of the deeper leakage in the ONH. The circle in plate (**J**) is 500 μm. Data for Figure 3 is reprinted with permission from [16]. 2021 PLOS-One.

2.3. ONH Edema-Based Expansion Predicts rNAION Severity

While very early biomarkers of severity remain to be found, edema development in the intraocular portion of the ONH at 1–2d post-induction using (mean) ONH diameter has proven to be a useful indicator of ultimate RGC loss [14,16]. The mean diameter of the intraocular portion of the uninduced rat ONH for current purposes, is defined as the mean distance between the two margins of the inner nuclear layers on either side of the optic nerve head, and is 310 ± 38.2 μm [16]. A 6-s laser induction generates ONH ICG leakage, edema, with ONH expansion to a mean of 347.5 ± 13.6 μm. However, this level of edema does not result in discernable RGC loss. Following a 9–11-s induction time, mean ONH diameter increased with a range between 355 μ to >650 μm [16]. RGC loss was only consistently seen when ONH diameter was >510 μm [16]. The majority of ONH edema develops by 1 day, with a minimal amount of additional edema between 1 day and 2 days post-induction.

ONH expansion to >510 um post-induction is predictive of significant RGC loss. This suggests that, in preclinical trials of neuroprotective agents for NAION, OCT can be used to either identify and segregate animals for analysis in neuroprotection treatment studies with long time window effects (>1 d), or to identify agents that effectively suppress post-induction edema 1–2 days post-rNAION induction. The use of the 510 um cutoff is also useful for identifying individuals that can be included in neuroregeneration studies, since these treatments are typically given later (=days) post-induction.

2.4. RGC Quantification

Many RGC neuroprotection analyses use estimation of the number of surviving RGCs. Rats have only a single layer of RGCs, unlike primates. Thus, randomized statistically valid cell analysis (stereology) of RGCs can be performed easily on retinal flat-mount preparations by immunohistochemistry. Antibodies against Brn3a(+) identify RGC nuclei, whereas anti-RPBMS labels RGC soma. While retrograde labeling of RGC soma can be performed using either intracerebral injection of fluorogold into the superior colliculus or application of the fluorescent dye DiI onto the cut section of the ON, these latter approaches may not consistently label all RGCs or even the same region of RGCs. Previous studies have revealed that to achieve 90–95% RGC fluorogold labeling, the superior colliculus must be covered with fluorogold-soaked gelfoam (M. Vidal-Sanz, personal communication).

2.5. Measuring Visual Function Loss following rNAION Induction

We currently evaluate visual function using a device which combines contrast sensitivity and optokinetic nystagmus (Optomotry). The optomotry device can evaluate visual acuity in each eye of an animal. Visual function in mice and rats is fairly coarse (mice: 0.5 cycles/degree; Long-Evans pigmented rats: 1 cycle/degree; ~20/500) [17]. This relatively low acuity is likely based on a lack of strong evolutionary pressure for high-level visual function in rodents compared with their motor skills. Visual acuity of albino rat strains is even lower (~0.5 cycles/degree) [18]. Thus, attempts to identify subtle degrees of subjective visual acuity improvement resulting from various neuroreparative therapies other than simple quantification of RGC numbers before and after treatment are likely to be problematic.

Visual function also is quantifiable using objective measures such as the visual-evoked potential (VEP), which evaluates signal received at the visual cortex, the photopic negative response (phNR), and the pattern electroretinogram (pERG) [19,20], the latter being able to evaluate the degree of RGC activity within the retina itself, rather than as an action potential to the brain. We previously demonstrated that in pNAION, the VEP and pERG were significantly correlated ($r = 0.80$, $p = 0.0002$ [12]. VEPs also may be useful in evaluating the degree of ON functional preservation distinct from simple RGC preservation. We found that administration of a monoclonal antibody (11c7mAb) that targeted the NOGO receptor in degenerate myelin did not improve either ONH edema or RGC counts following induction of rNAION, but flash VEP amplitudes were significantly preserved ($p = 0.01$

vs. vehicle; $n = 8$ animals) in 11C7mab-treated animals compared with mAb (anti-ragweed IgG) treated controls [21]. There was also reduced inflammatory cell infiltration. This suggests that treatments targeting functional preservation, distinct from simple RGC survival, may be an effective neuroregenerative strategy.

2.6. RGC Loss Variability in rNAION Using Different Induction Times

Generally, we use an 11-s laser exposure at 50mW laser power to induce rNAION. Power output is measured at the point of exposure, using a thermocouple power meter. These induction parameters result in few uninduced animals or unwanted intraretinal complications.

We evaluated the relative efficiency of laser exposure to induce rNAION and the corresponding severity of subsequent RGC loss (Figure 4). A 9-s laser induction ($n = 7$) yielded a mean RGC loss of 35.8 ± 17.9% (mean ± sem) (Figure 4A). The range varied from <5% to >76% RGC loss (Figure 4B). The severity variability of the 9- and 10-s-induced animals is strongly correlated with the degree of ONH edema produced. This suggests the rNAION model exhibits a threshold effect, in which low levels of ONH edema may not produce sufficient ONH compression to generate RGC loss. An 11-s induction time ($n = 10$) generated a mean 71.4 ± 2.4% (sem) RGC loss (Figure 4A) with a range of 60% to >84% loss (Figure 4B). Although these data support the idea of a threshold effect, longer exposure times were associated with a greater number of unwanted intraretinal complications; eg, branch retinal vein occlusions (BRVOs) and central retinal vein occlusions (CRVOs). Intraretinal complications can skew interpretation of neuroprotective approaches for rNAION, since retinal neuroprotective mechanisms (which include activity of Mueller cells) also may be considerably different from the astrocyte-driven mechanisms of the ON. This is confirmed by the number of agents known to be retina-neuroprotective but which fail to induce optic nerve neuroprotection. Therefore, identification and elimination of animals with retinal ischemic complications by both visual (retinal-fundus) examination and SD-OCT imaging is important in designing relevant treatment trials, especially those with fewer animals. As previously mentioned, ganzfeld electroretinography also can be helpful in identifying animals with large degrees of retinal ischemia.

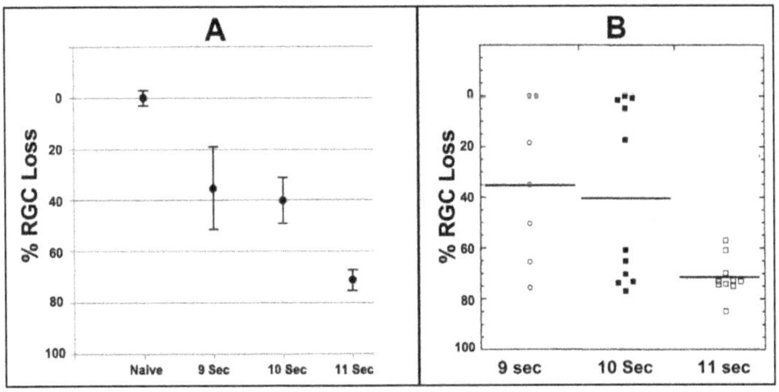

Figure 4. RGC loss patterns with increasing amounts of laser exposure. (**A**). Comparison of mean RGC loss in rNAION with increasing exposure times using a 532nm laser at constant power and spot size (50 mW power; 500 um spot size). (**B**). Induction times compared against the range of individual animal RGC loss values. Low induction times (9 s) result in a wide range of RGC loss values, including a number of animals without any RGC loss as well as animals with minimal levels of RGC loss. An intermediate induction time (10 s) results in identification of two animal subgroups suggestive of a threshold effect, with subthreshold- (low levels of RGC loss) and threshold- animals (high-level RGC loss). A further increase in exposure time to 11 s results in the majority of animals having significant RGC loss (threshold). Data for Figure 4 is reprinted with permission from [16]. 2021 PLOS-One.

2.7. Early Ischemic Stress-Related Changes in RGCs

Following rNAION induction, RGCs with axon dysfunction begin to show significant stress. cfos elevation is detected as soon as 5 h post-induction, which was the earliest time analyzed (see Figure 7a in [5]). In an early experiment, we used Affymetrix microarray analysis to evaluate early stress-related retinal gene expression changes at 1-day and 3 days post-induction from pooled (n = 3 retinae) Poly (A+) RNA from each condition, with two replicates (Table 1). Complete Affymetrix chip data is shown in Supplementary Table S1.

Table 1. Changes in retinal and ONH gene expression post-rNAION induction. Retinal expression data are derived from Affymetrix U34A genechips (Data from Supplemental Table S1, this report), whereas the ONH (in red) gene expression data are derived from Illumina sequencing and previously reported in Supplementary Materials in [22]. Retinal ratios are generated from individual assay results between comparison sets. ONH ratio data are generated from a single sample of six pooled rNAION ONHs from 1d post-induction, divided by the mean results from five individual naïve ONHs. Genes evaluated for protein expression (seen in Figure 4) are indicated in **bold**. Lipocalin-2 mRNA expression was elevated >6 fold at 1 day and decreased to >2 fold by 3 days post-rNAION. Crh expression did not increase in the first 3 days.

Gene ID	Gene Symbol	Gene Name	1d Post-rNAION Ratio (R1/L1) (Retina)	3d Post-rNAION Ratio (R3/L3) (Retina)	1d Post-rNAION Ratio (R3/L3) (ONH)
M14656	Spp1/osteopontin	Secreted phosphoprotein 1	3.432111001	1.417575157	1.530076555
AA892553	Stat 1	STAT1	10.43670886	4.104424779	1.080385971
U66707	Densin-180/Lrrc7	Densin-180	1.713261649	2.555331992	1.093128466
AF030089	Ania-4/Dclk1	neurotransmitter early gene 4 (ania-4)	8.987133516	1.700414108	0.975284552
J02722	hmox1	Heme Oxygenase-1	3.646239554	1.928571429	1.132401488
L33869	Cp	Ceruloplasmin	2.937233461	2.498855835	1.000494963
AF008650	SLC-1/SSTR1	Somatostatin receptor-1	3.253018661	2.729357798	0.954323595
D28508	JAK3	Jak-3 protein kinase	8.614443084	1.719766472	1.142099095
AI045030	CELF	CELF protein	4.181425486	1.86818377	1.027053789
M19651	Fra-1 fosl1	Fos-related antigen	5.223048327	1.319474836	1.174091099
AI176456	MT-2a	Metallothionein 2a	6.331651318	1.597822606	0.971216928
M29866	C3	Complement 3c	4.054368932	3.743093923	0.939352616
AI169327	TIMP1	Tissue inhibitor-metalloproteinases-1	25.57614679	1.648916117	1.223379175
U53184	Litaf	Lipoprotein inducing TNF factor	2.894752945	1.301528426	1.016124153
AA946503	**Lcn2**	**Lipocalin-2**	**6.955862534**	**2.376604473**	**1.038533352**
AA893280	Plin2	Perilipin 2	6.457792208	2.39125239	1.104502556

Table 1. *Cont.*

Gene ID	Gene Symbol	Gene Name	1d Post-rNAION Ratio (R1/L1) (Retina)	3d Post-rNAION Ratio (R3/L3) (Retina)	1d Post-rNAION Ratio (R3/L3) (ONH)
M54987	**CRF/Crh**	**Corticotropin releasing hormone**	**0.923984891**	**1.05511811**	**0.933884278**
U92081	RTI40/PDPN	RNRTI1-podoplanin	4.873994638	1.848832659	0.999564836
U56407	Ube2d4	ubiquitin conjugating enzyme	4.523255814	4.270042194	0.915009744
M11597	Calca	alpha-type calcitonin gene-related peptide	4.830188679	2.294117647	1.559015745
X61381	IFITM3	Interferon induced mRNA	3.532416331	0.916807529	1.048079385
U09228	TCF4	Deaconess E-box binding factor	3.228754366	1.075950771	1.041957282
D00753	Cpi-26	contrapsin-like prot. inhibitor (CPi-26)	4.660706861	2.730576441	Not Found
X06769	cFos	cFos mRNA	2.259195894	0.880295098	1.076489824
AF082125	AHR	Aryl hydrocarbon receptor	4.016318205	1.222446237	1.077670043
U01344	NAT1	N-Acetyl Transferase	3.98401066	1.263825929	1.025181547
X17053	MCP-1/CCL2	Monocyte chemoattractive protein-1	3.333156499	1.466160658	1.12708558
X17163	**cJun**	**c-jun oncogene**	**1.38262668**	**1.140383102**	**1.043633554**

The most dramatic changes in gene expression compared with contralateral uninduced eyes were found at 1d post-induction (Timp1: 25-fold induction; Stat1: 10-fold induction, and Lipocalin-2: 7-fold induction). STAT1 and lipocalin-2 expression declined to 4-fold and 2.4-fold, respectively, by 3 days. The decline in retinal TIMP1 expression was even greater, to 1.6-fold at 3 days post-induction, suggesting that there are distinct retinal requirements associated with early RGC stress.

Affymetrix-derived retinal results following rNAION-induced stress were compared against results obtained from changes in ischemic ONH gene expression obtained by illumina deep sequencing. Sequence data was obtained from total RNA from isolated ONHs from naïve vs. 3d post-rNAION induced animals (previously reported in [22]). Using the combined datasets, we then evaluated protein expression and RGC localization for a number of candidate RGC stress genes. These included Lipocalin-2, Jun-phosphorylation (pJun) and Corticotrophin releasing factor/releasing hormone (CRF/CRH). cJun phosphorylation is closely associated with neuronal ischemic stress [23]. CRF was chosen bibliographically because although this gene is known to be constitutively expressed in retinal amacrine neurons [24], it is upregulated in neurons after ischemia [25]. We confirmed expression in RGCs using Brn3a colocalization (Figure 5).

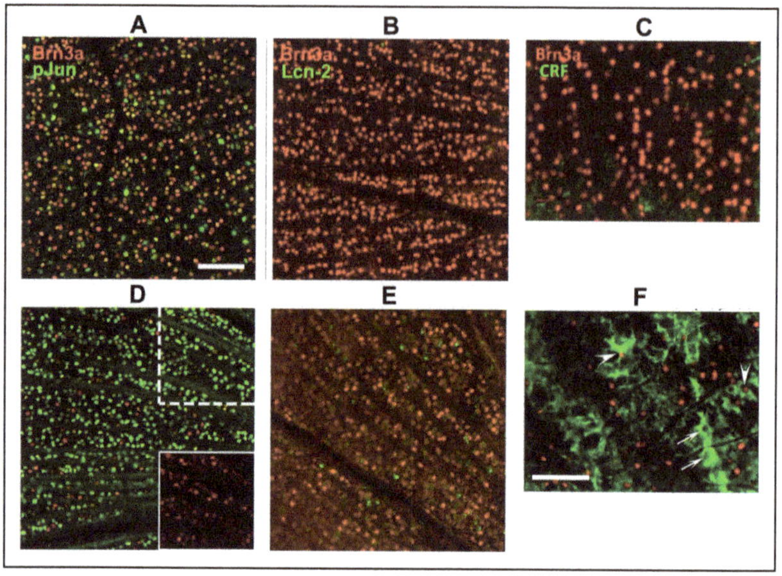

Figure 5. RGC stress protein expression after axon ischemic stress. A-C: RGC responses 1d post-rNAION induction. D-E: RGC responses 3d post-rNAION induction. F. RGC responses 7d post-rNAION induction. (**A**,**D**): Phospho-Jun (pJun). The majority of RGC nuclei (Brn3a(+) nuclei; in red) colocalize with pJun (in green) within 1 day of induction. (**D**). pJun expression is demonstrable in nearly every RGC nucleus in an affected region by 3d post-induction. The upper (dashed line-outlined actual area) and lower (inset: solid line) indicated areas reveal the relative decrease in Brn3(+) expression in RGCs by 3d post-induction. (**B**,**E**): Lipocalin-2. There is little signal at 1 day, despite high levels of lipocalin-2 mRNA. Lipocalin-2 protein signal is present in the majority of affected RGCs by 3d post-induction. (**C**,**F**): CRF. CRF expression is minimal in RGCs at one day (**C**), while in (**F**) Strong expression is seen 7 days post-induction. Expression is prominent in cells that have lost their nuclear Brn3a expression (arrows), but also in nuclei with persistent Brn3a (arrowheads). Scalebars in (**A**,**F**): 50 uM.

RGCs whose axons are undergoing ischemic stress rapidly upregulate cJun phosphorylation, likely via retrograde signaling through the double leucine zipper kinase (DLK), a member of the JNK signaling pathway [26]. One day post-rNAION induction, nearly all RGC nuclei express some degree of pJun signal, although the signal varies in intensity (Figure 5A). In contrast, while strong lcn-2 upregulation is seen at the mRNA level in Table 1, lipocalin-2 protein signal is low (Figure 5B). However, 3 days post-induction, lcn2 expression is clearly detectable in nearly all RGCs, as defined by coexpression of green (lcn2) and Brn3a(+) (red) nuclei (Figure 5E). There is also a significant reduction in the intensity of Brn3a(+) signal at this time (Figure 5E; compare red signal with Brn3(+) signal in 5B). RGC stress is also confirmed by the strong expression of pJun at 3 days (Figure 5D; green nuclei), with few RGC nuclei still expressing strong Brn3a(+) signal (Figure 5D; red nuclei). Individual confocal channels reveal that, while most RGC nuclei still express Brn3a, few RGCs have the same signal level seen in naïve retinae, suggesting a shutdown of Brn3a-homeodomain-related gene functions by this time. The timing of these events provides an indirect estimation of the potential window of neuroprotective treatment opportunities in NAION.

2.8. Soluble and Cellular Inflammatory ONH Responses

It is not surprising that a robust inflammatory response quickly follows the induction of an ischemic axonopathy. Nevertheless, the existence of post-NAION inflammation was debated for years, until the rNAION model became available. This was simply because of a lack of relevant clinical material, since NAION is not associated with acute mortality. Post-rNAION inflammatory responses include both soluble cytokine/chemokine changes in the lesion site within a day, as well as inflammatory cell migration (both extracellular macrophages and microglia) within 3 days post-lesion.

We performed deep sequencing on both naïve rat ONH and pooled ONH tissue from 1d post-rNAION induced eyes (n = 6). These results are shown in Table 2, and the data is derived from the Supplementary Materials previously deposited [22]. IL6 showed the greatest increase 1d post-induction (1.66 ± 1.0 fold in rNAION/Naïve), followed by CCL17 and CCL9 (1.46 ± 1.0 and 1.40 ± 0.85 fold, respectively).

Table 2. ONH-Interleukin and chemokine responses in early (1d) rNAION), compared with naïve tissue. Mean naïve is the average of five individual samples (Naïve 1–5), whereas rNAION is a pooled sample containing ONH-RNA from six eyes 1d post-induction. IL6 showed the greatest overall increase at 1 day.

Gene Symbol	Gene Name	Naive_1	Naive_2	Naive_3	Naïve_4	Naive_5	Mean Naïve	rNAION	rNAION /Naïve
	Interleukins								
Il6	interleukin 6	3.66	4.85	3.66	4.37	6.01	4.51	7.50	**1.66**
Il27	interleukin 27	4.77	5.05	3.66	4.93	3.66	4.41	5.72	**1.30**
Il24	interleukin 24	3.66	3.66	3.66	3.66	3.66	3.66	4.70	**1.28**
Il10	interleukin 10	3.66	3.66	3.66	3.66	3.66	3.66	4.49	**1.23**
Il3	interleukin 3	3.66	3.66	3.66	3.66	3.66	3.66	4.49	**1.23**
Il1b	interleukin 1 beta	6.35	5.67	5.79	5.62	7.05	6.10	7.43	**1.22**
Il11	interleukin 11	5.52	5.73	7.38	5.09	10.46	6.84	8.26	**1.21**
	Chemokines								
Ccl17	C-C motif chemokine ligand 17	3.66	3.66	3.66	4.79	6.00	4.35	6.34	**1.46**
Ccl9	chemokine (C-C motif) ligand 9	3.66	4.51	3.66	4.69	5.72	4.45	6.25	**1.40**
Cxcr3	C-X-C motif chemokine receptor 3	3.66	5.62	3.66	5.37	3.66	4.39	5.95	**1.35**
Cxcl11	C-X-C motif chemokine ligand 11	4.55	5.25	3.66	6.44	6.62	5.31	7.10	**1.34**
Cxcl3	chemokine (C-X-C motif) ligand 3	3.66	3.66	3.66	3.66	6.10	4.15	5.50	**1.33**
Ccl22	C-C motif chemokine ligand 22	4.92	4.51	3.66	3.66	6.03	4.56	5.95	**1.31**
Ccr7	C-C motif chemokine receptor 7	5.71	4.51	5.76	4.99	4.70	5.13	6.67	**1.30**
Cxcl10	C-X-C motif chemokine ligand 10	6.91	6.74	7.41	7.34	8.75	7.43	9.62	**1.29**
Ccl3	C-C motif chemokine ligand 3	6.10	5.48	3.66	5.73	7.46	5.69	7.36	**1.29**
Ccl4	C-C motif chemokine ligand 4	5.12	5.19	3.66	5.21	7.04	5.24	6.76	**1.29**
Ccl11	C-C motif chemokine ligand 11	5.98	6.00	5.24	6.27	8.80	6.46	8.03	**1.24**
Ccr4	C-C motif chemokine receptor 4	3.66	3.66	3.66	4.37	3.66	3.80	4.70	**1.23**
Ccl21	C-C motif chemokine ligand 21	3.66	3.66	3.66	3.66	5.98	4.13	5.06	**1.23**
Ccr8	C-C motif chemokine receptor 8	3.66	3.66	3.66	3.66	3.66	3.66	4.49	**1.23**
Cxcl17	C-X-C motif chemokine ligand 17	6.20	5.81	3.66	5.84	5.92	5.48	6.66	**1.21**
Cxcl6	C-X-C motif chemokine ligand 6	5.26	4.96	6.17	5.40	6.61	5.68	6.81	**1.20**

Within the lesion itself, early release (1d) of inflammatory proteins include multiple pro-inflammatory cytokines, such as osteopontin/SPP1 (see Table 1) and interleukin-6 (IL6; see Table 2) (rNAION/naïve = 1.53 and 1.66-fold, respectively) [22]. IL6 is a cytokine with pleotropic (multiple actions) activity. It is important in induction of acute-phase inflammation-related proteins, but also in the transition to chronic inflammation [27,28]. Additional changes include inflammatory prostaglandins (PGE_2) and thromboxanes A1 and A2. Post-rNAION, the retina and ONH also express pro-inflammatory TNFα and IL-1β mRNAs, with levels peaking by the first day and declining thereafter.

2.9. Neuroprotective Treatment Approaches to rNAION

2.9.1. Edema/Vascular

ONH edema is a key factor in NAION pathology. Early edema reduction would thus would seem to be an effective approach to NAION treatment. The caveats with respect to this approach are: (1) treatment needs to be effective after initiation of the edema-inducing insult, but before irreversible ischemic axon damage occurs, and (2) treatment must be effective before irreversible death-associated signaling occurs in the RGCs.

1. PGJ_2. 15-Deoxy *delta* 12,14-Prostaglandin J_2 (PGJ_2) is a natural, non-enzymatically generated product of prostaglandin D2 (PGD_2). We selected this prostaglandin because early studies revealed that PGD synthase gene expression declined dramatically after rNAION induction and then rebounded to supernormal levels precisely when post-stroke edema resolved, suggesting that the loss of either PGD_2 or one of its metabolites might play a major role in edema development and its rebound have a role in edema resolution.

PGJ_2 administered in pharmacological doses (100 ug/kg) up to 5 h post-induction reduced ONH edema (see Figure 1 in [29]) and also reduced RGC loss in rats with rNAION [29], and in a model of old-world primates [30]. Ultrastructural studies revealed that PGJ_2 likely reduces early intraneural edema by inhibiting endothelial vesicular fluid transport after rNAION induction [29]. This probably occurs by PGJ_2's suppression of NFκB activation in disc vasculature [31]. Late (>1d) treatment with PGJ_2 alone did not notably affect the levels of late ONH edema and did not improve RGC survival. This suggests that PGJ_2's major neuroprotective effect in rNAION occurs by early edema suppression.

2. TRPM4/Sur-1 inhibition. Following CNS ischemia, astrocytes express the transient receptor potential cation-family M/sulfonylurea receptor-1 (TRPM4/SUR1). This results in opening of a water channel, with resulting intracellular astrocytic edema contributing to ischemic damage. SUR1 inhibitors such as glibenclamide have been shown to be neuroprotective after hemorrhagic and ischemic strokes as well as after spinal cord injury in humans [32–34]. Interestingly, SUR-1 is not expressed in early (<1d) ONH exhibiting edema after rNAION induction [35], and there is minimal elevation in ONH-SUR1 mRNA expression even 3d post-induction compared with naïve ONH (DS-Seq: naïve 9.34 vs. 3d post-induction: 9.85). We performed a limited sighting study ($n = 4$ animals), utilizing rNAION induction in both eyes of each animal, with each animal serving as its own induction control. Animals were induced in one eye (11 s/50 mW/1 mg/kg 2.5 mM rose Bengal). Immediately following induction, we administered glibenclamide (50 ug/kg) daily via intraperitoneal injection for the next 5 days. One week post-induction of the first eye, the contralateral eye was induced to an identical level, and vehicle (PBS) was administered intraperitoneally. ONH edema was evaluated using SD-OCT at 2d post-induction in each eye (Figure 6A). We also evaluated RGC survival in both eyes of all animals. Because of the small number of animals used, no statistically valid analysis was possible.

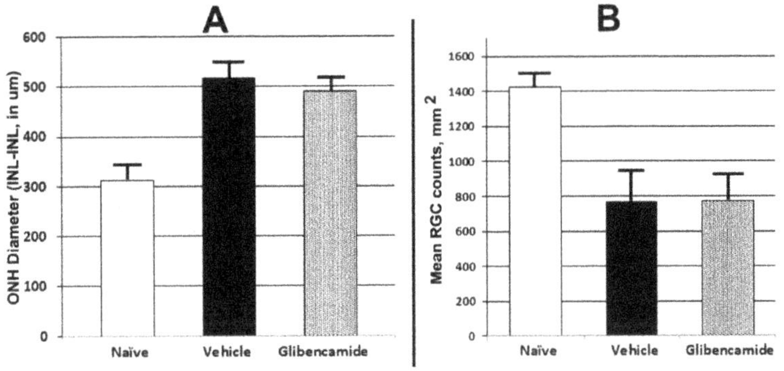

Figure 6. Effects of an astrocytic TRPM4/SUR1 (white matter edema inhibitor) on ONH edema and RGC survival post-rNAION. Adult rats were administered glibenclamide (40 ug/kg) immediately after rNAION induction and daily for 4 subsequent days via intraperitoneal injection. (**A**). ONH edema 2d post-induction. Minimal reduction was seen in glibenclamide-treated animals (ONH mean values 516 ± 17μm in vehicle-treated vs. 492 ± 20μm s.e.m in glibenclamide-treated animals; $n = 4$). (**B**). RGC survival post-rNAION induction. Brn3a(+)-RGC counts in naïve retinae yielded a ratio of 1423.2 ± 19.3 cells/unit area ($n = 10$ animals). Retinae 30d post-induction yielded a mean of 767.6 ± 167.6 cells/unit area for vehicle treatment vs. 775.7 ± 149.1 cells/unit area for glibenclamide treatment.

Glibenclamide treatment resulted in only a small reduction in ONH edema, compared with the vehicle-treated animals (Figure 6A). RGC quantification 30d post-induction revealed essentially no difference in RGC survival in glibenclamide-treated vs. vehicle-treated animals (775.7 ± 149.1 glibenclamide vs. 767.6 ± 167.6 cells sem for vehicle; Figure 6B). Interestingly, astrocytic SUR-1 induction takes about 1 day post-injury in the CNS (Gerzanich, personal communication), suggesting that TRPM4/SUR-1 suppression is not likely to be neuroprotective in sudden ON edema-associated damage. Nevertheless, other non-SUR1-dependent astrocytic mechanisms responsible for ON edema may still be responsive to edema reductive therapies.

2.9.2. Other rNAION-Neuroprotective Mechanisms

1. Astrocyte-associated neuroprotective mechanisms. Astrocytes exert neuroprotective effects directly via both edema-related mechanisms [36–38] and mechanisms related to ischemic preconditioning and that are associated with A1-Adenosine agonist activity [39]. In addition to TRPM4/SUR-1-mediated channels, Adenosine receptor-1 and -3 (A1R, A1e) agonists have been shown to be neuroprotective in cerebral ischemia [40] and are expressed in A2B5(+) glia, which include astrocytes [41]. A1R are also strongly expressed in RGCs [42,43]. Activation of A1Rs is at least partially responsible for neuroprotection associated with ischemic preconditioning [44]. Deep sequencing of rat ONH reveals moderately high levels of the A1R and nearly 8-fold less of A3Rs (Ds-Seq analysis in naïve ONH 12.53 (A1R) vs. 3.84 (A3R)(data provided on mdpi website https://www.mdpi.com/article/10.3390/cells10061440/s1, accessed on 5 June 2022 Table S1). This suggests that A1 or A1R agonists might be useful in RGC neuroprotection. We evaluated topical administration of Trabodenoson, a highly selective, topical A1R agonist. Although Trabodenoson only moderately suppressed ONH edema (564 ± 14.52 um sem for vehicle vs. 512.15 ±20.12 um sem for Trabodenoson; $n = 13$), the difference was significant (two-tailed t-test: $p = 0.05$). Even more importantly, however, Trabodenoson was potently RGC neuroprotective, with RGC loss reduced from 53.2 ± 7.1% sem in vehicle-treated animals to 27.9 ± 6.5% sem RGC loss in animals treated with Trabodenoson (Figure 7B; data derived from [45]). These results also were statistically significant (two-tailed t-test; $p = 0.01$) and suggest

that adenosine receptor agonism is potently neuroprotective, with effects only partly exerted through edema reduction. It should be noted that Trabodenoson treatment in this study was begun 3d before rNAION induction. Thus, the ability of A1 agonists to exert a neuroprotective effect in post-ischemic events is still an open question. We are now evaluating the ability of other A1 agonists to exert neuroprotective effects post-rNAION.

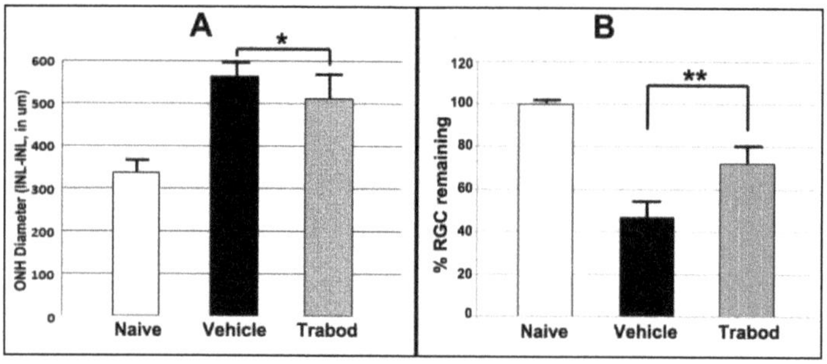

Figure 7. Adenosine A1 agonist effects on ONH edema and RGC survival. Trabodenoson drops were administered twice daily for 3 days prior to rNAION induction and for 2 weeks post-induction. (**A**). ONH edema. There is a statistically significant 15.4% reduction in ONH edema in Trabodenoson-treated eyes compared with vehicle-treated eyes. Two-tailed *t* test: * $p = 0.049$. (**B**). RGC preservation. Trabodenoson treatment resulted in a 62.1 ± 6.5% (sem) RGC survival 30d post-rNAION induction compared with 46.8 ± 7.1 % (sem) RGC survival in vehicle-treated eyes. Two-tailed *t* test: ** $p = 0.015$.

Following rNAION, cellular inflammatory invasion is present by 3 days post-induction [46], with late increases in a number of chemokines and inflammatory factors. Our lab and others have also evaluated compounds that can suppress or modify cellular inflammation, using multiple inflammatory pathways.

2. Corticosteroids. An initial clinical report suggested that immune suppression in clinical NAION treatment could be beneficial using high-dose/chronic glucocorticoids [47], but this was based on a retrospective study. In current clinical practice, some neuroophthalmologists either give no treatment or, based on the previous report, utilize corticosteroids (with its associated side effects, including steroid dependent glaucoma, diabetes and hip fractures). Most later prospective studies using steroids in clinical NAION did not show visual improvement effects [48,49]. These studies included patients diagnosed within a month of symptom onset. One study utilizing a modified steroid early in treatment suggested some effect [50], but the time from onset of symptoms to beginning treatment was not discussed. Multiple investigators have explored the use of inflammatory suppression to reduce rNAION-associated damage [51], with mixed results. Glucocorticoids were reported to be neuroprotective in a single report involving the rodent NAION model [52], but we have not seen this effect in our own study nor in other reported studies utilizing both methylprednisolone and triamcinolone [53]. No studies have combined corticosteroid administration and other inflammation- or edema-related therapies, such as the tetracyclines (see paragraph below) or PGJ_2. This is a reasonable area for further research, and the rNAION model would appear to be ideal for this.
3. Tetracycline derivatives. Minocycline is a CNS-penetrating tetracycline derivative with CNS neuroprotective effects in some models [54], but not in others, such as closed head trauma [55]. For ON injury, minocycline was reported to preserve RGCs at 2 weeks post-ON transection and at 4 weeks in model of glaucoma [56]. Minocycline treatment begun 3 days prior to rNAION was also reported to be RGC neuroprotective [57]. However, we did not see any neuroprotective effect when minocycline was

begun after rNAION induction [58]. This suggests that treatments designed to inhibit inflammation need to be started early in the course of the process.

2.9.3. Potentiated and Synergistic Treatment Approaches

As previously noted, no currently available treatment has been shown to be consistently clinically effective in human NAION. This may be because: (1) Multiple damage mechanisms (soma, axon, inflammation, post-stroke demyelination) are activated. (2) Late recognition of clinical NAION typically limits treatment opportunities to neuroregeneration as the window of survival for many RGC subtypes and their axons may have passed by the time NAION is diagnosed. However, recent studies have demonstrated that approaches using multiple reparative and/or regenerative mechanisms can exert a potentiated (one drug does not elicit a response on its own but enhances the response to another drug) or synergistic effect (the combined effect of two drugs is greater than the sum of their separated effects). Thus, combinatorial treatments for ON repair can potentiate ON regeneration effectiveness [59]. The rNAION model enables effective evaluation of multiple factors as well as multiple approaches; ie, combinatorial approaches with anti-inflammatory + growth factors, cell death suppression agents, etc.

We have evaluated a number of dual-treatment approaches, including the multispecific tyrosine kinase inhibitor sunitinib (Sutent), which was reported to enhance RGC survival in ex vivo culture as well as in vivo models of ON injury [60]. However, combining Sutent 10 mg/kg with PGJ_2 did not enhance overall RGC survival compared with PGJ_2 alone in our rNAION model, suggesting that the neuroprotective effects of suppressing nonspecific receptor tyrosine kinase activity and NFkB activity (anti-inflammatory) may mechanistically overlap. A recent approach of inhibiting **all** prostaglandin synthesis while simultaneously administering one anti-inflammatory prostaglandin (PGJ_2), was unsuccessful due to incomplete prostaglandin suppression by a monoacylglycerol lipase (MAGL) inhibitor [22]. These results reveal some of the complexities of multiple treatment approaches, as well some of the potential drawbacks.

3. Discussion

The rNAION model system has enabled recognition of a vast number of variables that are potentially associated with clinical ischemic optic neuropathies such as NAION. Although simply inhibiting ONH edema can be effective in early stages of lesion development, this is not likely to prove effective in clinical practice. An awareness of the significant differences in rNAION-associated RGC survival between pre- and post-treatment therapies is also essential; pre-treatments for NAION are not likely to be effective unless they are being considered as long-term adjuncts to prevent NAION from occurring in the contralateral eye of at-risk patients or in situations where there is high risk of precipitating NAION, such as cardiac surgery with cardiopulmonary bypass.

The rNAION model can be useful to help decipher the individual contributions to pathophysiology made by vascular leakage, as well as by the individual ONH cellular components such as astrocyte-associated inflammation and neuroprotection, RGC somatic and axon response times and stress resistance mechanisms, and potential neural progenitor cell contributions to ischemic stress resistance [61]. There is also a great opportunity to identify early biomarkers to both confirm the presence of disease and to predict disease severity.

As previously noted, no currently available treatment has been shown to be consistently clinically effective in human NAION. This is likely because: (1) Multiple damage mechanisms (soma, axon, inflammation, post-stroke demyelination) are activated and (2) The recognition of NAION typically limits neuroprotection treatment opportunities to inflammatory suppression or neuroregeneration as the window of survival for many RGC subtypes and their axons may have passed by the time NAION is diagnosed. However, recent studies have demonstrated that approaches using multiple reparative and/or regenerative mechanisms can exert a potentiated (one drug does not elicit a response on its own but enhances the response to another drug) or synergistic effect (the combined effect of two drugs is greater than the sum of their separated effects). Thus, combinatorial treatments for ON repair can potentiate ON regeneration effectiveness [60]. The rNAION model enables effective evaluation of multiple factors as well as multiple approaches; ie, combinatorial approaches with anti-inflammatory + growth factors, cell death suppression agents, etc.

The rNAION model may also be valuable for determining the potential time windows for treatment opportunities and identifying mechanisms that may extend these windows, both in terms of RGC survival, axonal survival and inflammatory pathways. Using the rNAION model to evaluate strategies for enhancing RGC and axonal survival by modulating multiple independent pathways is an exciting possibility, which may potentially extend the effective treatment time windows. The rNAION model's mechanistic similarity with the primate NAION model also provides an invaluable bridge to understanding primate responses in ischemic optic neuropathy, and ultimately the rapid evaluation of potential therapeutics and strategies for treatment of the human disease.

4. Materials and Methods

While the data in the majority of this report is based on other research we have previously reported on (Sections 2.1–2.6, 2.8 and 2.9), the data reported in Figure 4 and Table 1 in Section 2.7 and Figure 6 in Section 2.9 have never been reported before. Thus, we include the materials and methods for these experiments.

Animals: All animal protocols were approved by the UMB institutional animal care and use committee (IACUC).

Affymetrix gene expression analysis: Three Male Sprague Dawley rats (225–250 g) were used for each pooled mRNA preparation. Following unilateral rNAION induction, retinae were pooled from 3 individual eyes treated similarly, and the contralateral uninduced eyes were used as controls. Tissue was obtained from animals following induction at 1 and 3 days. Total RNA was purified using Qiaprep RNAeasy micro kit, and poly(A)RNA further isolated using oligo d(T) cellulose columns. 500 ng of total RNA was used for each pooled cDNA probe. Complementary DNA (cDNA) was generated from pooled poly (A+) RNA using a genechip one cycle cDNA synthesis kit for synthesis of double stranded cDNA with a T7 RNA polymerase promotor. Biotinylated complementary RNA (cRNA) probes were then generated for reaction to the genechips using a one- or two cycle in vitro transcription (IVT) reaction kit.

Two RNA preps were used for analysis of each timepoint and contralateral controls, with two U34A rat genome genechips (total of 4 chips). cRNA was loaded onto an Affymetrix U34A total genechip array, containing >24,000 genes and EST clusters, with ~7000 known genes (rat gene expression). The chips were reacted/hybridized with the biotinylated probes and processed on an Affymetrix fluidics station 400 platform according to manufacturer's protocols, and following genechip scanning, the resulting data was analyzed using Genechip sequence analysis software at the DC Children's hospital core sequencing facility. These results are seen in Table 1 results in Section 2.7.

Immunohistochemical analysis of rNAION-associated early RGC stress. To confirm early RGC stress following rNAION, we induced rNAION (11 s/50 mW/500 uM/532 nm) spot size in one eye each of three Long-Evans (L-E) male rats. L-E pigmented rats are preferred over albino strains for visual function studies and have largely replaced our use of the SD strain. Animals were euthanized at 1, 3 and 7 days post-induction, and tissue post-fixed in 4% paraformaldehyde-phosphate-buffered saline pH 7.4 (PF-PBS). Whole retinae were isolated, fixed overnight in PF-PBS, and the inner limiting membranes were permeabilized by brief (−70 °C) freezing in PBS, followed by incubation in 10% normal donkey serum/0.3% Triton X-100 with primary antibodies. Tissues were treated with primary antbodies. These included rabbit monoclonal antibody to lipocalin 2 (Lcn2)-purchased from Abcam (ab41105). Polyclonal goat antibody to Brn 3a (Santa Cruz Chemicals, Santa Cruz, CA). Rabbit monoclonal antibody to phospho-Jun (pJun; Cat # 3270/D47G9; Cell Signaling Technologies, Danvers, MA). Rabbit Polyclonal antibody to CRF/CRH (CRF;

Thermofisher/Bioss (BS-0328R)). Tissues were washed and incubated with fluorescent-labeled secondary donkey antibodies (Jackson Immunoresearch, West Grove PA), and examined using confocal microscopy on a Leica 4 channel confocal microscope.

Glibenclamide treatment for ONH edema. 4 male Long-Evans (LE) rats (225–250 g) were used as a sighting study to determine whether ONH edema is suppressible using glibenclamide, an FDA approved anti-glycosemic drug which, even at low doses, inhibits opening of astrocytic sulfonylurea receptor-1 (SUR1)-water associated channel [34], and suppresses cerebral edema. Animals were induced with 11 s laser (50 mW/532 nm/ 500 um spot size) 30 s post-injection with rose Bengal (2.5 mM solution' 1 ml/kg). Both eyes utilized in this sighting study; Animals were treated with subcutaneous (SC) saline for 5 days post-induction of the first eye. Following induction of the second eye, animals were SC injected with glibenclamide (50 ug/kg) immediately after induction and daily for five days thereafter. We evaluated ONH edema using OCT at two days post-induction of each eye [16], and quantified RGCs by stereology using Brn3a(+) immunopositivity of flat mounted retinae, at 30d post-induction of the second eye, as previously reported [14]. These results are seen in results Section 2.9.

5. Patents

The use of PGJ_2 in the treatment of NAION is covered by US patent US 8,106,096 B2 'Compositions and methods for treatment of optic nerve diseases (SLB).

Supplementary Materials: The following supporting information can be downloaded at: https://www.mdpi.com/article/10.3390/ijms232415604/s1.

Author Contributions: Conceptualization, S.L.B. and N.R.M.; methodology, Z.M., S.L.B. and Y.G.; validation, Z.M. and Y.G.; formal analysis, S.L.B., Z.M. and Y.G.; investigation, S.L.B., Y.G., Z.M. and N.R.M.; resources, S.L.B. and N.R.M.; data curation, S.L.B., Y.G. and Z.M.; writing—original draft preparation, S.L.B., writing—review and editing, S.L.B., Z.M., Y.G. and N.R.M.; funding acquisition, S.L.B. and N.R.M. All authors have read and agreed to the published version of the manuscript.

Funding: This work was funded by NIH RO1-EY105304 (SLB) and an unrestricted gift from the Hillside Foundation.

Institutional Review Board Statement: This animal study was conducted in accordance with the Declaration of Helsinki, and approved by the Institutional Animal Care and Use Committee of the University of Maryland at Baltimore (protocol number 062005, date of approval 8 December 2020) for studies involving animals.

Data Availability Statement: Data from Table 1 can be obtained from Supplementary Table S1 (S1) in this paper. Data from Table 2 can be obtained from Supplementary Materials previously deposited in figshare: https://doi.org/10.3390/cells10061440, and previously published in [22]. Accessed on 6 June 2022.

Acknowledgments: The authors would like to thank Marc Simard and Vladimir Gerzanich (UMB Department of Neurosurgery) for advice on the use and dosing of glibenclamide.

Conflicts of Interest: The authors declare no conflict of interest.

References

1. Tesser, R.A.; Niendorf, E.R.; Levin, L.A. The morphology of an infarct in nonarteritic anterior ischemic optic neuropathy. *Ophthalmology* **2003**, *110*, 2031–2035. [CrossRef] [PubMed]
2. Salomon, O.; Huna-Baron, R.; Kurtz, S.; Steinberg, D.M.; Moisseiev, J.; Rosenberg, N.; Yassur, I.; Vidne, O.; Zivelin, A.; Gitel, S.; et al. Analysis of prothrombotic and vascular risk factors in patients with nonarteritic anterior ischemic optic neuropathy. *Ophthalmology* **1999**, *106*, 739–742. [CrossRef]
3. Miller, N.R.; Arnold, A.C. Current concepts in the diagnosis, pathogenesis and management of nonarteritic anterior ischaemic optic neuropathy. *Eye* **2014**, *29*, 65–79. [CrossRef] [PubMed]
4. Killer, H.E. Compartment syndromes of the optic nerve and open-angle glaucoma. *J. Glaucoma.* **2013**, *22* (Suppl. 5), S19–S20. [CrossRef] [PubMed]
5. Bernstein, S.L.; Guo, Y.; Kelman, S.E.; Flower, R.W.; Johnson, M.A. Functional and cellular responses in a novel rodent model of anterior ischemic optic neuropathy. *Investig. Ophthalmol. Vis. Sci.* **2003**, *44*, 4153–4162. [CrossRef] [PubMed]

6. Goldenberg-Cohen, N.; Guo, Y.; Margolis, F.L.; Miller, N.R.; Cohen, Y.; Bernstein, S.L. Oligodendrocyte Dysfunction Following Induction of Experimental Anterior Optic Nerve Ischemia. *Investig. Ophthalmol. Vis. Sci.* **2005**, *46*, 2716–2725. [CrossRef]
7. Chen, C.S.; Johnson, M.A.; Flower, R.A.; Slater, B.J.; Miller, N.R.; Bernstein, S.L. A Primate Model of Nonarteritic Anterior Ischemic Optic Neuropathy (pNAION). *Investig. Ophthalmol. Vis. Sci.* **2008**, *49*, 2985–2992. [CrossRef]
8. Gibbs, R.A.; Weinstock, G.M.; Metzker, M.L.; Muzny, D.M.; Sodergren, E.J.; Scherer, S.; Scott, G.; Steffen, D.; Worley, K.C.; Burch, P.E.; et al. Genome sequence of the Brown Norway rat yields insights into mammalian evolution. *Nature* **2004**, *428*, 493–521. [CrossRef]
9. Stys, P.K. White matter injury mechanisms. *Curr. Mol. Med.* **2004**, *4*, 113–130. [CrossRef]
10. Horn, J.; Limburg, M. Calcium antagonists for ischemic stroke: A systematic review. *Stroke* **2001**, *32*, 570–576. [CrossRef]
11. Bernstein, S.L.; Guo, Y.; Peterson, K.; Wistow, G. Expressed sequence tag analysis of adult human optic nerve for NEIBank: Identification of cell type and tissue markers. *BMC Neurosci.* **2009**, *10*, 121. [CrossRef] [PubMed]
12. Johnson, M.A.; Miller, N.R.; Nolan, T.; Bernstein, S.L. Peripapillary Retinal Nerve Fiber Layer Swelling Predicts Peripapillary Atrophy in a Primate Model of Nonarteritic Anterior Ischemic Optic Neuropathy. *Investig. Ophthalmol. Vis. Sci.* **2016**, *57*, 527–532. [CrossRef] [PubMed]
13. Bernstein, S.L.; Guo, Y. Changes in cholinergic amacrine cells after rodent anterior ischemic optic neuropathy (rAION). *Investig. Ophthalmol. Vis. Sci.* **2011**, *52*, 904–910. [CrossRef] [PubMed]
14. Kapupara, K.; Huang, T.-L.; Wen, Y.-T.; Huang, S.-P.; Tsai, R.-K. Optic nerve head width and retinal nerve fiber layer changes are proper indexes for validating the successful induction of experimental anterior ischemic optic neuropathy. *Exp. Eye Res.* **2019**, *181*, 105–111. [CrossRef] [PubMed]
15. Contreras, I.; Rebolleda, G.; Noval, S.; Munoz-Negrete, F.J. Optic Disc Evaluation by Optical Coherence Tomography in Nonarteritic Anterior Ischemic Optic Neuropathy. *Investig. Ophthalmol. Vis. Sci.* **2007**, *48*, 4087–4092. [CrossRef] [PubMed]
16. Guo, Y.; Mehrabian, Z.; Johnson, M.A.; Miller, N.R.; Henderson, A.D.; Hamlyn, J.; Bernstein, S.L. Biomarkers of lesion severity in a rodent model of nonarteritic anterior ischemic optic neuropathy (rNAION). *PLoS ONE* **2021**, *16*, e0243186. [CrossRef] [PubMed]
17. Prusky, G.T.; West, P.W.R.; Douglas, R.M. Behavioral assessment of visual acuity in mice and rats. *Vis. Res.* **2000**, *40*, 2201–2209. [CrossRef]
18. Prusky, G.T.; Harker, K.T.; Douglas, R.M.; Whishaw, I.Q. Variation in visual acuity within pigmented, and between pigmented and albino rat strains. *Behav. Brain Res.* **2002**, *136*, 339–348. [CrossRef]
19. Yun, H.; Lathrop, K.L.; Yang, E.; Sun, M.; Kagemann, L.; Fu, V.; Stolz, D.B.; Schuman, J.S.; Du, Y. A Laser-Induced Mouse Model with Long-Term Intraocular Pressure Elevation. *PLoS ONE* **2014**, *9*, e107446. [CrossRef]
20. Koilkonda, R.; Yu, H.; Talla, V.; Porciatti, V.; Feuer, W.J.; Hauswirth, W.W.; Chiodo, V.; Erger, K.E.; Boye, S.L.; Lewin, A.S.; et al. LHON Gene Therapy Vector Prevents Visual Loss and Optic Neuropathy Induced by G11778A Mutant Mitochondrial DNA: Biodistribution and Toxicology Profile. *Investig. Ophthalmol. Vis. Sci.* **2014**, *55*, 7739–7753. [CrossRef]
21. Johnson, M.A.; Mehrabian, Z.; Guo, Y.; Ghosh, J.; Brigell, M.G.; Bernstein, S.L. Anti-NOGO Antibody Neuroprotection in a Rat Model of NAION. *Transl. Vis. Sci. Technol.* **2021**, *10*, 12. [CrossRef] [PubMed]
22. Mehrabian, Z.; Guo, Y.; Miller, N.R.; Henderson, A.D.; Roth, S.; Bernstein, S.L. Approaches to Potentiated Neuroprotective Treatment in the Rodent Model of Ischemic Optic Neuropathy. *Cells* **2021**, *10*, 1440. [CrossRef] [PubMed]
23. Eshraghi, A.A.; Lang, D.M.; Roell, J.; Van De Water, T.R.; Garnham, C.; Rodrigues, H.; Guardiola, M.; Gupta, C.; Mittal, J. Mechanisms of programmed cell death signaling in hair cells and support cells post-electrode insertion trauma. *Acta Oto-Laryngol.* **2015**, *135*, 328–334. [CrossRef]
24. Park, S.J.H.; Pottackal, J.; Ke, J.-B.; Jun, N.Y.; Rahmani, P.; Kim, I.-J.; Singer, J.H.; Demb, J.B. Convergence and Divergence of CRH Amacrine Cells in Mouse Retinal Circuitry. *J. Neurosci.* **2018**, *38*, 3753. [CrossRef] [PubMed]
25. Wong, M.L.; Loddick, S.A.; Bongiorno, P.B.; Gold, P.W.; Rothwell, N.J.; Licinio, J. Focal cerebral ischemia induces CRH mRNA in rat cerebral cortex and amygdala. *Neuroreport* **1995**, *6*, 1785–1788. [CrossRef]
26. Duque Escobar, J.; Kutschenko, A.; Schröder, S.; Blume, R.; Köster, K.A.; Painer, C.; Lemcke, T.; Maison, W.; Oetjen, E. Regulation of dual leucine zipper kinase activity through its interaction with calcineurin. *Cell Signal* **2021**, *82*, 109953. [CrossRef]
27. Avraham, B.C.; Dotan, G.; Hasanreisoglu, M.; Kramer, M.; Monselise, Y.; Cohen, Y.; Weinberger, D.; Goldenberg-Cohen, N. Increased plasma and optic nerve levels of IL-6, TNF-alpha, and MIP-2 following induction of ischemic optic neuropathy in mice. *Curr. Eye Res.* **2008**, *33*, 395–401. [CrossRef]
28. Tanaka, T.; Narazaki, M.; Kishimoto, T. IL-6 in inflammation, immunity, and disease. *Cold Spring Harb. Perspect. Biol.* **2014**, *6*, a016295. [CrossRef]
29. Nicholson, J.D.; Puche, A.C.; Guo, Y.; Weinreich, D.; Slater, B.J.; Bernstein, S.L. PGJ_2 Provides Prolonged CNS Stroke Protection by Reducing White Matter Edema. *PLoS ONE* **2012**, *7*, e50021. [CrossRef]
30. Miller, N.R.; Johnson, M.A.; Nolan, T.; Guo, Y.; Bernstein, A.M.; Bernstein, S.L. Sustained Neuroprotection from a Single Intravitreal Injection of PGJ_2 in a Non-Human Primate Model of Nonarteritic Anterior Ischemic Optic Neuropathy. *Investig. Ophth. Vis. Sci.* **2014**, *55*, 7047–7056. [CrossRef]
31. Straus, D.S.; Pascual, G.; Li, M.; Welch, J.S.; Ricote, M.; Hsiang, C.H.; Sengchanthalangsy, L.L.; Ghosh, G.; Glass, C.K. 15-deoxy-delta 12,14-prostaglandin J2 inhibits multiple steps in the NF-kappa B signaling pathway. *Proc. Natl. Acad. Sci. USA* **2000**, *97*, 4844–4849. [CrossRef] [PubMed]

32. Kunte, H.; Schmidt, S.; Eliasziw, M.; del Zoppo, G.J.; Simard, J.M.; Masuhr, F.; Weih, M.; Dirnagl, U. Sulfonylureas improve outcome in patients with type 2 diabetes and acute ischemic stroke. *Stroke* **2007**, *38*, 2526–2530. [CrossRef] [PubMed]
33. Simard, J.M.; Woo, S.K.; Bhatta, S.; Gerzanich, V. Drugs acting on SUR1 to treat CNS ischemia and trauma. *Curr. Opin. Pharmacol.* **2008**, *8*, 42–49. [CrossRef] [PubMed]
34. Gerzanich, V.; Stokum, J.A.; Ivanova, S.; Woo, S.K.; Tsymbalyuk, O.; Sharma, A.; Akkentli, F.; Imran, Z.; Aarabi, B.; Sahuquillo, J.; et al. Sulfonylurea Receptor 1, Transient Receptor Potential Cation Channel Subfamily M Member 4, and KIR6.2:Role in Hemorrhagic Progression of Contusion. *J. Neurotrauma* **2019**, *36*, 1060–1079. [CrossRef] [PubMed]
35. Nicholson, J.D.; Guo, Y.; Bernstein, S.L. SUR1-Associated Mechanisms Are Not Involved in Ischemic Optic Neuropathy 1 Day Post-Injury. *PLoS ONE* **2016**, *11*, e0148855. [CrossRef]
36. Neves, J.; Zhu, J.; Sousa-Victor, P.; Konjikusic, M.; Riley, R.; Chew, S.; Qi, Y.; Jasper, H.; Lamba, D.A. Immune modulation by MANF promotes tissue repair and regenerative success in the retina. *Science* **2016**, *353*, aaf3646. [CrossRef]
37. Livne-Bar, I.; Wei, J.; Liu, H.H.; Alqawlaq, S.; Won, G.J.; Tuccitto, A.; Gronert, K.; Flanagan, J.G.; Sivak, J.M. Astrocyte-derived lipoxins A4 and B4 promote neuroprotection from acute and chronic injury. *J. Clin. Investig.* **2017**, *127*, 4403–4414. [CrossRef]
38. Sun, D.; Moore, S.; Jakobs, T.C. Optic nerve astrocyte reactivity protects function in experimental glaucoma and other nerve injuries. *J. Exp. Med.* **2017**, *214*, 1411. [CrossRef]
39. Pugliese, A.M.; Latini, S.; Corradetti, R.; Pedata, F. Brief, repeated, oxygen-glucose deprivation episodes protect neurotransmission from a longer ischemic episode in the in vitro hippocampus: Role of adenosine receptors. *Br. J. Pharmacol.* **2003**, *140*, 305–314. [CrossRef]
40. Liston, T.E.; Hama, A.; Boltze, J.; Poe, R.B.; Natsume, T.; Hayashi, I.; Takamatsu, H.; Korinek, W.S.; Lechleiter, J.D. Adenosine A1R/A3R (Adenosine A1 and A3 Receptor) Agonist AST-004 Reduces Brain Infarction in a Nonhuman Primate Model of Stroke. *Stroke* **2022**, *53*, 238–248. [CrossRef]
41. Othman, T.; Yan, H.; Rivkees, S.A. Oligodendrocytes express functional A1 adenosine receptors that stimulate cellular migration. *Glia* **2003**, *44*, 166–172. [CrossRef] [PubMed]
42. Braas, K.; Zarbin, M.; Snyder, S. Endogenous adenosine and adenosine receptors localized to ganglion cells of the retina. *Proc. Natl. Acad. Sci. USA* **1987**, *84*, 3906–3910. [CrossRef] [PubMed]
43. Zhang, S.; Li, H.; Li, B.; Zhong, D.; Gu, X.; Tang, L.; Wang, Y.; Wang, C.; Zhou, R.; Li, Y.; et al. Adenosine A1 Receptors Selectively Modulate Oxygen-Induced Retinopathy at the Hyperoxic and Hypoxic Phases by Distinct Cellular Mechanisms. *Investig. Ophthalmol. Vis. Sci.* **2015**, *56*, 8108–8119. [CrossRef] [PubMed]
44. Hu, S.; Dong, H.; Zhang, H.; Wang, S.; Hou, L.; Chen, S.; Zhang, J.; Xiong, L. Noninvasive limb remote ischemic preconditioning contributes neuroprotective effects via activation of adenosine A1 receptor and redox status after transient focal cerebral ischemia in rats. *Brain Res.* **2012**, *1459*, 81–90. [CrossRef]
45. Guo, Y.; Mehrabian, Z.; Johnson, M.A.; Albers, D.S.; Rich, C.C.; Baumgartner, R.A.; Bernstein, S.L. Topical Trabodenoson Is Neuroprotective in a Rodent Model of Anterior Ischemic Optic Neuropathy (rNAION). *Transl. Vis. Sci. Technol.* **2019**, *8*, 47. [CrossRef]
46. Zhang, C.; Guo, Y.; Miller, N.R.; Bernstein, S.L. Optic nerve infarction and post-ischemic inflammation in the rodent model of anterior ischemic optic neuropathy (rAION). *Brain Res.* **2009**, *1264*, 67–75. [CrossRef]
47. Hayreh, S.S.; Zimmerman, M.B. Non-arteritic anterior ischemic optic neuropathy: Role of systemic corticosteroid therapy. *Graefes Arch. Clin. Exp. Ophthalmol.* **2008**, *246*, 1029–1046. [CrossRef]
48. Rebolleda, G.; Perez-Lopez, M.; Casas-Llera, P.; Contreras, I.; Munoz-Negrete, F.J. Visual and anatomical outcomes of non-arteritic anterior ischemic optic neuropathy with high-dose systemic corticosteroids. *Graefes Arch. Clin. Exp. Ophthalmol.* **2013**, *251*, 255–260. [CrossRef]
49. Saxena, R.; Singh, D.; Sharma, M.; James, M.; Sharma, P.; Menon, V. Steroids versus No Steroids in Nonarteritic Anterior Ischemic Optic Neuropathy: A Randomized Controlled Trial. *Ophthalmology* **2018**, *125*, 1623–1627. [CrossRef]
50. Prokosch, V.; Thanos, S. Visual outcome of patients following NAION after treatment with adjunctive fluocortolone. *Restor. Neurol. Neurosci.* **2014**, *32*, 381–389. [CrossRef]
51. Wen, Y.T.; Huang, T.L.; Huang, S.P.; Chang, C.H.; Tsai, R.K. Early applications of granulocyte colony-stimulating factor (G-CSF) can stabilize the blood-optic-nerve barrier and ameliorate inflammation in a rat model of anterior ischemic optic neuropathy (rAION). *Dis. Model Mech.* **2016**, *9*, 1193–1202. [CrossRef] [PubMed]
52. Huang, T.L.; Wen, Y.T.; Chang, C.H.; Chang, S.W.; Lin, K.H.; Tsai, R.K. Early Methylprednisolone Treatment Can Stabilize the Blood-Optic Nerve Barrier in a Rat Model of Anterior Ischemic Optic Neuropathy (rAION). *Investig. Ophthalmol. Vis. Sci.* **2017**, *58*, 1628–1636. [CrossRef] [PubMed]
53. Pereira, L.S.; Ávila, M.P.; Salustiano, L.X.; Paula, A.C.; Arnhold, E.; McCulley, T.J. Intravitreal Triamcinolone Acetonide Injection in a Rodent Model of Anterior Ischemic Optic Neuropathy. *J. Neuroophthalmol.* **2018**, *38*, 561–565. [CrossRef] [PubMed]
54. Hailer, N.P. Immunosuppression after traumatic or ischemic CNS damage: It is neuroprotective and illuminates the role of microglial cells. *Prog. Neurobiol.* **2008**, *84*, 211–233. [CrossRef] [PubMed]
55. Hanlon, L.A.; Raghupathi, R.; Huh, J.W. Differential effects of minocycline on microglial activation and neurodegeneration following closed head injury in the neonate rat. *Exp. Neurol.* **2017**, *290*, 1–14. [CrossRef] [PubMed]
56. Levkovitch-Verbin, H.; Kalev-Landoy, M.; Habot-Wilner, Z.; Melamed, S. Minocycline delays death of retinal ganglion cells in experimental glaucoma and after optic nerve transection. *Arch. Ophthalmol.* **2006**, *124*, 520–526. [CrossRef]

57. Fel, A.; Froger, N.G.; Simonutti, M.; Bernstein, N.R.; Bodaghi, B.; Lehoang, P.; Picaud, S.A.; Paques, M.; Touitou, V. Minocycline as a neuroprotective agent in a rodent model of NAION. *Investig. Ophth. Vis. Sci.* **2014**, *55*, 5736. [CrossRef]
58. Mehrabian, Z.; Guo, Y.; Weinreich, D.; Bernstein, S.L. Oligodendrocyte death, neuroinflammation, and the effects of minocycline in a rodent model of nonarteritic anterior ischemic optic neuropathy (rNAION). *Mol. Vis.* **2017**, *23*, 963–976.
59. Lim, J.-H.A.; Stafford, B.K.; Nguyen, P.L.; Lien, B.V.; Wang, C.; Zukor, K.; He, Z.; Huberman, A.D. Neural activity promotes long-distance, target-specific regeneration of adult retinal axons. *Nat. Neurosci.* **2016**, *19*, 1073. [CrossRef]
60. Welsbie, D.S.; Ziogas, N.K.; Xu, L.; Kim, B.J.; Ge, Y.; Patel, A.K.; Ryu, J.; Lehar, M.; Alexandris, A.S.; Stewart, N.; et al. Targeted disruption of dual leucine zipper kinase and leucine zipper kinase promotes neuronal survival in a model of diffuse traumatic brain injury. *Mol. Neurodegener.* **2019**, *14*, 44. [CrossRef]
61. Bernstein, S.L.; Guo, Y.; Kerr, C.; Fawcett, R.W.; Stern, J.H.; Temple, S.; Mehrabyan, Z. The optic nerve lamina region is a neural progenitor cell niche. *Proc. Natl. Acad. Sci. USA* **2020**, *117*, 11. [CrossRef] [PubMed]

International Journal of *Molecular Sciences*

MDPI

Article

Secondary Degeneration of Oligodendrocyte Precursor Cells Occurs as Early as 24 h after Optic Nerve Injury in Rats

Lillian M. Toomey [1,2], Melissa G. Papini [1], Thomas O. Clarke [3], Alexander J. Wright [1], Eleanor Denham [1], Andrew Warnock [1], Terry McGonigle [1], Carole A. Bartlett [3], Melinda Fitzgerald [1,2] and Chidozie C. Anyaegbu [1,2,]*

1 Curtin Health Innovation Research Institute, Curtin University, Bentley, WA 6102, Australia
2 Perron Institute for Neurological and Translational Science, Sarich Neuroscience Research Institute Building, 8 Verdun St., Nedlands, WA 6009, Australia
3 Experimental and Regenerative Neurosciences, School of Biological Sciences, The University of Western Australia, Perth, WA 6009, Australia
* Correspondence: chidozie.anyaegbu@curtin.edu.au; Tel.: +61-8-6457-0505

Abstract: Optic nerve injury causes secondary degeneration, a sequela that spreads damage from the primary injury to adjacent tissue, through mechanisms such as oxidative stress, apoptosis, and blood-brain barrier (BBB) dysfunction. Oligodendrocyte precursor cells (OPCs), a key component of the BBB and oligodendrogenesis, are vulnerable to oxidative deoxyribonucleic acid (DNA) damage by 3 days post-injury. However, it is unclear whether oxidative damage in OPCs occurs earlier at 1 day post-injury, or whether a critical 'window-of-opportunity' exists for therapeutic intervention. Here, a partial optic nerve transection rat model of secondary degeneration was used with immunohistochemistry to assess BBB dysfunction, oxidative stress, and proliferation in OPCs vulnerable to secondary degeneration. At 1 day post-injury, BBB breach and oxidative DNA damage were observed, alongside increased density of DNA-damaged proliferating cells. DNA-damaged cells underwent apoptosis (cleaved caspase3+), and apoptosis was associated with BBB breach. OPCs experienced DNA damage and apoptosis and were the major proliferating cell type with DNA damage. However, the majority of caspase3+ cells were not OPCs. These results provide novel insights into acute secondary degeneration mechanisms in the optic nerve, highlighting the need to consider early oxidative damage to OPCs in therapeutic efforts to limit degeneration following optic nerve injury.

Keywords: oligodendrocyte precursor cells; secondary degeneration; oxidative stress; DNA damage; proliferation; blood-brain barrier; CNS injury; optic nerve injury

Citation: Toomey, L.M.; Papini, M.G.; Clarke, T.O.; Wright, A.J.; Denham, E.; Warnock, A.; McGonigle, T.; Bartlett, C.A.; Fitzgerald, M.; Anyaegbu, C.C. Secondary Degeneration of Oligodendrocyte Precursor Cells Occurs as Early as 24 h after Optic Nerve Injury in Rats. *Int. J. Mol. Sci.* **2023**, *24*, 3463. https://doi.org/10.3390/ijms24043463

Academic Editors: Neil R. Miller and Rongkung Tsai

Received: 22 December 2022
Revised: 6 February 2023
Accepted: 7 February 2023
Published: 9 February 2023

1. Introduction

Injury to the central nervous system (CNS) involves two components of damage: the initial mechanical insult and a subsequent cascade of spreading damage called secondary degeneration [1]. The initial primary injury typically manifests as axonal shearing, contusions, and hemorrhage or hematoma [1,2]. Secondary degeneration occurs as pathological factors released by injured neurons and glia spread to the surrounding tissue, causing additional self-propagating damage [3]. Glaucoma and other optic neuropathies follow similar sequelae, where axonal injury to retinal ganglion cells triggers a plethora of degenerative mechanisms that spread throughout the visual system to progressively impair visual function [4]. Hypoxia-induced vascular dysfunction can reduce blood flow to the optic nerve head, contributing to axonal injury and vision loss in optic neuropathies [5,6]. The BBB, comprising endothelial cells, neurons, astrocytes, pericytes, and OPCs, is a key component of vascular function [7].

The rodent partial optic nerve transection model is especially useful for characterizing mechanisms of secondary damage in the optic nerve, facilitating spatial segregation between primary and secondary injury. Only the dorsal aspect of the right optic nerve is partially transected thus leaving the ventral aspect vulnerable solely to secondary degenerative processes [8]. Within the initially spared tissue, a multitude of secondary degeneration mechanisms occur, including oxidative stress, BBB dysfunction, reactive gliosis, axonal damage, dysmyelination, and oligodendrocyte death, associated with functional deficits post-injury [9,10]. Such secondary damage can spread as far into the brain as the superior colliculus via the visual pathways, to elicit a remote degenerative response following optic nerve injury [11].

A key feature of secondary degeneration that exacerbates acute pathology is oxidative stress. Oxidative stress occurs when the rate of reactive oxygen species production increases and overwhelms the detoxification capacity of the antioxidant system [12]. Excessive levels of reactive oxygen species can cause damage to a variety of cellular structures, including lipids, proteins, and DNA [13]. One form of oxidative DNA damage is nucleobase modifications, such as the guanine oxidation by-product 8-hydroxy-2-deoxyguanosine (8OHDG). Nucleobase modifications can cause particularly harmful effects by either modifying the genetic code or blocking DNA replication [14].

Within 5 min of a partial optic nerve transection, astrocytes are oxidatively stressed and become hypertrophic by 3 h [15]. No changes in Olig2+ oligodendroglia are observed by 24 h. However, at day 3, oligodendroglia, including OPCs, are significantly more likely to become oxidatively DNA damaged than other cell types within the ventral optic nerve [16]. The heightened vulnerability of OPCs is likely due in part to increased concentrations of Ca^{2+}-permeable $P2X_7$ receptors and α-amino-3-hydroxy-5-methyl-4-isoxazolepropionic acid (AMPA) receptors [17,18], increased intracellular iron levels [19], and decreased concentrations of antioxidant defenses [19,20]. Similarly, a specific subpopulation of newly derived mature oligodendrocytes has been identified to have elevated oxidative DNA damage compared to their pre-existing counterparts at this same time point [16]. The newly derived oligodendrocyte subpopulation was also less likely to become apoptotic than pre-existing oligodendrocytes, but instead demonstrated a decreased long-term capacity for myelination [16]. The concurrent death of pre-existing oligodendrocytes alongside the reduced myelination capacity of newly derived, DNA-damaged oligodendrocytes likely contributes to chronic deficits in myelination observed at 1, 3, and 6 months after optic nerve injury [21–23]. However, the specific vulnerability of oligodendroglia to this oxidative DNA damage at the earlier 1 day timepoint, is yet to be investigated. It is possible that a therapeutic window exists prior to 3 days, where oligodendroglia show signs of oxidative damage but are not yet proliferative or apoptotic.

To address this knowledge gap, this study assessed the vulnerability of OPCs to oxidative DNA damage at an acute 1 day timepoint following a partial optic nerve transection. Within the ventral nerve susceptible to secondary degeneration, 8OHDG DNA damage increased and correlated to the extent of BBB dysfunction. DNA-damaged cells showed increased proliferation with injury and increased apoptosis. While OPCs accounted for the majority of proliferating, DNA-damaged cells, these were not the largest population of apoptotic cells.

2. Results

2.1. Secondary Degeneration in the Ventral Optic Nerve following Partial Injury

At 1 day following a partial optic nerve transection, the ventral nerve was immunohistochemically assessed for 8OHDG, immunoglobulin G (IgG) and 5′Ethynyl-2-deoxyuridine (EdU) to quantify oxidative DNA damage, BBB dysfunction and cellular proliferation respectively. There was a significant effect of injury on both the area ($t(4.448) = 17$, $p = 0.0004$, Figure 1A) and mean intensity ($t(4.197) = 17$, $p = 0.0006$, Figure 1B) of 8OHDG immunoreactivity relative to sham controls, indicating increased oxidative DNA damage post-injury (Figure 1C). Similarly, the mean area of IgG immunoreactivity significantly increased with injury compared to sham controls ($Mdn_{sham} = 2.018$, $Mdn_{injured} = 0.00825$, $U = 0$, $p < 0.0001$, Figure 1D,F). The observed increase in IgG extravasation indicates an injury-induced breach of the BBB. A strong and significant positive monotonic relationship between the mean areas of IgG and 8OHDG immunoreactivities was also observed ($r_s = 0.752$, $p = 0.0003$, Figure 1E), suggesting that animals with increased DNA damage in the ventral optic nerve typically experience greater levels of BBB dysfunction.

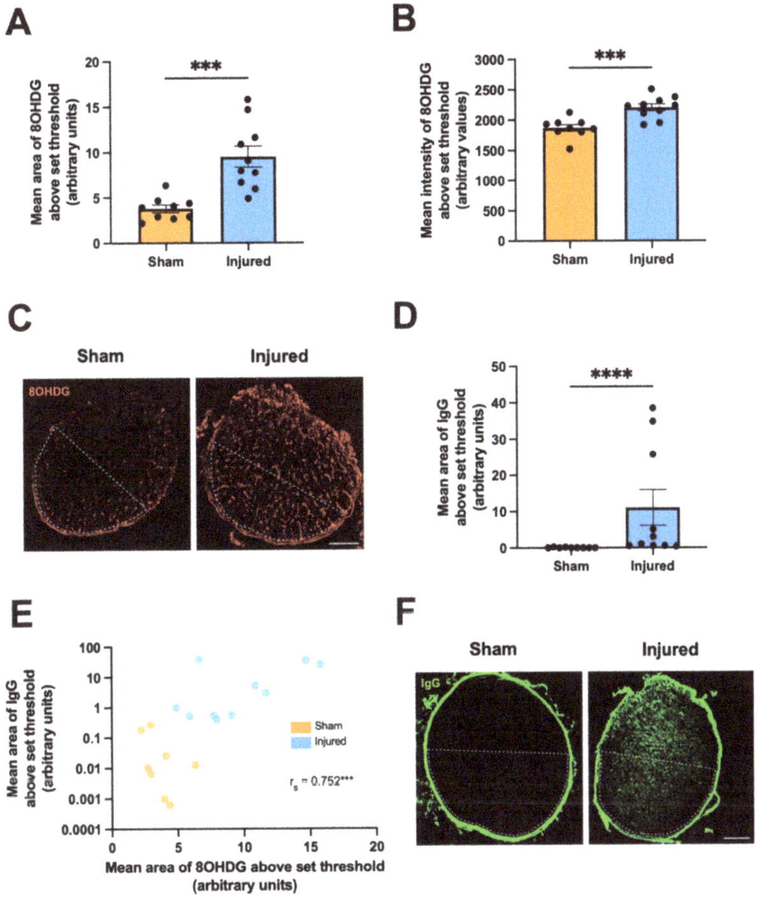

Figure 1. Effect of injury on oxidative DNA damage and BBB dysfunction within the ventral optic nerve, relative to sham injury. Area (**A**) and mean intensity (**B**) of 8OHDG immunoreactivity within the ventral optic nerve were assessed to determine the level of oxidative DNA damage. Graphs display individual data points overlaid on a bar displaying the mean ± SEM. n = 9–10 rats per group. Statistical analysis by t-tests. (**D**) Area of IgG immunointensity within the ventral nerve was assessed to determine the extent of BBB breach. Graph displays individual data points overlaid on a bar displaying the mean ± SEM. Statistical analysis by Mann-Whitney test. n = 9–10 rats per group. (**E**) The area of IgG immunointensity was correlated to the area of 8OHDG using Spearman's correlation, with the r_s value and corresponding p-value displayed on the graph. The mean area of IgG immunointensity was plotted on a log scale to best illustrate the overall relationship between IgG and 8OHDG on the scatterplot. Each data point on the graph represents an individual animal. n = 8–10 rats per group. (**C**,**F**) Representative images of both 8OHDG and IgG immunoreactivity in sham and injured rats are shown, scale bars = 100 μm. Area of the ventral nerve is denoted by dotted lines. All areas above threshold measurements are presented in arbitrary units as the data have been normalized to the total area of the ventral nerve for each animal. No outliers were removed for any outcome measure. Significant differences are indicated by *** $p \leq 0.001$, **** $p \leq 0.0001$.

The effect of partial optic nerve transection on cellular proliferation as indicated by EdU+ staining in the ventral nerve was also assessed. There was a trend towards an increased density of EdU+ cells with injury compared to sham controls, although this difference did not reach statistical significance (t(2.072) = 17, $p = 0.0538$, Figure 2A). EdU+ cells were then categorized based on colocalization with 8OHDG above a set threshold and a two-way ANOVA was used to compare the densities of proliferating cells either with or without oxidative DNA damage ($F(1,34) = 2.947$, Figure 2B,D). A significant difference was observed by Tukey *post-hoc* comparisons in the density of EdU+ 8OHDG+ cells with injury compared to the sham group ($p = 0.0264$). There were no differences in the density of EdU+ 8OHDG− cells with injury compared to those without injury ($p > 0.05$). A weak but significant positive monotonic relationship between the mean area of IgG immunointensity and EdU+ densities was also observed ($r_s = 0.489$, $p = 0.0394$, Figure 2C).

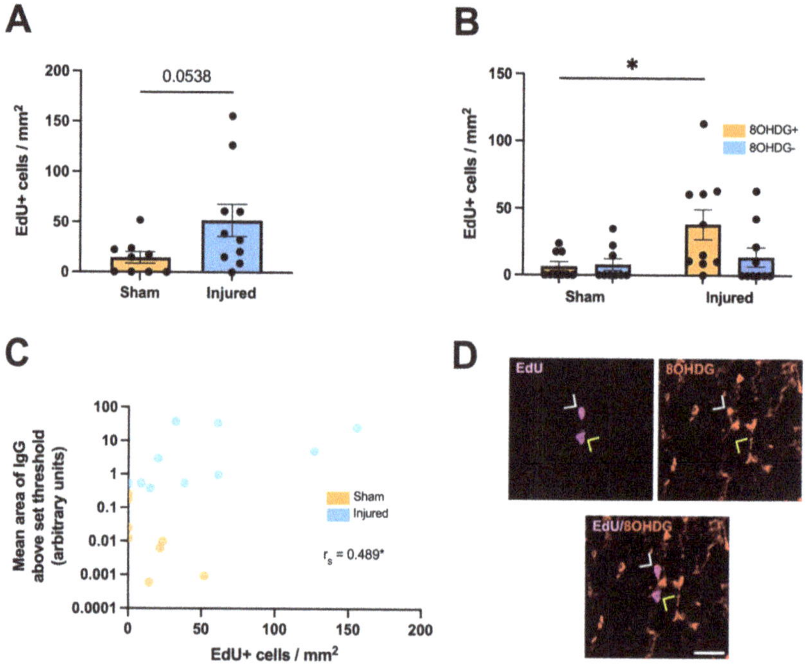

Figure 2. Effect of injury on cellular proliferation within the ventral optic nerve. (**A**) The density of EdU+ cells was quantified in the ventral optic nerve following partial optic nerve transection or sham injury. Graphs display individual data points overlaid on a bar displaying the mean ± SEM. $n = 9$–10 rats per group. Statistical analysis by *t*-test. (**B**) The relative densities of EdU+ 8OHDG+ and EdU+ 8OHDG− cells were quantified. Statistical analysis by two-way ANOVA and Tukey *post-hoc* tests. Graphs display individual data points overlaid on a bar displaying the mean ± SEM. $n = 9$–10 rats per group. (**C**) The area of IgG immunointensity was correlated to the density of EdU+ cells using Spearman's correlation, with the r_s value and corresponding *p*-value displayed on the graph. The mean area of IgG immunointensity was plotted on a log scale to best illustrate the overall relationship between IgG and EdU on the scatterplot. Each data point on the graph represents an individual animal. $n = 8$–10 rats per group. (**D**) Representative image of both an EdU+ 8OHDG+ cell (white arrow head) and an EdU+ 8OHDG− cell (yellow arrow head) is shown, scale bar = 25 μm. No outliers were removed for any outcome measure. Significant differences are indicated by * $p \leq 0.05$.

Additionally, the effect of partial optic nerve transection on apoptosis was assessed by detecting Cleaved Caspase3, the proteolytically-cleaved and functionally-active form of Caspase3 [24]. A significant increase was observed in the overall density of Cleaved Caspase3+ cells with injury compared to sham controls in the ventral nerve (t(5.064) = 16, $p = 0.0001$, Figure 3A). Cleaved Caspase3+ cells were then categorized based on colocalization with 8OHDG above a set threshold and a two-way ANOVA was used to compare the densities of apoptotic cells either with or without oxidative DNA damage ($F(1,32) = 25.64$, Figure 3B,D). A significant difference was observed by Tukey post hoc comparisons in the density of Cleaved Caspase3+ 8OHDG+ cells with injury compared to Cleaved Caspase3+ 8OHDG+ cells in the sham group ($p < 0.0001$). A significant increase was also found between Cleaved Caspase3+ cells with and without 8OHDG+ in both the injured ($p < 0.0001$) and sham groups ($p < 0.0001$). No differences were observed in the density of Cleaved Caspase3+ 8OHDG− cells with injury compared to Cleaved Caspase3+ 8OHDG− cells without injury ($p > 0.05$). A moderate and significant positive monotonic relationship between the mean area of IgG immunointensity and Cleaved Caspase3+ densities was also observed ($r_s = 0.694$, $p = 0.003$, Figure 3C).

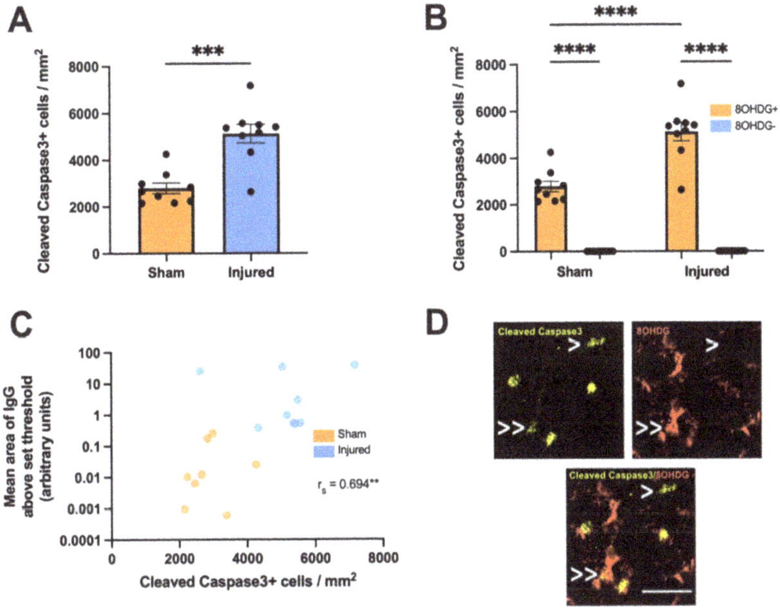

Figure 3. Effect of injury on apoptosis within the ventral optic nerve. (**A**) The density of Cleaved Caspase3+ cells was quantified in the ventral optic nerve following partial optic nerve transection or sham injury. Graphs display individual data points overlaid on a bar displaying the mean ± SEM. $n = 9$ rats per group. Statistical analysis by t-test. (**B**) The relative densities of Cleaved Caspase3+ 8OHDG+ and Cleaved Caspase3+ 8OHDG− cells were quantified. Statistical analysis by two-way ANOVA and Tukey post hoc tests. Graphs display individual data points overlaid on a bar displaying the mean ± SEM. $n = 9$ rats per group. (**C**) The area of IgG immunointensity was correlated to the density of Cleaved Caspase3+ cells using Spearman's correlation, with the r_s value and corresponding p-value displayed on the graph. The mean area of IgG immunointensity was plotted on a log scale to best illustrate the overall relationship between IgG and Cleaved Caspase3+ on the scatterplot. Each data point on the graph represents an individual animal. $n = 8$–9 rats per group. (**D**) Representative image of both a Cleaved Caspase3+ 8OHDG+ cell (indicated by >>) and a Cleaved Caspase3+ 8OHDG− cell (indicated by >) is shown, scale bar = 25 μm. No outliers were removed for any outcome measure. Significant differences are indicated by ** $p \leq 0.01$, *** $p \leq 0.001$, **** $p \leq 0.0001$.

2.2. Heightened Vulnerability of OPCs to Oxidative DNA Damage

To identify oxidatively damaged OPCs, antibodies detecting neural/glial antigen 2 (NG2) [25] or platelet-derived growth factor receptor α (PDGFRα) [26] were utilized. Within NG2+ glia specifically, the mean intensity of 8OHDG immunoreactivity significantly increased compared to sham controls ($t(2.161) = 15$, $p = 0.0472$, Figure 4A,B). Correspondingly, there was a significant increase with injury in the mean intensity of 8OHDG within PDGFRα+ glia ($t(3.992) = 17$, $p = 0.0007$, Figure 4C,D).

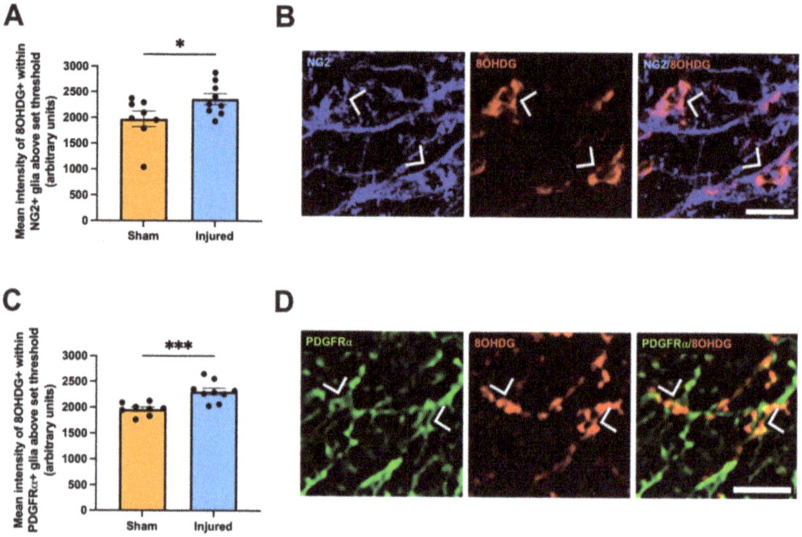

Figure 4. Effect of injury on oxidative DNA damage within NG2+ glia and PDGFRα+ glia. The mean immunointensity of 8OHDG was specifically quantified in NG2+ glial cells (**A**) and PDGFRα+ glia cells (**C**) in the ventral nerve. Graphs display individual data points overlaid on a bar displaying the mean ± SEM. $n = 8$–10 rats per group. Statistical analysis by *t*-tests. Representative images of NG2+ glia (**B**) and PDGFRα+ glia (**C**) with 8OHDG+ DNA damage are shown, indicated with arrow heads, scale bars = 20 μm. No outliers were removed for any outcome measure. Significant differences are indicated by * $p \leq 0.05$, *** $p \leq 0.001$.

2.3. Proliferative and Apoptotic Status of OPCs with Oxidative DNA Damage

The proliferative status of oxidatively DNA-damaged OPCs was then assessed within the ventral nerve. The EdU+ population was first identified as either PDGFRα+ or PDGFRα− cells and analyzed using a two-way ANOVA ($F(1,36) = 1.457$, Figure 5A). Tukey post hoc comparisons revealed a significant increase in the density of EdU+ PDGFRα+ OPCs with injury compared to sham ($p = 0.0466$). No significant difference was observed in the density of EdU+ PDGFRα− cells with injury ($p > 0.05$). The EdU+ PDGFRα+ and EdU+ PDGFRα− populations were further classified by colocalization with 8OHDG DNA damage and analyzed via a three-way ANOVA with Tukey post hoc comparisons ($F(1, 64) = 1.958$, Figure 5B,C). There was a significant increase with injury in the density of EdU+ PDGFRα+ 8OHDG+ cells compared to sham ($p = 0.0115$). Interestingly, the densities of EdU+ PDGFRα+ 8OHDG+ cells were also significantly higher than EdU+ PDGFRα+ 8OHDG− cells within injured animals ($p = 0.0033$). No significant differences were observed with injury for EdU+ PDGFRα+ 8OHDG− OPCs ($p > 0.05$), or EdU+ PDGFRα− 8OHDG+ ($p > 0.05$) or EdU+ PDGFRα− 8OHDG− ($p > 0.05$) cells compared to sham. Altogether, this suggests that OPCs are the major proliferating, DNA-damaged cell type at 1 day following injury to the optic nerve.

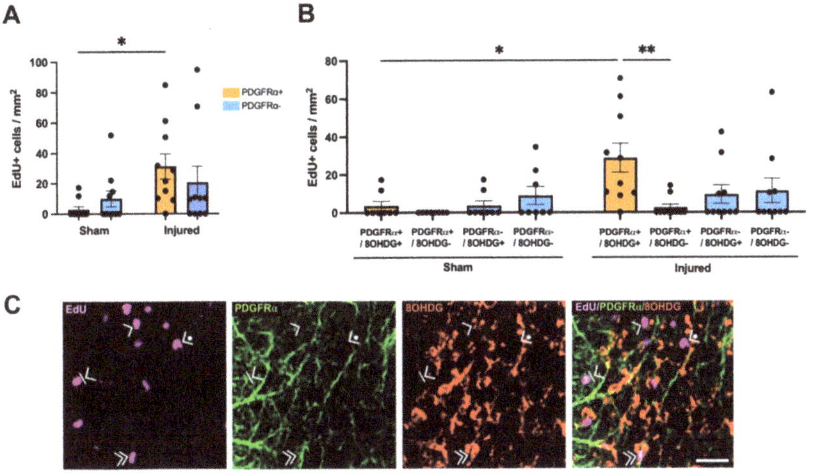

Figure 5. Effect of injury on proliferation and oxidative DNA damage within OPCs. (**A**) The relative densities of EdU+ PDGFRα+ and EdU+ PDGFRα− OPCs were quantified. Statistical analysis by two-way ANOVA and Tukey post hoc tests. (**B**) The relative densities of EdU+ cells colocalized with PDGFRα and 8OHDG were quantified. Statistical analysis by three-way ANOVA with Tukey post hoc tests. Graphs display individual data points overlaid on a bar displaying the mean ± SEM. $n = 8$–10 rats per group. (**C**) Representative images illustrating EdU+ PDGFRα+ 8OHDG+ OPCs (indicated by >>), EdU+ PDGFRα+ 8OHDG− OPCs (indicated by >|), EdU+ PDGFRα− 8OHDG+ cells (indicated by >), EdU+ PDGFRα− 8OHDG− cells (indicated by •>) are shown, scale bar = 25 µm. No outliers were removed for any outcome measure. Significant differences are indicated by * $p \leq 0.05$, ** $p \leq 0.01$.

The apoptotic status of oxidatively DNA-damaged OPCs was also assessed within the ventral nerve. The Cleaved Caspase3+ population was initially identified as either PDGFRα+ or PDGFRα− cells and analyzed using a two-way ANOVA ($F(1,32) = 5.611$, Figure 6A). Tukey post hoc comparisons revealed no significant increase in the density of Cleaved Caspase3+ PDGFRα+ OPCs with injury compared to sham ($p > 0.05$). A significant difference was observed in the density of Cleaved Caspase3+ PDGFRα− cells with injury ($p < 0.0001$). There was also a significant increase in the density of Cleaved Caspase3+ PDGFRα− cells compared to Cleaved Caspase3+ PDGFRα+ cells within both injured ($p < 0.0001$) and sham groups ($p < 0.0001$). The Cleaved Caspase3+ PDGFRα+ and Cleaved Caspase3+ PDGFRα− populations were further classified by colocalization with 8OHDG DNA damage and analyzed via a three-way ANOVA with Tukey *post-hoc* comparisons ($F(1, 64) = 33.37$, Figure 6B,C). There was a significant increase with injury in the density of both Cleaved Caspase3+ PDGFRα+ 8OHDG+ OPCs ($p = 0.0304$) and Cleaved Caspase3+ PDGFRα− 8OHDG+ cells ($p < 0.0001$) compared to sham. Within the sham group, there were significantly more Cleaved Caspase3+ PDGFRα− 8OHDG+ cells than Cleaved Caspase3+ PDGFRα+ 8OHDG+ OPCs ($p < 0.0001$), Cleaved Caspase3+ PDGFRα+ 8OHDG− OPCs ($p < 0.0001$) and Cleaved Caspase3+ PDGFRα− 8OHDG− cells ($p < 0.0001$). Similarly, within the injured group, there were significantly more Cleaved Caspase3+ PDGFRα− 8OHDG+ cells than OPCs that were Cleaved Caspase3+ PDGFRα+ 8OHDG+ ($p < 0.0001$) or Cleaved Caspase3+ PDGFRα+ 8OHDG− ($p < 0.0001$) or Cleaved Caspase3+ PDGFRα− 8OHDG− cells ($p < 0.0001$). In addition, there was a significant increase in the density of Cleaved Caspase3+ PDGFRα+ 8OHDG+ OPCs compared to both Cleaved Caspase3+ PDGFRα+ 8OHDG− OPCs ($p = 0.0019$) and Cleaved Caspase3+ PDGFRα− 8OHDG− cells ($p = 0.0019$) within the injured group. These data indicate an increase in apoptosis of DNA-damaged OPCs at 1 day following injury to the optic nerve, though these cells do not form the majority of the overall apoptotic cell population.

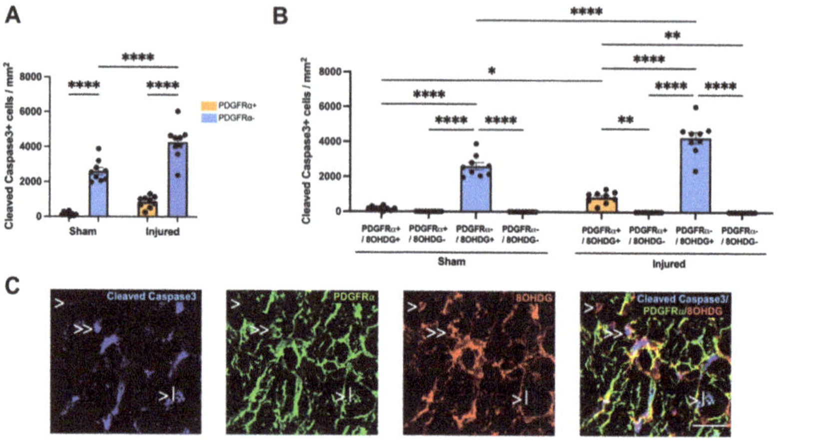

Figure 6. Effect of injury on apoptosis and oxidative DNA damage of OPCs. (**A**) The relative densities of Cleaved Caspase3+ PDGFRα+ and Cleaved Caspase3+ PDGFRα− OPCs were quantified. Statistical analysis by two-way ANOVA and Tukey post hoc tests. (**B**) The relative densities of Cleaved Caspase3+ cells colocalized with PDGFRα and 8OHDG were quantified. Statistical analysis by three-way ANOVA with Tukey post hoc tests. Graphs display individual data points overlaid on a bar displaying the mean ± SEM. $n = 9$ rats per group. (**C**) Representative image illustrating Cleaved Caspase3+ PDGFRα+ 8OHDG+ cells (indicated by >>), Cleaved Caspase3+ PDGFRα+ 8OHDG− cells (indicated by > |) and Cleaved Caspase3+ PDGFRα− 8OHDG+ cells (indicated by >) is shown. Cleaved Caspase3+ PDGFRα− 8OHDG− cells were not observed in the ventral nerve. Scale bar = 25μm. No outliers were removed for any outcome measure. Significant differences are indicated by * $p \leq 0.05$, ** $p \leq 0.01$, **** $p \leq 0.0001$.

3. Discussion

This study investigated the role of oxidative DNA damage to OPCs following optic nerve injury at an acute 1 day timepoint. Early pathological changes induced within the ventral nerve were indicative of secondary degeneration mechanisms, with observed increases in BBB dysfunction and 8OHDG DNA damage, as well as increased cellular proliferation specifically in DNA-damaged cells. Heightened DNA damage was also specifically identified within both NG2+ glia and PDGFRα+ glia, indicating a vulnerability of OPCs to oxidative DNA damage. Apoptotic cells were DNA damaged, and associated with BBB breach. Finally, this study demonstrated that while the PDGFRα+ OPC population was the major proliferating, DNA-damaged cell type following injury to the optic nerve, most of the apoptotic cells were not OPCs. While additional research is needed to further delineate the role of oxidative damage post-injury, these novel results provide valuable insights into early mechanisms that underpin secondary degeneration of the optic nerve at 1 day following injury.

In line with previous work that assessed outcomes at 1 day following a partial optic nerve transection, this study found significant increases in DNA damage and BBB dysfunction in the ventral optic nerve vulnerable to secondary degeneration [10,27]. A strong and significant relationship between the extent of oxidative DNA damage and BBB breach was also uncovered and observed across animals in both sham and injured groups. Though oxidative stress had already been closely associated with BBB dysfunction in a variety of CNS diseases and injuries [28], a direct relationship between the two has not been previously investigated within the partial optic nerve transection model. Taken together with the increased oxidative damage to OPCs, this direct relationship suggests that the observed increase in parenchymal IgG relates to a breakdown of the OPC component of the BBB and not due to transcellular transport [29]. The density of DNA-damaged cells undergoing proliferation significantly increased with injury. Meanwhile, there was no change in the density of proliferating cells without DNA damage as indicated by 8OHDG immunoreactivity. This finding suggests a relationship between oxidative DNA damage and cellular proliferation that requires further elucidation. Additionally, it will be important to determine whether oxidative damage is driving, or is a consequence of, secondary pathological mechanisms.

Consistent with previous studies [25,30], this study used NG2 and PDGFRα separately to identify OPCs. In our hands, immunohistochemical detection reliably allowed quantification of one cell identifying marker together with the functional indicators 8OHDG and Cleaved Caspase3. We, therefore, identified OPCs using a combination of their expression of NG2 or PDGFRα and known morphology (i.e., round features with small processes; in line with several other studies [25,31]). The majority of the PDGFRα+ cells in this study were most likely OPCs, as OPCs have the most abundant expression of PDGFRα in the CNS [26] and PDGFRα is the best singular marker for OPCs [25]. PDGFRα and NG2 likely identified a similar population of OPCs in this study, as the distribution and morphology of PDGFRα+ cells coincide with NG2+ cells in the brain [30,32], and PDGFRα+ and NG2+ cells showed a similar pattern of oxidative damage.

OPCs have previously been shown to be vulnerable to DNA damage at 3 days following a partial optic nerve transection [16]. The present study showed that this pathology occurs as early as 1 day after injury, with increases in oxidative DNA damage specifically observed within both NG2+ glia and PDGFRα+ glia. The PDGFRα+ OPC population was the major proliferating and DNA-damaged cell type. This finding builds on previous work in this model which showed that approximately 54% of proliferating cells were NG2+ Olig2+ OPCs at 1 day post-injury [33]. This early proliferative response of OPCs to injury occurs prior to the onset of cell death at 7 days, with OPC loss continuing out to 3 months post-injury [33]. Therefore, the observed early proliferation does not prevent a chronic depletion of OPCs later in the pathological sequelae. Combined with the observed increase in the proliferation of OPCs with oxidative DNA damage specifically within the injured nerve, these data suggest that proliferation could be an early indicator of OPC damage and dysfunction following optic nerve injury. However, whether increased OPC proliferation is actively induced by DNA damage or whether already proliferating OPCs are inherently more vulnerable to oxidative stress mechanisms post-injury is not yet known. Indeed, not all of the cells that are proliferating post-injury are OPCs, with a variety of cells known to proliferate following CNS injury, including astrocytes and microglia [34,35]. Nevertheless, the data suggest that oxidatively damaged OPCs drive the majority of cellular proliferation acutely post-injury.

As OPCs differentiate into mature oligodendrocytes post-injury, a peak ratio of proliferating to non-proliferating OPCs occurs at 3 days post-injury before these EdU+ OPCs differentiate through the stages of the oligodendroglial lineage towards mature myelinating oligodendrocytes [16]. By 3 days following a partial optic nerve transection, there is also a specific subpopulation of newly derived mature oligodendrocytes that have increased levels of DNA damage compared to their pre-existing counterparts [16]. Therefore, it is highly likely that a proportion of the identified proliferating and DNA-damaged OPC population at 1 day post-injury may differentiate into mature oligodendrocytes at later timepoints. This subpopulation of DNA-damaged, newly derived mature oligodendrocytes are less likely to become apoptotic than pre-existing oligodendrocytes but demonstrate a decreased long-term capacity for myelination [16]. The decreased apoptosis of newly derived and proliferating oligodendrocytes suggests that proliferation and differentiation may have been protective against the cell death associated with DNA damage post-injury. Nevertheless, the concurrent death of pre-existing oligodendrocytes alongside the reduced myelination capacity of newly derived, DNA-damaged oligodendrocytes likely contributes to chronic deficits in myelination following injury.

Heterogeneity within the overall OPC population [36] could convey varying degrees of susceptibility to oxidative damage. For example, some OPCs colocalize and interact with blood vessels, whilst others reside solely in the brain parenchyma [37]. OPCs with an intermediate phenotype have also been observed, whereby they are both simultaneously perivascular and parenchymal [38], suggesting a spectrum of OPC phenotypes based on association with the vasculature. Functional differences between OPC subpopulations identified here remain to be investigated. However, it may be that a portion of the observed DNA-damaged OPCs modulated detrimental effects at the BBB. OPCs located at the vasculature have already been found to play a key role in BBB integrity under pathological conditions, such as cerebral hypoperfusion [39] and MS [40,41]. Therefore, future studies should determine the relative vulnerability of OPC subpopulations to oxidative DNA damage to elucidate any potential contribution of perivascular OPC damage in pathological BBB dysfunction. It is also important to note that OPCs do not exist in isolation, and cross-talk between OPCs and other cells, both in the parenchyma and at the perivascular regions, is likely to contribute to outcomes.

Female rats were used in this study to enable initial comparison with our previously published work and to address the disproportionate overrepresentation of male animals within neuroscience literature. Future studies will include both male and female rats to identify possible sex-dependent changes. However, it is noteworthy that differences were observed between injured and uninjured female rats, indicating that any potential effect of female hormones does not preclude the detection of injury-induced changes in these animals.

This study identified OPCs as the major proliferating, DNA-damaged cells acutely following optic nerve injury. The observed early oxidative damage to this cell type likely plays a key role in exacerbating pathology post-injury, further highlighting oxidative stress as a therapeutic target worthy of future investigation. Pharmacological modulation of glial components of the BBB, such as the aquaporin-4 water channel on astrocytes, has been shown to reduce vasogenic edema and improve function in rats with CNS injury [42]. Given the importance of OPCs for BBB and CNS function, therapeutic interventions that attenuate oxidative DNA damage in OPCs are likely to mitigate the progression of secondary degeneration to axonal and functional loss after injury. Computer-aided, high-throughput drug screening platforms that investigate up to a hundred thousand compounds per day have the potential to accelerate the discovery or repurposing of drugs that effectively target oxidative stress-induced OPC dysfunction [43]. High-resolution imaging of OPCs and associated cells in humanized, self-organized 3D organoids or microvessel-on-a-chip platforms would facilitate the robust assessment of drug candidates likely to be effective in humans [44,45].

4. Materials and Methods

4.1. Animal Procedures and Study Design

Twenty adult, female PVG rats (180 g) were obtained from the Animal Resource Centre in Murdoch, Western Australia. All procedures were in accordance with the principles of the National Health and Medical Research Council (NHMRC) of Australia Code of Practice for use of Animals for Scientific Purposes and were approved by the Animal Ethics Committee of The University of Western Australia (RA/3/100/1485) and the Animal Ethics Committee of Curtin University (ARE2017-4). The rats were provided ad libitum access to both food and water and were housed under a 12 h light/dark cycle. Rats were also given a 1 week acclimatization period to the holding facility prior to commencing the experimental period. The cohort consisted of two experimental groups: a sham control group (n = 10) and an injured group (n = 10).

4.2. Surgical Procedures

Partial optic nerve transections were performed as previously described [8], under anesthesia with intraperitoneal Ketamine (Ketamil, 50 mg/kg, Troy Laboratories,

Glendenning, Australia) and Xylazine (Ilium Xylazil, 10 mg/kg, Troy Laboratories). In brief, the right optic nerve was surgically exposed about 1 mm behind the eye and the dorsal aspect of the nerve was partially lesioned to approximately 200 μm using a diamond radial keratotomy knife (Geuder, Heidelberg, Germany). Rats that underwent a sham injury received all surgical procedures except the cut in the surrounding nerve sheath and the partial transection into the optic nerve. Post-operative analgesia (Carprofen, 2.8 mg/kg, Norbook, Newry, UK) and sterile phosphate-buffered saline (PBS, 1 mL) were administered subcutaneously following surgery. To label cells actively undergoing the cell cycle, EdU (20 mg/kg, Invitrogen, Waltham, MA, USA) was delivered via intraperitoneal injection twice, once immediately following the surgical procedures during post-operative care and once the following morning at least 2 h prior to euthanasia. The total number of sham control animals was reduced to $n = 9$ due to $n = 1$ rat being resistant to the anesthesia necessary for surgery and thus omitted from the study. There were no deaths from the surgical procedure.

4.3. Tissue Processing

At 1 day post-injury, rats were euthanized with pentobarbitone sodium (160 mg/kg, Delvet) prior to being transcardially perfused with 0.9% saline followed by 4% paraformaldehyde (Sigma-Aldrich, St. Louis, MO, USA). The injured right optic nerves were dissected and immersed in a 4% paraformaldehyde solution overnight. The following day, the nerves were transferred to 5% sucrose (ChemSupply Australia, Bedford, South Australia, Australia), 0.1% sodium azide (Sigma-Aldrich) in PBS for cryoprotection. The optic nerves were then cryosectioned transversely at 14 μm, collected onto Superfrost Plus glass microscope slides, and stored at −80 °C prior to immunohistochemical analysis.

4.4. Multiplex Immunohistochemistry

Prior to commencing immunohistochemical analysis, the back surface of each slide was placed unsubmerged in PBS within an electrophoresis tank for 1 h at 70 V to reinforce the electrostatic bond between the tissue and slide, mitigating the risk of tissue detachment during the multiple wash steps involved in the protocol. Slides were then dried in a 37 °C oven for 10 min. Antigen retrieval involved heating the slides in 10 mM Tris-EDTA-0.5 M NaCl (pH 9.0) solution in the microwave for 2 min and 20 s, followed by a 20 min cooling period at room temperature. Slides were washed in a PBS bath prior to the application of a hydrophobic barrier around the tissue, using a PAP pen (Merck, Advanced PAP Pen, Darmstadt, Germany). Sections were washed with PBS three times before incubation with Peroxidazed 1 solution (0.3% H_2O_2, PX968M, 121219-2, Biocare Medical, Pacheco, CA, USA) for 10 min at room temperature. Slides were washed three times in PBS after the application period for each reagent was complete. Non-specific background was blocked using 3% bovine serum albumin solution (Merck, 12657) for 20 min at room temperature.

Primary antibodies used recognized: 8OHDG (1:250, 4 μg/mL, mouse, Abcam, ab62623, GR3284216-13), rat Immunoglobulin G (IgG, 1:150, 10 μg/mL, goat, BA-9400, ZG0108, Vector Laboratories, Burlingame, CA, USA), NG2 (1:50, 20 μg/mL, rabbit, AB5320B, 3218879, Merck), Cleaved Caspase3 (Asp175, 1:150; rabbit, D3E9, #9579, Lot 1, Cell Signaling Technology, Danvers, MA, USA) and PDGFRα (1:250, 4 μg/mL, rabbit, PA516571, VJ2870528A, ThermoFisher, Waltham, MA, USA). Primary antibodies were diluted in PBS and applied overnight at 4 °C. Target markers were detected sequentially in three separate combinations of antibodies/detection systems—Combination 1: PDGFRα, 8OHDG, EdU; Combination 2: PDGFRα, 8OHDG, Cleaved Caspase3; and Combination 3: NG2, 8OHDG. A separate section was used for each combination. IgG was detected alone on a separate section.

Fluorescence labeling of PDGFRα, 8OHDG, and Cleaved Caspase3 was performed using the following secondary antibodies, respectively: AF488-conjugated anti-rabbit IgG antibody (1:400; 5 μg/mL, donkey, A21206, 2289872, ThermoFisher), AF647-conjugated anti-mouse IgG antibody (1:100; 20 μg/mL, donkey, A31571, 2136787, ThermoFisher) and

AF555-conjugated anti-rabbit IgG antibody (1:400; 5 μg/mL, donkey, A31572, 1945911, ThermoFisher). Secondary antibodies were diluted in PBS and applied for 2 h at room temperature. To minimize cross-reactivity between the two anti-rabbit secondary antibodies for each combination, anti-rabbit IgG (H+L) antibody (1:100, 15 μg/mL, horse, BA-1100-1.5, ZH0421, Vector Laboratories) was applied for 1 h at room temperature after the full detection of the first rabbit antibody (i.e., after primary and secondary antibody application steps). The anti-rabbit IgG (H+L) antibody saturates the remaining binding sites for rabbit-specific secondary antibodies on the Fc region of the preceding rabbit primary antibody, restricting off-target binding when the next rabbit-specific secondary antibody is applied. The biotinylated NG2 and IgG antibodies were fluorescently labeled using the VECTASTAIN® Elite® ABC-HRP Kit (1:100, PK-6100, ZG0312, Vector Laboratories) in conjunction with a TSA FLUORESCEIN REAGENT PACK (NEL701A001KT, 191230019, Akoya Biosciences, Marlborough, MA, USA) according to manufacturers' instructions. To detect EdU+ cells, the Click-iT EdU AlexaFluor-647 Imaging Kit (C10340, 2284610, ThermoFisher) was utilized according to the manufacturer's instructions. Finally, sections were washed with PBS three times and coverslipped using Fluoromount-G (Thermo Fisher).

4.5. Imaging and Analysis

For each analysis, the entire optic nerve was visualized using a Nikon A1 confocal microscope (Nikon Corporation, Sydney, Australia) or a Dragonfly High Speed Confocal Microscope System (Andor Technology, Belfast, UK). A series of images were taken at 0.5 μm increments along the z-axis with consistent capture settings across all images for each outcome, at a magnification of 20× and numerical aperture of 0.75. Image analysis was performed using Fiji/ImageJ image processing software (National Institutes of Health, Bethesda, MD, USA).

The area of the ventral nerve region was segmented and quantified. Representative immunointensity thresholds for each outcome measure were determined to distinguish positive signals from the background prior to analyses within the ventral nerve. Using the most in-focus visual z-slice and the defined intensity thresholds, the mean area and intensity of immunoreactivity for IgG and 8OHDG were then semi-quantified. The areas above threshold measurements were normalized to the total area of the ventral nerve region. The number of EdU+ and Cleaved Caspase3+ cells was counted within the ventral nerve, normalized against the total ventral area, and expressed as the mean number of cells/mm^2. Both EdU+ 8OHDG+ and Cleaved Caspase3+ 8OHDG+ cells were detected by the colocalization of either EdU+ or Cleaved Caspase3+ cells with 8OHDG immunointensity above the set threshold similarly quantified.

Using the defined thresholds to identify NG2+ glia and PDGFRα+ glia, the intensity of 8OHDG was then also measured within the identified glia to assess the levels of DNA damage specifically within these cell types. EdU+ and Cleaved Caspase3+ cells were categorized into PDGFRα+ and PDGFRα− subpopulations based on immunoreactivity and cellular morphology. These subpopulations were further categorized via the colocalized detection of 8OHDG DNA damage.

4.6. Statistics

The obtained data were analyzed and plotted using GraphPad PRISM 9 software. All outcome measures, except for the area of IgG immunointensity, satisfied the assumption of normality according to a Kolmogorov–Smirnov test. Therefore, a t-test, two-way ANOVA with Tukey's post hoc or three-way ANOVA with Tukey's post hoc were used as appropriate. Given the area of IgG immunointensity did not satisfy the assumption of normality, the non-parametric Mann–Whitney test was used to assess the statistical difference between sham and injury for this outcome measure. A Spearman's correlation was used to assess the monotonic relationship between IgG and either 8OHDG, EdU or Cleaved Caspase3. Any reductions in final n's reflect a loss of tissue from slides during immunohistochemical analyses or the exclusion of sections that had become damaged during tissue processing and analysis in a way that precluded reliable quantification of outcomes. Statistical significances shown on graphs are hypothesis-driven and may not display all significant differences obtained. Specifically, only significant differences in comparable cell types between the sham control and injured groups are shown, as well as any differences found between cells within each group. No data outliers were removed for any outcome measures.

Author Contributions: Conceptualization, L.M.T., M.G.P., T.O.C., M.F. and C.C.A.; methodology, L.M.T., M.G.P., T.O.C., E.D., M.F. and C.C.A.; software, L.M.T. and C.C.A.; validation, L.M.T., M.G.P., T.O.C., A.J.W., E.D. and C.C.A.; formal analysis, L.M.T. and C.C.A.; investigation, L.M.T., M.G.P., T.O.C., A.J.W., E.D., A.W., T.M., C.A.B. and C.C.A.; resources, M.F.; data curation, L.M.T. and C.C.A.; writing—original draft preparation, L.M.T. and C.C.A.; writing—review and editing, L.M.T., M.G.P., T.O.C., A.J.W., E.D., A.W., T.M., C.A.B., M.F. and C.C.A.; visualization, L.M.T. and C.C.A.; supervision, M.F. and C.C.A.; project administration, L.M.T., M.G.P., T.O.C., E.D., M.F. and C.C.A.; funding acquisition, M.F. and C.C.A. All authors have read and agreed to the published version of the manuscript.

Funding: This work was supported by the National Health and Medical Research Fund (APP1160691). L.M.T. was supported by an MS Research Australia Postgraduate Scholarship and a Byron Kakulas Prestige Scholarship from the Perron Institute for Neurological and Translational Science.

Institutional Review Board Statement: The animal study protocol was approved by the Animal Ethics Committee of The University of Western Australia (RA/3/100/1485, approved 30 September 2016) and the Animal Ethics Committee of Curtin University (ARE2017-4, approved 28 April 2017).

Data Availability Statement: The datasets generated during this study are available from the corresponding author upon request.

Conflicts of Interest: The authors declare no conflict of interest. The funders had no role in the design of the study; in the collection, analyses, or interpretation of data; in the writing of the manuscript; or in the decision to publish the results.

References

1. Werner, C.; Engelhard, K. Pathophysiology of Traumatic Brain Injury. *Br. J. Anaesth.* **2007**, *99*, 4–9. [CrossRef] [PubMed]
2. Kaur, P.; Sharma, S. Recent Advances in Pathophysiology of Traumatic Brain Injury. *Curr. Neuropharmacol.* **2018**, *16*, 1224–1238. [CrossRef] [PubMed]
3. Li, H.-Y.; Ruan, Y.-W.; Ren, C.-R.; Cui, Q.; So, K.-F. Mechanisms of Secondary Degeneration after Partial Optic Nerve Transection. *Neural Regen. Res.* **2014**, *9*, 565–574. [CrossRef] [PubMed]
4. Tezel, G. Multifactorial Pathogenic Processes of Retinal Ganglion Cell Degeneration in Glaucoma towards Multi Target Strategies for Broader Treatment Effects. *Cells* **2021**, *10*, 1372. [CrossRef] [PubMed]
5. Chidlow, G.; Wood, J.P.M.; Casson, R.J. Investigations into Hypoxia and Oxidative Stress at the Optic Nerve Head in a Rat Model of Glaucoma. *Front. Neurosci.* **2017**, *11*, 478. [CrossRef]
6. Osborne, N.N.; Melena, J.; Chidlow, G.; Wood, J.P.M. A Hypothesis to Explain Ganglion Cell Death Caused by Vascular Insults at the Optic Nerve Head: Possible Implication for the Treatment of Glaucoma. *Br. J. Ophthalmol.* **2001**, *85*, 1252–1259. [CrossRef]
7. Cash, A.; Theus, M.H. Mechanisms of Blood-Brain Barrier Dysfunction in Traumatic Brain Injury. *Int. J. Mol. Sci.* **2020**, *21*, 3344. [CrossRef]
8. Bartlett, C.; Fitzgerald, M. Partial Transection of Adult Rat Optic Nerve as a Model of Secondary Degeneration in the Central Nervous System. *Bio-Protocol.* **2018**, *8*, e3118. [CrossRef]
9. Warnock, A.; Toomey, L.M.; Wright, A.J.; Fisher, K.; Won, Y.; Anyaegbu, C.; Fitzgerald, M. Damage Mechanisms to Oligodendrocytes and White Matter in Central Nervous System Injury: The Australian Context. *J. Neurotrauma* **2020**, *37*, 739–769. [CrossRef]
10. Smith, N.M.; Gachulincova, I.; Ho, D.; Bailey, C.; Bartlett, C.A.; Norret, M.; Murphy, J.; Buckley, A.; Rigby, P.J.; House, M.J.; et al. An Unexpected Transient Breakdown of the Blood Brain Barrier Triggers Passage of Large Intravenously Administered Nanoparticles. *Sci. Rep.* **2016**, *6*, 22595. [CrossRef]
11. Smith, N.M.; Giacci, M.K.; Gough, A.; Bailey, C.; McGonigle, T.; Black, A.M.; Clarke, T.O.; Bartlett, C.A.; Swaminathan Iyer, K.; Dunlop, S.A.; et al. Inflammation and Blood-Brain Barrier Breach Remote from the Primary Injury Following Neurotrauma. *J. Neuroinflammation* **2018**, *15*, 201. [CrossRef]
12. Cornelius, C.; Crupi, R.; Calabrese, V.; Graziano, A.; Milone, P.; Pennisi, G.; Radak, Z.; Calabrese, E.J.; Cuzzocrea, S. Traumatic Brain Injury: Oxidative Stress and Neuroprotection. *Antioxid. Redox Signal.* **2013**, *19*, 836–853. [CrossRef]
13. Ischiropoulos, H.; Beckman, J.S. Oxidative Stress and Nitration in Neurodegeneration: Cause, Effect, or Association? *J. Clin. Investig.* **2003**, *111*, 163–169. [CrossRef]

14. Laval, J.; Jurado, J.; Saparbaev, M.; Sidorkina, O. Antimutagenic Role of Base-Excision Repair Enzymes upon Free Radical-Induced DNA Damage. *Mutat. Res.* **1998**, *402*, 93–102. [CrossRef]
15. Fitzgerald, M.; Bartlett, C.A.; Harvey, A.R.; Dunlop, S.A. Early Events of Secondary Degeneration after Partial Optic Nerve Transection: An Immunohistochemical Study. *J. Neurotrauma* **2010**, *27*, 439–452. [CrossRef]
16. Giacci, M.K.; Bartlett, C.A.; Smith, N.M.; Iyer, K.S.; Toomey, L.M.; Jiang, H.; Guagliardo, P.; Kilburn, M.R.; Fitzgerald, M. Oligodendroglia Are Particularly Vulnerable to Oxidative Damage after Neurotrauma In Vivo. *J. Neurosci.* **2018**, *38*, 6491–6504. [CrossRef]
17. Matute, C.; Torre, I.; Pérez-Cerdá, F.; Pérez-Samartín, A.; Alberdi, E.; Etxebarria, E.; Arranz, A.M.; Ravid, R.; Rodríguez-Antigüedad, A.; Sánchez-Gómez, M.V.; et al. P2X7 Receptor Blockade Prevents ATP Excitotoxicity in Oligodendrocytes and Ameliorates Experimental Autoimmune Encephalomyelitis. *J. Neurosci.* **2007**, *27*, 9525–9533. [CrossRef]
18. Borges, K.; Ohlemeyer, C.; Trotter, J.; Kettenmann, H. AMPA/Kainate Receptor Activation in Murine Oligodendrocyte Precursor Cells Leads to Activation of a Cation Conductance, Calcium Influx and Blockade of Delayed Rectifying K+ Channels. *Neuroscience* **1994**, *63*, 135–149. [CrossRef]
19. Thorburne, S.K.; Juurlink, B.H. Low Glutathione and High Iron Govern the Susceptibility of Oligodendroglial Precursors to Oxidative Stress. *J. Neurochem.* **1996**, *67*, 1014–1022. [CrossRef]
20. Butts, B.D.; Houde, C.; Mehmet, H. Maturation-Dependent Sensitivity of Oligodendrocyte Lineage Cells to Apoptosis: Implications for Normal Development and Disease. *Cell Death Differ.* **2008**, *15*, 1178–1186. [CrossRef]
21. Fitzgerald, M.; Bartlett, C.A.; Evill, L.; Rodger, J.; Harvey, A.R.; Dunlop, S.A. Secondary Degeneration of the Optic Nerve Following Partial Transection: The Benefits of Lomerizine. *Exp. Neurol.* **2009**, *216*, 219–230. [CrossRef] [PubMed]
22. Payne, S.C.; Bartlett, C.A.; Harvey, A.R.; Dunlop, S.A.; Fitzgerald, M. Chronic Swelling and Abnormal Myelination during Secondary Degeneration after Partial Injury to a Central Nervous System Tract. *J. Neurotrauma* **2011**, *28*, 1077–1088. [CrossRef] [PubMed]
23. Payne, S.C.; Bartlett, C.A.; Harvey, A.R.; Dunlop, S.A.; Fitzgerald, M. Myelin Sheath Decompaction, Axon Swelling, and Functional Loss during Chronic Secondary Degeneration in Rat Optic Nerve. *Investig. Ophthalmol. Vis. Sci.* **2012**, *53*, 6093–6101. [CrossRef]
24. Nicholson, D.W.; Ali, A.; Thornberry, N.A.; Vaillancourt, J.P.; Ding, C.K.; Gallant, M.; Gareau, Y.; Griffin, P.R.; Labelle, M.; Lazebnik, Y.A.; et al. Identification and Inhibition of the ICE/CED-3 Protease Necessary for Mammalian Apoptosis. *Nature* **1995**, *376*, 37–43. [CrossRef]
25. Akay, L.A.; Effenberger, A.H.; Tsai, L.H. Cell of All Trades: Oligodendrocyte Precursor Cells in Synaptic, Vascular, and Immune Function. *Genes Dev.* **2021**, *35*, 180–198. [CrossRef] [PubMed]
26. Bergles, D.E.; Richardson, W.D. Oligodendrocyte Development and Plasticity. *Cold Spring Harb. Perspect. Biol.* **2016**, *8*, a020453. [CrossRef]
27. O'Hare Doig, R.L.; Bartlett, C.A.; Maghzal, G.J.; Lam, M.; Archer, M.; Stocker, R.; Fitzgerald, M. Reactive Species and Oxidative Stress in Optic Nerve Vulnerable to Secondary Degeneration. *Exp. Neurol.* **2014**, *261*, 136–146. [CrossRef]
28. Grammas, P.; Martinez, J.; Miller, B. Cerebral Microvascular Endothelium and the Pathogenesis of Neurodegenerative Diseases. *Expert Rev. Mol. Med.* **2011**, *13*, e19. [CrossRef]
29. Salman, M.M.; Kitchen, P.; Halsey, A.; Wang, M.X.; Törnroth-Horsefield, S.; Conner, A.C.; Badaut, J.; Iliff, J.J.; Bill, R.M. Emerging Roles for Dynamic Aquaporin-4 Subcellular Relocalization in CNS Water Homeostasis. *Brain* **2022**, *145*, 64–75. [CrossRef]
30. Nishiyama, A.; Lin, X.H.; Giese, N.; Heldin, C.H.; Stallcup, W.B. Co-Localization of NG2 Proteoglycan and PDGF α-Receptor on O2A Progenitor Cells in the Developing Rat Brain. *J. Neurosci. Res.* **1996**, *43*, 299–314. [CrossRef]
31. Jakovcevski, I.; Filipovic, R.; Mo, Z.; Rakic, S.; Zecevic, N. Oligodendrocyte Development and the Onset of Myelination in the Human Fetal Brain. *Front. Neuroanat.* **2009**, *3*, 5. [CrossRef]
32. Li, P.; Li, H.X.; Jiang, H.Y.; Zhu, L.; Wu, H.Y.; Li, J.T.; Lai, J.H. Expression of NG2 and Platelet-Derived Growth Factor Receptor Alpha in the Developing Neonatal Rat Brain. *Neural Regen. Res.* **2017**, *12*, 1843. [CrossRef]
33. Payne, S.C.; Bartlett, C.A.; Savigni, D.L.; Harvey, A.R.; Dunlop, S.A.; Fitzgerald, M. Early Proliferation Does Not Prevent the Loss of Oligodendrocyte Progenitor Cells during the Chronic Phase of Secondary Degeneration in a CNS White Matter Tract. *PLoS ONE* **2013**, *8*, 65710–65720. [CrossRef]
34. Karve, I.P.; Taylor, J.M.; Crack, P.J. The Contribution of Astrocytes and Microglia to Traumatic Brain Injury. *Br. J. Pharmacol.* **2016**, *173*, 692–702. [CrossRef]
35. Loane, D.J.; Byrnes, K.R. Role of Microglia in Neurotrauma. *Neurotherapeutics* **2010**, *7*, 366–377. [CrossRef]
36. Beiter, R.M.; Rivet-Noor, C.; Merchak, A.R.; Bai, R.; Johanson, D.M.; Slogar, E.; Sol-Church, K.; Overall, C.C.; Gaultier, A. Evidence for Oligodendrocyte Progenitor Cell Heterogeneity in the Adult Mouse Brain. *Sci. Rep.* **2022**, *12*, 12921. [CrossRef]
37. Maki, T. Novel Roles of Oligodendrocyte Precursor Cells in the Developing and Damaged Brain. *Clin. Exp. Neuroimmunol.* **2017**, *8*, 33–42. [CrossRef]
38. Maki, T.; Maeda, M.; Uemura, M.; Lo, E.K.; Terasaki, Y.; Liang, A.C.; Shindo, A.; Choi, Y.K.; Taguchi, A.; Matsuyama, T.; et al. Potential Interactions between Pericytes and Oligodendrocyte Precursor Cells in Perivascular Regions of Cerebral White Matter. *Neurosci. Lett.* **2015**, *597*, 164–169. [CrossRef]
39. Seo, J.H.; Miyamoto, N.; Hayakawa, K.; Pham, L.D.D.; Maki, T.; Ayata, C.; Kim, K.W.; Lo, E.H.; Arai, K. Oligodendrocyte Precursors Induce Early Blood-Brain Barrier Opening after White Matter Injury. *J. Clin. Investig.* **2013**, *123*, 782–786. [CrossRef]

40. Girolamo, F.; Errede, M.; Longo, G.; Annese, T.; Alias, C.; Ferrara, G.; Morando, S.; Trojano, M.; De Rosbo, N.K.; Uccelli, A.; et al. Defining the Role of NG2-Expressing Cells in Experimental Models of Multiple Sclerosis. A Biofunctional Analysis of the Neurovascular Unit in Wild Type and NG2 Null Mice. *PLoS ONE* **2019**, *14*, e0213508. [CrossRef]
41. Niu, J.; Tsai, H.H.; Hoi, K.K.; Huang, N.; Yu, G.; Kim, K.; Baranzini, S.E.; Xiao, L.; Chan, J.R.; Fancy, S.P.J. Aberrant Oligodendroglial–Vascular Interactions Disrupt the Blood–Brain Barrier, Triggering CNS Inflammation. *Nat. Neurosci.* **2019**, *22*, 709–718. [CrossRef] [PubMed]
42. Kitchen, P.; Salman, M.M.; Halsey, A.M.; Clarke-Bland, C.; MacDonald, J.A.; Ishida, H.; Vogel, H.J.; Almutiri, S.; Logan, A.; Kreida, S.; et al. Targeting Aquaporin-4 Subcellular Localization to Treat Central Nervous System Edema. *Cell* **2020**, *181*, 784–799.e19. [CrossRef] [PubMed]
43. Aldewachi, H.; Al-Zidan, R.N.; Conner, M.T.; Salman, M.M. High-Throughput Screening Platforms in the Discovery of Novel Drugs for Neurodegenerative Diseases. *Bioengineering* **2021**, *8*, 30. [CrossRef] [PubMed]
44. Papaspyropoulos, A.; Tsolaki, M.; Foroglou, N.; Pantazaki, A.A. Modeling and Targeting Alzheimer's Disease With Organoids. *Front. Pharmacol.* **2020**, *11*, 396. [CrossRef]
45. Salman, M.M.; Marsh, G.; Kusters, I.; Delincé, M.; Di Caprio, G.; Upadhyayula, S.; de Nola, G.; Hunt, R.; Ohashi, K.G.; Gray, T.; et al. Design and Validation of a Human Brain Endothelial Microvessel-on-a-Chip Open Microfluidic Model Enabling Advanced Optical Imaging. *Front. Bioeng. Biotechnol.* **2020**, *8*, 1077. [CrossRef]

International Journal of *Molecular Sciences*

MDPI

Article

Sera of Neuromyelitis Optica Patients Increase BID-Mediated Apoptosis in Astrocytes

Omri Zveik [1,2], Ariel Rechtman [1,2], Nitzan Haham [1,2], Irit Adini [3], Tamar Canello [1,2,4], Iris Lavon [1,2,4], Livnat Brill [1,2,†] and Adi Vaknin-Dembinsky [1,2,*,†]

1 Department of Neurology and Laboratory of Neuroimmunology, The Agnes-Ginges Center for Neurogenetics, Hadassah-Hebrew University Medical Center, Jerusalem 91120, Israel; omrizv@gmail.com (O.Z.); arielrechtman@gmail.com (A.R.); nitzan.haham@mail.huji.ac.il (N.H.); tamarcanello@gmail.com (T.C.); irisl@hadassah.org.il (I.L.); livnatb1@gmail.com (L.B.)

2 Faculty of Medicine, Hebrew University of Jerusalem, Jerusalem 91120, Israel

3 Department of Surgery, Harvard Medical School, Center for Engineering in Medicine & Surgery, Massachusetts General Hospital, 51 Blossom Street, Boston, MA 02114, USA; iadini@mgh.harvard.edu

4 Leslie and Michael Gaffin Center for Neuro-Oncology, Hadassah-Hebrew University Medical Center, Jerusalem 91120, Israel

* Correspondence: adembinsky@gmail.com; Tel.: +972-2-677-7741

† These authors contributed equally to this work.

Abstract: Neuromyelitis optica (NMO) is a rare disease usually presenting with bilateral or unilateral optic neuritis with simultaneous or sequential transverse myelitis. Autoantibodies directed against aquaporin-4 (AQP4-IgG) are found in most patients. They are believed to cross the blood–brain barrier, target astrocytes, activate complement, and eventually lead to astrocyte destruction, demyelination, and axonal damage. However, it is still not clear what the primary pathological event is. We hypothesize that the interaction of AQP4-IgG and astrocytes leads to DNA damage and apoptosis. We studied the effect of sera from seropositive NMO patients and healthy controls (HCs) on astrocytes' immune gene expression and viability. We found that sera from seropositive NMO patients led to higher expression of apoptosis-related genes, including BH3-interacting domain death agonist (BID), which is the most significant differentiating gene ($p < 0.0001$), and triggered more apoptosis in astrocytes compared to sera from HCs. Furthermore, NMO sera increased DNA damage and led to a higher expression of immunological genes that interact with BID (TLR4 and NOD-1). Our findings suggest that sera of seropositive NMO patients might cause astrocytic DNA damage and apoptosis. It may be one of the mechanisms implicated in the primary pathological event in NMO and provide new avenues for therapeutic intervention.

Keywords: NMO; astrocytes; apoptosis; BID; inflammation; neuroimmunology

Citation: Zveik, O.; Rechtman, A.; Haham, N.; Adini, I.; Canello, T.; Lavon, I.; Brill, L.; Vaknin-Dembinsky, A. Sera of Neuromyelitis Optica Patients Increase BID-Mediated Apoptosis in Astrocytes. *Int. J. Mol. Sci.* **2022**, *23*, 7117. https://doi.org/10.3390/ijms23137117

Academic Editors: Rongkung Tsai and Neil R. Miller

Received: 31 May 2022
Accepted: 23 June 2022
Published: 27 June 2022

Publisher's Note: MDPI stays neutral with regard to jurisdictional claims in published maps and institutional affiliations.

1. Introduction

Acute optic neuritis (ON) is the most common optic neuropathy affecting young adults [1]. It is characterized by reduced visual acuity, color desaturation, scotoma, and may induce ocular pain [2]. ON is present at onset in more than 50% of patients with Neuromyelitis optica (NMO) [3,4], a rare autoimmune inflammatory demyelinating syndrome of the central nervous system (CNS) [3]. The detection of antibodies against the astrocytic water channel aquaporin-4 (AQP4-IgG) distinguished NMO from other demyelinating disorders and re-defined NMO as an antibody-mediated autoimmune disease [5–8].

In the brain, AQP4 is mainly concentrated in astrocyte end-feet at pial and ependymal surfaces in contact with the cerebrospinal fluid (CSF) and blood vessels [9]. Astrocytes are critically important in the formation and maintenance of the blood–brain barrier (BBB), in maintaining ion and water homeostasis, neurotransmitter recycling, formation and maintenance, as well as the regulation of neural synaptogenesis [10–15]. They are known for their roles in immune response as well, including: the expression of immune-related receptors [16], synthesis of the complement components, and production of both immunomodulatory and immunopathogenic cytokines and chemokines [17–19].

AQP4-IgG primarily targets astrocytes in the CNS, resulting in secondary demyelination [20–22], which frequently leads to severe neurological deficits, including blindness and paraplegia [23,24]. It is thought that AQP4-IgG enters the CNS through areas of increased BBB permeability and binds selectively to AQP4 on astrocytes. The binding of the autoantigen is followed by complement activation and astrocyte destruction, leading to massive infiltration of leukocytes, particularly T and B lymphocytes, eosinophils, and neutrophils [25–27]. Although the role of autoantibodies and B cells remains the key factor in NMO pathogenesis, the primary pathological event remains elusive [21,26–28].

Here, we examined the effect of sera from seropositive NMO patients and healthy controls (HCs) on astrocytes' immune gene expression and viability. The ability to identify the pathological changes astrocytes undergo upon exposure to sera of NMO patients is of interest, as this may lead to the development of novel therapies in NMO patients.

2. Results

2.1. *Immunological Gene Expression Profiling of Human Astrocytes Cultured with NMO Sera*

In order to study the effect of sera of seropositive NMO patients on astrocytes, we performed a large-scale gene expression array of 580 immune-related genes using the NanoString nCounter code set panel. Human astrocytes were cultured with human sera (10% of media) of either seropositive NMO patients or HCs for 24 h ($n = 4$ for each group).

Out of 580 genes, we identified 73 genes that differentiate significantly (padj < 0.1) between the two groups (NMO vs. HCs, Figure 1a and Table S1). Functional and enrichment analyses of the differently expressed genes were performed using DAVID [29]. Top significant Gene Ontology (GO) terms related to the apoptotic process, Toll-like receptor (TLR) signaling pathway, regulation of Interleukin (IL)-6 production, and antigen processing and presentation (Figure 1b). In addition, among the 73 significantly differentiating genes are complement-related genes such as CR2 and C7, which are known to be involved in NMO pathogenesis [30].

2.2. *BID Pathway in Neuromyelitis Optica*

2.2.1. Increased *BID* Expression in Astrocytes Following Exposure to Sera of Seropositive NMO Patients

BH3-interacting domain death agonist (*BID*) is the most significant differentiating gene between the two groups as found in the nCounter analysis (NMO: 131.4 ± 9.3 nCounts, HCs: 73.7 ± 8.0 nCounts, $p < 0.0001$, Figure 2a). In a validation experiment performed on primary astrocytes of mice and a larger group of patients (NMO: $n = 18$, HCs: $n = 15$) using rt-QPCR analysis, we confirmed that the expression level of *BID* was significantly increased in astrocytes cultured with sera of seropositive NMO patients compared to HCs (1.02 ± 0.6 RQ and 0.54 ± 0.22 RQ, $p = 0.0037$, Figure 2b).

BID is an essential member of the apoptotic process [31]. Also, it is involved in the regulation of DNA damage [32], and the regulation of innate immunity and inflammation via TLR and nucleotide-binding oligomerization domain containing (NOD)-1 signaling and IL-6 production [33,34]. Thus, we next analyzed these pathways in astrocytes cultured with sera obtained from patients with NMO.

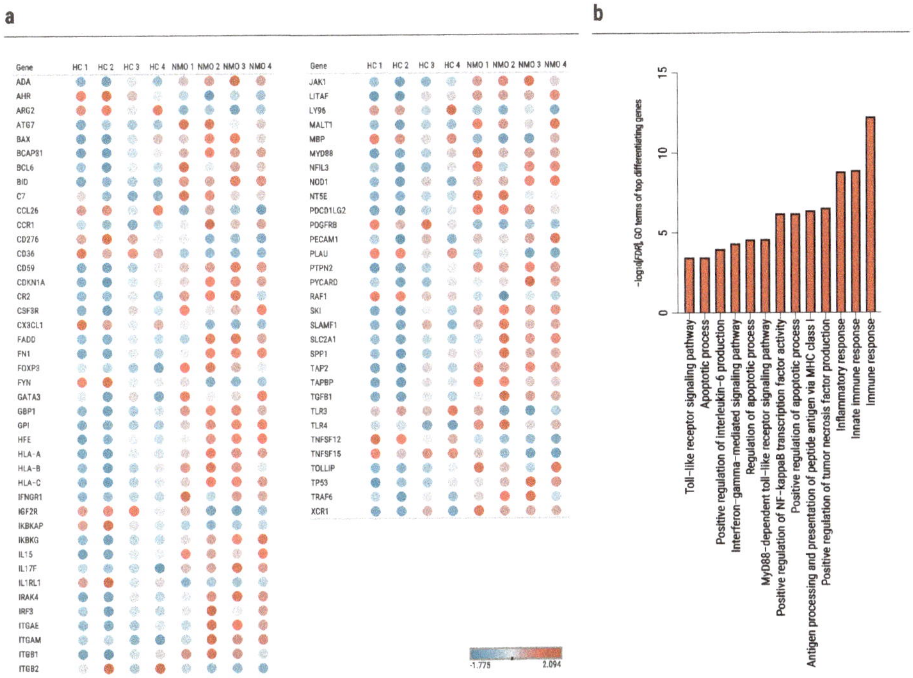

Figure 1. Immunological gene expression profiling in human primary astrocytes cultured with NMO sera. NanoString nCounter analysis of astrocytes cultured with human sera from HCs ($n = 4$) and NMO ($n = 4$) patients. (**a**) Dot plot illustrating top 73 differentially expressed genes: blue denotes low expression, red denotes high expression (padj < 0.1), (**b**) analysis of top 73 differentially expressed genes in NMO cultured astrocytes versus HC cultured astrocytes. Plot of the top enriched gene ontology (GO) terms (focus on 'function' in GOrilla), sorted by –log10[FDR].

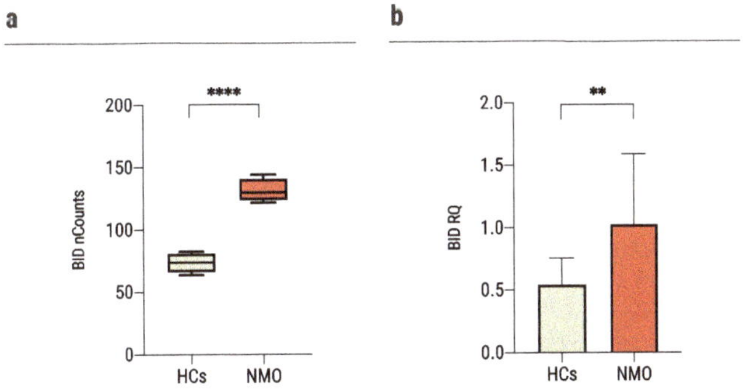

Figure 2. Exposure of astrocytes to sera of NMO patients increased *BID* expression. (**a**) The expression of *BID* increased significantly in human astrocytes cultured with sera of NMO patients (131.4 ± 9.3, $n = 4$) compared to astrocytes cultured with sera of HCs (73.7 ± 8.0, $n = 4$), as was determined with NanoString nCounter technology, (**b**) The expression of *BID* increased significantly in mouse astrocytes cultured with sera of NMO patients (1.02 ± 0.6, $n = 18$) compared to the HCs (0.54 ± 0.22, $n = 15$), as was determined using rt-QPCR. Each assay was repeated independently at least three times. Significance was determined by unpaired two-tailed student's t-test (p ** ≤ 0.01, **** ≤ 0.0001). Error bars in all graphs represent standard deviation.

2.2.2. Sera of NMO Patients Increase DNA Damage Response in Astrocytes

Tumor protein P53 (tp53) is an essential regulator of DNA damage, cell-cycle arrest, and the apoptotic process. It is known to regulate important genes that may initiate the intrinsic apoptotic pathway, such as *BID* [35,36]. In the nCounter analysis, *tp53* was significantly upregulated in NMO compared to HCs (2224.3 ± 139.3 nCounts and 1923.2 ± 150.9 nCounts, $p = 0.026$, Figure 3a). In a validation experiment performed using rt-QPCR, we found that the expression level of *tp53* is significantly increased in astrocytes cultured with seropositive NMO sera compared to sera of HCs (1.6 ± 0.6 RQ and 0.64 ± 0.4 RQ, respectively, $p < 0.0001$, Figure 3b).

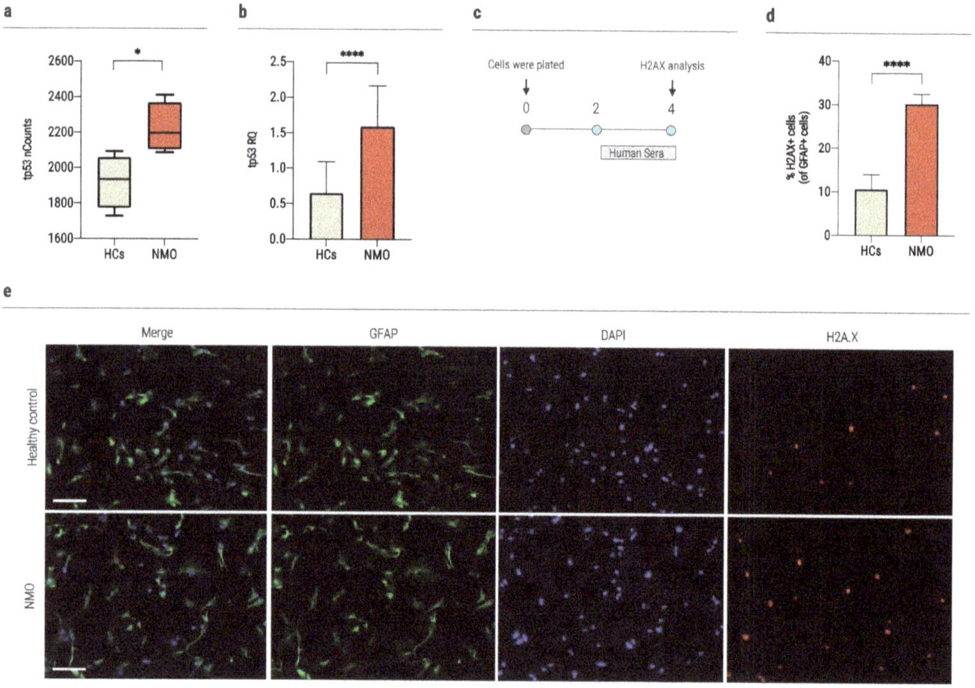

Figure 3. Sera of AQP4+NMO patients increase DNA damage response in astrocytes. (**a**) The expression of *tp53* increased significantly in the human astrocytes cultured with sera of NMO patients (2224.3 ± 139.3, $n = 4$) compared to the HCs (1923.2 ± 150.9, $n = 4$), as was determined with NanoString nCounter technology, (**b**) the expression of *tp53* increased significantly in the astrocytes cultured with sera of NMO patients (1.6 ± 0.6, $n = 15$) vs. 0.64 ± 0.4 ($n = 12$) of the HCs, as was determined using rt-QPCR, (**c**) time-course experiments of H2AX expression. Mouse primary astrocytes were cultured with human sera (20% of media) for 48 h, followed by evaluation of nuclear H2AX expression using immunofluorescence staining, (**d**) nuclear expression of H2AX was determined after culture of 48 h: HCs: 10.6 ± 3.4%; NMO: 30.3 ± 2.2%. Data are means ± SD ($n = 9$ for each group), (**e**) representative immunofluorescence analysis of primary astrocytes cultured with sera from seropositive NMO patient or HC for 48 h (scale bar = 60 μm). Each assay was repeated independently at least three times. Significance was determined by unpaired two-tailed student's *t*-test (p * ≤ 0.05, **** ≤ 0.0001,). Error bars in all graphs represent standard deviation.

To address DNA damage response, we examined histone family member X (H2AX) expression in primary astrocytes of mice following exposure to sera of AQP4+ patients. Immunofluorescence staining was performed following exposure to human sera (20% of media) for 48 h (Figure 3c). Exposure of astrocytes to sera from seropositive NMO patients resulted in significantly higher percentages of H2AX-expressing cells compared with the exposure to sera of HCs and no sera (30.3 ± 2.2%, 10.6 ± 3.4%, and 1.7 ± 0.6%, $p < 0.0001$, Figure 3d,e).

2.2.3. Increased Apoptosis of Astrocytes Following Exposure to NMO Sera

In response to pro-apoptotic signaling, BID interacts with other Bcl-2 family proteins, such as BCL2 Associated X (BAX), to initiate the apoptotic process [31]. *BAX* was found to be significantly upregulated in astrocytes cultured with NMO sera compared to HCs in the nCounter analysis (7680.1 ± 449.7 nCounts and 6270.4 ± 712.7 nCounts, $p = 0.038$). This was established in a validation experiment as described above (NMO: 1.11 ± 0.62 RQ, HCs: 0.56 ± 0.24 RQ, $p = 0.0059$, Figure 4a).

In order to assess the apoptosis level, we performed annexin staining of mouse primary astrocytes following exposure to sera of AQP4+ NMO patients or HCs. Astrocytes were cultured with human sera (20% of media) for 72 h. Then, we evaluated the astrocytes' apoptosis using flow cytometry (Figure 4b). Exposure of astrocytes to sera of NMO patients resulted in significantly higher annexin staining compared to the exposure to sera of HCs (13.34 ± 4.03% vs. 5.7 ± 3.3%, $p = 0.0002$, Figure 4c,d).

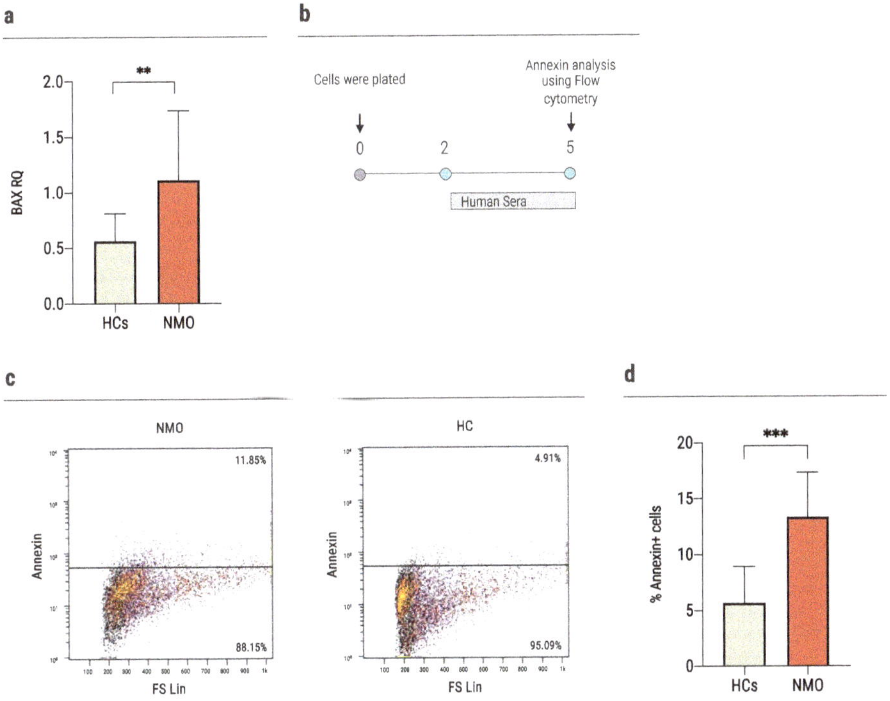

Figure 4. Exposure of NMO sera increased apoptosis in astrocytes. (**a**) The expression of *BAX* increased significantly in the astrocytes cultured with sera of NMO patients (1.11 ± 0.62, $n = 17$) vs. 0.56 ± 0.24 ($n = 13$) of the HCs, as was determined using rt-QPCR, (**b**) time-course experiments of annexin levels. Primary astrocytes were cultured with human sera (20% of media) for 72 h, followed by evaluation of apoptosis expression using flow cytometry, (**c**) representative flow cytometry analysis of apoptotic astrocytes upon culture with sera obtained from seropositive NMO patients or HCs, (**d**) higher levels of apoptosis among astrocytes cultured with sera of NMO patients (13.34 ± 4.03%, $n = 10$), compared to HCs (5.7 ± 3.3%, $n = 10$), as evaluated using annexin staining. Each assay was repeated independently at least three times. Significance was determined by unpaired two-tailed student's *t*-test (p ** ≤ 0.01, *** ≤ 0.001). Error bars in all graphs represent standard deviation.

2.2.4. Volumetric Brain Loss Correlates with *BID* and Annexin Levels of Astrocytes Cultured with Sera of NMO Patient

We analyzed the volume of 14 different brain structures using the Volbrain platform. We assessed the correlation of each patient's volumetric data and the effect of the same patient's sera on mouse astrocytes, as measured by *BID* expression and annexin levels.

We found a significant negative correlation between *BID* expression levels of mouse astrocytes cultured with sera of NMO patient and total cerebrum (r = −0.62, p = 0.0412, Figure 5a) and cerebellum volume (r = −0.88, p = 0.0003, Figure 5b) of the same patient. Furthermore, we assessed the correlation between brain volume and annexin levels of mouse astrocytes cultured with sera of NMO patient. We found a significant negative correlation between annexin levels and cerebellum volume (r = −0.78, p = 0.0068, Figure 5c) and brainstem volume (r = −0.81, p = 0.0038, Figure 5d) of the same patient.

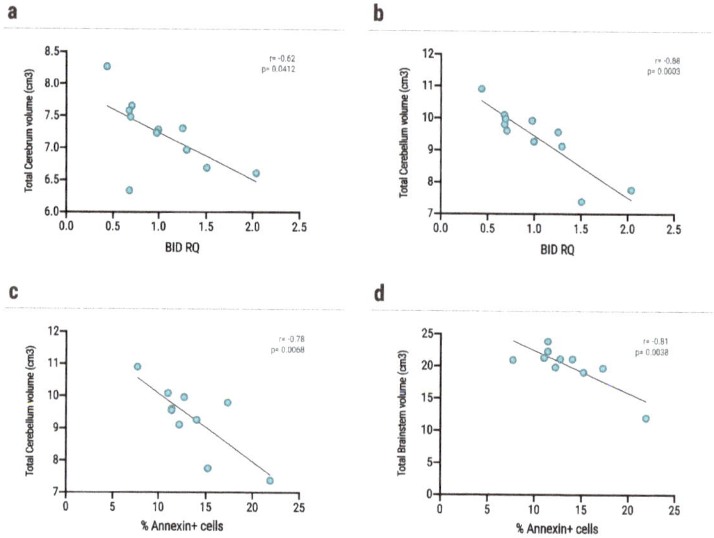

Figure 5. Correlation between *BID* and annexin levels in sera-cultured astrocytes and brain volume. (**a**,**b**) Correlation between *BID* RQ expression levels of mouse astrocytes following culture with sera of AQP4+ patients and (**a**) total cerebrum volume (r = −0.62, p = 0.0412), (**b**) total cerebellum volume (r = −0.88, p = 0.0003), (**c**,**d**) correlation between annexin levels of mouse astrocytes following culture with sera of AQP4+ patients and (**c**) total cerebellum volume (r = −0.78, p = 0.0068), (**d**) total brainstem volume (=−0.81, p = 0.0038). Correlation was determined by Pearson correlation test. Differences were considered significant at $p < 0.05$.

2.3. *Increased Pro-Inflammatory Gene Expression upon Exposure of Astrocytes to Sera of NMO Patients*

To better understand the immune effect of NMO sera on astrocytes, we validated two representative genes that were found to differ significantly between the groups.

One of the major signaling pathways was TLR signaling pathway (Figure 1b). TLR4 is known for its roles in pathogen recognition and activation of innate immunity [37], but also for its involvement in autoimmune disorders such as multiple sclerosis [38]. Additionally, TLR4 interacts with BID both in innate immune pathways [33] and the apoptotic pathway [39]. In nCounter analysis, the expression of *TLR4* was significantly higher among astrocytes exposed to sera of seropositive NMO patients (1597.1 ± 146.7 nCounts) compared to sera of HCs (1218.9 ± 136.3 nCounts). These findings were further validated on mouse primary astrocytes and a larger group of patients using rt-QPCR analysis (NMO: 1.9 ± 0.6 RQ, HCs: 1.26 ± 0.4 RQ, p = 0.0003, Figure 6a).

NOD-1 plays a key role in innate immune [40] and activated TLR4 signaling [41] pathways. It is also regulated by BID, and their interactions may eventually lead to NF-kB activation [33]. BID is required to activate host defense mechanisms to control bacterial infections but may also exacerbate immune-mediated inflammatory disease [33]. In nCounter analysis, *NOD-1* expression levels were significantly higher among astrocytes exposed to NMO sera compared to HCs (188.11 ± 17.01 nCounts, and 127.4 ± 28.0 nCounts, respectively, $p = 0.009$). These findings were further validated as described above (NMO: 1.8 ± 0.9 RQ, HCs: 0.66 ± 0.62 RQ, $p = 0.002$, Figure 6b).

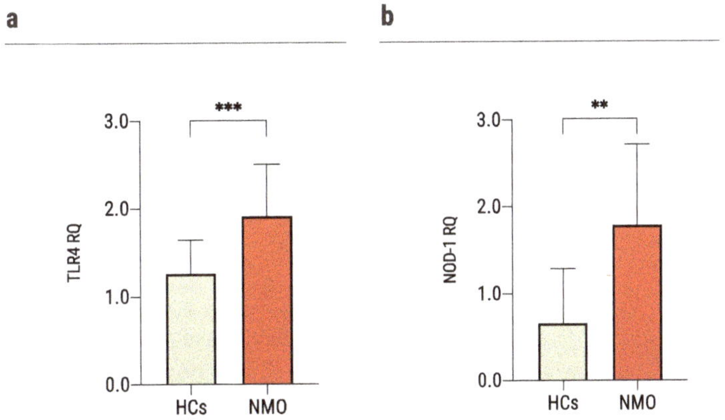

Figure 6. Increased pro-inflammatory gene expression upon exposure of astrocytes to sera of NMO patients. Quantitative PCR gene expression analysis of: (**a**) the expression of *TLR4* increased significantly in astrocytes cultured with sera of NMO patients (1.9 ± 0.6, $n - 19$) vs. 1.26 ± 0.4 ($n = 19$) of astrocytes cultured with sera of HCs, (**b**) the expression of *NOD-1* increased significantly in astrocytes cultured with sera of NMO patients (1.8 ± 0.9, $n = 15$) vs. 0.66 ± 0.62 ($n = 11$) of astrocytes cultured with sera of HCs. Each assay was repeated independently at least three times. Significance was determined by unpaired two-tailed student's *t*-test (p ** ≤ 0.01, *** ≤ 0.001). Error bars in all graphs represent standard deviation.

2.4. Sera of NMO Patients Stimulates a Repair Process

Following our observation that sera of seropositive NMO patients increased the expression of both genes involved in apoptosis and the TLR signaling pathway, we explored two immunological genes involved in synaptogenesis and known to reduce neuronal damage.

IL-15 is known to be upregulated in the CNS after injury [42–46]. Its expression is known to be related to NMO progression: high expression is implicated in reduced lesion size, attenuation of BBB leakage and tight junctions lost, reduced brain infiltration of immune cell subsets, and promotion of astrocytes survival [47]. IL-15 induces the activation of JAK1. Studies suggested that this cytokine may increase the expression of apoptosis inhibitor BCL2L1/BCL-x(L) [48]. Both *IL-15* and *JAK-1* were significantly upregulated among astrocytes exposed to NMO sera compared to HCs (*IL-15*: 185.8 ± 13.4 nCounts vs. 137.6 ± 24.7 nCounts; *JAK-1*: 4356.9 ± 175.1 nCounts vs. 3818.1 ± 130.02 nCounts). In validation experiments as described above, we found that the expression levels of *IL-15* and *JAK-1* were significantly increased in astrocytes cultured with NMO sera compared to HCs (*IL-15*: 1.1 ± 0.5 RQ vs. 0.72 ± 0.3 RQ, $p = 0.0008$; and *JAK-1*: 1.1 ± 0.4 RQ vs. 0.86 ± 0.4 RQ, $p = 0.029$, Figure 7a,b).

Taken together, these data suggest that exposure of astrocytes to NMO sera triggers not only a damaging cascade but also a repair process, which may eventually serve as a therapeutic target.

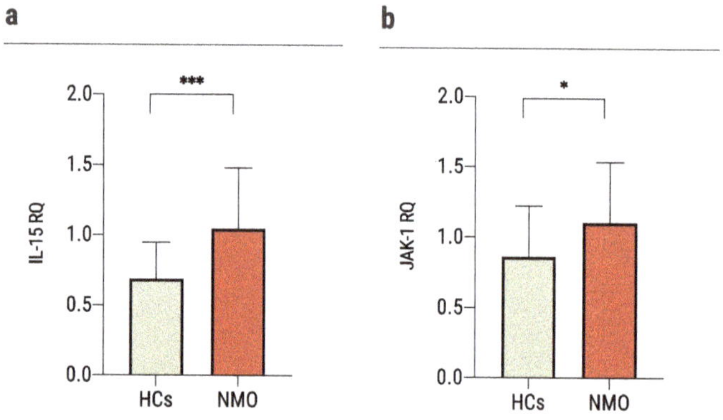

Figure 7. Sera of NMO patients stimulates repair process. Quantitative PCR gene expression analysis of: (**a**) the expression of *IL-15* increased significantly in astrocytes cultured with sera of NMO patients (1.1 ± 0.5, $n = 31$) vs. 0.72 ± 0.3 ($n = 24$) of astrocytes cultured with sera of HCs, (**b**) the expression of *JAK-1* increased significantly in astrocytes cultured with sera of NMO patients (1.1 ± 0.4, $n = 32$) vs. 0.86 ± 0.4 ($n = 24$) of astrocytes cultured with sera of HCs. Each assay was repeated independently at least three times. Significance was determined by unpaired two-tailed student's *t*-test (p * ≤ 0.05, *** ≤ 0.001). Error bars in all graphs represent standard deviation.

3. Discussion

In the current study, we found that sera from NMO patients have a differential effect on astrocytes' immune gene expression. Sera from NMO patients led to increased apoptosis of astrocytes compared to sera from HCs. In addition, it also led to higher expression of DNA damage marker, H2AX, and higher expression of immunological genes, such as *TLR4* and *NOD-1*.

Although NMO has been studied extensively, it is still not entirely clear what the primary pathological event is [21,26–28]. One accepted theory is that complement activation is initiated upon binding to the autoantigen, leading to astrocyte destruction and secondary demyelination and axonal damage [25–27]. It is in line with our result of higher expression of complement-related genes such as CR2 and C7 in human astrocytes cultured with sera of NMO patients. Other studies suggested that astrocyte damage may produce a toxic bystander effect on oligodendrocytes which can lead eventually to demyelination [49–51]. An additional possible explanation may be that following the primary event of the interaction of AQP4-IgG and astrocytes, there is an increase in DNA damage, increased expression of *BID*, and a higher level of apoptosis. The increased expression of *BID* also leads to higher expression of *TLR4* and *NOD-1*. Understanding the mechanisms leading to NMO pathology may promote the development of new therapeutic interventions.

Another question regarding NMO pathology is why NMO lesions localize to the optic nerve. Previous works suggested that the restricted diffusion of AQP4 and other pro-inflammatory factors in the optic nerve may increase their concentration [52,53]. Also, the unique anatomy of the optic nerve is exceptional in myelinated tracks, which may provide another explanation for ON as well [54]. Furthermore, the high expression of AQP4 on astrocytes in the optic nerve compared to the brain remains the main reason for the susceptibility of the optic nerve in NMO patients [55].

Initially, we chose to focus on the apoptotic process. *BID*, the most significant differentiating gene in the nCounter analysis, is a pro-apoptotic member of the Bcl-2 protein family [31]. We assessed apoptosis in astrocytes exposed to NMO and HCs sera using annexin staining. We found higher levels of apoptotic astrocytes (2.34 time-fold) among the NMO group compared to the HCs. These observations align with a previous work by Brill et al., which showed an increase in apoptosis and *BID* expression levels in peripheral blood mononuclear cells (PBMCs) of NMO patients compared to HCs [56]. Additionally, we found a significant negative correlation between annexin levels or *BID* expression of mouse astrocytes cultured with sera of NMO patients and their volumetric MRI data. Liu et al. observed lower brain volume in NMO patients compared to HCs [57]. Previous works suggested a correlation between brain atrophy and cognitive impairment in NMO patients [58,59]. Our data show that sera of seropositive NMO patients induce more apoptosis of astrocytes in vitro and suggest that a mechanism of programmed astrocytic death by apoptosis might be implicated in the pathology of NMO.

BID is a regulator of the apoptotic process. In response to apoptotic signaling, BID interacts with other Bcl-2 family proteins, such as BAX. We found higher expression of *BAX* in astrocytes cultured with sera of NMO patients compared to HCs. BAX has previously been implicated in mediating nitric oxide-induced apoptosis in astrocytes of the cerebral cortex and the optic nerve through a tp53-dependent pathway [60–62]. To initiate apoptosis and activate BAX, BID must be trunked into trunked(t)-BID [63]. It can be due to cues from the extrinsic pathway (such as FADD), the granzyme B pathway, or due to DNA damage response [64]. Our data showed a higher expression of *tp53* in astrocytes cultured with sera of NMO patients compared to HCs. Using H2AX staining, we found that sera of NMO patients led to higher levels of DNA damage in astrocytes compared to sera of HCs. It is possible that one of the signals leading to higher apoptosis in astrocytes cultured with NMO sera is DNA damage (Figure 8). DNA damage leads to activation of cell-cycle regulator tp53, which might lead to BID activation and initiation of the intrinsic pathway.

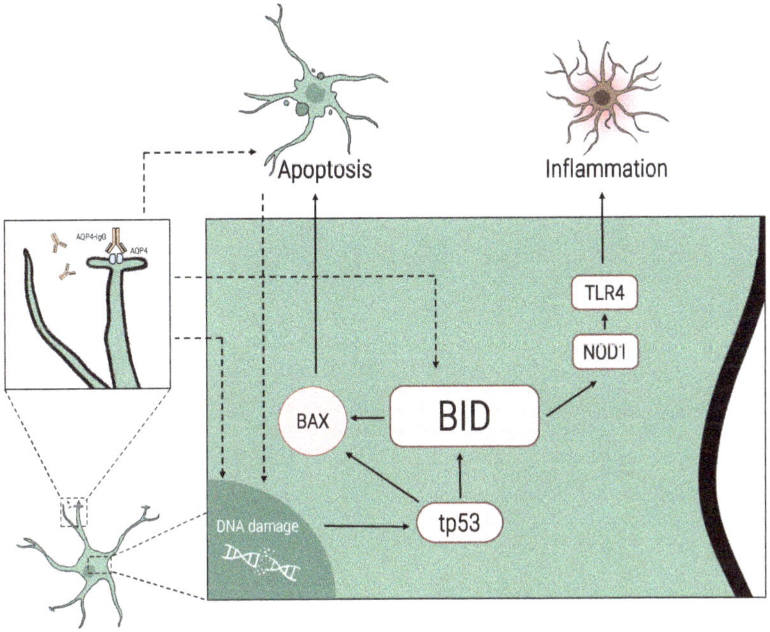

Figure 8. Proposed scheme for BID-mediated apoptosis in astrocytes in NMO. Following culture of astrocytes with sera of NMO patients, we found an increase in the expression of *BID*, *tp53*, *BAX*, *NOD-1*, and *TLR4*. Increased *BID* levels may be linked to NMO pathogenesis through several pathways: The increase in *BID* can mediate the inflammation process in NMO by increasing *NOD-1* and *TLR4*. The interaction of AQP4-IgG and AQP4 receptors on astrocytes leads to complement activation, necrosis/apoptosis, and DNA damage, which in turn may activate cell-cycle regulator *tp53*, leading to BID-mediated apoptosis. Other inflammatory factors in the sera of NMO patients can directly activate the BID pathway or indirectly by increasing DNA damage.

BID also has a role in inflammation and innate immunity [33]. It is suggested that BID is important for the ability to respond to local or systemic exposure to infection [33]. To do so, BID interacts directly with NOD-1 and activates nuclear factor kappa B (NFκB) and ERK pathways [33]. NOD-1 acts as a pattern-recognition receptor that binds bacterial peptidoglycans and initiates inflammation [65,66]. Previous work has shown that activation of NOD-1 in PBMCs of NMO patients increased IL-6 levels [67]. We found that *NOD-1* is upregulated in astrocytes cultured with NMO sera compared to HCs. Once activated, NOD-1 can interact with TLR4 and is involved in innate immune activation [33,40,41]. Interestingly, three of the leading pathways found in the nCounter analysis are TLR signaling pathway, IL-6 production, and apoptotic process.

Our data reveal that *TLR4* is upregulated in astrocytes cultured with sera of NMO patients at the mRNA expression level. It was previously reported that using bacterial lipopolysaccharide (LPS), a typical TLR4 activator, astrocytes are activated and induce a complex set of molecular reactions mediated by NFκB, mitogen-activated protein kinase (MAPK), and Jak1/Stat1 signaling pathways [68]. This cascade may lead to both pro-inflammatory and anti-inflammatory signals. The use of TLR4 agonist has shown to lead to higher secretion of pro-inflammatory mediators (such as IL-6, IL-17, and IL-1b) and to impede secretion of anti-inflammatory IL-10 in PBMCs of NMO patients [69,70]. Haase et al. showed that macrophages deficient for TLR4 diminished Yersinia-induced apoptosis [39]. They also showed that the extended stimulation of overexpressed TLR4 elicited cellular death in epithelial cells. These suggest the implication of TLR4 not only in the immune response but also in the apoptotic process.

Demyelination and oligodendrocytes loss are two of the most important pathological processes leading to disability in NMO patients [30]. Both pathological events are considered secondary damage to astrocyte dysfunction or inflammatory bystander damage [71]. The crosstalk of astrocytes and oligodendrocytes in the CNS is complex and may lead to different outcomes [72]. Astrocytes can secrete detrimental factors (such as hyaluronan or fibronectin), which may halt remyelination and differentiation of oligodendrocyte progenitor cells into mature myelinating oligodendrocytes [73–76]. On the other hand, astrocytes play a major role in the homeostatic support of oligodendrocytes and secrete beneficial factors to promote remyelination (such as CXCL12 and IGF-1) [77,78]. We suggest that astrocytic apoptosis may lead to a breach of the homeostatic balance and support of oligodendrocytes, thus, eventually leading to loss of oligodendrocytes and failure of remyelination. Theoretically, it is plausible that following damage and apoptosis, astrocytes are secreting detrimental factors that lead to apoptosis of oligodendrocytes. Moreover, the same BID-mediated apoptosis pathway may occur not only in astrocytes but also in oligodendrocytes of NMO patients. This hypothesis is difficult to assess due to the lack of an animal model for NMO and the technical difficulties in co-culture experiments of both cells.

Upon injury, astrocytes may increase the expression of anti-inflammatory or pro-synaptogenesis genes. We found that *IL-15* is highly expressed in NMO-cultured astrocytes compared to HCs. Its expression is known to be related to NMO progression: high expression is implicated in reduced lesion size, attenuation of BBB leakage and tight junctions lost, reduced brain infiltration of immune cell subsets, and promotion of astrocytes survival [47]. IL-15 induces the activation of JAK1. Studies suggested that this cytokine may increase the expression of apoptosis inhibitor BCL2L1/BCL-x(L) [48]. These data suggest that exposure of astrocytes to NMO sera prompts not only damage cascade, but also a repair process, which may eventually serve as a therapeutic target. Targeting astrocytes with treatments that may induce IL-15 expression may serve as a potential treatment for ON and NMO [79,80].

Further potential therapeutic intervention may be the inhibition of astrocytic apoptosis. Inhibition of cysteine cathepsin B and L in astrocytes was reported to contribute to neuroprotection against cerebral ischemia via blocking the t-BID-mitochondrial apoptotic pathway [81]. Other small molecules such as BI-6C9 or idebenone were previously suggested as inhibitors of BID or BAX-induced apoptosis [61,82]. However, there is a potential risk in inhibiting programmed apoptosis instead of targeting the reason that initiated the process.

The limitations of this study are the relatively small cohort and the use of mouse primary astrocytes. Although, we used both human and mouse cells for the immunological expression data.

In conclusion, we showed that following exposure to sera from seropositive NMO patients, there is an increased expression of both immunological and apoptosis-related genes in astrocytes. Astrocytes undergo more apoptosis and gain DNA damage upon exposure to NMO sera. Our data contribute to the current knowledge regarding astrocytic destruction in NMO pathology, suggesting apoptosis as one of the implicated mechanisms in the primary pathology in NMO. These findings may provide new avenues for therapeutic intervention and furnish a better understanding of disease pathogenesis.

4. Materials and Methods

4.1. Approvals

The Hadassah Medical Organization Ethics Committee approved this study. All subjects provided written informed consent (0589-08-HMO). The research reported in this study complied with all relevant ethical regulations for animal testing and research and was approved by the Hebrew University Institutional Animal Care and Use Committee (MD-20-16227-1).

4.2. Subjects

The patients cohort included 35 NMO patients (26 females, 9 males; mean age at diagnosis 41.9 $\pm$ 16.9 years; disease duration 9.4 $\pm$ 5.2 years; EDSS 4.47 $\pm$ 2.4) and 28 healthy individuals who served as controls (16 females, 10 males; mean age 40.5 $\pm$ 15.9 years). All patients were followed at the Neurology clinic in the Neurology Department of Hadassah Medical Center, Jerusalem, Israel. The participants' characteristics were obtained from medical files from the Neurology clinic. All NMO patients were diagnosed according to 2015 diagnostic criteria [5], and were tested positive to anti-AQP4.

4.3. Gene Expression Array and Bioinformatics Analysis

A large-scale gene expression array was performed by utilizing NanoString nCounter technology (NanoString Technologies Inc., Seattle, WA, USA). Total RNA was extracted from human astrocytes (LONZA, Haifa, Israel) cultured with sera of NMO patients and HCs using Tri Reagent BD (Sigma–Aldrich, Rehovot, Israel). Samples were analyzed for 580 immunology genes with the nCounter code set panel (NanoString Technologies Inc., Seattle, WA, USA). The assay is based on direct digital detection of mRNA molecules of interest with the aid of target-specific, color-coded probe pairs, without the use of reverse transcription or amplification. Raw data (following control and reference gene normalization) is analyzed with nsolver analysis software. Following hierarchical clustering, GO pathway enrichment analysis is used to define pathways related to these genes [83]. The Database for Annotation, Visualization and Integrated Discovery (DAVID) [29] was used to study shared biological processes of significant differential genes (https://david.ncifcrf.gov, RRID:SCR_001881, Date: 31 May 2022).

4.4. Mouse Primary Astrocytes Culture

Mouse primary astrocytes were isolated from naïve P0 to P1 neonatal *C57/BL6* mice cortices as previously described by Chen et al. [84], with minor modifications [85,86]. Briefly, a mixed glial culture isolated from neonatal mice was grown for 8 days in Dulbecco's modified Eagle's medium (DMEM) low glucose (Biological Industries, Kibbutz Beit-Haemek, Israel) supplemented with 5% fetal bovine serum (Biological Industries, Kibbutz Beit-Haemek, Israel), 1 mM sodium pyruvate (Biological Industries, Kibbutz Beit-Haemek, Israel), 1 mM L-glutamine (Sigma–Aldrich, Rehovot, Israel) and 0.6% Gentamycin

Sulfate (Biological Industries, Kibbutz Beit-Haemek, Israel). Culture medium was replaced every 2 days. After 8 days, microglia were detached by 30 min shaking at 140 rpm using an orbital shaker. After medium was removal, a new fresh culture medium was added, and OPCs at the top of the astrocyte monolayer were detached by shaking for 18 h at 200 rpm. Media was replaced and astrocytes were grown for further 7 days. Cells were detached from flasks using TrypLE (Thermo Fisher Scientific, Waltham, MA, USA). All cultures expressed high level of GFAP (mean of 96.6% GFAP+ cells, Figure S1).

4.5. Apoptosis Assay

Cells were seeded in plates for 24 h. Then, media was replaced for DMEM low glucose (Biological Industries, Kibbutz Beit-Haemek, Israel) supplemented with 1 mM sodium pyruvate (Biological Industries, Kibbutz Beit-Haemek, Israel), 1 mM L-glutamine (Sigma–Aldrich, Rehovot, Israel) and 0.6% Gentamycin Sulfate (Biological Industries, Kibbutz Beit-Haemek, Israel). Human sera of either NMO patients or HCs (20% of media) were added into mouse primary astrocytes media for 72 h. Apoptosis was assessed by Annexin V detection kit (Cat# BG-62700, EMELCA Bioscience, Clinge, The Netherlands). All fluorescence-activated cell sorting (FACS) samples were analyzed in a Beckman coulter FC500 apparatus using the CXP software. Each assay was repeated independently at least three times.

4.6. DNA Damage Assay

Cells were seeded in plates for 24 h. Then, media was replaced for DMEM low glucose (Biological Industries, Kibbutz Beit-Haemekm Israel) supplemented with 1 mM sodium pyruvate (Biological Industries, Kibbutz Beit-Haemek, Israel), 1 mM L-glutamine (Sigma–Aldrich, Rehovot, Israel) and 0.6% Gentamycin Sulfate (Biological Industries, Kibbutz Beit-Haemek, Israel). Human sera of either NMO patients or HCs (20% of media) were added into mouse primary astrocytes media for 48 h. Then, DNA damage response was evaluated using anti-H2AX (Cat# sc-517348, Santa Cruz biotechnology Inc., Dallas, TX, USA, 1:100). Each assay was repeated independently at least three times.

4.7. RNA Isolation and Reverse Transcription

Mouse primary astrocytes were cultured with 10% human CSF for 24 h. RNA was extracted from cultured astrocytes using Tri-reagent (Sigma–Aldrich, Rehovot, Israel) as previously described [87,88]. The cDNA was synthesized from 250 ng total RNA using the qScript cDNA Synthesis Kit (Quanta Biosciences, Gaithersburg, MD, USA). Quantitative polymerase chain reaction (PCR) was performed using PerfeCTa SYBR Green FastMix Rox (Quanta Biosciences, Gaithersburg, MD, USA). Gene amplification was carried out using the StepOnePlus real-time PCR system (Applied Biosystems, Waltham, MA, USA). The threshold cycle value ($2^{-\Delta CT}$) was used for statistical analysis. All target mRNAs were normalized to the Hypoxanthine-guanine phosphoribosyltransferase (HPRT) reference gene. At least three independent experiments were performed; expression of each gene was evaluated in triplicate and is presented as mean mRNA relative quantification ± SD.

Primers used (Agentek, Yakum, Israel):

HPRT F: 5′ CATGGACTGATTATGGACGGAC R: 5′ ACAGAGGGCCACAATGT-GATG

BH3-Interacting Domain Death Agonist (BID) F: 5′ GGCTCCTCAGTCCATCTGGTT R: 5′ GCCAGTCACGCACCATCT

Tp53 F: R: F: 5′ GAGGGAGCTCGAGGCTGATAT F: 5′ TTCTCCGAAGACTGGAT-GACTG

Nucleotide-Binding Oligomerization Domain Containing (NOD)-1 F: 5′ TGAGGAG-CAACCTAGGACAAAG R: 5′ CAGCCATAACAGAGATTTGTCTC

Interleukin (IL-)15 F: 5′ AGCCTACAGGAGGCCAAGAA R: 5′ AATGCCCAGGTAA-GAGCTTCAA

Janus Kinase 1 (JAK1) F: 5′ GCTCCACTACCGCATGAGGTT R: 5′ TGGAGAAT-GTCGCCATACAGAC

TLR-4: F: 5′ TGATGACATTCCTTCTTCAACCA R: 5′ TGGTTGAAGAAGGAATGT-CATCA

BCL2 Associated X (BAX): F: 5′ AGTGCACAGGGCCTTGAG R: 5′ GCGTGGTTGCC-CTCTICT

4.8. Immunostaining

For intra-cellular markers, staining was performed on living cells followed by fixation and permeabilization. Anti-Glial fibrillary acidic protein (GFAP; Cat# Z0334, RRID: AB_10013382, Agilent, Santa Clara, CA, USA, 1:50) was used to identify astrocytes, anti-H2AX (Cat# sc-517348, RRID:AB_2783871, Santa Cruz biotechnology Inc., Dallas, TX, USA, 1:100) was used for evaluation of DNA damage response. Goat anti-rabbit Alexa Fluor 488 (Cat# A-11034, RRID: AB_2576217, Invitrogen, Thermo Fisher Scientific, Waltham, MA, USA, 1:200) and goat anti-mouse Alexa Fluor 555 (Cat# A28180, RRID:AB_2536164, Invitrogen, Thermo Fisher Scientific, Waltham, MA, USA, 1:200) were used as secondary antibodies appropriately. Nuclei were counterstained with 4′,6-diamidino-2-phenylindole (DAPI; Cat# H-1200, RRID:AB_2336790, Vector Laboratories, Burlingame, CA, USA). Quantification was performed using ImageJ software (NIH, public domain software) by measuring positively stained cells relative to total DAPI. Quantifications are represented as mean percentages from total DAPI+ cells $\pm$ SD and are from at least 15 random fields captured in three or more independent experiments.

4.9. MRI Data Acquisition, Processing, and Analysis

Brain MRIs were acquired using demyelination protocol [89]. T1-weighted images were acquired using MRI scanners at Hadassah Ein Kerem medical center as described before [90]. Volumetric data were extracted using volBrain (http://volbrain.upv.es, Date: 1 December 2021) platform. VolBrain software contains advanced pipelines and automatically provides volumetric information of the brain MR images at different scales [91]. Volbrain provide volumes of total brain, total white matter, total gray matter, cerebrum, cerebellum, brainstem, lateral ventricles, caudate, putamen, thalamus, globus pallidus, hippocampus, amygdala, and nucleus accumbens.

4.10. Statistical Analyses

Unpaired two-tailed student's t-test, one-way ANOVA with Tukey's multiple comparisons post hoc test, Mann–Whitney, and Pearson correlation tests were performed. Specific tests are noted in figure legends with significance level annotations. Values are provided as mean $\pm$ SD, or as described for each figure. All error bars represent standard deviation.

Supplementary Materials: The following supporting information can be downloaded at: https://www.mdpi.com/article/10.3390/ijms23137117/s1.

Author Contributions: Conceptualization, O.Z., L.B. and A.V.-D.; Methodology, O.Z., L.B. and A.V.-D.; Validation, O.Z.; Formal Analysis, O.Z., L.B., A.R., N.H., T.C. and I.L.; Investigation, O.Z., L.B., A.R., N.H., T.C. and I.L.; Data Curation, O.Z.; Writing—Original Draft Preparation, O.Z., I.A., L.B. and A.V.-D.; Writing—Review & Editing, O.Z., I.A., L.B. and A.V.-D.; Visualization, O.Z.; Supervision, L.B. and A.V.-D. All authors have read and agreed to the published version of the manuscript.

Funding: This research received no external funding.

Institutional Review Board Statement: The study was conducted according to the guidelines of the Declaration of Helsinki, and approved by the Institutional Ethics Committee of Hadassah Medical Organization (0589-08-HMO). The research reported in this study complied with all relevant ethical regulations for animal testing and research and was approved by the Hebrew University Institutional Animal Care and Use Committee (MD-20-16227-1).

Informed Consent Statement: Informed consent was obtained from all subjects involved in the study.

Data Availability Statement: Not applicable.

Conflicts of Interest: The authors declare no conflict of interest.

References

1. Toosy, A.T.; Mason, D.F.; Miller, D.H. Optic neuritis. *Lancet Neurol.* **2014**, *13*, 83–99. [CrossRef]
2. Beck, R.W.; Sellers, B.J.; Cleary, P.A.; Backlund, J.Y.C.; Becker, D.; Kenny, D.; Dunbar, J.; Optic Neuritis Study Group. The Clinical Profile of Optic Neuritis. *Arch. Ophthalmol.* **1991**, *109*, 1673–1678. [CrossRef]
3. Jarius, S.; Ruprecht, K.; Kleiter, I.; Borisow, N.; Asgari, N.; Pitarokoili, K.; Pache, F.; Stich, O.; Beume, L.A.; Hümmert, M.W.; et al. MOG-IgG in NMO and related disorders: A multicenter study of 50 patients. Part 2: Epidemiology, clinical presentation, radiological and laboratory features, treatment responses, and long-term outcome. *J. Neuroinflamm.* **2016**, *13*, 280. [CrossRef]
4. Jarius, S.; Ruprecht, K.; Wildemann, B.; Kuempfel, T.; Ringelstein, M.; Geis, C.; Kleiter, I.; Kleinschnitz, C.; Berthele, A.; Brettschneider, J.; et al. Contrasting disease patterns in seropositive and seronegative neuromyelitis optica: A multicentre study of 175 patients. *J. Neuroinflamm.* **2012**, *9*, 14. [CrossRef]
5. Wingerchuk, D.M.; Banwell, B.; Bennett, J.L.; Cabre, P.; Carroll, W.; Chitnis, T.; De Seze, J.; Fujihara, K.; Greenberg, B.; Jacob, A.; et al. International consensus diagnostic criteria for neuromyelitis optica spectrum disorders. *Neurology* **2015**, *85*, 177–189. [CrossRef]
6. Lennon, P.V.A.; Wingerchuk, D.M.; Kryzer, T.J.; Pittock, S.J.; Lucchinetti, C.F.; Fujihara, K.; Nakashima, I.; Weinshenker, B.G. A serum autoantibody marker of neuromyelitis optica: Distinction from multiple sclerosis. *Lancet* **2004**, *364*, 2106–2112. [CrossRef]
7. Bradl, M.; Misu, T.; Takahashi, T.; Watanabe, M.; Mader, S.; Reindl, M.; Adzemovic, M.; Bauer, J.; Berger, T.; Fujihara, K.; et al. Neuromyelitis optica: Pathogenicity of patient immunoglobulin in vivo. *Ann. Neurol.* **2009**, *66*, 630–643. [CrossRef]
8. Oh, J.; Levy, M. Neuromyelitis Optica: An Antibody-Mediated Disorder of the Central Nervous System. *Neurol. Res. Int.* **2012**, *2012*, 460825. [CrossRef]
9. Nielsen, S.; Nagelhus, E.A.; Amiry-Moghaddam, M.; Bourque, C.; Agre, P.; Ottersen, O.P. Specialized Membrane Domains for Water Transport in Glial Cells: High-Resolution Immunogold Cytochemistry of Aquaporin-4 in Rat Brain. *J. Neurosci.* **1997**, *17*, 171–180. [CrossRef]
10. Psenicka, M.W.; Smith, B.C.; Tinkey, R.A.; Williams, J.L. Connecting Neuroinflammation and Neurodegeneration in Multiple Sclerosis: Are Oligodendrocyte Precursor Cells a Nexus of Disease? *Front. Cell. Neurosci.* **2021**, *15*, 221. [CrossRef]
11. Allen, N.J.; Bennett, M.; Foo, L.C.; Wang, G.; Chakraborty, C.; Smith, S.J.; Barres, B.A. Astrocyte glypicans 4 and 6 promote formation of excitatory synapses via GluA1 AMPA receptors. *Nature* **2012**, *486*, 410–414. [CrossRef]
12. Alvarez, J.I.; Dodelet-Devillers, A.; Kebir, H.; Ifergan, I.; Fabre, P.J.; Terouz, S.; Sabbagh, M.; Wosik, K.; Bourbonnière, L.; Bernard, M.; et al. The Hedgehog Pathway Promotes Blood-Brain Barrier Integrity and CNS Immune Quiescence. *Science* **2011**, *334*, 1727–1731. [CrossRef]
13. Chung, W.-S.; Clarke, L.E.; Wang, G.X.; Stafford, B.K.; Sher, A.; Chakraborty, C.; Joung, J.; Foo, L.C.; Thompson, A.; Chen, C.; et al. Astrocytes mediate synapse elimination through MEGF10 and MERTK pathways. *Nature* **2013**, *504*, 394–400. [CrossRef]
14. Molofsky, A.V.; Kelley, K.W.; Tsai, H.-H.; Redmond, S.A.; Chang, S.M.; Madireddy, L.; Chan, J.R.; Baranzini, S.E.; Ullian, E.M.; Rowitch, D.H. Astrocyte-encoded positional cues maintain sensorimotor circuit integrity. *Nature* **2014**, *509*, 189–194. [CrossRef]
15. Tsai, H.-H.; Li, H.; Fuentealba, L.C.; Molofsky, A.V.; Taveira-Marques, R.; Zhuang, H.; Tenney, A.; Murnen, A.T.; Fancy, S.P.J.; Merkle, F.; et al. Regional Astrocyte Allocation Regulates CNS Synaptogenesis and Repair. *Science* **2012**, *337*, 358–362. [CrossRef]
16. Farina, C.; Aloisi, F.; Meinl, E. Astrocytes are active players in cerebral innate immunity. *Trends Immunol.* **2007**, *28*, 138–145. [CrossRef]
17. Chakraborty, S.; Kaushik, D.K.; Gupta, M.; Basu, A. Inflammasome signaling at the heart of central nervous system pathology. *J. Neurosci. Res.* **2010**, *88*, 1615–1631. [CrossRef]
18. Carpentier, P.A.; Begolka, W.S.; Olson, J.K.; Elhofy, A.; Karpus, W.J.; Miller, S.D. Differential activation of astrocytes by innate and adaptive immune stimuli. *Glia* **2004**, *49*, 360–374. [CrossRef]
19. Oh, J.-W.; Schwiebert, L.M.; Benveniste, E.N. Cytokine regulation of CC and CXC chemokine expression by human astrocytes. *J. Neurovirol.* **1999**, *5*, 82–94. [CrossRef]
20. Paul, S.; Mondal, G.P.; Bhattacharyya, R.; Ghosh, K.C.; Bhat, I.A. Neuromyelitis optica spectrum disorders. *J. Neurol. Sci.* **2021**, *420*, 117225. [CrossRef]
21. Jarius, S.; Wildemann, B. AQP4 antibodies in neuromyelitis optica: Diagnostic and pathogenetic relevance. *Nat. Rev. Neurol.* **2010**, *6*, 383–392. [CrossRef]
22. Jarius, S.; Paul, F.; Franciotta, D.; Waters, P.; Zipp, F.; Hohlfeld, R.; Vincent, A.; Wildemann, B. Mechanisms of Disease: Aquaporin-4 antibodies in neuromyelitis optica. *Nat. Clin. Pract. Cardiovasc. Med.* **2008**, *4*, 202–214. [CrossRef]
23. Hardy, T.A.; Reddel, S.W.; Barnett, M.H.; Palace, J.; Lucchinetti, C.F.; Weinshenker, B.G. Atypical inflammatory demyelinating syndromes of the CNS. *Lancet Neurol.* **2016**, *15*, 967–981. [CrossRef]
24. Asgari, N.; Lillevang, S.T.; Skejoe, H.P.B.; Falah, M.; Stenager, E.; Kyvik, K.O. A population-based study of neuromyelitis optica in Caucasians. *Neurology* **2011**, *76*, 1589–1595. [CrossRef]
25. Wingerchuk, D.M.; Lennon, V.A.; Lucchinetti, C.F.; Pittock, S.J.; Weinshenker, B.G. The spectrum of neuromyelitis optica. *Lancet Neurol.* **2007**, *6*, 805–815. [CrossRef]

26. Jasiak-Zatonska, M.; Kalinowska-Lyszczarz, A.; Michalak, S.; Kozubski, W. The Immunology of Neuromyelitis Optica—Current Knowledge, Clinical Implications, Controversies and Future Perspectives. *Int. J. Mol. Sci.* **2016**, *17*, 273. [CrossRef]
27. Levy, M.; Wildemann, B.; Jarius, S.; Orellano, B.; Sasidharan, S.; Weber, M.S.; Stuve, O. Immunopathogenesis of Neuromyelitis Optica. *Adv. Immunol.* **2014**, *121*, 213–242. [CrossRef]
28. Lucchinetti, C.F.; Mandler, R.N.; McGavern, D.; Bruck, W.; Gleich, G.; Ransohoff, R.M.; Trebst, C.; Weinshenker, B.; Wingerchuk, D.; Parisi, J.E.; et al. A role for humoral mechanisms in the pathogenesis of Devic's neuromyelitis optica. *Brain* **2002**, *125*, 1450–1461. [CrossRef]
29. Huang, D.W.; Sherman, B.T.; Lempicki, R.A. Systematic and integrative analysis of large gene lists using DAVID bioinformatics resources. *Nat. Protoc.* **2009**, *4*, 44–57. [CrossRef]
30. Jarius, S.; Paul, F.; Weinshenker, B.G.; Levy, M.; Kim, H.J.; Wildemann, B. Neuromyelitis Optica. *Nat. Rev. Dis. Primers* **2020**, *6*, 85. [CrossRef]
31. Wang, K.; Yin, X.M.; Chao, D.T.; Milliman, C.L.; Korsmeyer, S.J. BID: A novel BH3 domain-only death agonist. *Genes Dev.* **1996**, *10*, 2859–2869. [CrossRef]
32. Zinkel, S.S.; Hurov, K.E.; Ong, C.; Abtahi, F.M.; Gross, A.; Korsmeyer, S.J. A Role for Proapoptotic BID in the DNA-Damage Response. *Cell* **2005**, *122*, 579–591. [CrossRef]
33. Yeretssian, G.; Correa, R.; Doiron, K.; Fitzgerald, P.; Dillon, C.P.; Green, D.; Reed, J.C.; Saleh, M. Non-apoptotic role of BID in inflammation and innate immunity. *Nature* **2011**, *474*, 96–99. [CrossRef]
34. Nachbur, U.; Vince, J.E.; O'Reilly, L.A.; Strasser, A.; Silke, J. Is BID required for NOD signalling? *Nature* **2012**, *488*, E4–E6. [CrossRef]
35. Schuler, M.; Green, D.R. Mechanisms of p53-dependent apoptosis. *Biochem. Soc. Trans.* **2001**, *29*, 684–688. [CrossRef]
36. Sax, J.K.; Fei, P.; Murphy, M.E.; Bernhard, E.; Korsmeyer, S.J.; El-Deiry, W.S. BID regulation by p53 contributes to chemosensitivity. *Nat. Curell Biol.* **2002**, *4*, 842–849. [CrossRef]
37. Tatematsu, M.; Yoshida, R.; Morioka, Y.; Ishii, N.; Funami, K.; Watanabe, A.; Saeki, K.; Seya, T.; Matsumoto, M. Raftlin Controls Lipopolysaccharide-Induced TLR4 Internalization and TICAM-1 Signaling in a Cell Type–Specific Manner. *J. Immunol.* **2016**, *196*, 3865–3876. [CrossRef]
38. Marta, M. Toll-like Receptors in Multiple Sclerosis Mouse Experimental Models. *Ann. N. Y. Acad. Sci.* **2009**, *1173*, 458–462. [CrossRef]
39. Haase, R.; Kirschning, C.J.; Sing, A.; Schröttner, P.; Fukase, K.; Kusumoto, S.; Wagner, H.; Heesemann, J.; Ruckdeschel, K. A Dominant Role of Toll-Like Receptor 4 in the Signaling of Apoptosis in Bacteria-Faced Macrophages. *J. Immunol.* **2003**, *171*, 4294–4303. [CrossRef]
40. Correa, R.G.; Milutinovic, S.; Reed, J.C. Roles of NOD1 (NLRC1) and NOD2 (NLRC2) in innate immunity and inflammatory diseases. *Biosci. Rep.* **2012**, *32*, 597–608. [CrossRef]
41. Farzi, A.; Reichmann, F.; Meinitzer, A.; Mayerhofer, R.; Jain, P.; Hassan, A.; Fröhlich, E.E.; Wagner, K.; Painsipp, E.; Rinner, B.; et al. Synergistic effects of NOD1 or NOD2 and TLR4 activation on mouse sickness behavior in relation to immune and brain activity markers. *Brain Behav. Immun.* **2014**, *44*, 106–120. [CrossRef] [PubMed]
42. Gomez-Nicola, D.; Valle-Argos, B.; Pita-Thomas, D.W.; Nieto-Sampedro, M. Interleukin 15 expression in the CNS: Blockade of its activity prevents glial activation after an inflammatory injury. *Glia* **2008**, *56*, 494–505. [CrossRef] [PubMed]
43. Li, H.-D.; Li, M.; Shi, E.; Jin, W.-N.; Wood, K.; Gonzales, R.; Liu, Q. A translocator protein 18 kDa agonist protects against cerebral ischemia/reperfusion injury. *J. Neuroinflamm.* **2017**, *14*, 151. [CrossRef] [PubMed]
44. Li, M.; Li, Z.; Ren, H.; Jin, W.-N.; Wood, K.; Liu, Q.; Sheth, K.N.; Shi, F.-D. Colony stimulating factor 1 receptor inhibition eliminates microglia and attenuates brain injury after intracerebral hemorrhage. *J. Cereb. Blood Flow Metab.* **2016**, *37*, 2383–2395. [CrossRef]
45. Li, M.; Li, Z.; Yao, Y.; Jin, W.-N.; Wood, K.; Liu, Q.; Shi, F.-D.; Hao, J. Astrocyte-derived interleukin-15 exacerbates ischemic brain injury via propagation of cellular immunity. *Proc. Natl. Acad. Sci. USA* **2017**, *114*, E396–E405. [CrossRef]
46. Saikali, P.; Antel, J.P.; Pittet, C.L.; Newcombe, J.; Arbour, N. Contribution of Astrocyte-Derived IL-15 to CD8 T Cell Effector Functions in Multiple Sclerosis. *J. Immunol.* **2010**, *185*, 5693–5703. [CrossRef]
47. Li, Z.; Han, J.; Ren, H.; Ma, C.-G.; Shi, F.-D.; Liu, Q.; Li, M. Astrocytic Interleukin-15 Reduces Pathology of Neuromyelitis Optica in Mice. *Front. Immunol.* **2018**, *9*, 523. [CrossRef]
48. Zheng, X.; Wang, Y.; Wei, H.; Ling, B.; Sun, R.; Tian, Z. Bcl-xL is associated with the anti-apoptotic effect of IL-15 on the survival of CD56dim natural killer cells. *Mol. Immunol.* **2008**, *45*, 2559–2569. [CrossRef]
49. Domercq, M.; Etxebarria, E.; Pérez-Samartín, A.; Matute, C. Excitotoxic oligodendrocyte death and axonal damage induced by glutamate transporter inhibition. *Glia* **2005**, *52*, 36–46. [CrossRef]
50. Wilke, S.; Thomas, R.; Allcock, N.; Fern, R. Mechanism of Acute Ischemic Injury of Oligodendroglia in Early Myelinating White Matter: The Importance of Astrocyte Injury and Glutamate Release. *J. Neuropathol. Exp. Neurol.* **2004**, *63*, 872–881. [CrossRef]
51. Hinson, S.R.; Roemer, S.F.; Lucchinetti, C.F.; Fryer, J.P.; Kryzer, T.J.; Chamberlain, J.L.; Howe, C.; Pittock, S.J.; Lennon, V.A. Aquaporin-4–binding autoantibodies in patients with neuromyelitis optica impair glutamate transport by down-regulating EAAT 2. *J. Exp. Med.* **2008**, *205*, 2473–2481. [CrossRef] [PubMed]
52. Papadopoulos, M.C.; Kim, J.K.; Verkman, A. Extracellular Space Diffusion in Central Nervous System: Anisotropic Diffusion Measured by Elliptical Surface Photobleaching. *Biophys. J.* **2005**, *89*, 3660–3668. [CrossRef] [PubMed]

53. Hickman, S.J.; Toosy, A.T.; Jones, S.J.; Altmann, D.R.; Miszkiel, K.A.; MacManus, D.; Barker, G.; Plant, G.T.; Thompson, A.J.; Miller, D.H. Serial magnetization transfer imaging in acute optic neuritis. *Brain* **2003**, *127*, 692–700. [CrossRef]
54. Ludwin, S.K. Phagocytosis in the rat optic nerve following Wallerian degeneration. *Acta Neuropathol.* **1990**, *80*, 266–273. [CrossRef]
55. Saini, H.; Fernandez, G.; Kerr, D.; Levy, M. Differential expression of aquaporin-4 isoforms localizes with neuromyelitis optica disease activity. *J. Neuroimmunol.* **2010**, *221*, 68–72. [CrossRef] [PubMed]
56. Brill, L.; Lavon, I.; Vaknin-Dembinsky, A. Reduced expression of the IL7Ra signaling pathway in Neuromyelitis optica. *J. Neuroimmunol.* **2018**, *324*, 81–89. [CrossRef]
57. Liu, Y.; Fu, Y.; Schoonheim, M.M.; Zhang, N.; Fan, M.; Su, L.; Shen, Y.; Yan, Y.; Yang, L.; Wang, Q.; et al. Structural MRI substrates of cognitive impairment in neuromyelitis optica. *Neurology* **2015**, *85*, 1491–1499. [CrossRef]
58. Cao, G.; Duan, Y.; Zhang, N.; Sun, J.; Li, H.; Li, Y.; Li, Y.; Zeng, C.; Han, X.; Zhou, F.; et al. Brain MRI characteristics in neuromyelitis optica spectrum disorders: A large multi-center retrospective study in China. *Mult. Scler. Relat. Disord.* **2020**, *46*, 102475. [CrossRef]
59. Hyun, J.-W.; Park, G.; Kwak, K.; Jo, H.-J.; Joung, A.; Kim, J.-H.; Lee, S.H.; Kim, S.-H.; Lee, J.-M.; Kim, H.J. Deep gray matter atrophy in neuromyelitis optica spectrum disorder and multiple sclerosis. *Eur. J. Neurol.* **2016**, *24*, 437–445. [CrossRef]
60. Yung, H.W.; Bal-Price, A.K.; Brown, G.C.; Tolkovsky, A.M. Nitric oxide-induced cell death of cerebrocortical murine astrocytes is mediated through p53- and Bax-dependent pathways. *J. Neurochem.* **2004**, *89*, 812–821. [CrossRef]
61. Kernt, M.; Arend, N.; Buerger, A.; Mann, T.; Haritoglou, C.; Ulbig, M.W.; Kampik, A.; Hirneiss, C. Idebenone Prevents Human Optic Nerve Head Astrocytes From Oxidative Stress, Apoptosis, and Senescence by Stabilizing BAX/Bcl-2 Ratio. *J. Glaucoma* **2013**, *22*, 404–412. [CrossRef] [PubMed]
62. Giffard, R.G.; Swanson, R.A. Ischemia-induced programmed cell death in astrocytes. *Glia* **2005**, *50*, 299–306. [CrossRef] [PubMed]
63. Zhai, D.; Luciano, F.; Zhu, X.; Guo, B.; Satterthwait, A.C.; Reed, J.C. Humanin Binds and Nullifies Bid Activity by Blocking Its Activation of Bax and Bak. *J. Biol. Chem.* **2005**, *280*, 15815–15824. [CrossRef] [PubMed]
64. Renshaw, S.; Dempsey, C.E.; Barnes, F.A.; Bagstaff, S.M.; Dower, S.K.; Bingle, C.; Whyte, M.K.B. Three Novel Bid Proteins Generated by Alternative Splicing of the Human Bid Gene. *J. Biol. Chem.* **2004**, *279*, 2846–2855. [CrossRef]
65. Strober, W.; Murray, P.J.; Kitani, A.; Watanabe, T. Signalling pathways and molecular interactions of NOD1 and NOD2. *Nat. Rev. Immunol.* **2006**, *6*, 9–20. [CrossRef]
66. Chamaillard, M.; Hashimoto, M.; Horie, Y.; Masumoto, J.; Qiu, S.; Saab, L.; Ogura, Y.; Kawasaki, A.; Fukase, K.; Kusumoto, S.; et al. An essential role for NOD1 in host recognition of bacterial peptidoglycan containing diaminopimelic acid. *Nat. Immunol.* **2003**, *4*, 702–707. [CrossRef]
67. Wang, H.; Wang, K.; Wang, C.; Xu, F.; Qiu, W.; Hu, X. Increased Plasma Interleukin-32 Expression in Patients with Neuromyelitis Optica. *J. Clin. Immunol.* **2013**, *33*, 666–670. [CrossRef]
68. Gorina, R.; Font-Nieves, M.; Márquez-Kisinousky, L.; Santalucia, T.; Planas, A.M. Astrocyte TLR4 activation induces a proinflammatory environment through the interplay between MyD88-dependent NFκB signaling, MAPK, and Jak1/Stat1 pathways. *Glia* **2010**, *59*, 242–255. [CrossRef]
69. Barros, P.O.; Linhares, U.C.; Teixeira, B.; Kasahara, T.M.; Ferreira, T.B.; Alvarenga, R.; Hygino, J.; Silva-Filho, R.G.; Bittencourt, V.C.B.; Andrade, R.M.; et al. High in vitro immune reactivity to Escherichia coli in neuromyelitis optica patients is correlated with both neurological disabilities and elevated plasma lipopolysaccharide levels. *Hum. Immunol.* **2013**, *74*, 1080–1087. [CrossRef]
70. Dias, A.S.; Sacramento, P.M.; Lopes, L.M.; Sales, M.C.; Castro, C.; Araújo, A.C.R.; Ornelas, A.M.; Aguiar, R.S.; Silva-Filho, R.G.; Alvarenga, R.; et al. TLR-2 and TLR-4 agonists favor expansion of CD4+ T cell subsets implicated in the severity of neuromyelitis optica spectrum disorders. *Mult. Scler. Relat. Disord.* **2019**, *34*, 66–76. [CrossRef]
71. Tradtrantip, L.; Yao, X.; Su, T.; Smith, A.J.; Verkman, A.S. Bystander mechanism for complement-initiated early oligodendrocyte injury in neuromyelitis optica. *Acta Neuropathol.* **2017**, *134*, 35–44. [CrossRef] [PubMed]
72. Domingues, H.; Portugal, C.; Socodato, R.; Relvas, J.B. Oligodendrocyte, Astrocyte, and Microglia Crosstalk in Myelin Development, Damage, and Repair. *Front. Cell Dev. Biol.* **2016**, *4*, 71. [CrossRef] [PubMed]
73. Sloane, J.A.; Batt, C.; Ma, Y.; Harris, Z.M.; Trapp, B.; Vartanian, T. Hyaluronan blocks oligodendrocyte progenitor maturation and remyelination through TLR2. *Proc. Natl. Acad. Sci. USA* **2010**, *107*, 11555–11560. [CrossRef]
74. Back, S.A.; Tuohy, T.M.F.; Chen, H.; Wallingford, N.; Craig, A.; Struve, J.; Luo, N.L.; Banine, F.; Liu, Y.; Chang, A.; et al. Hyaluronan accumulates in demyelinated lesions and inhibits oligodendrocyte progenitor maturation. *Nat. Med.* **2005**, *11*, 966–972. [CrossRef] [PubMed]
75. Šišková, Z.; Yong, V.W.; Nomden, A.; van Strien, M.; Hoekstra, D.; Baron, W. Fibronectin attenuates process outgrowth in oligodendrocytes by mislocalizing MMP-9 activity. *Mol. Cell. Neurosci.* **2009**, *42*, 234–242. [CrossRef]
76. Stoffels, J.M.J.; de Jonge, J.C.; Stancic, M.; Nomden, A.; van Strien, M.E.; Ma, D.; Šišková, Z.; Maier, O.; Ffrench-Constant, C.; Franklin, R.J.M.; et al. Fibronectin aggregation in multiple sclerosis lesions impairs remyelination. *Brain* **2013**, *136*, 116–131. [CrossRef]
77. Patel, J.R.; Williams, J.L.; Muccigrosso, M.M.; Liu, L.; Sun, T.; Rubin, J.B.; Klein, R.S. Astrocyte TNFR2 is required for CXCL12-mediated regulation of oligodendrocyte progenitor proliferation and differentiation within the adult CNS. *Acta Neuropathol.* **2012**, *124*, 847–860. [CrossRef]

78. Zeger, M.; Popken, G.; Zhang, J.; Xuan, S.; Lu, Q.R.; Schwab, M.H.; Nave, K.-A.; Rowitch, D.; D'Ercole, A.J.; Ye, P. Insulin-like growth factor type 1 receptor signaling in the cells of oligodendrocyte lineage is required for normalin vivo oligodendrocyte development and myelination. *Glia* **2006**, *55*, 400–411. [CrossRef]
79. Colpitts, S.L.; Stoklasek, T.A.; Plumlee, C.R.; Obar, J.J.; Guo, C.; Lefrançois, L. Cutting Edge: The Role of IFN-α Receptor and MyD88 Signaling in Induction of IL-15 Expression In Vivo. *J. Immunol.* **2012**, *188*, 2483–2487. [CrossRef]
80. DePaolo, R.W.; Abadie, V.; Tang, F.; Fehlnerpeach, H.; Hall, J.A.; Wang, W.; Marietta, E.V.; Kasarda, D.D.; Waldmann, T.A.; Murray, J.A.; et al. Co-adjuvant effects of retinoic acid and IL-15 induce inflammatory immunity to dietary antigens. *Nature* **2011**, *471*, 220–224. [CrossRef]
81. Xu, M.; Yang, L.; Rong, J.-G.; Ni, Y.; Gu, W.-W.; Luo, Y.; Ishidoh, K.; Katunuma, N.; Li, Z.-S.; Zhang, H.-L. Inhibition of cysteine cathepsin B and L activation in astrocytes contributes to neuroprotection against cerebral ischemia via blocking the tBid-mitochondrial apoptotic signaling pathway. *Glia* **2014**, *62*, 855–880. [CrossRef] [PubMed]
82. Becattini, B.; Sareth, S.; Zhai, D.; Crowell, K.J.; Leone, M.; Reed, J.C.; Pellecchia, M. Targeting Apoptosis via Chemical Design: Inhibition of Bid-Induced Cell Death by Small Organic Molecules. *Chem. Biol.* **2004**, *11*, 1107–1117. [CrossRef] [PubMed]
83. Tsang, H.-F.; Xue, W.; Koh, S.-P.; Chiu, Y.-M.; Ng, L.P.-W.; Wong, S.-C.C. NanoString, a novel digital color-coded barcode technology: Current and future applications in molecular diagnostics. *Expert Rev. Mol. Diagn.* **2016**, *17*, 95–103. [CrossRef] [PubMed]
84. Chen, Y.; Balasubramaniyan, V.; Peng, J.; Hurlock, E.C.; Tallquist, M.; Li, J.; Lu, Q.R. Isolation and culture of rat and mouse oligodendrocyte precursor cells. *Nat. Protoc.* **2007**, *2*, 1044–1051. [CrossRef]
85. Barateiro, A.; Fernandes, A. Temporal oligodendrocyte lineage progression: In vitro models of proliferation, differentiation and myelination. *Biochim. Biophys. Acta* **2014**, *1843*, 1917–1929. [CrossRef]
86. Zveik, O.; Fainstein, N.; Rechtman, A.; Haham, N.; Ganz, T.; Lavon, I.; Brill, L.; Vaknin-Dembinsky, A. Cerebrospinal fluid of progressive multiple sclerosis patients reduces differentiation and immune functions of oligodendrocyte progenitor cells. *Glia* **2022**, *70*, 1191–1290. [CrossRef]
87. Rio, D.C.; Ares, M., Jr.; Hannon, G.J.; Nilsen, T.W. Purification of RNA Using TRIzol (TRI Reagent). *Cold Spring Harb. Protoc.* **2010**, *2010*, pdb-prot5439. [CrossRef]
88. Ganz, T.; Fainstein, N.; Elad, A.; Lachish, M.; Goldfarb, S.; Einstein, O.; Ben-Hur, T. Microbial pathogens induce neurodegeneration in Alzheimer's disease mice: Protection by microglial regulation. *J. Neuroinflamm.* **2022**, *19*, 5. [CrossRef]
89. Simon, J.H.; Li, D.; Traboulsee, A.; Coyle, P.K.; Arnold, D.L.; Barkhof, F.; Frank, J.A.; Grossman, R.; Paty, D.W.; Radue, E.W.; et al. STATEMENT Standardized MR Imaging Protocol for Multiple Sclerosis: Consortium of MS Centers Consensus. *Am. J. Neuroradiol.* **2006**, *27*, 455–461.
90. Rechtman, A.; Brill, L.; Zveik, O.; Uliel, B.; Haham, N.; Bick, A.S.; Levin, N.; Vaknin-Dembinsky, A. Volumetric Brain Loss Correlates With a Relapsing MOGAD Disease Course. *Front. Neurol.* **2022**, *13*, 867190. [CrossRef]
91. Manjón, J.V.; Coupé, P. volBrain: An Online MRI Brain Volumetry System. *Front. Neuroinform.* **2016**, *10*, 30. [CrossRef] [PubMed]

International Journal of *Molecular Sciences*

MDPI

Article

Candidate Modifier Genes for the Penetrance of Leber's Hereditary Optic Neuropathy

Hui-Chen Cheng [1,2,3,4,5], Sheng-Chu Chi [2], Chiao-Ying Liang [6], Jenn-Yah Yu [4,5] and An-Guor Wang [2,3,*]

1 Program in Molecular Medicine, College of Life Sciences, National Yang Ming Chiao Tung University, Taipei 11221, Taiwan
2 Department of Ophthalmology, Taipei Veterans General Hospital, 201 Sec. 2, Shih-Pai Rd., Taipei 11217, Taiwan
3 Department of Ophthalmology, School of Medicine, National Yang Ming Chiao Tung University, Taipei 11221, Taiwan
4 Department of Life Sciences and Institute of Genome Sciences, College of Life Sciences, National Yang Ming Chiao Tung University, Taipei 11221, Taiwan
5 Brain Research Center, National Yang Ming Chiao Tung University, Taipei 11221, Taiwan
6 Department of Ophthalmology, Taichung Veterans General Hospital, Taichung 40705, Taiwan
* Correspondence: agwang@vghtpe.gov.tw; Tel.: +886-2-2875-7325; Fax: +886-2-2876-1351

Abstract: Leber's hereditary optic neuropathy (LHON) is a maternally transmitted disease caused by mitochondria DNA (mtDNA) mutation. It is characterized by acute and subacute visual loss predominantly affecting young men. The mtDNA mutation is transmitted to all maternal lineages. However, only approximately 50% of men and 10% of women harboring a pathogenic mtDNA mutation develop optic neuropathy, reflecting both the incomplete penetrance and its unexplained male prevalence, where over 80% of patients are male. Nuclear modifier genes have been presumed to affect the penetrance of LHON. With conventional genetic methods, prior studies have failed to solve the underlying pathogenesis. Whole exome sequencing (WES) is a new molecular technique for sequencing the protein-coding region of all genes in a whole genome. We performed WES from five families with 17 members. These samples were divided into the proband group (probands with acute onset of LHON, $n = 7$) and control group (carriers including mother and relative carriers with mtDNSA 11778 mutation, without clinical manifestation of LHON, $n = 10$). Through whole exome analysis, we found that many mitochondria related (MT-related) nuclear genes have high percentage of variants in either the proband group or control group. The MT genes with a difference over 0.3 of mutation percentage between the proband and control groups include AK4, NSUN4, RDH13, COQ3, and FAHD1. In addition, the pathway analysis revealed that these genes were associated with cofactor metabolism pathways. Family-based analysis showed that several candidate MT genes including METAP1D (c.41G > T), ACACB (c.1029del), ME3 (c.972G > C), NIPSNAP3B (c.280G > C, c.476C > G), and NSUN4 (c.4A > G) were involved in the penetrance of LHON. A GWAS (genome wide association study) was performed, which found that ADGRG5 (Chr16:575620A:G), POLE4 (Chr2:7495872T:G), ERMAP (Chr1:4283044A:G), PIGR (Chr1:2069357C:T;2069358G:A), CDC42BPB (Chr14:102949A:G), PROK1 (Chr1:1104562A:G), BCAN (Chr 1:1566582C:T), and NES (Chr1:1566698A:G,1566705T:C, 1566707T:C) may be involved. The incomplete penetrance and male prevalence are still the major unexplained issues in LHON. Through whole exome analysis, we found several MT genes with a high percentage of variants were involved in a family-based analysis. Pathway analysis suggested a difference in the mutation burden of MT genes underlining the biosynthesis and metabolism pathways. In addition, the GWAS analysis also revealed several candidate nuclear modifier genes. The new technology of WES contributes to provide a highly efficient candidate gene screening function in molecular genetics.

Keywords: Leber's hereditary optic neuropathy; LHON; whole exome sequencing; nuclear modifier genes

Citation: Cheng, H.-C.; Chi, S.-C.; Liang, C.-Y.; Yu, J.-Y.; Wang, A.-G. Candidate Modifier Genes for the Penetrance of Leber's Hereditary Optic Neuropathy. *Int. J. Mol. Sci.* **2022**, *23*, 11891. https://doi.org/10.3390/ijms231911891

Academic Editors: Rongkung Tsai and Neil R. Miller

Received: 17 August 2022
Accepted: 4 October 2022
Published: 6 October 2022

1. Introduction

Leber's hereditary optic neuropathy (LHON) is a maternally transmitted disease characterized by acute and subacute visual loss predominantly affecting young men [1–3]. It usually onsets between 15 and 35 years of age, with a male predominance [1,4]. The course of visual loss is usually acute or subacute. The optic disc becomes hyperemic and is associated with peripapillary telangiectasia. The retinal nerve fiber layers are swollen. Over months, the disc edema subsides and becomes pale and atrophic. Visual acuity deteriorates to the degree of less than 20/200, commonly accompanied by a cecocentral scotoma [1]. Both eyes are involved with or without intervals [1]. Three primary mitochondrial DNA (mtDNA) mutations underlie the main pathogenesis of LHON. The first association of a mtDNA 11778 mutation with LHON was reported by Wallace and colleagues in 1988 [5]. These three primary mutations of mtDNA 11778, 14484, and 3460 encodes the NADH dehydrogenase subunit 4, subunit 6, and subunit 1 of Complex I of the respiratory chain, respectively [5–8].

Despite intense studies on the clinical and molecular aspects of LHON from 1988, the pathogenesis is still unclear, especially in the area of gender prevalence and penetrance. The mtDNA mutation is transmitted to all maternal lineages. However, only approximately 50% of men and 10% of women harboring a pathogenic mtDNA mutation develop optic neuropathy, reflecting both the incomplete penetrance and the gender prevalence difference [1]. LHON is well-known for its male prevalence, where over 80% of patients are male [1,2]. This male predominance exists in different mutation groups with a male to female ratio of 3:1, 4–6:1, and 8:1 in patients harboring the 3460, 11778, and 14484 mutations, respectively [1,4]. The reason for this male predominance remains unknown.

The penetrance in LHON is incomplete and variable, where a positive family history was found in 50% of patients with the 11778 mutation, 71% with the 3460 mutations, and 100% with the 14484 mutation [1,9]. The penetrance of LHON is variable, even with the same mutation in homoplasmic fashion within the same family in a different pedigree branch [1,10]. All of these features cannot be explained by a single point mutation of mtDNA alone. Thus, genetic and epigenetic factors have been presumed to be involved in the penetrance of the LHON. Previously investigated genetic modifiers include heteroplasmy [11–14], secondary mtDNA mutations [15,16], mtDNA haplogroup [17–19], X-linked modifying gene or susceptibility locus [20–22], and other nuclear genes [23]. Tobacco and alcohol consumption have been proposed to be related to the onset of LHON, but the results are controversial from different studies [24,25].

Whole exome sequencing (WES) is a molecular technique for sequencing the protein-coding region of all genes in a whole genome. As humans have about 180,000 exons, constituting about 1% of the human genome, to sequence the exonic DNA, one needs to use high-throughput next generation DNA sequencing technology. WES may help to identify genetic mutations that alter protein sequences in either Mendelian and common polygenic diseases. It could be performed at a much lower cost than whole-genome sequencing. Thus, whole exome sequencing has been used in different fields of basic research and clinical practice [26].

The pathogenesis of incomplete penetrance and male prevalence in LHON is still unclear [1]. The comparative genomic hybridization (CGH) technique detects the chromosomal copy number changes. With the CGH technique, we did not detect any chromosomal abnormalities in LHON patients or in unaffected relatives [27]. The male predominance suggests that an X-linked modifying gene acts in concert with the pathogenic mtDNA mutation [20,22]. However, many other previous studies have failed to support an X-linked susceptibility locus based on linkage analysis [10], X-inactivation analysis or skewed X-inactivation in the affected tissues [28], or meiotic breakpoint mapping [29]. There have been many other studies investigating LHON susceptibility nuclear genes such as NDUFA-1, EPHX1 . . . etc. [30,31] by using conventional genetic approaches. However, no conclusive evidence supports the pathogenic role of these genetic candidates.

With the new technology of whole exome sequencing (WES), Jiang PP et al. searched the nuclear modifier gene in a LHON family with four family members, and presumed

YARS2 as the candidate gene [32]. YARS2 gene is yet to be verified by further study for its role in the LHON penetrance, since it came from a single family only.

In this study, we aimed to identify the LHON susceptibility allele(s) in the nuclear genomes by using whole exome sequencing technology. We intended to examine multiple LHON families including the LHON proband (11778 G > A mutation), adult sibling carrier, and the proband's mother. By taking advantage of a larger cohort with multiple LHON families, we might be able to find the nuclear modifier gene responsible for the disease penetrance.

2. Results

A total of five families with the mt11778G > A mutation including seven patients and 10 relative carriers were enrolled in this study (Figure 1B).

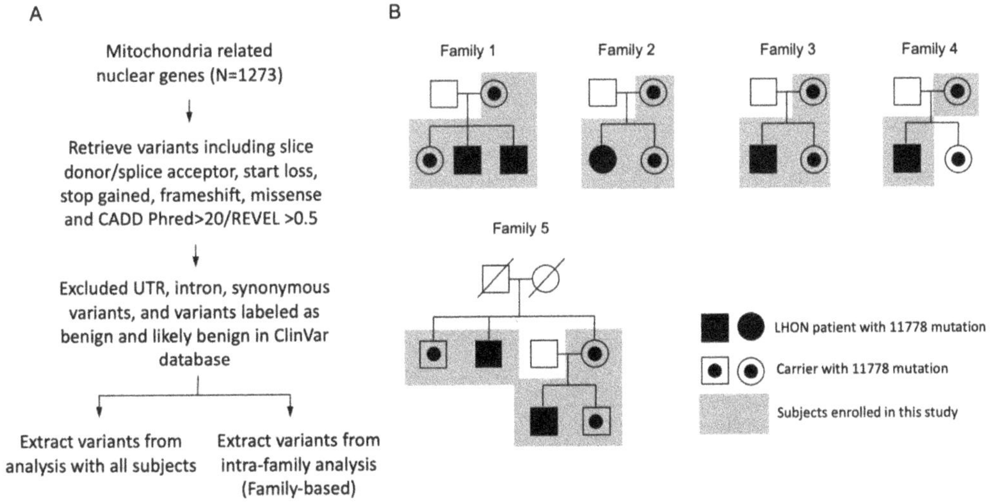

Figure 1. (**A**) Summary of exome sequencing in this study. (**B**) Five Chinese pedigrees with LHON. Vision-impaired individuals are indicated by blackened symbols.

The mean age of the LHON patients was significant younger than the carrier group (mean age, 30.71 years in the LHON vs. 50.40 years in the carrier group, $p = 0.005$). There was a significant male predominance in the LHON group compared to female predominance in the carrier group (male percentage, 86% in the LHON vs. 20% in the carrier group, $p = 0.01$). The LHON patients had significantly worse BCVA compared to the carrier group (mean logMAR, 1.80 in the LHON vs. 0.02 in the carrier, $p < 0.001$). Regarding the other ocular examinations, the LHON patients had worse VF and a thinner peripapillary RNFL and GCIPL thickness on OCT compared to the carrier group (all $p < 0.05$) (Table 1).

2.1. *Identification of Nuclear Modifier Genes*

To identify the nuclear modifier gene for the phenotypic penetrance of the mtDNA 11778 mutation associated LHON, we performed exome sequencing of DNA from five families with 17 members. These samples were divided into the proband group (probands with acute onset of LHON, $n = 7$) and control group (carriers including mother and relative carriers with the mtDNA 11778 mutation, without clinical manifestation of LHON, $n = 10$).

Table 1. The basic characteristics of patients with Leber's hereditary optic neuropathy (LHON) and their relative carrier with the mitochondrial 11778 mutation.

	LHON Patient (*n* = 7)	Relative Carrier (*n* = 10) *	*p* Value #
Age in years, mean (SD)	30.71 (11.32)	50.40 (12.87)	0.005
Gender			
Male, *n* (%)	6 (86%)	2 (20%)	0.01
Female, *n* (%)	1 (14%)	8 (80%)	
Best-corrected visual acuity			<0.001
logMAR, mean (SD) [range]	1.80 (0.68) [0.6~2.8]	0.02 (0.08) [−0.18~0.22]	
Snellen visual acuity [range]	[LP~0.3]	[0.6~1.5]	
RNFL thickness, mean (SD)	60.82 (11.69)	101.43 (5.92)	<0.001
GCIPL thickness, mean (SD)	50.42 (3.15)	76.33 (8.94)	<0.001
MD of VF in dB, mean (SD)	−17.19 (12.52)	−1.11 (2.08)	0.03

* One patient in the carrier group had poor BCVA due to cataract. # *t*-test for continuous variables and Fisher's exact test for categorical variables. GCIPL, ganglion cell-inner plexiform layer; MD, mean deviation; logMAR, the logarithm of the minimum angle of resolution; RNFL, retinal nerve fiber layer; SD, standard deviation; VF, visual field.

We found that many MT genes had a high percentage of variants in either the proband group or control group, with missense mutation as the major mutation type (Figure 2). Based on the gene burden method, we calculated the affected sample rate of genes for the control and proband groups. Then, we compared the difference of the affected sample rate between the control and proband groups. We focused on the top difference and a short list of genes due to these genes providing more correlations and more potential to be a key regulator between the control and proband groups. The difference of 0.3 gave us around ten genes, which is in accordance with our expectations. Therefore, the MT genes with a difference over 0.3 of mutation percentage between the proband and control groups are shown in Table 2.

We next asked whether these genes were involved in any pathway. To answer this question, we conducted the pathway analysis for the genes in Table 2. Notably, the pathway analysis revealed that these genes were associated with the cofactor metabolism pathways (Table 3) [33]. Collectively, these data suggest a difference in the mutation burden of MT genes between the controls and probands, underlining the cofactor metabolism pathways. The complete list of variants in this study are available from the corresponding author, A.-G.W., upon reasonable request.

2.2. Family-Based Analysis for MT Genes

Next, we conducted family-based analysis and performed intra-family genotype filtering analysis. After the initial analysis, an inter-family comparison was conducted. We found several interesting candidate MT genes, but conflicting results existed in different families (Table 4). METAP1D (c.41G > T), ACACB (c.1029del), ME3 (c.972G > C), NIPSNAP3B (c.280G > C, c.476C > G), and NSUN4 (c.4A > G) seem to be involved in the penetrance of LHON.

2.3. GWAS (Genome Wide Association Study) Analysis

A GWAS (genome wide association study) was performed with the strategy of the Cochran–Armitage trend test. The Cochran–Armitage trend test was used with the proband versus the control as having a "trend", which depends on the count of the minor/alternate allele D/A, which is zero within genotype dd/rr, one within genotype Dd/Ar, and two within genotype DD/AA. We found that ADGRG5 (Chr16:575620A:G), POLE4 (Chr2:7495872T:G), ERMAP (Chr1:4283044A:G), PIGR (Chr1:2069357C:T;2069358G:A), CDC 42BPB (Chr14:102949A:G), PROK1 (Chr1:1104562A:G), BCAN (Chr 1:1566582C:T), NES

(Chr1:1566698A:G,1566705T:C, 1566707T:C) may be involved in the clinical penetrance of LHON (Table 5).

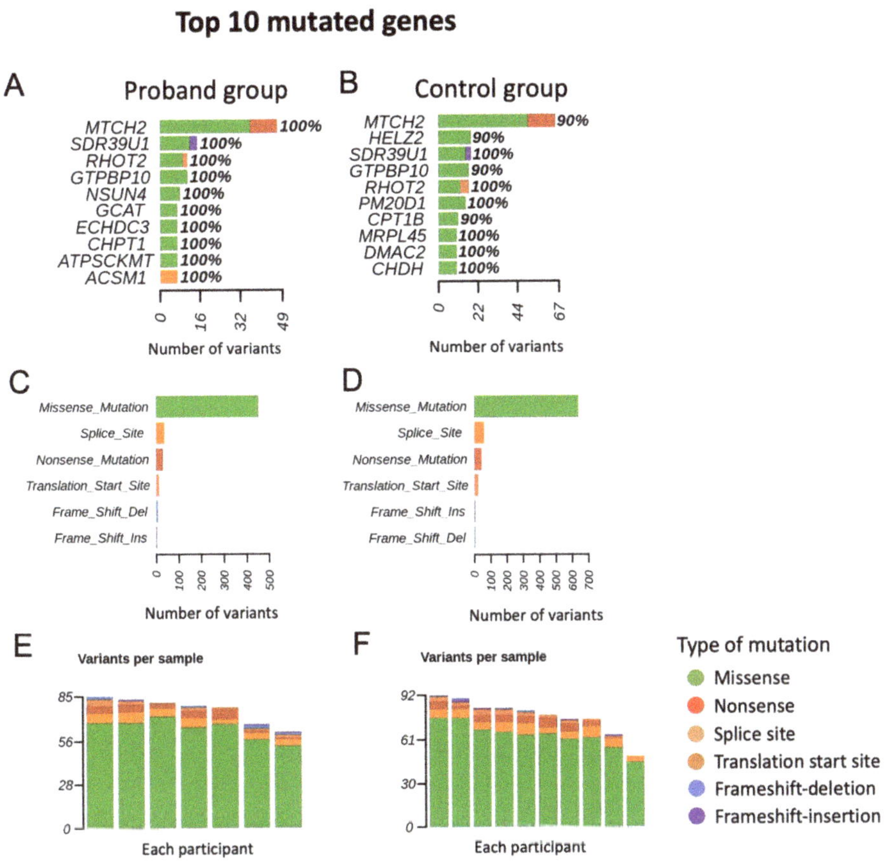

Figure 2. Mitochondria-related nuclear genes with variants in the proband and control group. The top 10 mutated genes are shown for the proband (**A**) and control group (**B**). The percentage indicates the ratio of mutation in all samples. Counts of consequences of variants for the proband (**C**) and control group (**D**). Counts of variants per sample for the proband (**E**) and control group (**F**). The color of the bars indicates the consequences of the variants while each bar presents a sample. We found that many MT genes had a high percentage of variants in either the proband group or control group, with missense mutation as the major mutation type. Forty percent of the top 10 mutated genes in the control group were the same as in the proband group, which may be related to a similar genetic background, since our controls were the proband's relatives. The colors green, red, orange, international orange, sky blue, and violet indicate the missense, nonsense, splice site, translation start site, frameshift deletion, and frameshift insertion, respectively.

Table 2. Mitochondria-related nuclear genes with aa difference over 0.3 of variant percentage between the proband and control groups.

Symbol	Chromosome	Variant Percentage		Differences
		Control	Proband	
AK4	chr1	0.70	0.29	−0.41
NSUN4	chr1	0.60	1	0.40
RDH13	chr19	0.50	0.14	−0.36
COQ3	chr6	0.50	0.86	0.36
FAHD1	chr16	0.10	0.43	0.33
CHPT1	chr12	0.70	1.00	0.30
METAP1D	chr2	0.70	1.00	0.30
MRM1	chr17	0.30	0	−0.30
NCOA6	chr20	0.30	0	−0.30
TOP3A	chr17	0.30	0	−0.30

Chr, chromosome.

Table 3. Pathway analysis of the mitochondria-related nuclear genes with a difference over 0.3 of variant percentage between the proband and control groups.

Pathway	Symbol	Adjusted *p* Value
Biosynthesis of cofactors *	AK4/RDH13/COQ3	0.000628845
Ubiquinone and other terpenoid-quinone biosynthesis	COQ3	0.030532282
Thiamine metabolism	AK4	0.030532282

* Biosynthesis of cofactors: A metabolism of essential cofactors used by the minimal cell starting with precursors such as nicotinamide, riboflavin, thiamine, pyridoxal, pantothenic acid, methionine, and folic acid [33].

Table 4. Family-based analysis of mitochondria-related nuclear genes between the proband and control groups.

Gene Symbol	Chromosome	Family	Description
METAP1D	Chr2	1	Heterozygous c.41G > T in proband
		2	Homozygous c.41G > T proband, heterozygous in control
ACACB	Chr12	1	Heterozygous c.1029del in 2 probands
		3	Missense variant found in control
		4	Heterozygous c.1951G > A in proband
ME3	Chr11	2	Heterozygous c.972G > C in proband
		4	Homozygous c.972G > C in proband, heterozygous in control
NIPSNAP3B	Chr9	3	Homozygous c.280G > C, c.476C > G in proband, heterozygous in control
		4	Heterozygous c.280G > C, c.476C > G in proband
NSUN4	Chr1	4	Homozygous c.4A > G in proband, heterozygous in control
		5	Heterozygous c.4A > G in proband

Table 5. The genome wide association study (GWAS) analysis of the proband and control groups.

Symbol	Gene ID	SNP	HGVSc	*p* Value
ADGRG5	221188	chr16:57562087:A:G	NM_001304376.3: c.-7A > G	0.001
POLE4	56655	chr2:74958729:G:T	NM_019896.4: c.50G > T	0.002
ERMAP	114625	chr1:42830447:G:A	NM_001017922.2: c.-2G > A	0.005
PIGR	5284	chr1:206935771:C:T	NM_002644.4: c.1093G > A	0.006
		chr1:206935822:G:A	NM_002644.4: c.1046-4C > T	0.006
CDC42BPB	9578	chr14:102949759:G:A	NM_006035.4: c.3449 + 6C > T	0.006
PROK1	84432	chr1:110456232:G:A	NM_032414.3: c.199G > A	0.007
BCAN	63827	chr1:156658204:T:C	NM_021948.5: c.2370T > C	0.008
NES	10763	chr1:156669844:G:A	NM_006617.2: c.4344C > T	0.008
		chr1:156670516:C:T	NM_006617.2: c.3672G > A	0.008
		chr1:156670711:C:T	NM_006617.2: c.3477G > A	0.008

HGVSc, Human Genome Variation Society notation in the cDNA; SNP, single nucleotide polymorphism.

3. Discussion

LHON is the major hereditary optic neuropathy in Taiwan [1]. It has a minimum point prevalence for the mtDNA LHON mutation of 11.82 per 100,000 subjects and the minimum point prevalence of visual failure due to LHON of 3.22 per 100,000 subjects in adults under 65 years of age in Northeast England [1,34]. It may cause bilateral blindness in a young adult and cause severe disability. Thus, it is of utmost importance to understand this disease. Even though it has not been difficult to diagnose since the development of molecular diagnosis, there are few treatments available for this disease.

The incomplete penetrance and male prevalence are still the major unexplained issues in LHON. Nuclear modifier genes have been presumed to affect the penetrance of LHON-associated mtDNA mutations. Through whole exome analysis, we found that many mitochondria related (MT-related) genes had a high percentage of variants in either the proband group or control group (Figure 2). Forty percent of the top 10 mutated genes in the control group were the same as in the proband group, which may be related to a similar genetic background, since our controls were the proband's relatives. However, all of the participants in the control group did not have an abnormal phenotype at the current stage. Therefore, the impact of these variants on the participants in the control group was not determined and need further follow-up. The MT genes with a difference over 0.3 of mutation percentage between the proband and control groups include AK4, NSUN4, RDH13, COQ3, and FAHD1. AK4 (Adenylate Kinase 4) encodes the enzymes of the adenylate kinase family, which localize to the mitochondrial matrix [35]. It is related to the metabolism of nucleotides, which can catalyze the reversible transfer of the phosphate group among the adenine and guanine nucleotides (www.genecards.org, accessed date: 28 July 2022) [35–39]. NSUN4 (NOP2/Sun RNA Methyltransferase 4) encodes 5-methylcytosine rRNA methyltransferase NSUN4 in humans, which methylates mitochondrial 12S rRNA and is probably involved in mitochondrial ribosome small subunit (SSU) maturation and mitochondrial ribosome assembly [36,40,41]. RDH13 (Retinol Dehydrogenase 13) encodes a mitochondrial short-chain dehydrogenase/reductase, which localizes at the entrance to the mitochondrial matrix [42]. It may aid retinoic acid production and protect the mitochondria against oxidative stress [35,36,42]. COQ3 (Coenzyme Q3, methyltransferase) encodes mitochondrial ubiquinone biosynthesis O-methyltransferase, which catalyzes the 2 O-methylation steps in the ubiquinone biosynthetic pathway [36,40,43]. FAHD1 (Fumarylacetoacetate Hydrolase Domain Containing 1) encodes mitochondrial aC.-Y.L.pyruvase FAHD1, which is able to hydrolyze fumarylpyruvate and acetylpyruvate in vitro [36,40,44,45]. It may also have oxaloacetate decarboxylase activity in eukaryotes [46]. Pathway analysis also supports the findings that these genes are associated with cofactor metabolism pathways (Table 3). As above-mentioned, AK4 encodes adenylate kinases, which catalyze the phosphorylation of AMP while using ATP/GTP as phosphate donors [35–39]. It may also be involved in thiamine metabolism [47–49]. RDH13 encodes a mitochondrial short-chain dehydrogenase/reductase that may protect the mitochondria against oxidative stress [35,36,42]. COQ3 encodes mitochondrial ubiquinone biosynthesis O-methyltransferase and is involved in the ubiquinone biosynthetic pathway, while ubiquinone is an important electron carrier in the mitochondrial respiratory chain [36,40,43]. All of these genes contribute to the biosynthesis of cofactors and help to maintain the essential functions of mitochondria. The malfunction of these genes may endanger the essential functions of mitochondria including the respiratory chain reaction, which is important for the pathophysiology of LHON.

Family-based analysis showed that several candidate MT genes including METAP1D (c.41G > T), ACACB (c.1029del), ME3 (c.972G > C), NIPSNAP3B (c.280G > C, c.476C > G), and NSUN4 (c.4A > G) seem to be involved in the penetrance of LHON (Table 3). METAP1D (methionyl aminopeptidase type 1D, mitochondrial) is a gene encoding the mitochondrial aminopeptidase responsible for removing the N-terminal methionine from many proteins [50]. METAP1D gene mutation has been associated with spinocerebellar ataxia (www.genecards.org, accessed date: 28 July 2022) [36]. ACACB (acetyl-CoA carboxylase beta) is a biotin-containing enzyme that catalyzes the carboxylation of acetyl-CoA to malonyl-CoA, the rate-limiting step in fatty acid synthesis [36]. ME3 (malic enzyme 3) encodes an isoform of mitochondrial NADP (+)-dependent malic enzyme, which catalyzes the oxidative decarboxylation of malate to pyruvate using NADP+ as a cofactor [36]. NIPSNAP3B protein belongs to a vesicular trafficking-related protein family [51], and seems to be associated with type I 3-methylglutaconic aciduria and anemia of prematurity [36]. In family-based analysis, the results showed some differences between different families. However, there seemed to be a trend of dose-effect. For example, homozygous in the proband vs. heterozygous in the control and heterozygous in the proband vs. null in the control. Therefore, we still believe that these variants may contribute to the penetrance of LHON.

A GWAS (genome wide association study) was performed, which found that ADGRG5 (Chr16:575620A:G), POLE4 (Chr2:7495872T:G), ERMAP (Chr1:4283044A:G), PIGR (Chr1:2069357C:T;2069358G:A), CDC42BPB (Chr14:102949A:G), PROK1 (Chr1:1104562A:G), BCAN (Chr 1:1566582C:T), and NES (Chr1:1566698A:G,1566705T:C,1566707T:C) may be involved (Table 4). ADGRG5 (adhesion G protein-coupled receptor G5) encodes a member of the adhesion family of G-protein coupled receptors. They may play a role in the immune system as well as in the central nervous system [36]. POLE4 (DNA polymerase epsilon 4, accessory subunit) is a histone-fold protein that interacts with other histone-fold proteins to bind DNA in a sequence-independent manner [36]. ERMAP (erythroblast membrane associated protein) is a cell surface transmembrane protein that may act as an erythroid cell receptor, possibly as a mediator of cell adhesion [36]. PIGR (polymeric immunoglobulin receptor) is a member of the immunoglobulin superfamily [36]. CDC42BPB (CDC42 binding protein kinase beta) encodes a member of the serine/threonine protein kinase family containing a Cdc42/Rac-binding p21 binding domain resembling that of PAK kinase [36]. The PROK1 (prokineticin 1) protein may induce proliferation, migration, and fenestration (the formation of membrane discontinuities) in the capillary endothelial cells derived from endocrine glands [41]. BCAN (brevican) encodes a member of the lectican family of chondroitin sulfate proteoglycans, specifically expressed in the central nervous system. It is developmentally regulated and may function in the formation of the brain extracellular matrix [36]. NES (nestin) encodes a member of the intermediate filament protein family and is expressed primarily in nerve cells [36].

Although the clinical studies disclose a male predilection in LHON, we did not find a significant change in sex chromosome in our studies [1,52]. The mystery of gender bias in LHON may need more investigation to unravel.

This study was limited to the small sample size. However, we collected both the proband and carriers in the same family and established the family-based analysis. We believe that a family-based strategy could help to avoid the confounding factor from population stratification in genetic studies. In addition, we included only mitochondria-related nuclear genes for efficacious analysis, which may miss other genes that might also contribute to clinical penetrance. Moreover, we did not have a prediction model regarding the structural/functional alterations of the variants, and further investigations including verifying these candidate genes are required. Although it has many limitations, this study provides a new profile of candidate nuclear modifier genes for the clinical penetrance of LHON.

In summary, the incomplete penetrance and male prevalence are still the major unexplained issues in LHON. Through whole exome analysis, we found that several MT genes with a high percentage of variants were involved in a family-based analysis. A difference in the mutation burden of MT genes underlining the cofactor metabolism pathways was suggested by pathway analysis. In addition, the GWAS analysis also revealed several candidate nuclear modifier genes. The new technology of WES contributes to providing a highly efficient candidate gene screening function in molecular genetics. However, these candidate modifier genes need further verification for their modifying effect on the clinical penetrance in a larger cohort as well as more in-depth investigation of their biologic mechanism.

4. Materials and Methods

This prospective cross-sectional study was conducted from 6 January 2020 to 31 December 2021 at Taipei Veterans General Hospital. Eligible LHON patients with mitochondrial(mt) 11778 mutation G > A and their relatives who also carried the mt11778G > A mutation were invited to participate in this study consecutively. The study was approved by the institutional review board of Taipei Veterans General Hospital and the study protocol adhered to the tenets of the Declaration of Helsinki. Written informed consent was obtained from each participant after the goals and methods of the study were fully explained.

4.1. Families and Subjects

DNA samples used for this investigation were obtained from members of families who carried the mtDNA 11778G > A mutation including the probands, proband's mother, and adult relative carriers. The genomic DNA of the probands and family members will be extracted from the peripheral blood for WES. Ophthalmic examinations and other clinical evaluations of probands and other members of these families were conducted.

Subjects who did not have genetic-proved mtDNA 11778G > A mutation had no comparable relative carriers or who could not cooperate with the ophthalmic examinations were excluded from the study.

4.2. Ophthalmic Examinations

The best-corrected visual acuity (BCVA) was examined with the Snellen visual acuity chart. Other ophthalmic examinations included intraocular pressure, slit-lamp examination, fundoscopy, visual field (VF) with the Humphrey 30-2 SITA-standard protocol (Humphrey Field Analyzer 3, Carl Zeiss Meditec, Dublin, CA, USA), and optical coherence tomography (OCT) (Avanti RTVue XR, Optovue, Inc., Fremont, CA, USA) for the peripapillary retinal nerve fiber layer (RNFL) and ganglion cell-inner plexiform layer (GCIPL) thickness was conducted if feasible.

4.3. Sample Collection and DNA Extraction

Peripheral blood (10 mL) was collected from each participant after obtaining their informed consent. DNA was extracted using Nucleospin Blood Mini (MACHEREY-NAGEL, Düren, Germany) according to the manufacturer's instructions. Briefly, 20 μL Proteinase K and 200 μL blood were mixed, and 200 μL B3 buffer was added for 15 min of incubation at 70 °C. Next, 210 μL of ethanol was added to the lysate from the last step and mixed thoroughly. Then, the sample was transferred to the NucleoSpin® Blood Column and centrifuged for 1 min at 11,000× *g* for DNA binding. For the silica membrane wash, 500 μL of Buffer BW was added to the column and centrifuged for 1 min at 11,000× *g* twice, followed by silica membrane dry spinning for 1 min at 11,000× *g*. The purified DNA was obtained by adding 100 μL preheated Buffer BE to the column and incubating for 1 min, followed by 1 min at 11,000× *g* centrifuge.

4.4. Whole Exome Sequencing

Whole exome sequencing was performed according to the referenced paper as follows [53]. WES was conducted on 500 ng of genomic DNA from the probands and their family members. Fragment libraries were prepared from the sheared samples by sonication and target enrichment was performed according to the manufacturer's protocols (Agilent SureSelect QXT ALL Human Exon V6 Kit or Roche KAPA HyperExome Kit). Captured DNA was amplified followed by solid-phase bridge amplification and paired-end sequenced on Illumina NovaSeq 6000 (Illumina, Inc., San Diego, CA, USA). Alignment of reads to the human reference sequence (hg38 assembly) and variant detection were performed using DRAGEN 3.7.5 (Illumina, Inc.) with the alt-aware configuration. The variant annotation information was obtained from Variant Effect Predictor (version 100) and Jannovar (version 0.35) with dbNSFP 4.1a. The novel variants were filtered against 1000 Genomes (1000 genomes release phase 3, http://www.1000genomes.org/, accessed date: 28 July 2022), dbSNP (http://www.ncbi.nlm.nih.gov/projects/SNP/snp_summary.cgi accessed date: 28 July 2022), and the Genome Aggregation Database (gnomad.broadinstitute.org accessed date: 28 July 2022) [54–56].

4.5. Mitochondria-Related Genes Analysis

The overview of the exome analysis is summarized as follows. First, we used the Msigdb mitochondria (MT)-related canonical pathway (CP) database with 838 genes and the MitoCarta3.0 database with 1135 genes to sort out a total of 1273 mitochondria-related nuclear genes (MT genes) as our target genes. Next, we excluded UTR, intron and synonymous variants, and also excluded those variants labeled as benign and likely benign in the ClinVar database. We filtered for variants including donor/splice acceptor, start loss, stop gained, frameshift, missense, and CADD Phred > 20/REVEL >0.5 (Figure 1A). Thereafter, we extracted the most significant variants from the analysis of all of the probands and controls. We also investigated the intra-family variants differences between the proband and carriers as our family-based analysis, which may help to find the variants important for penetrance for participants with the same genetic background (Figure 1A). The pathway analysis was performed using R package "clusterProfiler" with the ontology database of the Kyoto Encyclopedia of Genes and Genomes (KEGG) [47]. An adjusted p (Benjamini–Hochberg method) < 0.05 was considered as statistically significant for the pathway analysis.

4.6. GWAS Analysis

The input of GWAS was the exome sequencing data, which was converted to the PLINK format for the GWAS analysis. The GWAS analysis focuses on the correlation between the control and proband groups at a scale of SNP or the locus near SNP, while the gene burden analysis aims to look for candidate genes. We applied two different approaches intending to explore any genes or SNPs that potentially contribute to the pathogenesis of LHON. The gvcf files of all samples were combined and genotyped using the GATK bundle (4.2.0.0). The quality of cohort variants was evaluated by the Variant Quality Score Recalibration (VQSR) with the indel and SNP tranche of 99 and 99.8, respectively. The variants with GQ <20, depth of diploid <10, depth of haploid <5, allele fraction <0.2 and >0.8 for heterozygous or low inbreeding coefficient <−0.8 were excluded. The vcf format of the high-quality variants was converted to the PLINK (v1.90b6.24) bed format. Single SNPs had to meet the following criteria: minor allele frequencies (MAF) >10%, missing rate <10%, Hardy–Weinberg equilibrium (HWE) significance threshold <0.00001, otherwise, they were excluded from further analysis. The association analysis was conducted by using PLNK with the "–model" function. A $p < 0.05$ was considered as statistically significant.

4.7. Family-Based Analysis

The MT genes obtained from Section 4.5 were also used for family-based analysis (Figure 1A). We applied an intra-family filter that looked for variants that were either homozygous alternate in the proband and heterozygous alternate in the control, or heterozygous alternate in the proband and homozygous reference in the control. Then, we counted the concurrence of matched variants across families and reported variants with a concurrence count >1.

Author Contributions: Conceptualization, H.-C.C., S.-C.C., C.-Y.L., J.-Y.Y. and A.-G.W.; methodology, H.-C.C., S.-C.C., J.-Y.Y. and A.-G.W.; software, S.-C.C.; validation, H.-C.C., S.-C.C., C.-Y.L., J.-Y.Y. and A.-G.W.; formal analysis, H.-C.C. and A.-G.W.; investigation, H.-C.C. and A.-G.W.; resources, A.-G.W.; data curation, H.-C.C., S.-C.C., C.-Y.L., J.-Y.Y. and A.-G.W.; writing—original draft preparation, H.-C.C.; writing—review and editing, H.-C.C., S.-C.C., C.-Y.L., J.-Y.Y. and A.-G.W.; visualization, H.-C.C.; supervision, A.-G.W.; project administration, S.-C.C.; funding acquisition, H.-C.C. and A.-G.W. All authors have read and agreed to the published version of the manuscript.

Funding: This research was funded by Taipei Veterans General Hospital (grant no. VGH V110C-052, V111C-099) and the Ministry of Science and Technology of Taiwan (grant no. MOST 110-2314-B-075-054-MY3, MOST 111-2324-B-075-42). The APC was funded by Ministry of Science and Technology of Taiwan (grant no. MOST 110-2314-B-075-054-MY3).

Institutional Review Board Statement: The study was conducted in accordance with the Declaration of Helsinki, and approved by the Institutional Review Board of Taipei Veterans General Hospital (IRB-TPEVGH No.: 2020-01-002A and date of approval: Jan 06, 2020)." for studies involving humans.

Informed Consent Statement: Informed consent was obtained from all subjects involved in the study.

Data Availability Statement: The data presented in this study are available on request from the corresponding author, A.-G.W. The data are not publicly available due to ethical restrictions.

Acknowledgments: We thank Shao-Min Wu (Compassbioinfo Inc.) for the assistance and consultation of the WES data analysis.

Conflicts of Interest: The authors declare no conflict of interest.

References

1. Yen, M.Y.; Wang, A.G.; Wei, Y. Leber's hereditary optic neuropathy: A multifactorial disease. *Prog. Retin. Eye Res.* **2006**, *25*, 381–396. [CrossRef] [PubMed]
2. Newman, N.J.; Lott, M.T.; Wallace, D. The clinical characteristics of pedigrees of Leber's hereditary optic neuropathy with the 11778 mutation. *Am. J. Ophthalmol.* **1991**, *111*, 750–762. [CrossRef]
3. Newman, N. Leber's hereditary optic neuropathy. New genetic considerations. *Arch. Neurol.* **1993**, *50*, 540–548. [CrossRef] [PubMed]
4. Carelli, V.; Ross-Cisneros, F.N.; Sadun, A. Mitochondrial dysfunction as a cause of optic neuropathies. *Prog. Retin. Eye Res.* **2004**, *23*, 53–89. [CrossRef] [PubMed]
5. Wallace, D.C.; Singh, G.; Lott, M.T.; Hodge, J.A.; Schurr, T.G.; Lezza, A.M.; Elsas, L., 2nd; Nikoskelainen, E. Mitochondrial DNA mutation associated with Leber's hereditary optic neuropathy. *Science* **1988**, *242*, 1427–1430. [CrossRef] [PubMed]
6. Huoponen, K.; Vilkki, J.; Aula, P.; Nikoskelainen, E.K.; Savontaus, M. A new mtDNA mutation associated with Leber hereditary optic neuroretinopathy. *Am. J. Hum. Genet.* **1991**, *48*, 1147–1153.
7. Howell, N.; Bindoff, L.A.; McCullough, D.A.; Kubacka, I.; Poulton, J.; Mackey, D.; Taylor, L.; Turnbull, D. Leber hereditary optic neuropathy: Identification of the same mitochondrial ND1 mutation in six pedigrees. *Am. J. Hum. Genet.* **1991**, *49*, 939–950.
8. Mackey, D.; Howell, N. A variant of Leber hereditary optic neuropathy characterized by recovery of vision and by an unusual mitochondrial genetic etiology. *Am. J. Hum. Genet.* **1992**, *51*, 1218–1228.
9. Riordan-Eva, P.; Sanders, M.D.; Govan, G.G.; Sweeney, M.G.; Da Costa, J.; Harding, A. The clinical features of Leber's hereditary optic neuropathy defined by the presence of a pathogenic mitochondrial DNA mutation. *Brain* **1995**, *118 Pt 2*, 319–337. [CrossRef]
10. Charlmers, R.M.; Harding, A. A case-control study of Leber's hereditary optic neuropathy. *Brain* **1996**, *119 Pt 5*, 1481–1486. [CrossRef]
11. Smith, K.H.; Johns, D.R.; Heher, K.L.; Miller, N. Heteroplasmy in Leber's hereditary optic neuropathy. *Arch. Ophthalmol.* **1993**, *111*, 1486–1490. [CrossRef] [PubMed]
12. Jacobi, F.K.; Leo-Kottler, B.; Mittelviefhaus, K.; Zrenner, E.; Meyer, J.; Pusch, C.M.; Wissinger, B. Segregation patterns and heteroplasmy prevalence in Leber's hereditary optic neuropathy. *Investig. Ophthalmol. Vis. Sci.* **2001**, *42*, 1208–1214.

13. Howell, N.; Xu, M.; Halvorson, S.; Bodis-Wollner, I.; Sherman, J. A heteroplasmic LHON family: Tissue distribution and transmission of the 11778 mutation. *Am. J. Hum. Genet.* **1994**, *55*, 203–206.
14. Yen, M.Y.; Lee, H.C.; Wang, A.G.; Chang, W.L.; Liu, J.H.; Wei, Y.H. Exclusive homoplasmic 11778 mutation in mitochondrial DNA of Chinese patients with Leber's hereditary optic neuropathy. *Jpn. J. Ophthalmol.* **1999**, *43*, 196–200. [CrossRef]
15. Chinnery, P.F.; Howell, N.; Andrews, R.M.; Turnbull, D.M. Mitochondrial DNA analysis: Polymorphisms and pathogenicity. *J. Med. Genet.* **1999**, *36*, 505–510. [CrossRef]
16. Howell, N.; Mackey, D.A. Low-penetrance branches in matrilineal pedigrees with Leber hereditary optic neuropathy. *Am. J. Hum. Genet.* **1998**, *63*, 1220–1224. [CrossRef]
17. Brown, M.D.; Sun, F.; Wallace, D.C. Clustering of Caucasian Leber hereditary optic neuropathy patients containing the 11778 or 14484 mutations on an mtDNA lineage. *Am. J. Hum. Genet.* **1997**, *60*, 381–387.
18. Yu-Wai-Man, P.; Howell, N.; Mackey, D.A.; Norby, S.; Rosenberg, T.; Turnbull, D.M.; Chinnery, P.F. Mitochondrial DNA haplogroup distribution within Leber hereditary optic neuropathy pedigrees. *J. Med. Genet.* **2004**, *41*, e41.
19. Carelli, V.; Achilli, A.; Valentino, M.L.; Rengo, C.; Semino, O.; Pala, M.; Olivieri, A.; Mattiazzi, M.; Pallotti, F.; Carrara, F.; et al. Haplogroup effects and recombination of mitochondrial DNA: Novel clues from the analysis of Leber hereditary optic neuropathy pedigrees. *Am. J. Hum. Genet.* **2006**, *78*, 564–574. [CrossRef]
20. Bu, X.D.; Rotter, J.I. X chromosome-linked and mitochondrial gene control of Leber hereditary optic neuropathy: Evidence from segregation analysis for dependence on X chromosome inactivation. *Proc. Natl. Acad. Sci. USA* **1991**, *88*, 8198–8202. [CrossRef]
21. Hudson, G.; Keers, S.; Yu-Wai-Man, P.; Griffiths, P.; Huoponen, K.; Savontaus, M.L.; Nikoskelainen, E.; Zeviani, M.; Carrara, F.; Horvath, R.; et al. Identification of an X-chromosomal locus and haplotype modulating the phenotype of a mitochondrial DNA disorder. *Am. J. Hum. Genet.* **2005**, *77*, 1086–1091. [CrossRef]
22. Shankar, S.P.; Fingert, J.H.; Carelli, V.; Valentino, M.L.; King, T.M.; Daiger, S.P.; Salomao, S.R.; Berezovsky, A.; Belfort, R., Jr.; Braun, T.A.; et al. Evidence for a novel x-linked modifier locus for leber hereditary optic neuropathy. *Ophthalmic Genet.* **2008**, *29*, 17–24. [CrossRef]
23. Abu-Amero, K.K.; Jaber, M.; Hellani, A.; Bosley, T.M. Genome-wide expression profile of LHON patients with the 11778 mutation. *Br. J. Ophthalmol.* **2010**, *94*, 256–259. [CrossRef]
24. Sadun, A.A.; Carelli, V.; Salomao, S.R.; Berezovsky, A.; Quiros, P.A.; Sadun, F.; DeNegri, A.M.; Andrade, R.; Moraes, M.; Passos, A.; et al. Extensive investigation of a large Brazilian pedigree of 11778/haplogroup J Leber hereditary optic neuropathy. *Am. J. Ophthalmol.* **2003**, *136*, 231–238. [CrossRef]
25. Kerrison, J.B.; Miller, N.R.; Hsu, F.; Beaty, T.H.; Maumenee, I.H.; Smith, K.H.; Savino, P.J.; Stone, E.M.; Newman, N.J. A case-control study of tobacco and alcohol consumption in Leber hereditary optic neuropathy. *Am. J. Ophthalmol.* **2000**, *130*, 803–812. [CrossRef]
26. Gupta, S.; Chatterjee, S.; Mukherjee, A.; Mutsuddi, M. Whole exome sequencing: Uncovering causal genetic variants for ocular diseases. *Exp. Eye Res.* **2017**, *164*, 139–150. [CrossRef]
27. Yen, M.Y.; Chen, Y.J.; Lin, C.H.; Wang, A.G.; Wei, Y.H. Genetic analysis in Leber's hereditary optic neuropathy using the comparative genomic hybridization technique. *Clin. Exp. Ophthalmol.* **2003**, *31*, 435–438. [CrossRef]
28. Pegoraro, E.; Vettori, A.; Valentino, M.L.; Molon, A.; Mostacciuolo, M.L.; Howell, N.; Carelli, V. X-inactivation pattern in multiple tissues from two Leber's hereditary optic neuropathy (LHON) patients. *Am. J. Med. Genet. A* **2003**, *119A*, 37–40.
29. Handoko, H.Y.; Wirapati, P.J.; Sudoyo, H.A.; Sitepu, M.; Marzuki, S. Meiotic breakpoint mapping of a proposed X linked visual loss susceptibility locus in Leber's hereditary optic neuropathy. *J. Med. Genet.* **1998**, *35*, 668–671. [CrossRef]
30. Zhuchenko, O.; Wehnert, M.; Bailey, J.; Sun, Z.S.; Lee, C.C. Isolation, mapping, and genomic structure of an X-linked gene for a subunit of human mitochondrial complex I. *Genomics* **1996**, *37*, 281–288. [CrossRef] [PubMed]
31. Ishikawa, K.; Funayama, T.; Ohde, H.; Inagaki, Y.; Mashima, Y. Genetic variants of TP53 and EPHX1 in Leber's hereditary optic neuropathy and their relationship to age at onset. *Jpn. J. Ophthalmol.* **2005**, *49*, 121–126. [CrossRef] [PubMed]
32. Jiang, P.; Jin, X.; Peng, Y.; Wang, M.; Liu, H.; Liu, X.; Zhang, Z.; Ji, Y.; Zhang, J.; Liang, M.; et al. The exome sequencing identified the mutation in YARS2 encoding the mitochondrial tyrosyl-tRNA synthetase as a nuclear modifier for the phenotypic manifestation of Leber's hereditary optic neuropathy-associated mitochondrial DNA mutation. *Hum. Mol. Genet.* **2016**, *25*, 584–596. [CrossRef] [PubMed]
33. Gil, R.; Silva, F.J.; Pereto, J.; Moya, A. Determination of the core of a minimal bacterial gene set. *Microbiol. Mol. Biol. Rev.* **2004**, *68*, 518–537. [CrossRef]
34. Yu-Wai-Man, P.; Griffiths, P.G.; Brown, D.T.; Howell, N.; Turnbull, D.M.; Chinnery, P.F. The epidemiology of Leber hereditary optic neuropathy in the North East of England. *Am. J. Hum. Genet.* **2003**, *72*, 333–339. [CrossRef]
35. Maglott, D.; Ostell, J.; Pruitt, K.D.; Tatusova, T. Entrez Gene: Gene-centered information at NCBI. *Nucleic Acids Res.* **2005**, *33*, D54–D58. [CrossRef]
36. Safran, M.R.N.; Twik, M.; BarShir, R.; Iny Stein, T.; Dahary, D.; Fishilevich, S.; Lancet, D. The Gene Cards Suite Chapter. In *Practical Guide to Life Science Databases*; Springer: Singapore, 2022.
37. Liu, R.; Xu, H.; Wei, Z.; Wang, Y.; Lin, Y.; Gong, W. Crystal structure of human adenylate kinase 4 (L171P) suggests the role of hinge region in protein domain motion. *Biochem. Biophys. Res. Commun.* **2009**, *379*, 92–97. [CrossRef]
38. Panayiotou, C.; Solaroli, N.; Johansson, M.; Karlsson, A. Evidence of an intact N-terminal translocation sequence of human mitochondrial adenylate kinase 4. *Int. J. Biochem. Cell Biol.* **2010**, *42*, 62–69. [CrossRef]

39. Lanning, N.J.; Looyenga, B.D.; Kauffman, A.L.; Niemi, N.M.; Sudderth, J.; DeBerardinis, R.J.; MacKeigan, J.P. A mitochondrial RNAi screen defines cellular bioenergetic determinants and identifies an adenylate kinase as a key regulator of ATP levels. *Cell Rep.* **2014**, *7*, 907–917. [CrossRef]
40. UniProt, C. UniProt: The universal protein knowledgebase in 2021. *Nucleic Acids Res.* **2021**, *49*, D480–D489.
41. Camara, Y.; Asin-Cayuela, J.; Park, C.B.; Metodiev, M.D.; Shi, Y.; Ruzzenente, B.; Kukat, C.; Habermann, B.; Wibom, R.; Hultenby, K.; et al. MTERF4 regulates translation by targeting the methyltransferase NSUN4 to the mammalian mitochondrial ribosome. *Cell Metab.* **2011**, *13*, 527–539. [CrossRef]
42. Belyaeva, O.V.; Korkina, O.V.; Stetsenko, A.V.; Kedishvili, N.Y. Human retinol dehydrogenase 13 (RDH13) is a mitochondrial short-chain dehydrogenase/reductase with a retinaldehyde reductase activity. *FEBS J.* **2008**, *275*, 138–147. [CrossRef]
43. Jonassen, T.; Clarke, C.F. Isolation and functional expression of human COQ3, a gene encoding a methyltransferase required for ubiquinone biosynthesis. *J. Biol. Chem.* **2000**, *275*, 12381–12387. [CrossRef]
44. Manjasetty, B.A.; Niesen, F.H.; Delbruck, H.; Gotz, F.; Sievert, V.; Bussow, K.; Behlke, J.; Heinemann, U. X-ray structure of fumarylacetoacetate hydrolase family member Homo sapiens FLJ36880. *Biol. Chem.* **2004**, *385*, 935–942. [CrossRef]
45. Pircher, H.; Straganz, G.D.; Ehehalt, D.; Morrow, G.; Tanguay, R.M.; Jansen-Durr, P. Identification of human fumarylacetoacetate hydrolase domain-containing protein 1 (FAHD1) as a novel mitochondrial acylpyruvase. *J. Biol. Chem.* **2011**, *286*, 36500–36508. [CrossRef] [PubMed]
46. Pircher, H.; Von Grafenstein, S.; Diener, T.; Metzger, C.; Albertini, E.; Taferner, A.; Unterluggauer, H.; Kramer, C.; Liedl, K.R.; Jansen-Durr, P. Identification of FAH domain-containing protein 1 (FAHD1) as oxaloacetate decarboxylase. *J. Biol. Chem.* **2015**, *290*, 6755–6762. [CrossRef]
47. Kanehisa, M.; Furumichi, M.; Sato, Y.; Ishiguro-Watanabe, M.; Tanabe, M. KEGG: Integrating viruses and cellular organisms. *Nucleic Acids Res.* **2021**, *49*, D545–D551. [CrossRef]
48. Kanehisa, M.; Goto, S. KEGG: Kyoto encyclopedia of genes and genomes. *Nucleic Acids Res.* **2000**, *28*, 27–30. [CrossRef]
49. Kanehisa, M. Toward understanding the origin and evolution of cellular organisms. *Protein Sci.* **2019**, *28*, 1947–1951. [CrossRef]
50. Serero, A.; Giglione, C.; Sardini, A.; Martinez-Sanz, J.; Meinnel, T. An unusual peptide deformylase features in the human mitochondrial N-terminal methionine excision pathway. *J. Biol. Chem.* **2003**, *278*, 52953–52963. [CrossRef]
51. Buechler, C.; Bodzioch, M.; Bared, S.M.; Sigruener, A.; Boettcher, A.; Lapicka-Bodzioch, K.; Aslanidis, C.; Duong, C.Q.; Grandl, M.; Langmann, T.; et al. Expression pattern and raft association of NIPSNAP3 and NIPSNAP4, highly homologous proteins encoded by genes in close proximity to the ATP-binding cassette transporter A1. *Genomics* **2004**, *83*, 1116–1124. [CrossRef]
52. Poincenot, L.; Pearson, A.L.; Karanjia, R. Demographics of a Large International Population of Patients Affected by Leber's Hereditary Optic Neuropathy. *Ophthalmology* **2020**, *127*, 679–688. [CrossRef] [PubMed]
53. Qiao, F.; Wang, C.; Luo, C.; Wang, Y.; Shao, B.; Tan, J.; Hu, P.; Xu, Z. A De Novo heterozygous frameshift mutation identified in BCL11B causes neurodevelopmental disorder by whole exome sequencing. *Mol. Genet. Genom. Med.* **2019**, *7*, e897. [CrossRef] [PubMed]
54. The 1000 Genomes Project Consortium. A global reference for human genetic variation. *Nature* **2015**, *526*, 68–74. [CrossRef] [PubMed]
55. Sherry, S.T.; Ward, M.; Sirotkin, K. dbSNP-database for single nucleotide polymorphisms and other classes of minor genetic variation. *Genome Res.* **1999**, *9*, 677–679. [CrossRef]
56. Karczewski, K.J.; Francioli, L.C.; Tiao, G.; Cummings, B.B.; Alfoldi, J.; Wang, Q.; Collins, R.L.; Laricchia, K.M.; Ganna, A.; Birnbaum, D.P.; et al. The mutational constraint spectrum quantified from variation in 141,456 humans. *Nature* **2020**, *581*, 434–443. [CrossRef]

International Journal of
Molecular Sciences

MDPI

Article

Neuroprotective Effect of Azithromycin Following Induction of Optic Nerve Crush in Wild Type and Immunodeficient Mice

Ofira Zloto [1,2,†], Alon Zahavi [2,3,4,†], Stephen Richard [5], Moran Friedman-Gohas [2,4], Shirel Weiss [2,4] and Nitza Goldenberg-Cohen [4,5,6,*]

1 Goldschlager Eye Institute, Sheba Medical Center, Ramat Gan 5262000, Israel
2 Sackler Faculty of Medicine, Tel Aviv University, Tel Aviv 6997801, Israel
3 Department of Ophthalmology, Rabin Medical Center—Beilinson Hospital, Petach Tikva 4941492, Israel
4 The Krieger Eye Research Laboratory, Felsenstein Medical Research Center, Petach Tikva 4941492, Israel
5 The Krieger Eye Research Laboratory, Faculty of Medicine, Technion-Israel Institute of Technology, Haifa 3200003, Israel
6 Department of Ophthalmology, Bnai Zion Medical Center, Haifa 3339419, Israel
* Correspondence: ncohen1@gmail.com; Tel.: +972-34-8359554
† These authors contributed equally to this work.

Abstract: This study evaluated the potential neuroprotective effect of azithromycin (AZ) intraperitoneal injections in male C57Bl/6 (wild type, WT) and female NOD scid gamma (NSG) mice subjected to optic nerve crush (ONC) as a model for optic neuropathy. Histologically, reduced apoptosis and improved retinal ganglion cell (RGC) preservation were noted in the AZ-treated mice as shown by TUNEL staining—in the WT mice more than in the NSG mice. The increased microglial activation following ONC was reduced with the AZ treatment. In the molecular analysis of WT and NSG mice, similar trends were detected regarding apoptosis, as well as stress-related and inflammatory markers examining BCL2-associated X (*Bax*), heme oxygenase 1 (*Ho-1*), interleukin 1 beta (*Il1β*), superoxide dismutase 1 (*Sod1*), and nuclear factor-kappa B (*Nfkb*) levels. In the optic nerve, AZ increased the levels of expression of *Sod1* and *Nfkb* only in the WT mice and decreased them in the NSG mice. In the retinas of the WT and NSG mice, the *Bax* and *Ho-1* levels of expression decreased following the AZ treatment, while the *Sod1* and *Nfkb* expression decreased only in the WT mice, and remained stable near the baseline in the NSG mice. *Il1β* remained at the baseline in WT mice while it decreased towards the baseline in AZ-treated NSG mice. The neuroprotective effects demonstrated by the reduced RGC apoptosis in AZ-treated WT mice retinae, and in the optic nerves as stress-related and inflammatory gene expression increase. This did not occur in the immunodeficient NSG mice. AZ modulated the inflammatory reaction and microglial activation. The lack of an effect in NSG mice supports the assumption that AZ acts by immunomodulation, which is known to play a role in ONC damage. These findings have implications for the development and repurposing of drugs to preserve RGCs after acute optic neuropathies.

Keywords: optic nerve crush; neuroprotection; azithromycin; NAION; neural injury; neural ischemia; neural inflammation

Citation: Zloto, O.; Zahavi, A.; Richard, S.; Friedman-Gohas, M.; Weiss, S.; Goldenberg-Cohen, N. Neuroprotective Effect of Azithromycin Following Induction of Optic Nerve Crush in Wild Type and Immunodeficient Mice. *Int. J. Mol. Sci.* **2022**, *23*, 11872. https://doi.org/10.3390/ijms231911872

Academic Editors: Rongkung Tsai and Neil R. Miller

Received: 7 September 2022
Accepted: 4 October 2022
Published: 6 October 2022

1. Introduction

Ischemic optic neuropathy (ION) refers to the infarction of any portion of the optic nerve from the chiasm to the optic nerve head. Clinically, it may be divided into anterior and posterior forms [1]. The pathogenesis of non-arteritic anterior ION (NAION) is not fully understood. NAION has been associated with acute nocturnal hypotension, sleep apnea, microvascular diseases, and Phosphodiesterase-5 inhibitor usage, but in most cases, it is unpredictable and no direct trigger is found [2,3]. Salgado et al. [4] reported an inflammatory component in the pathogenesis of NAION. In animal studies, the mechanical crush of the optic nerve posterior to the globe often serves as a model for investigating the pathogenesis of optic neuropathy and possible neuroprotective treatments [5,6].

The anti-inflammatory effect of azithromycin has been reported, especially in the mouse model of cerebral infarction and retinal ischemia, and its neuroprotective effect has also been reported [7–12]. Immunological modifications may be involved in the neuroprotective effects of azithromycin.

The neuroprotective effect of azithromycin may be effective as a treatment for NAION. Although not a model for NAION, the purpose of this study is to verify the neuroprotective effect of azithromycin using an experimental system of optic nerve crush (ONC) in mice as a model for optic nerve disease and to further verify the involvement of immunological modification.

2. Results

2.1. Histological Analysis (Day 21): RGC Survival

At 21 days after ONC, the RGC count was significantly higher in AZ-treated than untreated WT mice (30.1 ± 0.3 vs. 26.3 ± 2.8 cells/field, respectively, $p = 0.01$) and significantly higher in AZ-treated than untreated NSG mice (31.4 ± 2.3 vs. 19.4 ± 4.9 cells/field, respectively, $p = 0.01$). There were no statistically significant differences in retinal thickness between the treated and untreated WT groups (212 μ ± 20 vs. 208 μ ± 10, respectively) and NSG groups (214 μ ± 12 vs. 202 μ ± 15, respectively).

2.2. Immunohistochemistry Analysis (Day 21): Gliosis (GFAP)

The analysis following ONC in WT and NSG mice demonstrated maximal reactive gliosis and RGC loss in WT mice without the AZ treatment and a reduction in gliosis following the AZ treatment in both groups. In addition, RGC preservation can be noted in AZ-treated mice as compared to non-treated mice (Figure 1A–H).

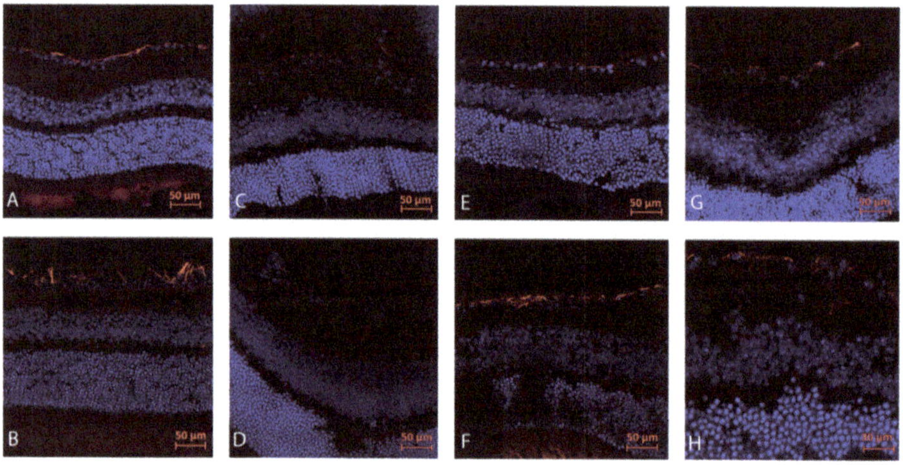

Figure 1. Immunohistochemistry analysis (day 21): Gliosis (GFAP). (**A**) The right eye of WT mouse following ONC and injected with AZ, demonstrating reduced gliosis and RGC preservation in comparison to right eye ONC without AZ treatment (**B**). The left eye of a WT mouse with AZ (**C**) as compared to the control left eye without AZ, (**D**) both demonstrating minimal gliosis. NSG mice following right eye ONC and systemic AZ injection demonstrates right moderate gliosis and RGC preservation, (**E**) as compared to right eye following ONC without AZ (**F**). Note that NSG mice following ONC demonstrate reduced gliosis both with (**E**) and without (**F**) AZ injection as compared to WT mice following ONC with AZ injection (**A**). NSG mice left control eye with (**G**) and without (**H**) AZ systemic injection.

2.3. TUNEL Staining (Day 1 and 3): Apoptosis

The TUNEL staining of retinal sections showed a reduction in the rate of RGC apoptosis in the AZ-treated than the untreated WT mice on day 1 (1.20 ± 0.4 vs. 2.00 ± 0.7 cells/field, respectively, p = 0.0081) and day 3 (4.40 ± 2.5 vs. 6.00 ± 3.7 cells/field, respectively, p = 0.028), respectively (Figure 2).

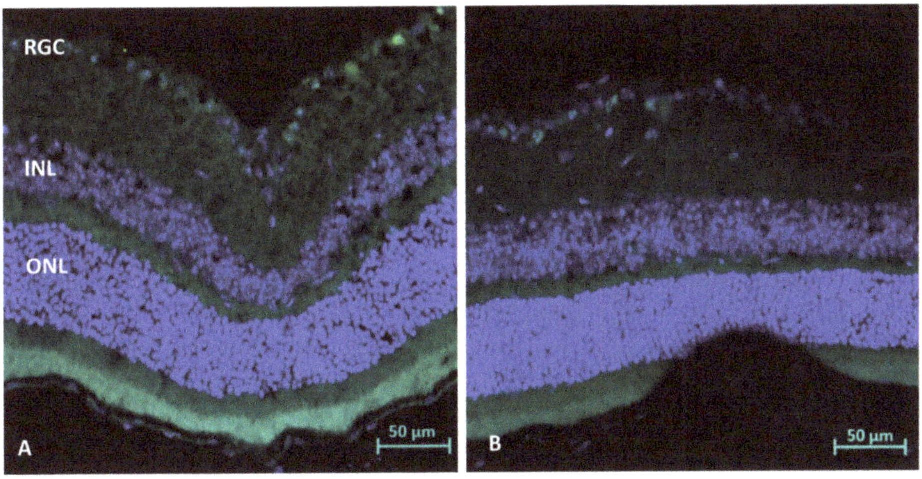

Figure 2. Immunohistochemistry analysis (day 3) for apoptosis (TUNEL). Note stained apoptotic RGC cells following ONC only (**A**), with reduced apoptosis following AZ treatment (**B**).

2.4. Immunohistochemistry Analysis (Day 3): Microglial Activation (Iba1)

The analysis following ONC in WT mice demonstrated reduced microglial activation in AZ-treated mice (Figure 3).

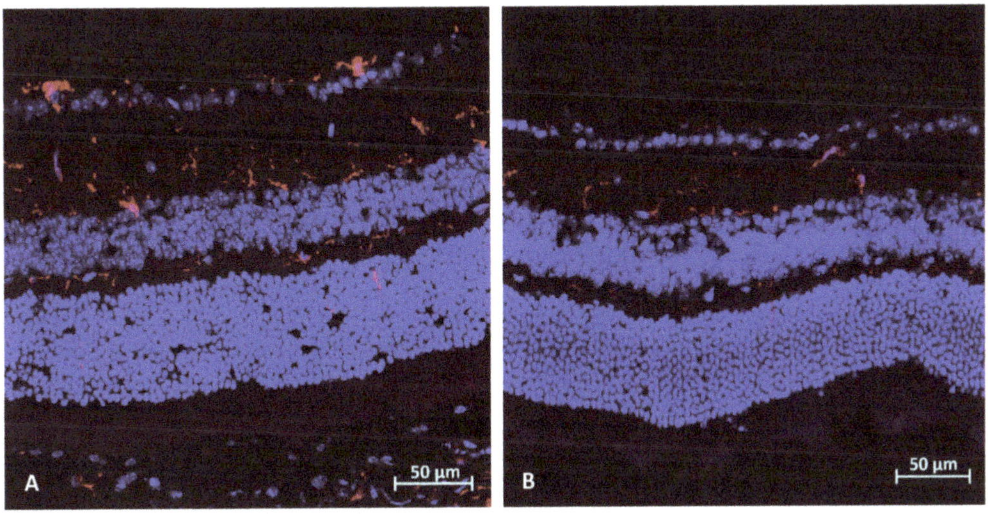

Figure 3. Immunohistochemistry analysis (day 3) for microglial activation (Iba1): (**A**) Right eye of WT mouse following ONC without treatment, showing increased microglial activation, as compared to AZ-treated RE ONC-induced eye (**B**), demonstrating reduced activation.

2.5. *Immunohistochemistry Analysis (Day 3): CD45*

The analysis following ONC in the WT mice was nonspecific.

2.6. *Molecular Analysis WT and NSG Mice (Day 3 after ONC): Optic Nerves*

Bax. WT mice: The *Bax* expression levels remained at the baseline without treatment (0.83 ± 0.21-fold, n = 3) and increased with the AZ treatment (3.77 ± 3.55-fold, $p = 0.17$, n = 4). NSG mice: The *Bax* expression levels remained at the baseline without treatment (0.813 ± 1.186-fold, n = 4) and increased with the AZ treatment (3.176 ± 2.262-fold, $p = 0.087$, n = 3) (Figure 4A).

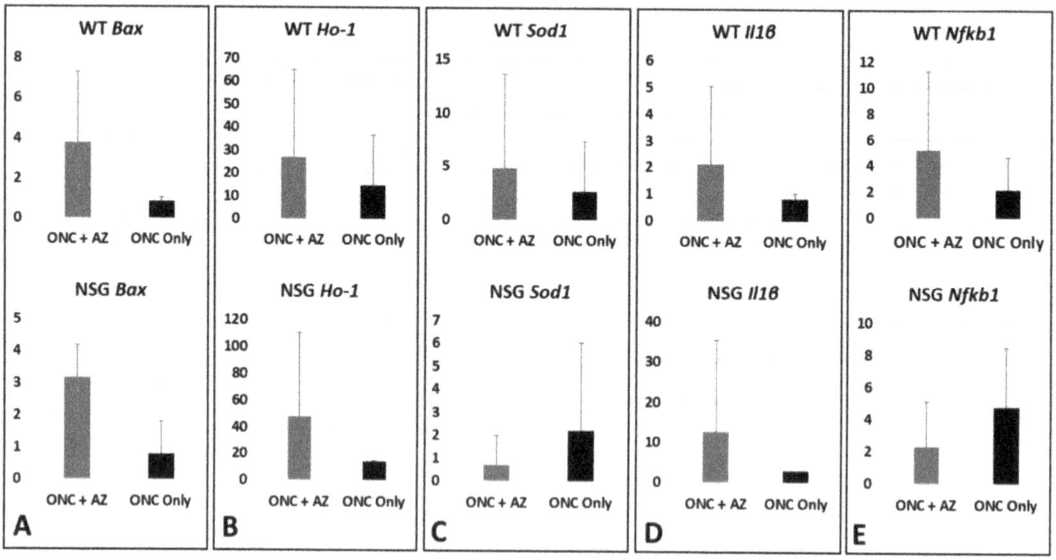

Figure 4. Molecular analysis of the optic nerves, day 3 after ONC. (**A**) *Bax* expression levels in WT and NSG mice remained at baseline without treatment and increased with AZ treatment. (**B**) *Ho-1* levels in WT and NSG mice increased without treatment and further increased with AZ treatment. (**C**) *Sod1* levels in WT mice increased without treatment and further increased with AZ treatment, while in NSG mice levels increased without treatment but decreased with AZ treatment. (**D**) *Il1β* levels in WT mice remained at baseline without treatment and increased with AZ treatment, while in NSG mice levels increased without treatment and further increased with AZ treatment. (**E**) *Nfkb1* levels in WT mice increased without treatment and further increased with AZ treatment, while in NSG mice levels increased without treatment with a relative decrease with AZ treatment.

Ho-1. WT mice: The *Ho-1* expression levels increased without treatment (14.42 ± 22.19-fold, n = 3) and further increased with the AZ treatment (27.22 ± 37.76-fold, $p = 0.64$, n = 6). NSG mice: The *Ho-1* expression levels increased without treatment (14.25 fold, n = 1) and further increased with the AZ treatment (47.73 ± 62.42-fold, n = 3) (Figure 4B).

Sod1. WT mice: The *Sod1* expression levels increased without treatment (2.64 ± 4.75-fold, n = 8) and further increased with the AZ treatment (4.83 ± 8.76-fold, $p = 0.46$, n = 9). NSG mice: The *Sod1* expression levels increased without treatment (2.22 ± 3.84-fold, n = 5) and decreased with the AZ treatment (0.73 ± 1.27-fold, $p = 0.386$, n = 4) (Figure 4C).

Il1β. WT mice: The *Il1β* expression levels remained at baseline without treatment (0.81 ± 0.23-fold, n = 4) and increased with the AZ treatment (2.12 ± 2.94-fold, $p = 0.82$, n = 7). NSG mice: The *Il1β* expression levels increased without treatment (2.94 fold, n = 1) and further increased with the AZ treatment (12.64 ± 22.81-fold, n = 4) (Figure 4D).

Nfkb1. WT mice: The *Nfkb1* expression levels increased without treatment (2.15 ± 2.54-fold, n = 7) and further increased with the AZ treatment (5.21 ± 6.10-fold, $p = 0.24$, n = 7).

NSG mice: The *Nfkb1* expression levels increased without treatment (4.811 ± 3.676-fold, n = 3), with a relative decrease with the AZ treatment (2.304 ± 2.845-fold; $p = 0.139$, n = 4) (Figure 4E).

2.7. Molecular Analysis WT and NSG Mice (Day 3 after ONC): Retinas

Bax. WT mice: The *Bax* expression levels increased without treatment (2.14 ± 1.98-fold, n = 5) and decreased with the AZ treatment (0.93 ± 0.69-fold, $p = 0.23$, n = 5). NSG mice: The *Bax* expression levels were reduced without treatment (0.766 ± 0.585-fold, n = 2) and further decreased with the AZ treatment (0.385±0.632-fold, $p = 0.149$, n = 3) (Figure 5A).

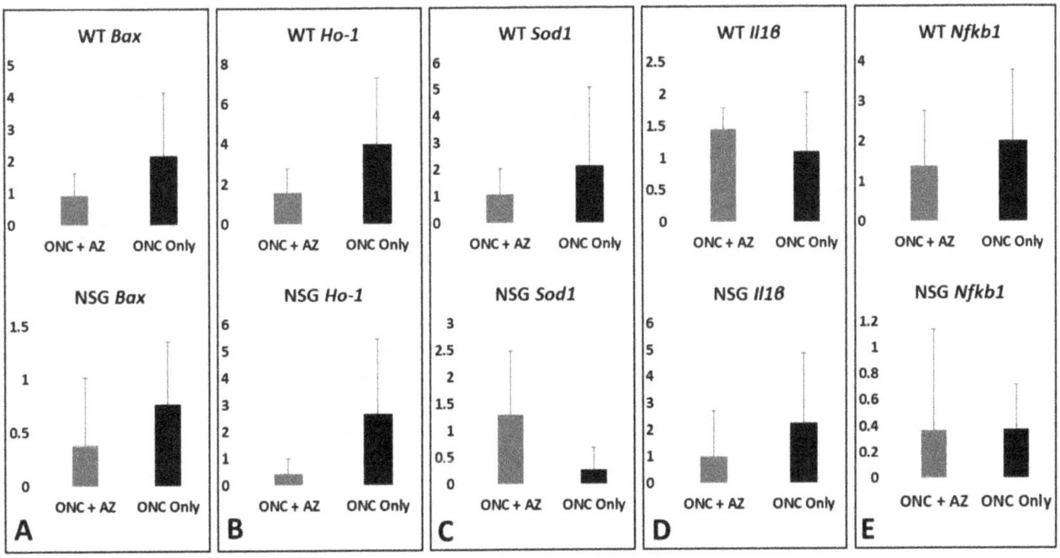

Figure 5. Molecular analysis of the retinas, day 3 after ONC. (**A**) *Bax* expression levels in WT mice increased without treatment and decreased with AZ treatment, while in NSG mice levels remained at baseline without treatment and decreased with AZ treatment. (**B**) *Ho-1* levels in both WT and NSG mice increased without treatment and decreased with AZ treatment. (**C**) *Sod1* levels in WT mice increased without treatment and decreased with AZ treatment, while levels in NSG mice decreased without treatment and increased with AZ treatment. (**D**) *Il1β* levels in WT mice slightly increased without and with treatment, while in NSG mice levels increased without treatment and decreased with AZ treatment. (**E**) *Nfkb1* levels in WT mice increased without treatment and decreased with AZ treatment, while in NSG mice levels decreased without and with treatment.

Ho-1. WT mice: The *Ho-1* expression levels increased without treatment (4.00 ± 3.26-fold, n = 3) and decreased with the AZ treatment (1.55 ± 1.20-fold, $p = 0.29$, n = 3). NSG mice: The *Ho-1* expression levels increased without treatment (2.66 ± 2.78-fold, n = 2) and decreased with the AZ treatment (0.412 ± 0.563-fold, $p = 0.379$, n = 2) (Figure 5B).

Sod1. WT mice: The *Sod1* expression levels increased without treatment (2.16 ± 2.92-fold, n = 5) and decreased with the AZ treatment (1.08 ± 0.96-fold, $p = 0.44$, n = 9). NSG mice: The *Sod1* expression levels decreased without treatment (0.256 ± 0.422-fold, n = 3) and increased with the AZ treatment (1.30 ± 1.188-fold, $p = 0.225$, n = 3) (Figure 5C).

Il1β. WT mice: The *Il1β* expression levels slightly increased without and with treatment, (1.1 ± 0.92-fold and 1.4 ± 0.33-fold, respectively; $p = 0.41$, n = 4, n = 5, respectively). NSG mice: The *Il1β* expression levels increased without treatment (2.236 ± 2.59-fold, n = 2) and decreased with the AZ treatment (0.986 ± 1.70-fold, $p = 0.283$, n = 3) (Figure 5D).

Nfkb1. WT mice: The *Nfkb1* expression levels increased without treatment (2.01 ± 1.77-fold, n = 5) and decreased with the AZ treatment (1.39 ± 1.37-fold, $p = 0.23$, n = 9). NSG mice:

The *Nfkb1* expression levels decreased without and with treatment (0.372 ± 0.343-fold and 0.367 ± 0.771-fold, respectively; $p = 0.158$, n = 3, n = 5, respectively) (Figure 5E).

3. Discussion

AZ is a macrolide that was recently found to have potential neuroprotective effects in animal models [13,14]. On the assumption that its mode of action which is still unclear is related to immunomodulation, we sought to evaluate the effect of AZ in an ONC model of WT and immunodeficient NSG mice. Histologically and in immunohistochemistry, we demonstrated a neuroprotective effect of AZ in both groups of mice, with no effect on retinal thickness. However, there was a difference between the WT and NSG mice in molecular expression, as the AZ effect was relevant only to the WT mice while the NSG mice were not influenced by stress-related or inflammatory-related gene expression levels. In both groups, the apoptosis-related gene *Bax* was reduced in the retinas following AZ treatment, also shown by TUNEL staining. The increased *Bax* levels in the optic nerves in both the WT and NSG mice can be associated with oligodendrocyte loss directly from ONC [15].

To support the possible neuroprotective effect of AZ via immunomodulation and to investigate the underlying pathophysiological mechanisms, we studied inflammation- and stress-related genes in WT and NSG immune deficient transgenic mice. The inclusion of the transgenic NSG mice, which lack B-, T-, and NK-cells, in the analysis was intended to obtain information on the role of the immune response, which has been implicated in ONC [16]. Our results demonstrated significant differences in the molecular expression levels between the WT and immunodeficient NSG mice only in stress-related and inflammatory-related gene expression, while the *Bax* and *Ho-1* levels behaved similarly in both the retina and optic nerve. These differences, as expected, support AZ's role as an immunomodulator. The major molecular effect was detected in the optic nerves and less so in the retina, while the microglial activation and apoptosis were clearly demonstrated in retinal immunostaining.

Nfkb1 expression increases when the tumor necrosis factor (TNF) pathway is activated. The role of the TNF pathway in the neuroprotection of RGC survival was established by Mac Nair et al. [17]. The present study showed that treatment with AZ activated the protective effect of *Nfkb1* following the ONC-induced inflammatory reaction, only in the optic nerves of WT mice.

Previous studies of stress-related genes showed that SOD1 enzymatic activity increases during oxidative stress, such as that induced by ischemia-reperfusion injury [18] or in optic neuropathies [19,20]. In the present study, *Sod1* levels were increased in the injured optic nerves of the WT and NSG mice compared to the healthy internal control nerves and further increased in the WT AZ treated mice, but not the NSG mice, suggesting that it may reduce stress-related damage. In the retina, AZ treatment was associated with *Sod1* return to baseline in both WT and NSG mice. In the present study, the difference in the ON expression levels of *Sod1* between the WT and NSG mice may suggest a different response to injury and AZ treatment, implying differences in the response to oxidative stress between WT and NSG mice.

The levels of *Ho-1*, another stress-related gene with an attributable neuroprotective role, have also been found to increase significantly during oxidative stress in the optic nerves, in line with published data related to optic nerve damage [21]. Kutty et al. [22] reported that *Ho-1* levels were barely detectable under normal circumstances in the retina, but increased markedly in mice exposed to intense visible light compared to unexposed controls. We found in the retina increased levels (4- and 2.6-fold, WT and NSG, respectively) which returned to baseline following the AZ treatment.

Previous studies from our group reported an increase in *Ho-1* expression in the retina under extreme stress (central retinal artery occlusion) [23–25] and its reduction following treatment with brimonidine [25]. In an ONC model, the *Ho-1* level increased on day 3 with a hyperbaric chamber treatment [26].

Inba et al. [14] examined several macrolides, including AZ, in transient cerebral ischemia, but they administered the treatment before the induction of the ischemic damage. We injected AZ intraperitoneally immediately after the ONC induction. Its significant effect suggested that ONC leads to an immediate lymphocyte/macrophage/microglia immune reaction that can be controlled or reduced by AZ. Preventive treatment for acute optic neuropathy is possible only under laboratory conditions and not in real-life clinical scenarios. Therefore, based on our findings, we assume that the earlier the treatment is given, the greater the effect. Under laboratory conditions, the treatment administered almost concurrently with the injury revealed the maximal therapeutic effect that might be achieved. Further studies are needed to determine whether neuroprotection is achieved when the injection is given one to three days after damage. Inba et al. [14] used immunodeficient Sprague–Dawley rats, similar to NSG mice, to examine the effect of AZ and reported a limited inflammatory response.

A similar study by Varano et al. [13] investigating the effect of intraperitoneal AZ on retinal ischemia in a male Wistar rat model found that it had a neuroprotective effect. Ours is the first study, to the best of our knowledge, to examine an ONC model in NSG mice, which are usually used to investigate cancer, not ischemic or inflammatory diseases [27–29]. We propose that NSG mice might also serve for the study of the latter conditions, as a neuroinflammatory response is relevant in a wide spectrum of ocular diseases, including diabetic retinopathy [30].

This study revealed the role of the inflammatory system in response to damage. By including the NSG mouse groups, we were able to compare the effect of AZ on ONC-induced damage in WT mice and isolate the immunomodulating effect. The lesser effect of AZ in NSG mice, especially in the gene expression of the optic nerves, may indicate that in the presence of a compromised immune system, the inflammatory damage caused by ONC was reduced due to a decreased immune response. The effect of AZ on RGC survival and gene expression in WT mice suggests that it acts not only as an immunomodulator but also as an anti-inflammatory and anti-apoptotic agent. The possible neuroprotective effect suggested in this study may lead to novel immunomodulation treatments for optic neuropathies.

This study has several limitations. Although we clearly showed a protective effect of AZ, not all changes in gene expression were statistically significant. Additionally, there was a limited number of NSG mice, and all were female, as opposed to WT males. Furthermore, additional pathways may be involved in the neuronal and RGC damage induced by ONC.

4. Materials and Methods

4.1. Animals

A total of 68 mice were included in the study: 44 male C57/Bl6 wild-type (WT) mice (weight 24–26 g) obtained from Envigo RMS Laboratories (Jerusalem, Israel) and 24 female immunodeficient NOD scid gamma (NSG) mice from a self-colony. All mice were maintained and handled in accordance with the ARVO Statement for the Use of Animals in Ophthalmic and Vision Research and the National Institute of Health guidelines. The animal protocols for the study were approved by the local institutional animal research committee (Rabin Medical Center, RMC-020619).

4.2. Experimental Design

ONC was induced in the right eyes of all the animals. Animals were placed under general anesthesia by intramuscular injection of combined ketamine/xylazine (80 and 4 mg/kg, respectively) supplemented with topical proparacaine hydrochloride 0.5%. Forceps were inserted ~2.5 to 3.0 mm posterior to the right globe, and the right optic nerve was crushed 3 times for 7 s each, separated by a 3 s interval, as previously described by our group [23]. Mice were divided into four groups: two treated with AZ (WT = 23, NSG = 12), and two untreated controls (WT = 21, NSG = 12) (Table 1). Immediately after ONC induction, mice allocated to the treated groups were given a single IP injection of AZ (Zithromax®, azithromycin dehydrated for injection; Pfizer, New York, NY, USA) dissolved in saline (0.9% NaCl) at a dose of 50 mg/kg, as reported elsewhere [31]. The control groups were injected with the same amount of saline only.

Table 1. Experimental design.

Procedure/Study	Analysis Method	C57Bl/6 Mice (n = 24)	NSG Mice (n = 24)
ONC	molecular	10	5
	IHC	11	7
ONC + AZ	molecular	10	5
	IHC	13	7

ONC = optic nerve crush, AZ = azithromycin, IHC = immunohistochemistry; NSG = NOD scid gamma.

4.3. Tissue Collection

Mice were euthanized by carbon dioxide asphyxiation at 3 or 21 days after ONC/treatment, and the eyes (globes and nerves) were enucleated for molecular and histological analysis.

4.4. Molecular Analysis (Day 3)

Three days following ONC induction, retinas and optic nerves were dissected from both eyes (WT = 5, NSG = 5) and placed in RNAlater solution (Invitrogen, Life Technologies, Carlsbad, CA, USA) at −80 °C. Total RNA was isolated using a reagent (TRIzol; Invitrogen, CA, USA) according to the manufacturer's protocol and then reverse-transcribed into cDNA using random hexamers (Bioline, London, UK) and Moloney murine leukemia virus (M-MLV)-reverse transcriptase (Promega, Madison, WI, USA).

Two-stage real-time quantitative polymerase chain reaction (PCR; sequence detection system, Prism 7900; Applied Biosystems, Foster City, CA, USA) was used to evaluate levels of mRNA expression of genes coding for proteins involved in apoptosis, ischemia, and oxidative stress: *Bax*, superoxide dismutase 1 (*Sod1*), heme oxygenase 1 (*Ho-1*), interleukin 1 beta (*Il1β*), and nuclear factor-kappa B 1 (*Nfkb1*). Mouse glyceraldehyde 3-phosphate dehydrogenase (*Gapdh*) was used to normalize cDNA input levels. The primers are listed in Table 2. Reactions were performed in a 20 μL volume containing 4 μL cDNA, 0.5 μM each of forward and reverse primers and buffer included in the master mix (SYBR Green I; Applied Biosystems, Foster City, CA, USA). Duplicate reactions were performed for each gene to minimize individual tube variability, and an average was taken for each time point. Threshold cycle efficiency corrections were calculated, and melting curves were obtained using cDNA for each gene PCR assay.

Table 2. List of primers for molecular studies.

*Sod1*_F	GCCCGGCGGATGAAGA
*Sod1*_R	CGTCCTTTCCAGCAGTCACA
*Bax*_F	CTGAGCTGACCTTGGAGC
*Bax*_R	GACTCCAGCCACAAAGATG
*Ho-1*_F	CAGGTGTCCAGAGAAGGCT
*Ho-1*_R	TCTTCCAGGGCCGTGTAGAT
Il1β _F	TGACAGTGATGAGAATGACCTGTTC
Il1β _R	GGACAGCCCAGGTCAAAGG
*Gapdh*_F	TGCCACTCAGAAGACTGTGGATG
*Gapdh*_R	GCCTGCTTCACCACCTTCTTGAT
*Nfkb1*_F	CCTGCAAAGGTTATCGTTCAGTT
*Nfkb1*_R	GCAAAGCCAACCACCATGT

PCR cycling conditions consisted of an initial denaturation step of 95 °C for 10 min followed by 40 cycles of 15 s of denaturation at 95 °C and 1 min of annealing and extension at 60 °C. Standard curves were obtained using untreated mouse cDNA for each gene PCR assay. The results were quantified using a comparative threshold cycle (Ct) method, also known as the $2-\Delta\Delta Ct$ method, where: $\Delta\Delta Ct = \Delta Ct$ (sample) $-$ ΔCt (reference gene).

Molecular analysis was performed comparing the right (ONC) and left (control) optic nerves and retinas with and without AZ treatment for each of the WT and transgenic NSG groups.

4.5. Histological Analysis

4.5.1. Hematoxylin and Eosin Staining (Day 21)

At 21 days after ONC induction, the eyes were enucleated and fixed in 4% formaldehyde for 1 h, washed in phosphate-buffered saline (PBS, 1X; Beit HaEmek, Israel), and placed in 15% and 20% sucrose dissolved in PBS for 1 h each. Eyes were then placed in 30% sucrose at 4 °C for 12 h and embedded in optimum cutting temperature compound (Sakura Tissue-Tek, Tokyo, Japan). Cryosections of the globes and optic nerve (6 μm) were mounted on slides and stained with hematoxylin and eosin (H&E), with three consecutive sections on each slide.

4.5.2. Retinal Ganglion Cell (RGC) Count and Retinal Thickness Measurement

H&E stained slides were examined under a light microscope (Ernst Leitz GMBH Wetzlar, Germany). RGC count was determined by counting the nuclei of the RGC in the RGC layer (horizontal counting) in three sections of every 10 slides (30 consecutive sections), for a total of 7 to 10 slides per eye. The percentage of cell loss was calculated as follows: retinal cell loss = 100 * (1 − [average left-eye cell count in the RGC layer/average right-eye cell count in the RGC layer]). Retinal thickness was measured in each section by drawing a vertical line under light microscopy guidance from the outer segment of the photoreceptors, avoiding artificial detachment from the retinal pigment epithelium to the retinal nerve fiber layer internal limiting membrane.

4.5.3. GFAP and CD45 Immunostaining

Cryosections of the enucleated eyes taken on day 21 were washed with PBS × 1, blocked with 2% BSA in PBS with 0.5% Triton X-100 for 15 min and incubated at 4 °C overnight with the primary antibody, rat anti-CD45 (1:100, Millipore, Temecula, CA, USA), and GFAP (1:200, Proteintech, Thermo Fisher Scientific, MA, USA). The sections were washed with 0.2% PBS with 0.5% Triton X-100 and incubated at room temperature for 1 h with the secondary antibody, goat anti-rat IgG Alexa Fluor 488 (1:200) (Molecular Probes, Invitrogen). The sections underwent nuclear counterstaining with DAPI (Invitrogen). Images were generated using a conventional fluorescence microscope (Fluoview X; Olympus, Tokyo, Japan). Excitation wavelengths were 405 nm for DAPI and 488 nm for Alexa.

4.5.4. In Situ TdT-Mediated dUTP Nick End-Labeling (TUNEL) Immunostaining

Retinal cryosections 10 μm thick were cut in the direction of the optic nerve axis on days 1 and 3 following ONC with or without AZ treatment and examined by in situ TdT-mediated dUTP nick end-labeling (TUNEL) assay (Roche Diagnostics GmbH, Germany, Cat. No: 11684795910) which is a fluorescein-tagged apoptosis detection system. Staining was performed according to the manufacturer's instructions. The sections underwent nuclear counterstaining with DAPI. Results were analyzed with a confocal fluorescence microscope (LSM 700 Inverted, Carl Zeiss, Oberkochen, Germany) equipped with appropriate filters. Excitation wavelengths used were 405 nm for DAPI and 488 nm for Cy2. The mean number of TUNEL-positive cells was determined in five different regions in the section and plotted as a column chart with standard deviation.

4.5.5. IBA1 Immunostaining

Cryosections of the enucleated eyes taken on day 3 were washed with PBS × 1, permeabilized with 1% Triton for 10 min, blocked with 5% Fetal calf serum in PBS for 60 min, and incubated at 4 °C overnight with the primary antibody, rabbit anti-IBA1 (1:500,

Abcam, Cat# ab178846). The sections were washed with PBS ×1 and incubated at room temperature for 1 h with the secondary antibody, goat anti-rabbit IgG H&L Alexa Fluor 647 (1:1000, Abcam, Cat# ab150079). The sections underwent nuclear counterstaining with DAPI (Sigma Aldrich Israel, Rehovot, Israel). Images were generated using an LSM 700 inverted confocal fluorescence microscope (Carl Zeiss, Oberkochen, Germany). Excitation wavelengths used were 405 nm for DAPI and 647 nm for Alexa Fluor.

4.6. Statistical Analysis

Differences between groups were analyzed using an unpaired Student's *t*-test. Significance was defined as $p < 0.05$.

5. Conclusions

This study demonstrated important differences between WT mice with a normal immune response and immunodeficient NSG mice subjected to ONC. AZ had a neuroprotective effect against ONC-induced damage that preserved the RGCs in the WT mice. This effect was not significant in the NSG mice, which had a lower (baseline) level of inflammatory markers following ONC. AZ treatment reduced the expression of stress-related genes and modulated the inflammatory reaction in the retina while increasing it in the optic nerves. This macrolide drug, already available and FDA-approved for infections, may potentially protect oxidative-stress-related acute optic neuropathies. We suggest that the neuroprotective effect is instigated by immunomodulation, as indicated by the improved response of the WT mice to the AZ treatment compared to the NSG mice.

Author Contributions: Conceptualization, N.G.-C.; methodology, N.G.-C., M.F.-G., S.W., O.Z., A.Z. and S.R.; validation, M.F.-G., S.W., A.Z., S.R. and N.G.-C.; formal analysis, M.F.-G., S.R. and N.G.-C.; investigation, O.Z., A.Z., M.F.-G., S.W. and S.R.; resources, N.G.-C.; writing—original draft preparation, O.Z., A.Z. and N.G.-C.; writing—review and editing, A.Z., S.R. and N.G.-C.; visualization, A.Z., S.R. and N.G.-C.; supervision, N.G.-C.; project administration, N.G.-C.; funding acquisition, N.G.-C. and O.Z. All authors have read and agreed to the published version of the manuscript.

Funding: This research was partially supported by the Recanati Foundation Herman Schauder Fund, Tel Aviv University, Tel Aviv, Israel (O.Z.) and by the Zanvyl and Isabelle Krieger Fund, Baltimore, Maryland, USA (N.G.C.).

Institutional Review Board Statement: The animal study protocol was approved by the local institutional animal research committee of Rabin Medical Center (protocol code RMC-020619, June 2019).

Informed Consent Statement: Not applicable.

Data Availability Statement: The data presented in this study are available on request from the corresponding author.

Acknowledgments: We thank Gloria Ginzach and Melanie Kave for their editorial assistance.

Conflicts of Interest: The authors declare no conflict of interest. The funders had no role in the design of the study; in the collection, analyses, or interpretation of data; in the writing of the manuscript, or in the decision to publish the results.

References

1. Biousse, V.; Newman, N.J. Ischemic optic neuropathies. *N. Engl. J. Med.* **2015**, *372*, 2428–2436. [CrossRef] [PubMed]
2. Chen, T.; Song, D.; Shan, G.; Wang, K.; Wang, Y.; Ma, J.; Zhong, Y. The association between diabetes mellitus and nonarteritic anterior ischemic optic neuropathy: A systematic review and meta-analysis. *PLoS ONE* **2013**, *8*, e76653. [CrossRef]
3. Fraser, C.L. Obstructive sleep apnea and optic neuropathy: Is there a link? *Curr. Neurol. Neurosci. Rep.* **2014**, *14*, 465. [CrossRef]
4. Salgado, C.; Vilson, F.; Miller, N.R.; Bernstein, S.L. Cellular inflammation in nonarteritic anterior ischemic optic neuropathy and its primate model. *Arch. Ophthalmol.* **2011**, *129*, 1583–1591. [CrossRef] [PubMed]
5. Rappoport, D.; Morzaev, D.; Weiss, S.; Vieyra, M.; Nicholson, J.D.; Leiba, H.; Goldenberg-cohen, N. Effect of intravitreal injection of bevacizumab on optic nerve head leakage and retinal ganglion cell survival in a mouse model of optic nerve crush. *Investig. Ophthalmol. Vis. Sci.* **2013**, *54*, 8160–8171. [CrossRef]

6. Morzaev, D.; Nicholson, J.D.; Caspi, T.; Weiss, S.; Hochhauser, E.; Goldenberg-Cohen, N. Toll-like receptor-4 knockout mice are more resistant to optic nerve crush damage than wild-type mice. *Clin. Exp. Ophthalmol.* **2015**, *43*, 655–665. [CrossRef]
7. Bosnar, M.; Čužić, S.; Bošnjak, B.; Nujić, K.; Ergović, G.; Marjanović, N.; Pašalić, I.; Hrvačić, B.; Polančec, D.; Glojnarić, I.; et al. Azithromycin inhibits macrophage interleukin-1β production through inhibition of activator protein-1 in lipopolysaccharide-induced murine pulmonary neutrophilia. *Int. Immunopharmacol.* **2011**, *11*, 424–434. [CrossRef]
8. Feola, D.J.; Garvy, B.A.; Cory, T.J.; Birket, S.E.; Hoy, H.; Hayes, D., Jr.; Murphy, B.S. Azithromycin alters macrophage phenotype and pulmonary compartmentalization during lung infection with Pseudomonas. *Antimicrob. Agents Chemother.* **2010**, *54*, 2437–2447. [CrossRef]
9. Parnham, M.J.; Erakovic Haber, V.; Giamarellos-Bourboulis, E.J.; Perletti, G.; Verleden, G.M.; Vos, R. Azithromycin: Mechanisms of action and their relevance for clinical applications. *Pharmacol. Ther.* **2014**, *143*, 225–245. [CrossRef] [PubMed]
10. Geudens, N.; Timmermans, L.; Vanhooren, H.; Vanaudenaerde, B.M.; Vos, R.; Van De Wauwer, C.; Verleden, G.M.; Verbeken, E.; Lerut, T.; Van Raemdonck, D.E. Azithromycin reduces airway inflammation in a murine model of lung ischaemia reperfusion injury. *Transpl. Int.* **2008**, *21*, 688–695. [CrossRef] [PubMed]
11. Amantea, D.; Certo, M.; Petrelli, F.; Tassorelli, C.; Micieli, G.; Corasaniti, M.T.; Puccetti, P.; Fallarino, F.; Bagetta, G. Azithromycin protects mice against ischemic stroke injury by promoting macrophage transition towards M2 phenotype. *Exp. Neurol.* **2016**, *275 Pt 1*, 116–125. [CrossRef]
12. Cercek, B.; Shah, P.K.; Noc, M.; Zahger, D.; Zeymer, U.; Matetzky, S.; Maurer, G.; Mahrer, P.; AZACS Investigators. Effect of short-term treatment with azithromycin on recurrent ischaemic events in patients with acute coronary syndrome in the Azithromycin in Acute Coronary Syndrome (AZACS) trial: A randomised controlled trial. *Lancet* **2003**, *361*, 809–813. [CrossRef]
13. Varano, G.P.; Parisi, V.; Adornetto, A.; Cavaliere, F.; Amantea, D.; Nucci, C.; Corasaniti, M.T.; Morrone, L.A.; Bagetta, G.; Russo, R. Post-ischemic treatment with azithromycin protects ganglion cells against retinal ischemia/reperfusion injury in the rat. *Mol. Vis.* **2017**, *23*, 911–921. [PubMed]
14. Inaba, T.; Katayama, Y.; Ueda, M.; Nito, C. Neuroprotective effects of pretreatment with macrolide antibiotics on cerebral ischemia reperfusion injury. *Neurol. Res.* **2015**, *37*, 514–524. [CrossRef] [PubMed]
15. Goldenberg-Cohen, N.; Guo, Y.; Margolis, F.; Cohen, Y.; Miller, N.R.; Bernstein, S.L. Oligodendrocyte dysfunction after induction of experimental anterior optic nerve ischemia. *Investig. Ophthalmol. Vis. Sci.* **2005**, *46*, 2716–2725. [CrossRef]
16. Zhang, C.; Guo, Y.; Miller, N.R.; Bernstein, S.L. Optic nerve infarction and post-ischemic inflammation in the rodent model of anterior ischemic optic neuropathy (rAION). *Brain Res.* **2009**, *1264*, 67–75. [CrossRef] [PubMed]
17. Mac Nair, C.E.; Fernandes, K.A.; Schlamp, C.L.; Libby, R.T.; Nickells, R.W. Tumor necrosis factor alpha has an early protective effect on retinal ganglion cells after optic nerve crush. *J. Neuroinflamm.* **2014**, *11*, 194. [CrossRef] [PubMed]
18. Eleutherio, E.C.A.; Silva Magalhães, R.S.; de Araújo Brasil, A.; Monteiro Neto, J.R.; de Holanda Paranhos, L. SOD1, more than just an antioxidant. *Arch. Biochem. Biophys.* **2021**, *697*, 108701. [CrossRef] [PubMed]
19. Levin, L.A. Superoxide generation explains common features of optic neuropathies associated with cecocentral scotomas. *J. Neuroophthalmol.* **2015**, *35*, 152–160. [CrossRef] [PubMed]
20. Kanamori, A.; Catrinescu, M.M.; Mahammed, A.; Gross, Z.; Levin, L.A. Neuroprotection against superoxide anion radical by metallocorroles in cellular and murine models of optic neuropathy. *J. Neurochem.* **2010**, *114*, 488–498. [CrossRef] [PubMed]
21. Himori, N.; Maruyama, K.; Yamamoto, K.; Yasuda, M.; Ryu, M.; Omodaka, K.; Shiga, Y.; Tanaka, Y.; Nakazawa, T. Critical neuroprotective roles of heme oxygenase-1 induction against axonal injury-induced retinal ganglion cell death. *J. Neurosci. Res.* **2014**, *92*, 1134–1142. [CrossRef] [PubMed]
22. Kutty, R.K.; Kutty, G.; Wiggert, B.; Chader, G.J.; Darrow, R.M.; Organisciak, D.T. Induction of heme oxygenase 1 in the retina by intense visible light: Suppression by the antioxidant dimethylthiourea. *Proc. Natl. Acad. Sci. USA* **1995**, *92*, 1177–1181. [CrossRef] [PubMed]
23. Dratviman-Storobinsky, O.; Hasanreisoglu, M.; Offen, D.; Barhum, Y.; Weinberger, D.; Goldenberg-Cohen, N. Progressive damage along the optic nerve following induction of crush injury or rodent anterior ischemic optic neuropathy in transgenic mice. *Mol. Vis.* **2008**, *14*, 2171–2179. [PubMed]
24. Goldenberg-Cohen, N.; Dadon, S.; Avraham, B.C.; Kramer, M.; Hasanreisoglu, M.; Eldar, I.; Weinberger, D.; Bahar, I. Molecular and histological changes following central retinal artery occlusion in a mouse model. *Exp. Eye Res.* **2008**, *87*, 327–333. [CrossRef] [PubMed]
25. Goldenberg-Cohen, N.; Dadon-Bar-El, S.; Hasanreisoglu, M.; Avraham-Lubin, B.C.; Dratviman-Storobinsky, O.; Cohen, Y.; Weinberger, D. Possible neuroprotective effect of brimonidine in a mouse model of ischaemic optic neuropathy. *Clin. Exp. Ophthalmol.* **2009**, *37*, 718–729. [CrossRef] [PubMed]
26. Avraham-Lubin, B.C.; Dratviman-Storobinsky, O.; Dadon-Bar El, S.; Hasanreisoglu, M.; Goldenberg-Cohen, N. Neuroprotective effect of hyperbaric oxygen therapy on anterior ischemic optic neuropathy. *Front. Neurol.* **2011**, *2*, 23. [CrossRef] [PubMed]
27. Scopim-Ribeiro, R.; Lizardo, M.M.; Zhang, H.F.; Dhez, A.C.; Hughes, C.S.; Sorensen, P.H. NSG mice facilitate ex vivo characterization of Ewing sarcoma lung metastasis using the PuMA model. *Front. Oncol.* **2021**, *11*, 645757. [CrossRef] [PubMed]
28. Kim, J.; Ryu, B.; Kim, U.; Kim, C.H.; Hur, G.H.; Kim, C.Y.; Park, J.H. Improved human hematopoietic reconstitution in HepaRG co-transplanted humanized NSG mice. *BMB Rep.* **2020**, *53*, 466–471. [CrossRef]

29. Skoda, J.; Neradil, J.; Staniczkova Zambo, I.; Nunukova, A.; Macsek, P.; Borankova, K.; Dobrotkova, V.; Nemec, P.; Sterba, J.; Veselska, R. Serial xenotransplantation in NSG mice promotes a hybrid epithelial/mesenchymal gene expression signature and stemness in rhabdomyosarcoma cells. *Cancers* **2020**, *12*, 196. [CrossRef] [PubMed]
30. Yu, Y.; Chen, H.; Su, S.B. Neuroinflammatory responses in diabetic retinopathy. *J. Neuroinflamm.* **2015**, *12*, 141. [CrossRef]
31. Azoulay-Dupuis, E.; Vallée, E.; Bedos, J.P.; Muffat-Joly, M.; Pocidalo, J.J. Prophylactic and therapeutic activities of azithromycin in a mouse model of pneumococcal pneumonia. *Antimicrob. Agents Chemother.* **1991**, *35*, 1024–1028. [CrossRef] [PubMed]

International Journal of *Molecular Sciences*

MDPI

Article

Specific Activation of Yamanaka Factors via HSF1 Signaling in the Early Stage of Zebrafish Optic Nerve Regeneration

Kayo Sugitani [1,*], Takumi Mokuya [1], Shuichi Homma [1], Minami Maeda [1], Ayano Konno [1] and Kazuhiro Ogai [2]

1 Department of Clinical Laboratory Science, Graduate School of Medical Science, Kanazawa University, 5-11-80 Kodatsuno, Kanazawa 920-0942, Japan
2 AI Hospital/Macro Signal Dynamics Research and Development Center, 5-11-80 Kodatsuno, Kanazawa 920-0942, Japan
* Correspondence: sugitani@staff.kanazawa-u.ac.jp; Tel.: +81-76-265-2599

Abstract: In contrast to the case in mammals, the fish optic nerve can spontaneously regenerate and visual function can be fully restored 3–4 months after optic nerve injury (ONI). However, the regenerative mechanism behind this has remained unknown. This long process is reminiscent of the normal development of the visual system from immature neural cells to mature neurons. Here, we focused on the expression of three Yamanaka factors (Oct4, Sox2, and Klf4: OSK), which are well-known inducers of induced pluripotent stem (iPS) cells in the zebrafish retina after ONI. mRNA expression of OSK was rapidly induced in the retinal ganglion cells (RGCs) 1–3 h after ONI. Heat shock factor 1 (HSF1) mRNA was most rapidly induced in the RGCs at 0.5 h. The activation of OSK mRNA was completely suppressed by the intraocular injection of HSF1 morpholino prior to ONI. Furthermore, the chromatin immunoprecipitation assay showed the enrichment of OSK genomic DNA bound to HSF1. The present study clearly showed that the rapid activation of Yamanaka factors in the zebrafish retina was regulated by HSF1, and this sequential activation of HSF1 and OSK might provide a key to unlocking the regenerative mechanism of injured RGCs in fish.

Keywords: HSF1; Klf4; Oct4; Sox2; Yamanaka factors; retina; optic nerve regeneration; zebrafish

Citation: Sugitani, K.; Mokuya, T.; Homma, S.; Maeda, M.; Konno, A.; Ogai, K. Specific Activation of Yamanaka Factors via HSF1 Signaling in the Early Stage of Zebrafish Optic Nerve Regeneration. *Int. J. Mol. Sci.* **2023**, *24*, 3253. https://doi.org/10.3390/ijms24043253

Academic Editors: Neil R. Miller and Rongkung Tsai

Received: 30 December 2022
Revised: 30 January 2023
Accepted: 3 February 2023
Published: 7 February 2023

1. Introduction

Neurons in the mammalian central nervous system (CNS) cannot regenerate after nerve injury and eventually die, whereas neurons in the fish CNS can regenerate and fully recover CNS function [1–3]. Since the work of Sperry in the 1950s, the fish visual system has been the most popular model of CNS regeneration [4–9]. For the past 20 years, we have examined the regeneration of fish optic nerves from nerve crush to the recovery of visual function by using modern neurobiological tools such as immunohistochemistry [10–12], cell and tissue culture systems [13–15], and three-dimensional image processing systems for behavioral analysis [11,16,17]. The obtained results revealed that fish optic nerve regeneration includes (i) an early preparation period at 0–4 days; (ii) a middle neurite outgrowth period at 5–30 days; and (iii) a late synaptic refinement period at 1–4 months after optic nerve injury (ONI). We were particularly interested in the early period (0–4 days) because molecular events arising in this period are the most mysterious and important for resolving the regenerative mechanism of adult fish retinal ganglion cells (RGCs) after ONI.

In the past 10 years, we have applied molecular genetics in the search for genes upregulated at this early stage using zebrafish. Some cell survival-related and anti-apoptotic factors were found to be induced in RGCs within 1–4 days after ONI such as insulin-like growth factor-I (IGF-I), Bcl-2, phospho-Akt (p-Akt), and phospho-Bad (p-Bad) [17,18]. Similarly, molecules such as purpurin [19], neuroglobin [20,21], and cellular factor XIII A subunit (cFXIII-A) [12,15] were induced in RGCs to activate neurite outgrowth. Heat shock factor 1 (HSF1) was most rapidly induced in RGCs at 0.5 h after ONI [22–24]. These molecules were shown to function to maintain the viability of the injured RGCs and activate neural budding in preparation for promoted neurite elongation in the next stage [22–24].

However, why adult fish RGCs can regenerate after ONI has remained unclear. In consideration of the similarity between the regenerative process of the fish optic nerve and the normal development of the visual system in embryogenesis, we hypothesize that the injured fish RGCs are initialized to immature RGCs as soon as possible at the early stage after ONI. These immature RGCs can easily regenerate, regrow their axons, and restore visual function.

In the present study, we investigated the expression of Yamanaka factor genes after ONI in zebrafish. The term "Yamanaka factors" originally referred to four transcription factors, Oct4, Sox2, Klf4, and c-Myc, which have the effect of inducing somatic cells to become induced pluripotent stem (iPS) cells [25,26]. Of these four Yamanaka factors, c-Myc was reported to not necessarily be essential for initiating cell reprogramming [27–29]. Therefore, we evaluated the expression of three Yamanaka factors, Oct4, Sox2, and Klf4 (OSK), and their relationship to optic nerve regeneration. We also focused on the interaction between the expression of OSK and HSF1 as the fastest acute-phase response molecule after ONI.

2. Results

2.1. Rapid Increase of HSF1 Gene Expression in Zebrafish Retina after ONI

We performed real-time PCR using gene-specific primers to examine how the expression of the *HSF1* gene changes in the retina after optic nerve crush. The upregulation of *HSF1* mRNA started at 0.5 h after ONI, peaked at 6 h, and decreased at 24 h (Figure 1a). However, HSF1 expression was still significantly higher at 24 h.

The same results were confirmed upon in situ hybridization of *HSF1* in zebrafish retina (Figure 1b). A prominent increase in *HSF1* signal was first observed in the ganglion cell layer (GCL) and the inner nuclear layer (INL) at 0.5 h after ONI (Figure 1b). These changes were subsequently enhanced and spread to all of the nuclear layers in the retina, peaking at 6 h after ONI. Similarly, immunohistochemical staining of the HSF1 protein in zebrafish retina detected positive signals in all nuclear layers 1–24 h after ONI (Figure 1c). These increases of HSF1 were accompanied by increases in four heat shock proteins (HSPs), *HSP25, HSP60, HSP70*, and *HSP90*, the target genes of HSF1 examined here by real-time PCR analysis (Figure S1).

2.2. Increase in OSK Gene Expression in Zebrafish Retina after ONI

Next, we performed real-time PCR to examine the expression of the three Yamanaka factors—*Oct4, Sox2*, and Klf4 (OSK)—in the injured retina with the optic nerve crushed using gene-specific primers (see Table S1). Figure 2a showed that the expression of these transcription factors increased significantly and rapidly in the retina within 1 h after ONI. *Klf4* responded most quickly, followed by *Oct4* and then *Sox2*. The localization of OSK was confirmed by in situ hybridization (Figure 2b). In situ hybridization showed the weak expression of Klf4 throughout the retina at 1 h, which then became restricted to the GCL at 3 h after ONI (Figure 2b, upper panel). Meanwhile, *Oct4* showed a prominent signal only in the GCL and INL at 3 h after ONI (Figure 2b, center panel), but this expression then expanded to all nuclear layers at 6 h. The expression of *Sox2* was observed in all nuclear layers including the outer nuclear layer (ONL), INL, and GCL, at 3–6 h after ONI (Figure 2b, lower panel). Immunohistochemical studies of OSK (Figure S2) revealed similar patterns in the real-time PCR and in situ hybridization.

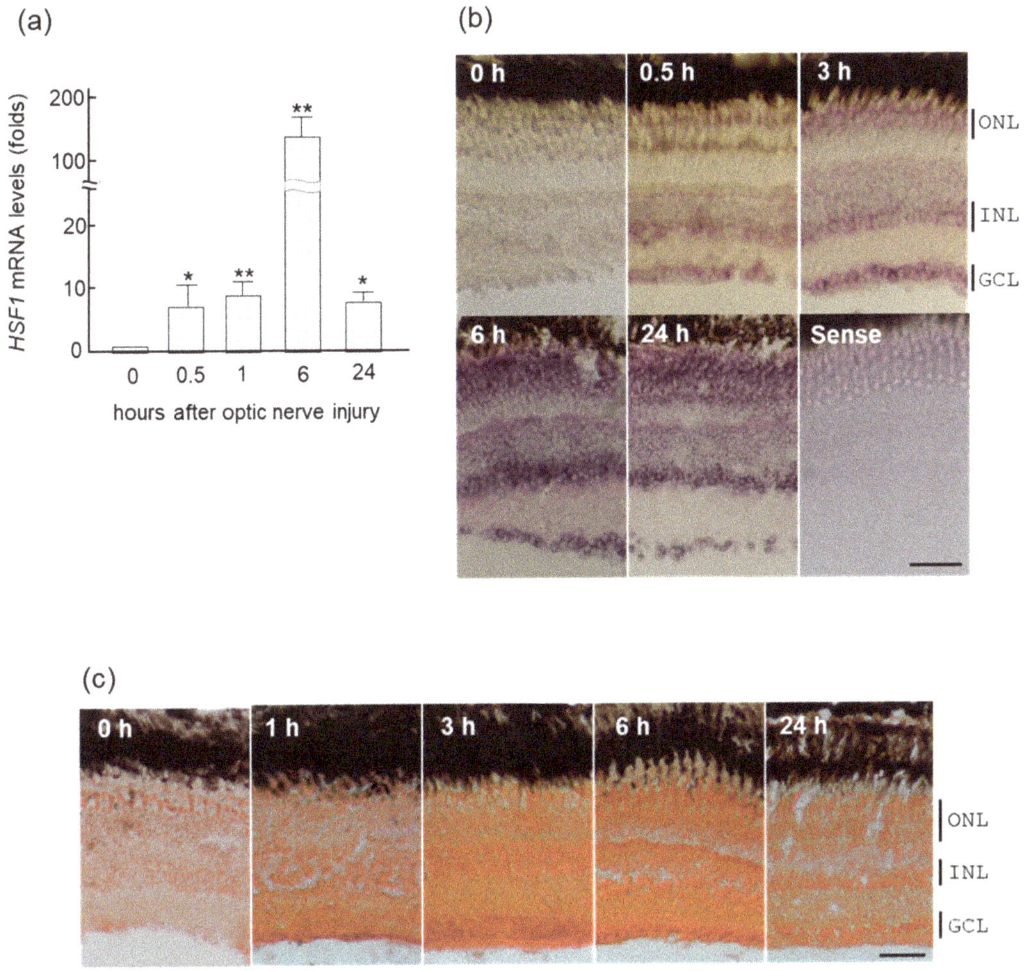

Figure 1. Upregulation of HSF1 (heat shock factor 1) mRNA in zebrafish retina after ONI (optic nerve injury). (**a**) *HSF1* mRNA expression levels after ONI were determined using quantitative real-time PCR. (**b**) In situ hybridization of *HSF1* in the zebrafish retina after nerve injury. *HSF1* mRNA started to increase in the retina for 0.5 h and peaked at 6 h after ONI. Its localization was first seen in the GCLs (ganglion cell layers) and after the INLs (inner nuclear layers). Then, these signals spread to all nuclear layers including the ONLs (outer nuclear layers) at 6 h and slightly decreased at 24 h after ONL. (**c**) Immunohistochemical staining of HSF1 in the zebrafish retina after ONI. Significant immunostaining peaked at 3 to 6 h in all nuclear layers after ONI. Data are expressed as the mean ± SEM of five independent experiments and analyzed by one-way ANOVA, followed by Scheffe's multiple comparisons. Statistical significance was set at * $p < 0.05$ or ** $p < 0.01$. Scale bar = 50 μm.

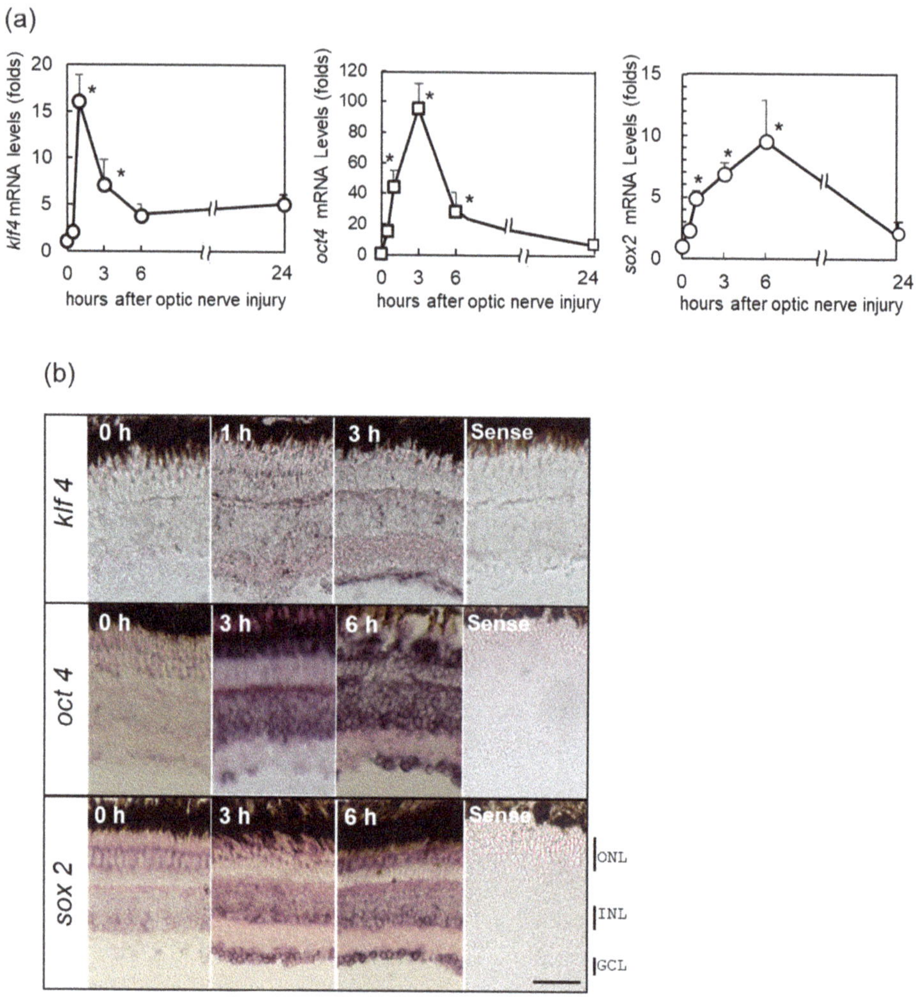

Figure 2. Upregulation of the Yamanaka factors (OSK) in zebrafish retina after ONI. (**a**) mRNA expression levels of OSK after ONI were determined by quantitative real-time PCR (left, klf4; center, oct4; right, sox2). (**b**) In situ hybridization of OSK in zebrafish retina after ONI. *Klf4* mRNA expression started to increase at 1 h and localized to the GCLs at 3 h after ONI. *Oct4* mRNA signal was observed in the GCL and strongly in the INL and ONL at 3 h, but this strong signal was seen in all nuclear layers at 6 h after ONI. *Sox2* mRNA expression was observed in all nuclear layers 3 h after ONI and more prominent at 6 h. No positive signals could be seen with the sense probe (Sense). Five to six experiments were repeated with different retinas under each experimental condition and produced the same results. Data are expressed as the mean ± SEM and analyzed by one-way ANOVA, followed by Scheffe's multiple comparisons. Statistical significance was set at * $p < 0.05$. Scale bar = 50 μm.

2.3. HSF1 Regulates Expression of OSK

We explored the relationship between HSF1 and the three Yamanaka factors, OSK, because the expression of these genes was induced so rapidly in the retina. *HSF1* mRNA expression was increased over 100 times at 6 h after ONI compared with the level in the control (Figure 1a). Therefore, we used morpholino (MO) to suppress *HSF1* expression by the method shown in Figure 3a. Intraocular injection of *HSF1*-specific MO was conducted

20 h before ONI completely suppressed the increase of *HSF1* mRNA in the retina 6 h after ONI (Figure 3b). In addition, treatment with *HSF1* MO completely suppressed the upregulation of *Klf4* mRNA (Figure 3c), *Oct4* mRNA (Figure 3d), and *Sox2* mRNA (Figure 3e). Intraocular injection of standard morpholino (Std. MO) was not effective at suppressing the ONI-induced increase in OSK mRNA (Figure 3b–e).

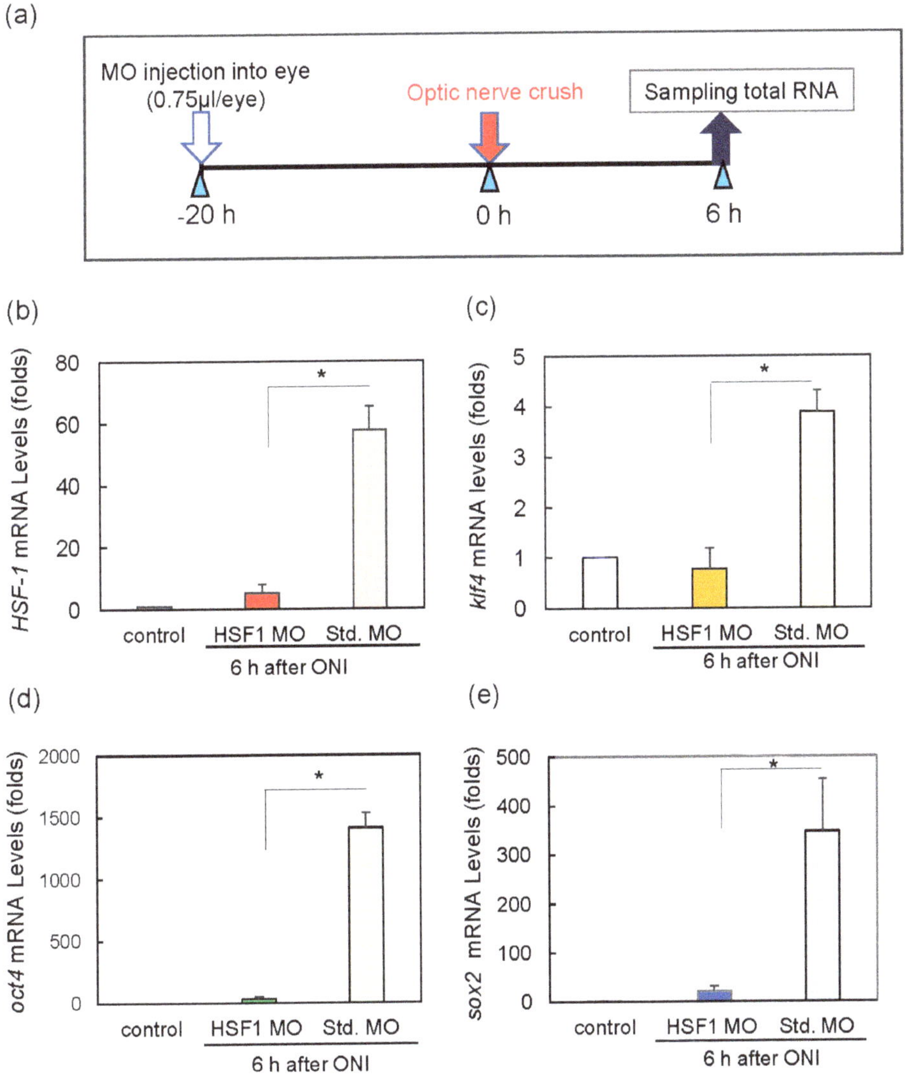

Figure 3. Treatment of HSF1 MO (morpholino) significantly reduced the mRNA expression of Klf4, Oct4, and Sox2 6 h after ONI. (**a**) HSF1 MO or standard MO (Std. MO) was injected intraocularly 20 h before ONI. (**b**) HSF1 MO-treated group suppressed HSF1 mRNA expression compared to the Std. MO-treated group. Under these conditions, the mRNA expression of Klf4 (**c**), Oct4 (**d**), and Sox2 (**e**) was inhibited compared to the control (Std. MO) groups. Five experiments were repeated under each experimental condition. Data are expressed as the mean ± SEM of independent experiments and analyzed by one-way ANOVA, followed by Scheffe's multiple comparisons. Statistical significance was set at * $p < 0.05$.

2.4. ChIP Assay of OSK in Response to HSF1

To confirm the correlation between the induction of HSF1 expression after ONI and the subsequent increase in OSK, we performed a ChIP assay by using retinal samples with anti-HSF antibodies. After ONI, DNA samples were extracted from the intact retina (0 h) or injured retina 6 h. These samples were immunoprecipitated with anti-HSF1 antibodies and purified. ChIP-enriched DNA samples were amplified with several primer sets for the encoding of OSK (Table S1), which have putative HSF1 binding regions (Figure S3). Anti-HSF1 antibodies precipitated approximately 10–20 times more of the specific DNA of each OSK gene than the IgG control did (Figure 4a, 6 h). No amplified products were detected in the IgG control-treated group (Figure 4b, IgG) or the intact group (Figure 4a, 0 h).

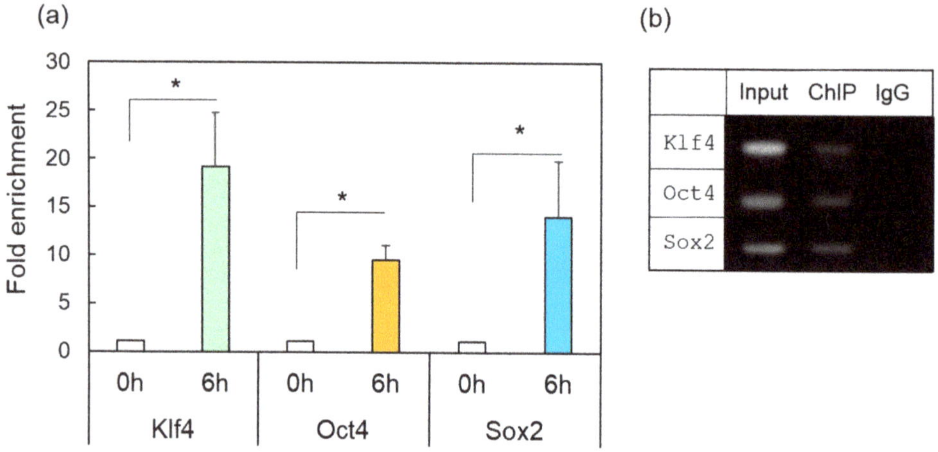

Figure 4. ChIP-enriched DNA was prepared using preimmune serum (IgG) or anti-HSF1 antibody from the control (0 h) or damaged zebrafish retina after ONI (6 h). (**a**) The immunoprecipitated DNA of *Klf4*, *Oct4*, and *Sox2* were analyzed by real-time PCR. Each ChIP signal was divided by the no-antibody signals (IgG), representing the ChIP signals as the fold increase in signals relative to the background signals. (**b**) Gel electrophoresis image using the ChIP samples. The input was used as an internal positive control for the ChIP assay. Five to six experiments were repeated with different retinas under each experimental condition. Data are expressed as the mean ± SEM of independent experiments and analyzed by one-way ANOVA, followed by Scheffe's multiple comparisons. Statistical significance was set at * $p < 0.05$.

3. Discussion

3.1. Rapid Activation of OSK via HSF1 Signaling in the Zebrafish Retina after ONI

We found that the gene expression of OSK was rapidly induced after ONI. Among these three factors, Klf4 was expressed transiently (1–3 h) and its expression peaked at 1 h. Meanwhile, Oct4 was expressed at 1–6 h and peaked at 3 h. Finally, Sox2 exhibited more long-lasting expression and peaked at 6 h. Regarding the localizations of these molecules, Klf4 was predominantly expressed in the GCL, while Oct4 and Sox2 were first localized in the GCL and INL, and later extended to all nuclear layers including the ONL. Since the gene expression of OSK was so rapidly activated within 1 h after ONI, we tested whether preceding HSF1 directly regulated OSK expression. Injection of the *HSF1*-specific MO into the eye before ONI markedly suppressed OSK gene expression (Figure 3). Furthermore, as the promoter regions of the OSK genes have a consensus sequence that binds to HSF1 (see Figure S3), we performed a ChIP assay. Results of the ChIP analysis with anti-HSF1 antibodies showed that enrichment genomic OSK bind to HSF1. Thus, both the *HSF1* MO treatment assay and the ChIP assay clearly showed that the OSK genes were all regulated by

HSF1 (Figures 3 and 4). It is well-known that HSF1 and its target heat shock proteins (HSPs) protect cells under various stresses [22,23,30–36]. However, a genome-wide study of the biological stress response highlighted novel target genes of HSF1 other than HSPs [30,31]. HSF1, as a master transcription factor, was recently shown to activate many genes related to various cell functions such as development, aging, and carcinogenesis [32–35]. It is possible that OSK may also be the target of HSF1. Therefore, we concluded that HSF1 directly regulated the gene expression of OSK in the fish retina 1 h after ONI.

3.2. Role of Yamanaka Factors in the Injured Retina at the Early Stage of Optic Nerve Regeneration

The serial activations of HSF1-OSK protect cells and maintain their viability after ONI stress. The gene expression of HSF1 started to increase at 0.5 h, peaked at over 100-fold at 6 h, and was still maintained 24 h after ONI. This rapid and widespread retinal expression of HSF1 is essential for cell survival in the acute phase after ONI. When *HSF1-MO* was pre-injected and the optic nerve was injured under conditions of suppressed HSF1 expression, numerous apoptotic cells were observed in all nuclear layers and the retinal layered structure was severely disrupted (Figure S4). The long-lasting HSF1 gene expression must induce the gene expression of cell survival factors such as IGF-1, Bcl-2, and p-Akt 1–5 days after ONI [10,12,14]. Furthermore, the gene expression of OSK was induced rapidly and at the same time after ONI (Figure 2). This rapid activation of Yamanaka factors in the injured retina is also necessary for initializing transformation and maintaining cell survival. Sox2 is a well-established marker of neural stem cells and progenitor cells [37–39]. In mammals, Sox2 is highly expressed in the neuroepithelium of the developing central nervous system [39]. In injured zebrafish RGCs, the gene expression of Sox2 could be seen at 1–24 h after ONI (Figure 2 and Figure S2). Retinal neurons have been reported to change their properties in this early stage of optic nerve regeneration. The electrophysiological data reported that spike activities were suddenly lost a few days after ONI [24,40], and then hypertrophic change occurred in fish RGCs [41,42]. These changes indicate that injured RGCs in fish may initiate neural stem cell-like transformation. The other INL and ONL cells also expressed Sox2 strongly, as late as 6 h after ONI (Figure 2 and Figure S2). At present, we think that all retinal neurons transformed into neural stem-like cells under strong HSF1 signals in all nuclear layers at 6 h after ONI. However, future studies are needed to confirm this. Recently, Lu et al. demonstrated that overexpression of the OSK genes in the mouse eye using a viral vector could increase the survival of RGCs, partially regenerate optic axons, and recover vision [43]. This is because the expression of OSK can reset DNA methylation of the gene, allowing the retinal neuron to regain its young state. Interestingly, they also showed that if one of the three OSK factors was missing, the regenerative effect was lost [43]. In our zebrafish retina, the genes encoding these Yamanaka factors were all spontaneously and rapidly activated at the same time of 1 h after ONI, but their expression peaks and durations were slightly different (Figure 2). An in vivo model of OSK activity/expression in the fish retina after ONI would be useful for the next step of addressing the relationship between OSK genes and their target gene expression. The present study clearly showed that the rapid serial activations of HSF1-Yamanaka factors contribute to cell survival and the induction of neuronal stem cells in injured fish retina immediately after ONI.

4. Materials and Methods

4.1. Animals

Adult zebrafish (Danio rerio; 3–4 cm in length) were used in this study. The zebrafish were anesthetized with 0.02% MS222 (Sigma-Aldrich, St. Louis, MO, USA) in 10 mM phosphate-buffered saline (PBS; pH 7.4). Under anesthesia, the optic nerves on both sides were carefully crushed with forceps 1 mm posterior to the eyeball to create an "injured retina". Then, the fish were reared in water at 28 °C until the appropriate timepoints. All animal care was performed in accordance with the guidelines for animal experiments of Kanazawa University. Special care was taken to minimize the suffering of the fish.

4.2. Tissue Preparation

Retinal samples were prepared for histological analysis at specific timepoints following ONI. Briefly, the eyes were enucleated, bisected, and fixed in 4% paraformaldehyde solution containing 0.1 M phosphate buffer (pH 7.4) and 5% sucrose for 2 h at 4 °C. After infiltration with increasing concentrations of sucrose (5–20%), followed by overnight incubation in 20% sucrose at 4 °C, the tissues were embedded in Optimal Cutting Temperature (OCT) compound (Sakura Fine Technical, Tokyo, Japan) and sectioned at a thickness of 12 μm.

4.3. Total RNA Extraction and cDNA Synthesis

Fish were killed by an overdose (0.1%) of MS222 in PBS at appropriate timepoints after ONI. For total RNA extraction, we used Isogen (Nippon Gene, Tokyo, Japan), in accordance with the manufacturer's instructions. Total RNA samples from each timepoint or treatment were subjected to first-strand cDNA synthesis using a Transcriptor High Fidelity cDNA Synthesis Kit (Roche, Mannheim, Germany).

4.4. Quantitative Real-Time PCR

Quantitative real-time PCR was performed with FastStart Essential DNA Probes Master or Green Master Mix (Roche, Mannheim, Germany) using a LightCycler 96 (Roche). On the basis of the zebrafish cDNA sequences (see Table S1), gene-specific primers were created by Probe Finder using Universal Probe Library (Roche, Mannheim, Germany). The expression levels were analyzed by the ΔΔCt method, using glyceraldehyde 3-phosphate dehydrogenase (GAPDH) as a reference gene. The accession numbers for the genes, DNA sequences of the primer pairs, and lengths of the PCR products used in each experiment are shown in Table S1.

4.5. Immunohistochemistry

Retinal sections from zebrafish were incubated at 121 °C for 10 min in 10 mM citrate buffer. Following washing and blocking, sections were incubated with primary antibodies overnight at 4 °C (HSF1, 1:300; Sox2, 1:500; Oct4, 1:500; Klf4, 1:200). Following incubation with a biotinylated secondary antibody (Vector Laboratories, Burlingame, CA, USA) for 2 h at room temperature, bound antibodies were detected using horseradish peroxidase (HRP)-conjugated streptavidin and 3-amino-9-ethyl carbazole (AEC; Nichirei Biosciences Inc., Tokyo, Japan).

4.6. In Situ Hybridization

In situ hybridization was carried out as previously described [15]. Briefly, tissue sections were rehydrated and treated with 5 mg/mL proteinase K (Invitrogen, CA, USA) at room temperature for 5 min. After acetylation and prehybridization, hybridization was performed with cRNA probes labeled with digoxigenin in a hybridization solution overnight at 42 °C. The following day, the sections were washed and treated with 20 mg/mL RNase A at 37 °C for 30 min. To detect the signals, the sections were incubated with an alkaline phosphatase-conjugated anti-digoxigenin antibody (Roche, Rotkreuz, Switzerland) overnight at 4 °C and visualized with tetrazolium-bromo-4-chloro-3-indolylphosphate (Roche) as the substrate.

4.7. Chromatin Immunoprecipitation

Chromatin immunoprecipitation (ChIP) was performed using the MAGnifity Chromatin Immunoprecipitation System (Thermo Fisher Scientific, Waltham, MA, USA), in accordance with the manufacturer's instructions. Briefly, retinal samples were homogenized and linked in 1% formaldehyde for 10 min at room temperature, and 100 mM glycine was added to stop the reaction, followed by washing with cold PBS three times. After centrifugation and ultrasonication using a Bioruptor ultrasonic homogenizer (BM Equipment Co. Ltd., Tokyo, Japan), samples were incubated with magnetic protein A/G beads conjugated with anti-HSF1 (Millipore, CA, USA) or normal IgG, and kept overnight at 4 °C. After immunoprecipitation and washing, the genomic DNA associated with HSF1 was purified and quantified by SYBR Green-based quantitative real-time PCR using the primer sets shown in Table S1. All primer sets were designed to contain the predicted HSF1 binding region. ChIP dilution buffer was used as a negative control and DNA from the total input was used as an internal positive control.

4.8. *Intraocular Injection of HSF1 Morpholino to Zebrafish Eye*

Vivo-Morpholino (MO) was designed to inhibit the expression of the zebrafish heat shock factor 1 gene via the following sequence: 5′-AGTTTAGTGATGATTTCTGACGGTA-3′. A standard vivo-MO (5′-CCTCTTACCTCAGTTACAATTTATA-3′) was used as a control. All MOs were purchased from GeneTools (Philomath, OR, USA). The MOs were injected into the eye with a Hamilton 33G neuron syringe. Twenty hours after the injection of 0.75 μL of MO solution (0.5 mM) into the eye, the optic nerve was crushed.

4.9. *Statistical Analysis*

To evaluate the mRNA expression of HSF1, Sox2, Oct4, and Klf4, their levels were expressed as the mean ± SEM and the significance of differences was evaluated by one-way ANOVA. Significance was determined at $p < 0.05$ with IBM SPSS Statistic software.

5. Conclusions

HSF1 mRNA was immediately upregulated in the zebrafish retina after ONI. The acute expression of HSF1 directly regulated the expression of Yamanaka factors, which might dedifferentiate retinal neurons at the early stage of optic nerve regeneration after ONI.

Supplementary Materials: The following supporting information can be downloaded at: https://www.mdpi.com/article/10.3390/ijms24043253/s1.

Author Contributions: Conceptualization, K.S.; Methodology, K.S. and K.O.; Formal analysis, T.M., S.H., M.M. and A.K.; Investigation, T.M., S.H., M.M., A.K. and K.S.; Data curation, K.S.; Writing—Review & Editing, K.S. All authors have read and agreed to the published version of the manuscript.

Funding: This work was supported by Grants-in-Aid for Scientific Research to K.S. (No. 17K01954, No. 20K05725) from the Ministry of Education, Culture, Sports, Science, and Technology, Japan.

Institutional Review Board Statement: All experimental procedures were approved by the Committee on Animal Experimentation of Kanazawa University (2 March 2022).

Informed Consent Statement: Not applicable.

Data Availability Statement: Not applicable.

Acknowledgments: We thank Mayumi Nagashimada (Kanazawa University) for assistance with apoptotic cell analysis.

Conflicts of Interest: The authors declare no conflict of interest.

References

1. Laha, B.; Stafford, B.K.; Huberman, A.D. Regenerating optic pathways from the eye to the brain. *Science* **2017**, *356*, 1031–1034. [CrossRef] [PubMed]
2. Williams, P.R.; Benowitz, L.I.; Goldberg, J.L.; He, Z. Axon Regeneration in the Mammalian Optic Nerve. *Annu. Rev. Vis. Sci.* **2020**, *6*, 195–213. [CrossRef] [PubMed]
3. Fague, L.; Liu, Y.A.; Marsh-Armstrong, N. The basic science of optic nerve regeneration. *Ann. Transl. Med.* **2021**, *15*, 1276. [CrossRef] [PubMed]
4. Attardi, D.G.; Sperry, R.W. Preferential selection of central pathways by regenerating optic fibers. *Exp. Neurol.* **1963**, *7*, 46–64. [CrossRef]
5. Sperry, R.W. Patterning of central synapses in regeneration of the optic nerve in teleosts. *Physiol. Zool.* **1948**, *21*, 351–361. [CrossRef]
6. Becker, T.; Becker, C.G. Axonal regeneration in zebrafish. *Curr. Opin. Neurobiol.* **2014**, *27*, 186–191. [CrossRef]
7. Lenkowski, J.R.; Raymond, P.A. Müller glia: Stem cells for generation and regeneration of retinal neurons in teleost fish. *Prog. Retin. Eye Res.* **2014**, *40*, 94–123. [CrossRef]

8. Goldman, D. Müller glial cell reprogramming and retina regeneration. *Nat. Rev. Neurosci.* **2014**, *15*, 431–442. [CrossRef]
9. Marques, I.J.; Lupi, E.; Mercader, N. Model systems for regeneration: Zebrafish. *Development* **2019**, *146*, dev167692. [CrossRef]
10. Sugitani, K.; Matsukawa, T.; Maeda, A.; Kato, S. Upregulation of transglutaminase in the goldfish retina during optic nerve regeneration. In *Retinal Degenerative Diseases. Advances in Experimental Medicine and Biology*; Springer: Boston, MA, USA, 2006; Volume 572, pp. 525–530. [CrossRef]
11. Kaneda, M.; Nagashima, M.; Nunome, T.; Muramatsu, T.; Yamada, Y.; Kubo, M.; Muramoto, K.; Matsukawa, T.; Koriyama, Y.; Sugitani, K.; et al. Changes of phospho-growth associated protein 43 (phospho-GAP43) in zebrafish retina after optic nerve injury: A long term observation. *Neurosci. Res.* **2008**, *61*, 281–288. [CrossRef]
12. Sugitani, K.; Koriyama, Y.; Ogai, K.; Furukawa, A.; Kato, S. Alternative Splicing for Activation of Coagulation Factor XIII-A in the Fish Retina After Optic Nerve Injury. *Adv. Exp. Med. Biol.* **2018**, *1074*, 387–393.
13. Sugitani, K.; Matsukawa, T.; Koriyama, Y.; Shintani, T.; Nakamura, T.; Noda, M.; Kato, S. Upregulation of retinal transglutaminase during the axonal elongation stage of goldfish optic nerve regeneration. *Neuroscience* **2006**, *142*, 1081–1092. [CrossRef] [PubMed]
14. Koriyama, Y.; Yasuda, R.; Homma, K.; Mawatari, K.; Nagashima, M.; Sugitani, K.; Matsukawa, T.; Kato, S. Nitric oxide-cGMP signaling regulates axonal elongation during optic nerve regeneration in the goldfish in vitro and in vivo. *J. Neurochem.* **2009**, *110*, 890–901. [CrossRef] [PubMed]
15. Sugitani, K.; Ogai, K.; Hitomi, K.; Nakamura-Yonehara, K.; Shintani, T.; Noda, M.; Koriyama, Y.; Tanii, H.; Matsukawa, T.; Kato, S. A distinct effect of transient and sustained upregulation of cellular factor XIII in the goldfish retina and optic nerve on optic nerve regeneration. *Neurochem. Int.* **2012**, *61*, 423–432. [CrossRef] [PubMed]
16. Kato, S.; Devadas, M.; Okada, K.; Shimada, Y.; Ohkawa, M.; Muramoto, K.; Takizawa, N.; Matsukawa, T. Fast and slow recovery phases of goldfish behavior after transection of the optic nerve revealed by a computer image processing system. *Neuroscience* **1999**, *93*, 907–914. [CrossRef] [PubMed]
17. Ogai, K.; Hisano, S.; Mawatari, K.; Sugitani, K.; Koriyama, Y.; Nakashima, H.; Kato, S. Upregulation of anti-apoptotic factors in upper motor neurons after spinal cord injury in adult zebrafish. *Neurochem. Int.* **2012**, *61*, 1202–1211. [CrossRef]
18. Koriyama, Y.; Homma, K.; Sugitani, K.; Higuchi, Y.; Matsukawa, T.; Murayama, D.; Kato, S. Upregulation of IGF-I in the goldfish retinal ganglion cells during the early stage of optic nerve regeneration. *Neurochem. Int.* **2007**, *50*, 749–756. [CrossRef]
19. Matsukawa, T.; Sugitani, K.; Mawatari, K.; Koriyama, Y.; Liu, Z.; Tanaka, M.; Kato, S. Role of purpurin as a retinol-binding protein in goldfish retina during the early stage of optic nerve regeneration: Its priming action on neurite outgrowth. *J. Neurosci.* **2004**, *24*, 8346–8353. [CrossRef]
20. Sugitani, K.; Koriyama, Y.; Ogai, K.; Wakasugi, K.; Kato, S. A Possible Role of Neuroglobin in the Retina After Optic Nerve Injury: A Comparative Study of Zebrafish and Mouse Retina. *Adv. Exp. Med. Biol.* **2016**, *854*, 671–675. [PubMed]
21. Sugitani, K.; Koriyama, Y.; Sera, M.; Arai, K.; Ogai, K.; Wakasugi, K. A novel function of neuroglobin for neuroregeneration in mice after optic nerve injury. *Biochem. Biophys. Res. Commun.* **2017**, *493*, 1254–1259. [CrossRef]
22. Nagashima, M.; Fujikawa, C.; Mawatari, K.; Mori, Y.; Kato, S. HSP70, the earliest-induced gene in the zebrafish retina during optic nerve regeneration: Its role in cell survival. *Neurochem. Int.* **2011**, *58*, 888–895. [CrossRef] [PubMed]
23. Fujikawa, C.; Nagashima, M.; Mawatari, K.; Kato, S. HSP 70 gene expression in the zebrafish retina after optic nerve injury: A comparative study under heat shock stresses. *Adv. Exp. Med. Biol.* **2012**, *723*, 663–668. [PubMed]
24. Kato, S.; Matsukawa, T.; Koriyama, Y.; Sugitani, K.; Ogai, K. A molecular mechanism of optic nerve regeneration in fish: The retinoid signaling pathway. *Prog. Retin. Eye Res.* **2013**, *37*, 13–30. [CrossRef] [PubMed]
25. Takahashi, K.; Yamanaka, S. Induction of pluripotent stem cells from mouse embryonic and adult fibroblast cultures by defined factors. *Cell* **2006**, *126*, 663–676. [CrossRef]
26. Takahashi, K.; Tanabe, K.; Ohnuki, M.; Narita, M.; Ichisaka, T.; Tomoda, K.; Yamanaka, S. Induction of pluripotent stem cells from adult human fibroblasts by defined factors. *Cell* **2007**, *131*, 861–872. [CrossRef] [PubMed]
27. Hofmann, J.W.; Zhao, X.; De Cecco, M.; Peterson, A.L.; Pagliaroli, L.; Manivannan, J.; Hubbard, G.B.; Ikeno, Y.; Zhang, Y.; Feng, B.; et al. Reduced expression of MYC increases longevity and enhances healthspan. *Cell* **2015**, *160*, 477–488. [CrossRef]
28. Nakagawa, M.; Koyanagi, M.; Tanabe, K.; Takahashi, K.; Ichisaka, T.; Aoi, T.; Okita, K.; Mochiduki, Y.; Takizawa, N.; Yamanaka, S. Generation of induced pluripotent stem cells without Myc from mouse and human fibroblasts. *Nat. Biotechnol.* **2008**, *26*, 101–106. [CrossRef]
29. Wernig, M.; Meissner, A.; Cassady, J.P.; Jaenisch, R. c-Myc is dispensable for direct reprogramming of mouse fibroblasts. *Cell Stem Cell* **2008**, *2*, 10–12. [CrossRef]
30. Pirkkala, L.; Nykänen, P.; Sistonen, L. Roles of the heat shock transcription factors in regulation of the heat shock response and beyond. *FASEB J.* **2001**, *15*, 1118–1131. [CrossRef]
31. Hu, Z.; Killion, P.J.; Iyer, V.R. Genetic reconstruction of a functional transcriptional regulatory network. *Nat. Genet.* **2007**, *39*, 683–687. [CrossRef]
32. Akerfelt, M.; Morimoto, R.I.; Sistonen, L. Heat shock factors: Integrators of cell stress, development and lifespan. *Nat. Rev. Mol. Cell Biol.* **2010**, *11*, 545–555. [CrossRef] [PubMed]
33. Fujimoto, M.; Nakai, A. The heat shock factor family and adaptation to proteotoxic stress. *FEBS J.* **2010**, *277*, 4112–4125. [CrossRef] [PubMed]
34. Anckar, J.; Sistonen, L. Regulation of HSF1 function in the heat stress response: Implications in aging and disease. *Annu. Rev. Biochem.* **2011**, *80*, 1089–1115. [CrossRef]

35. Vihervaara, A.; Sistonen, L. HSF1 at a glance. *J. Cell Sci.* **2014**, *127*, 261–266. [CrossRef]
36. Liu, W.; Xia, F.; Ha, Y.; Zhu, S.; Li., Y.; Folorunso, O.; Pashaei-Marandi, A.; Lin, P.Y.; Tilton, R.G.; Pierce, A.P.; et al. Neuroprotective Effects of HSF1 in Retinal Ischemia-Reperfusion Injury. *Invest. Ophthalmol. Vis. Sci.* **2019**, *60*, 965–977. [CrossRef]
37. Episkopou, V. SOX2 functions in adult neural stem cells. *Trends Neurosci.* **2005**, *28*, 219–221. [CrossRef] [PubMed]
38. Maucksch, C.; Jones, K.S.; Connor, B. Concise review: The involvement of SOX2 in direct reprogramming of induced neural stem/precursor cells. *Stem Cells Transl. Med.* **2013**, *2*, 579–583. [CrossRef] [PubMed]
39. Amador-Arjona, A.; Cimadamore, F.; Huang, C.T.; Wright, R.; Lewis, S.; Gage, F.H.; Terskikh, A.V. SOX2 primes the epigenetic landscape in neural precursors enabling proper gene activation during hippocampal neurogenesis. *Proc. Natl. Acad. Sci. USA* **2015**, *112*, 1936–1945. [CrossRef]
40. Northmore, D.P. Quantitative electrophysiological studies of regenerating visuotopic maps in goldfish-II. Delayed recovery of sensitivity to small light flashes. *Neuroscience* **1989**, *32*, 749–757. [CrossRef]
41. Murray, M.; Grafstein, B. Changes in the morphology and amino acid incorporation of regenerating goldfish optic neurons. *Exp. Neurol.* **1969**, *23*, 544–560. [CrossRef]
42. Devadas, M.; Sugawara, K.; Shimada, Y.; Sugitani, K.; Liu, Z.W.; Matsukawa, T.; Kato, S. Slow recovery of goldfish retinal ganglion cells' soma size during regeneration. *Neurosci. Res.* **2000**, *37*, 289–297. [CrossRef] [PubMed]
43. Lu, Y.; Brommer, B.; Tian, X.; Krishnan, A.; Meer, M.; Wang, C.; Vera, D.L.; Zeng, Q.; Yu, D.; Bonkowski, M.S.; et al. Reprogramming to recover youthful epigenetic information and restore vision. *Nature* **2020**, *88*, 124–129. [CrossRef] [PubMed]

International Journal of *Molecular Sciences*

MDPI

Article

Ligand-Induced Activation of GPR110 (ADGRF1) to Improve Visual Function Impaired by Optic Nerve Injury

Heung-Sun Kwon [1], Karl Kevala [1], Haohua Qian [2], Mones Abu-Asab [3], Samarjit Patnaik [4], Juan Marugan [4] and Hee-Yong Kim [1,*]

1 Laboratory of Molecular Signaling, NIAAA, National Institutes of Health, 5625 Fishers Lane Room 3S-02, Rockville, MD 20892-9410, USA
2 Visual Function Core, NEI, National Institutes of Health, Bethesda, MD 20892-0616, USA
3 Electron Microscopy Laboratory, Biological Imaging Core, NEI, National Institutes of Health, Bethesda, MD 20850-2510, USA
4 Division of Pre-Clinical Innovation, NCATS, National Institutes of Health, Rockville, MD 20817, USA
* Correspondence: hykim@nih.gov; Tel.: +1-301-402-8746; Fax: +1-301-594-0035

Abstract: It is extremely difficult to achieve functional recovery after axonal injury in the adult central nervous system. The activation of G-protein coupled receptor 110 (GPR110, ADGRF1) has been shown to stimulate neurite extension in developing neurons and after axonal injury in adult mice. Here, we demonstrate that GPR110 activation partially restores visual function impaired by optic nerve injury in adult mice. Intravitreal injection of GPR110 ligands, synaptamide and its stable analogue dimethylsynaptamide (A8) after optic nerve crush significantly reduced axonal degeneration and improved axonal integrity and visual function in wild-type but not *gpr110* knockout mice. The retina obtained from the injured mice treated with GPR110 ligands also showed a significant reduction in the crush-induced loss of retinal ganglion cells. Our data suggest that targeting GPR110 may be a viable strategy for functional recovery after optic nerve injury.

Keywords: synaptamide; A8; axonal degeneration; retinal ganglion cells; neuronal survival; optic nerve crush; visual evoked potential

Citation: Kwon, H.-S.; Kevala, K.; Qian, H.; Abu-Asab, M.; Patnaik, S.; Marugan, J.; Kim, H.-Y. Ligand-Induced Activation of GPR110 (ADGRF1) to Improve Visual Function Impaired by Optic Nerve Injury. *Int. J. Mol. Sci.* **2023**, *24*, 5340. https://doi.org/10.3390/ijms24065340

Academic Editors: Neil R. Miller and Rongkung Tsai

Received: 30 December 2022
Revised: 3 February 2023
Accepted: 1 March 2023
Published: 10 March 2023

1. Introduction

CNS injuries in adulthood are difficult to repair [1]. In particular, the inherently low axon growth capacity of mature neurons [2] along with neuronal cell death caused by injury [3,4] hinder the development of recovery strategies for functional restoration. Although limited, the regeneration and repair of the optic nerve system have been demonstrated by manipulating genes or signaling pathways to stimulate the intrinsic developmental program for axon growth or to promote neuronal survival [5–8]. In addition, the induction of cyclic adenosine monophosphate (cAMP) signaling has been proposed to be a promising strategy to stimulate axon growth [9–11]. We have demonstrated that *N*-docosahexaenoylethanolamine (synaptamide), an endogenous metabolite of docosahexaenoic acid (DHA, 22:6n-3), potently promotes neurite outgrowth and synaptogenesis in developing neurons by binding to the G-protein coupled receptor 110 (GPR110, ADGRF1) and increasing cAMP [12,13]. Recently, we have demonstrated that this developmental mechanism for neurite outgrowth is applicable to a repair strategy for axonal injury in the adult stage, as GPR110 is upregulated after injury [14,15]. For example, activating GPR110 using its ligands stimulated axonal extension following optic nerve injury [14] and improved the optic nerve axonal pathology and visual dysfunction caused by a traumatic brain injury (TBI) in adult mice [15]. In this study, we investigated whether ligand-induced GPR110 activation can improve visual function and axonal integrity impaired by crush-induced optic nerve injuries in adult mice.

2. Results

2.1. Synaptamide Stimulates Axon Regeneration after ONC

We have previously demonstrated that GPR110 ligands, synaptamide and A8 stimulate axon extension in injured optic nerves [14]. At 3 weeks after ONC, synaptamide treatment dose-dependently increased GAP43 staining, indicating that axon regeneration was stimulated (Figure 1A,B). CTB labeling was detected together with GAP43-positive staining in injured axons when treated with synaptamide, indicating that regenerating axons at least in part contributed to synaptamide-induced axon extension after the injury. The mass spectrometric analysis of synaptamide in the eye indicated that the synaptamide level decreased by 20% from the initially injected amount at 1 h after the injection, and further decreased by nearly 80% at 24 h (Figure 1C). Nevertheless, a single intravitreal injection of synaptamide at 2.5 mg/kg appeared to be effective to trigger axonal regeneration and extension during the subsequent 3 weeks of recovery in the injured animals (Figure 1A, bottom). A more stable and effective ligand, A8 [14,15], also showed a time-dependent decrease, but to a lesser extent.

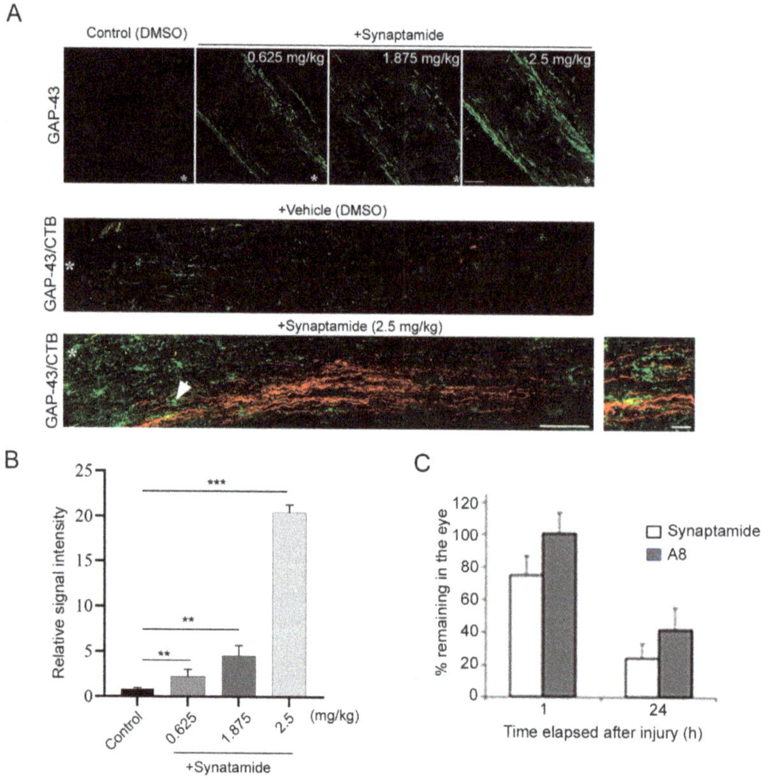

Figure 1. Intravitreal injection of synaptamide stimulates axon regeneration and extension after injury. (**A**). Synaptamide dose-dependent axon regeneration indicated by GAP43 staining of optic nerve (top), and synaptamide (2.5 mg/kg)-induced GAP43-positive regenerating axons (green) and axonal extension indicated by CTB labeling (red) at 3 weeks after ONC (bottom) compared to the vehicle-treated control (middle). Longitudinal sections through the optic nerve were collected at 3 weeks after ONC and regenerating axons were visualized by immunostaining for GPA-43, a regenerating axon marker (top). On the third day prior to euthanasia, the animals were injected with CTB-Alexa Fluor 555-conjugated cholera toxin subunit B (CTB, red) as an anterograde tracer to visualize axons

in the optic nerve originating from RGCs (bottom). Lesion sites were marked by asterisks (*). Scale bar, 100 µm. An enlarged view around the white arrow is shown as the boxed area, indicating overlapping signals of GAP-43 and CTB. Scale bar, 20 µm. (**B**). The fluorescent intensities of GAP-43 staining shown in ((**A**) top) were quantified by setting the whole captured image as the region of interest. The signal intensity was shown relative to the control group. Data are expressed as mean ± s.e.m. ($n = 3$ per group). ** $p < 0.01$, *** $p < 0.001$. (**C**). The time course of synaptamide and A8 detected in the eye. Synaptamide (2.5 mg/kg) or A8 (0.3 mg/kg) intravitreally injected were detected by tandem mass spectrometry. The data are expressed as mean ± SD ($n = 3$).

2.2. GPR110 Activation by Synaptamide or A8 Treatment Leads to Partial Restoration of Visual Activity Impaired by ONC

The functional outcome of GPR110 activation was determined by evaluating the effect of synaptamide and A8 treatment on visually evoked potentials (VEPs) [16]. At 12 weeks after ONC, a drastic reduction in VEP amplitude was observed in the animals treated with the vehicle, indicating that ONC caused vision impairment (Figure 2). Remarkably, a single intravitreal injection of synaptamide (2.5 mg/kg) or A8 (0.03 mg/kg) following injury improved their visual function, showing partial restoration of the VEP amplitude with a normalized VEP wave (Figure 2A). In *gpr110 KO* mice, however, synaptamide or A8 injection did not reverse the reduction in VEP amplitude caused by ONC (Figure 2B), indicating that the observed in vivo effect of synaptamide and A8 on the functional outcome was mediated by GPR110. The improvement of VEP amplitude was not shown when the injured WT mice were treated with OEA (2.5 mg/kg), which was used as a bio-inactive lipid control for synaptamide. The electroretinogram (ERG) of WT and *gpr110 KO* mice indicated no significant effect of either injury or treatment (Figure 2C).

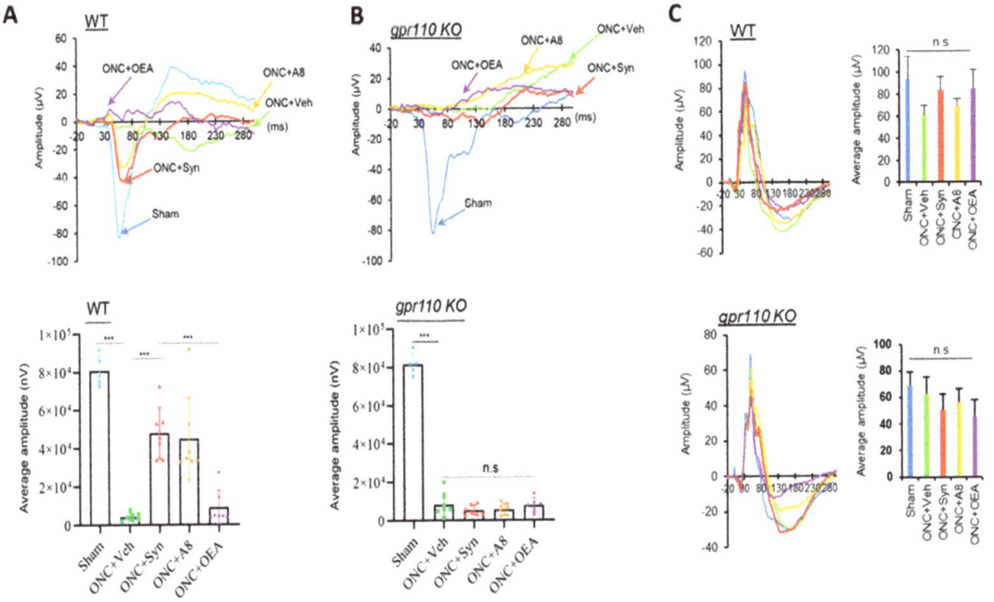

Figure 2. Intravitreal injection of synaptamide or A8 GPR110 dependently improved visual function impaired by ONC. (**A**,**B**), Representative VEP responses (top) and the mean amplitude (bottom) measured at 12 weeks after ONC in sham (blue), vehicle- (green), synaptamide- (red), A8-(orange) or OEA-injected (purple) C57BL/6 WT and gpr110 KO mice. ONC caused a drastic reduction in VEP compared to sham animals (83.3 ± 5.5 µV). At 12 weeks, WT mice injected with synaptamide (2.5 mg/kg) or A8 (0.03 mg/kg) showed improvement of VEP amplitude, but the gpr110 KO group

did not show the same improvement. The improvement in the VEP amplitude was not shown in OEA-injected WT mice. Full-field flash VEP was elicited under light-adapted conditions (10 cd·s/m^2). (**C**) ERG measurements at 12 weeks after ONC, showing no effects of the injury or treatment in either WT and gpr110 KO mice. Data are expressed as mean ± s.e.m. ($n = 7$), representing two independent experiments. *** $p < 0.001$. n.s., not significant.

2.3. ONC-Induced Loss of RGC Axons at the Brain Target was Partly Prevented by the Treatment with GPR110 Ligands

The observed partial recovery of VEP function by the treatment with GPR110 ligands suggests that at least some RGC axons successfully achieved or maintained target innervation in the brain. The axon innervation to the lateral geniculate nucleus (LGN), the brain target of RGC axons, was visualized by anterograde CTB labeling. At 12 weeks after injury, the axon labeling at LGN was clearly missing in animals injured by ONC (Figure 3), indicating that ONC caused the degeneration of distal axons. The axon labeling at the target partially reappeared after the treatment with synaptamide or A8 in WT, but this effect was not observed in *gpr110 KO*, which is consistent with the GPR110-dependent partial restoration of visual function observed in Figure 2.

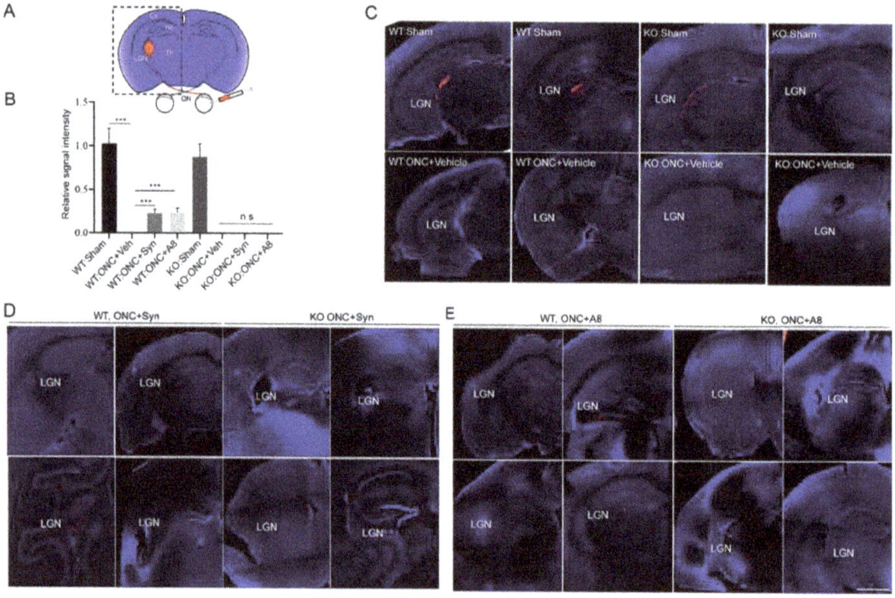

Figure 3. Intravitreal injection of GPR110 ligands partly prevented the ONC-induced loss of optic nerve axons at the target. (**A**) Schematic representation of a brain section depicting the visual system labeled by the CTB injection. The axons of retinal ganglion cells exit the eye via the optic nerve (ON) and project to the contralateral lateral geniculate nucleus (LGN) through the optic tract (OT). (**B**) The CTB fluorescent intensities were quantified by setting the whole captured image as the region of interest. The signal intensity was shown relative to the WT-sham group. Data are expressed as mean ± s.e.m. ($n = 4$ per group). *** $p < 0.001$. (**C–E**) Representative micrographs showing axon projection to the contralateral LGN region of the brain. Anterograde axon tracing of regenerated optic nerves was performed by injecting CTB conjugated to Alexa 555 on the third day prior to the scheduled euthanasia at 12 weeks after ONC. The CTB labelling that was not observed in the brains after ONC (**C**) was detected in synaptamide- or A8-injected injured WT (**D**), but not in gpr110 KO mice (**E**). The micrographs of four individual mouse brains per each group are shown with DAPI counterstaining. LGN, lateral geniculate nucleus. Cx, cortex. Th, thalamus. Hc, hippocampus. Scale bars, 100 μm. n.s., not significant.

2.4. Optic Nerve Myelination Status Degraded after ONC Was Improved by Synaptamide or A8 Treatment

To determine the integrity of the optic nerve in relation to the functional outcome, the myelination status was evaluated for the optic nerve tissues collected from the animals in which VEP and ERG were measured at the end of the 12-week recovery period (Figure 4). ONC appeared to cause myelin degradation, as the myelin basic protein (MBP) immunostaining in the cross-section of the optic nerve fibers was markedly decreased after ONC (Figure 4A,B). The level of oligodendrocyte marker proteins, MBP, CNPase and O2 in the optic nerve tissues was also significantly decreased after ONC (Figure 4C,D), indicating that ONC caused the degradation of oligodendrocytes that are responsible for the myelination of neuronal axons. The treatment with synaptamide or A8 partly, but significantly, prevented the loss of these proteins at 12 weeks post-injury, indicating that these GPR110 ligands improved the myelination status.

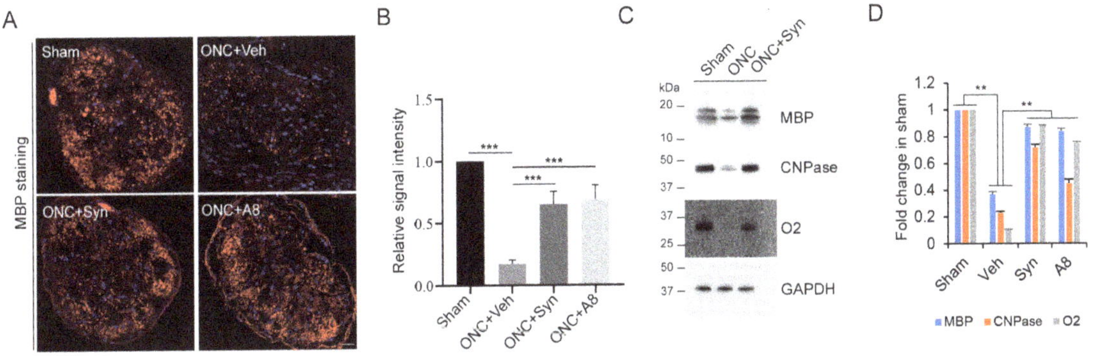

Figure 4. ONC-induced degradation of optic nerve myelination was partially prevented by synaptamide or A8 treatment. (**A**) Cross section of the optic nerve immunostained for MBP indicates the loss of the axon structure at 12 weeks after ONC, which is partially reversed by synaptamide or A8 injection. (**B**) The fluorescent intensities of MBP staining were quantified by setting the whole captured image as the region of interest. The signal intensity was shown relative to the sham control group. (**C**,**D**) Immunoblot of myelination marker proteins, MBP, CNPase and O2 from optic nerves collected at 12 weeks after ONC from sham and vehicle-, synaptamide- or A8-treated group (**C**), with quantitative results normalized by GAPDH from three mice per group (**D**). Data are expressed as mean ± s.e.m. ($n = 3$), representing two independent experiments. ** $p < 0.01$, *** $p < 0.001$. Scale bar, 10 µm.

2.5. GPR110 Ligands Improved Structural Integrity of Axons Deteriorated by ONC

Because myelin degradation has been shown to accompany cytoskeletal disintegration of distal axons after injury [17], we also examined the ultrastructure of the optic nerves by electron microscopy (Figure 5). The electron micrographs of the injured optic nerves showed a severely disorganized structure with a drastically reduced axon number and apparent penetration of astrocytic processes. Synaptamide or A8 treatment significantly increased the total axon numbers in WT, but not in *gpr110 KO* animals (Figure 5A,B). The thickness of the myelin sheath was also significantly decreased after ONC, as indicated by the increased *g*-ratio [18]. However, this increase in the *g*-ratio was reversed by synaptamide or A8 treatment (Figure 5C–E). These data indicated that the structural integrity of axons deteriorated by injury can be reversed by ligand-induced GPR110 activation.

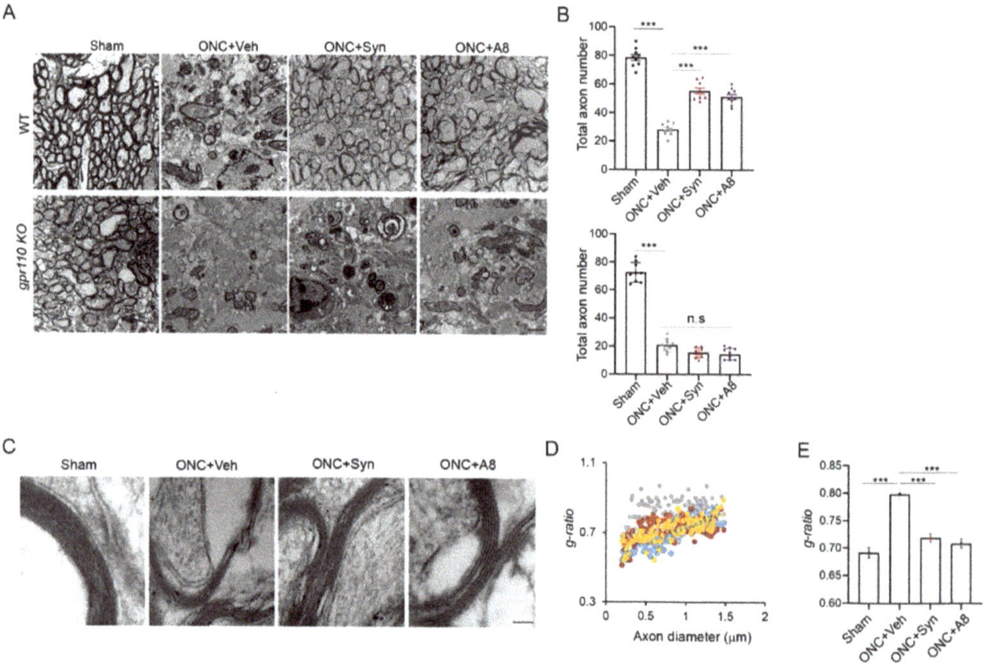

Figure 5. Structural integrity of axons deteriorated by ONC was improved by treatment with GPR110 ligands. (**A**,**B**) Transmission electron microscopic images show cross sections of the optic nerves from sham and vehicle-, synaptamide- or A8-treated WT or gpr110 KO mice at 12 weeks after ONC (**A**), and the quantitation of the total axon number per field (**B**). Data are expressed as mean ± s.e.m. of the total 9 sections (3 sections per mouse) from 3 mice per group. (**C**–**E**) Electron microscopic images show the thickness of the myelin sheath of the axon fibers at 12 weeks after ONC (**C**) and the scatter plot for the g-ratio (the ratio of the inner to the outer diameter of the myelin sheath) as a function of axon diameter (**D**), along with the average g-ratio for the sham (blue), ONC + vehicle (grey), ONC + synaptamide (red) and ONC + A8 (orange) groups (**E**). Data are expressed as mean ± s.e.m. of the total 114 axons from 6 mice per group. *** $p < 0.001$. Scale bars, 2 μm (**A**) and 100 nm (**C**). n.s., not significant.

2.6. RGC Loss after ONC Was Alleviated by Synaptamide or A8 Treatment

We also examined the surviving RGCs in the retina collected from the animals after VEP and ERG were measured at the end of the 12-week recovery period (Figure 6). The β-III tubulin-positive RGC neurons and neurites significantly decreased after ONC (Figure 6A,B), as has been reported earlier [19,20]. The ONC-induced loss of RGCs and neurites was partially rescued by the intravitreal injection of synaptamide or A8.

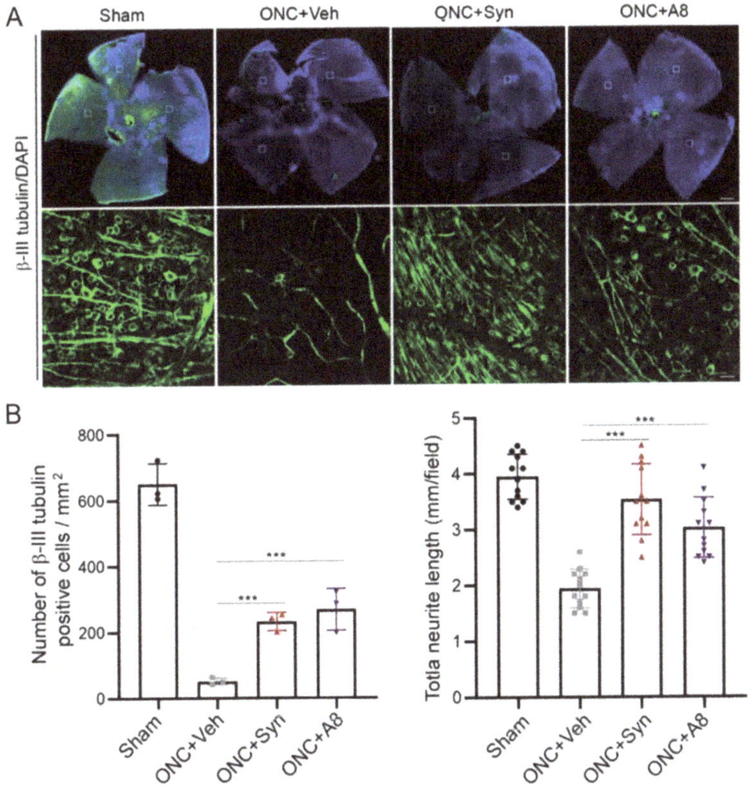

Figure 6. ONC-induced RGC loss was alleviated by synaptamide or A8 treatment. (**A**,**B**) Confocal images of whole mount retina where RGCs were visualized by b-III tubulin (green) and DAPI (blue) at 12 weeks post-ONC (**A**), indicating significantly greater numbers of neurons and neurites after synaptamide or A8 treatment compared to the vehicle-treated ONC control (**B**). A representative image from the red-outlined boxed region is also shown with higher magnification ((**A**), bottom). The number of b-III tubulin-positive RGC neurons and total neurite length were quantified for 4 fields (boxed regions) per retina from three animals (**B**). Scale bars in (**A**), 400 μm (top), 20 μm (bottom). *** $p < 0.001$.

3. Discussion

In this study, we demonstrated the GPR110-dependent restoration of the visual function impaired after optic nerve injury in adult mice. The treatment with GPR110 ligands after optic nerve crush injury at least partially prevented axonal degeneration and RGC loss, improving visual function.

GPR110, an adhesion GPCR that has recently been deorphanized as the target receptor of synaptamide [12], mediates neurogenic, neuritogenic and synaptogenic activity in developing neurons through the activation of cAMP/PKA signaling [21]. We have recently demonstrated that GPR110 expression in RGCs is rapidly induced after optic nerve injury, and that activating GPR110-mediated cAMP/PKA signaling, a developmental mechanism of stimulated axon growth, enables the extension of injured axons in adulthood [14]. Similarly, it has been previously shown that cAMP/PKA signaling can regulate neuronal regenerative capacity [22], and by priming with neurotrophins, the axon growth inhibitory signals derived from CNS glia around the injury site can be overcome in a cAMP- and PKA-dependent manner [23]. Axon regeneration observed after synaptamide treatment (Figure 1) is consistent with the reported cAMP-dependent regenerative capacity, since synaptamide is an endogenous ligand to GPR110 that activates cAMP/PKA signaling. Considering synaptamide's potent neuritogenic activity with IC50 at a low nanomolar range [12], a local concentration of synaptamide from a single injection of synaptamide at 2.5 mg/kg may be sufficient to trigger axon repair in the early stage of injury and stimulate axonal regeneration during the subsequent recovery period. The drastic reduction in VEP observed after ONC (Figure 2) was accompanied by the nearly absent optic nerve innervation at LGN, the target area for RGC axons in the brain (Figure 3), together with the significant degeneration of optic nerve axons (Figures 4 and 5). When injured animals were treated with GPR110 ligands, synaptamide or A8, the structural integrity of axons post injury was improved (Figures 4 and 5), and optic nerve axons were detected in LGN (Figure 3) in a GPR110-dependnet manner. The axonal degeneration alleviated through the activation of cAMP/PKA signaling by specifically targeting GPR110 may have facilitated the partial restoration of visual function. Given that GPR110 plays an important role in developmental neurite outgrowth, the lack of GPR110 may have affected RGC axonal outgrowth during development. However, the total RGC axon number per field (Figure 6A,B), as well as the VEP amplitude (Figure 2), appeared to be similar between WT and KO sham animals, suggesting that unlike the injury situation, other mechanisms for axonal outgrowth can compensate in the long run for the developmental deficit caused by the lack of GPR110 activation.

Axonal injury caused by ONC is known to be mild. It has been reported that RGC survival of greater than 40% can be achieved depending on the severity of the crush [24]. It has also been reported that the loss of RGC soma is not required for axon degeneration. We observed more than 10% of the total RGCs were still spared at 12 weeks after injury (Figure 6). It is noteworthy that GPR110 activation by its ligands improved the survival of RGC neurons after the optic nerve injury (Figure 6). In addition to stimulating axon growth after injury, it is possible that GPR110 activation that elevates the cAMP level may have a specific role in survival/death signaling to help preserve injured neurons, especially when target-derived trophic support is absent after ONC. Similarly, it has been reported that cAMP analogues can promote neuronal survival and neurite outgrowth independently of nerve growth factors [25]. The timely repair of injured axons by the activation of GPR110/cAMP signaling may have prevented the death of neurons traumatized by ONC, preserving their capacity to sprout neurites to form new synapses for signal transmission. In such a case, the rapid induction of GPR110 in RGCs after injury that has been previously observed [14] may be an intrinsic mechanism for preserving RGCs and stimulating axon growth through activating GPR110/cAMP signaling. Further studies will be required to fully understand the mechanisms underlying GPR110-derived trophic signals for RCG survival after injury.

The effect of synaptamide and its stable analogue A8 was observed with a single treatment after ONC, suggesting that GPR110 activation in an early stage of injury can mitigate RGC death (Figure 6) and axon degradation (Figures 4 and 5), and thus help preserve visual function (Figure 2). The partial restoration of VEP function observed in the present study (Figure 2) is a rare demonstration of successful functional recovery after CNS injury. After spinal cord injury, improvement of motor function has been demonstrated with pharmacologic intervention to decrease scarring using chondritinase ABC [26] or the microtubule-stabilizing drug epothilone B [27]. Although clinically inapplicable, combination treatment with the inflammation-inducer zymosan and a cAMP analog, along with *pten* deletion to reactivate the growth potential, was also shown to trigger partial restoration of functional responses after optic nerve injury [20]. To the best of our knowledge, the pharmacologic activation of GPR110 by its ligands represents the first demonstration of functional improvement with translational potential following optic nerve injury. It is also noteworthy that the activation of GPR110/cAMP signaling has been shown to suppress neuroinflammation caused by traumatic brain injury [15] or endotoxin administration [28], indicating the possibility that these GPR110 ligands may be similarly effective in ameliorating inflammation-associated neuropathological conditions such as ischemia and Alzheimer's disease. Further investigation is warranted to find an optimal and practical therapeutic time window for a treatment strategy based on ligand-induced GPR110 activation.

In summary, our data indicate that GPR110 activation by synaptamide or its stable analogue A8 promotes RGC survival after optic nerve injury, preserves axonal integrity and enables at least partial recovery of visual function. Our findings demonstrate a novel restoration strategy for injured axons by activating GPR110 using its ligands synaptamide or A8. We propose that synaptamide and its stable analogue may have therapeutic potential for patients who have suffered an optic nerve injury, offering a new translational possibility for CNS injuries.

4. Materials and Methods

4.1. Animals

Timed pregnant female C57BL/6 mice were obtained from the NIH-NCI animal production program or Charles River Laboratories (Portage, MI, USA), and GPR110 (adhesion G protein-coupled receptor F1: Adgrf1) heterozygous mice with a C57BL/6 background were generated by the Knockout Mouse Project (KOMP) Repository. The animals were housed in the SPF facility and *gpr110* KO mice and matching WT were generated by heterozygote mating in the NIAAA animal facility. All experiments were carried out in accordance with the guiding principles for the care and use of animals approved by the National Institute on Alcohol Abuse and Alcoholism (LMS-HK13).

4.2. Optic Nerve Crush (ONC)

Mice at 2 months of age were anesthetized by an injection of ketamine (100 mg/kg, i.p.) and xylazine (10 mg/kg, i.p.). Under a binocular operating scope, a small incision was made with spring scissors (cat. #RS-5619; Roboz, Gaithersburg, MD, USA) in the conjunctiva beginning inferior to the globe and around the eye temporally. Caution was taken, as making this cut too deep can result in cutting into the underlying musculature (inferior oblique, inferior rectus muscles or the lateral rectus) or the supplying vasculature. With micro-forceps (Dumont #5/45 forceps, cat. #RS-5005; Roboz), the edge of the conjunctiva next to the globe was grasped and retracted, rotating the globe nasally, which exposed the posterior aspect of the globe, allowing visualization of the optic nerve. The exposed optic nerve was grasped approximately 1–3 mm from the globe with Dumont #N7 cross-action forceps (cat. #RS-5027; Roboz) for 5 s to apply pressure on the nerve by the self-clamping action. The Dumont cross-action forceps were chosen because their spring action applied a constant and consistent force to the optic nerve. During the 5 s clamping, we were able to observe mydriasis. After 5 s, the pressure on the optic nerve was released and the forceps removed, allowing the eye to rotate back into place. The ONC operation was performed on one eye for each mouse.

4.3. Intravitreal Administration of Synaptamide or A8

Synaptamide (2.5 mg/kg), *N*-oleoylethanolamine (OEA, 2.5 mg/kg), A8 (0.03 mg/kg) or the vehicle (DMSO) were intravitreally injected immediately after ONC while the mice were still under anesthesia. The experimenter was blinded to the identity of the compounds, including the vehicle. Before the injection of the compounds, PBS was applied to clean the cornea. A pulled glass micropipette attached to a 10 μL Hamilton syringe was used to deliver 2 μL of a solution into the vitreous chamber of the eye, posterior to the limbus. Care was taken to prevent damage to the lens. The pipette was held in place for 3 s after the injection and slowly withdrawn from the eye to prevent reflux. Injections were performed under a surgical microscope to visualize pipette entry into the vitreous chamber and to confirm the delivery of the injected solution.

4.4. Anterograde Labeling

On the third day prior to euthanasia at 3 weeks after the injury or within a few days after testing visual function at 12 weeks post injury, the animals were intravitreally injected with CTB-Alexa Fluor 555-conjugated cholera toxin subunit B (CTB, Life Technologies, CA, USA) as an anterograde tracer to visualize axons in the optic nerve that originated from RGCs.

4.5. Visual-Evoked Potentials (VEP) and Electroretinogram (ERG)

The VEP and ERG were recorded using an Espion Electrophysiology System (Diagnosys, LLC, MA, USA), as described earlier [29]. At 12 weeks after ONC, the mice were anesthetized by an intraperitoneal injection of ketamine (100 mg/kg) and xylazine (10 mg/kg). Pupils were dilated with 1% tropicamide and 2.5% phenylephrine and mice were placed on a heated platform with their head covered by the Ganzfeld dome with the uninjured eye covered. A reference needle electrode was inserted in the lower lip, while the ground electrode was inserted in the tail. For VEP recording, the test electrode was subcutaneously inserted medially on the head such that it was in contact with the skull over the visual cortex. Eyes were stimulated by the flash stimuli of white light generated by the ColorDome Ganzfeld that had an intensity of 10 cd-s/m^2, with each set including 100 sweeps. Three sets of readings were recorded and averaged to obtain the amplitude and latency (implicit time) of the N1 component (the first negative peak: P1–N1). Standard ERG was recorded according to the photopic protocol [30], as described earlier [29]. After applying a drop of topical petroleum ophthalmic ointment, a gold wire loop electrode was placed in the center of the cornea, a reference electrode in the forehead, and a grounding electrode in the tail, and responses were recorded for 0.3 s after each stimulation. After the test, the electrodes were removed, and the mice were transferred to their home cage on a heating pad and allowed to regain consciousness and housed until further analysis.

4.6. Electron Microscopic Analysis

Shortly after the VEP measurements at 12 weeks after injury, the mice were anesthetized by an intraperitoneal injection of a lethal dose of ketamine/xylazine, and quickly perfused with a fixative that contained 4% paraformaldehyde, 2.5% glutaraldehyde, 0.13 N NaH_4PO_4, and 0.11 M NaOH, at pH 7.4. Optic nerve tissues were collected and fixed in PBS-buffered 2.5% glutaraldehyde and 0.5% osmium tetroxide, dehydrated, and embedded into Spurr's epoxy resin [31]. Ultrathin sections (90 nm) were taken from the optic nerve approximately 100–500 μm from the legion, double-stained with uranyl acetate and lead citrate, and viewed in a JEOL JEM 1010 transmission electron microscope equipped with a digital imaging camera. EM images were taken for samples from 6 mice per each group and analyzed by NIH Image J software. The *g*-ratio (quotient axon diameter/fiber diameter) of each axon was calculated by the perimeter of axons (inner) divided by the perimeter of the corresponding fibers (outer) [32].

4.7. Whole Mount Retina Staining and RGC Survival Quantification

Eyes were dissected from PFA-perfused animals and left in 4% PFA for an additional hour. Whole-mount immunostaining was performed using anti-β-III tubulin (Cell signaling, 1:500) with DAPI counterstaining. Retinas were mounted onto coverslips in mounting medium (FluorSave) and imaged with a Zeiss LSM700 confocal microscope and images were acquired from 4 representative fields per retina. For each field, 4 stacked images in each perpendicular direction were acquired. The number of RGCs and neurite length were measured using Metamorph and Image J software by an observer masked to the treatment and genotype.

4.8. Immunohistochemistry

At 3 or 12 weeks after ONC, tissues were collected after perfusion for immunostaining. Frozen sections (25 μm thickness) were prepared using a cryostat microtome (Leica, Deer

Park, IL, USA) and fixed in 4% PBS-buffered paraformaldhyde solution, and permeabilized using 0.3% Triton-X 100 and 3% goat serum in PBS for immunostaining. Tissue samples were incubated with primary antibodies diluted in PBS that contained 3% goat serum at 4 °C overnight. The primary antibodies used were rabbit anti-GAP43 (1:500, Cell Signaling, Denve, MA, USA), anti-β-III tubulin (1:500, Cell signaling) and anti-MBP (1:500, Cell signaling). After washing 3 times with PBS, the samples were incubated with Alexa Fluor 488 (1:200, green) or Alexa Fluor 555 secondary antibody (1:200, red) (Molecular Probes, Waltham, MA, USA) for 1 h at room temperature. The samples were mounted in fluoro mounting medium (Millipore, Burlington, MA, USA) and images were taken with a Zeiss LSM700 confocal microscope (Kuehnstrasse, Hamburg, Germany). The fluorescence images were analyzed using ImageJ from the National Institute of Health (Bethesda, MD, USA) to analyze the fluorescence intensities of the tissues compared with that of the control after subtracting the background value.

4.9. Western Blot

WT or *gpr110 KO* mice were intracardially perfused with phosphate-buffered saline (PBS) to clear their blood before the brains were removed. Optic nerve tissues were dissected out and homogenized in ice-cold solubilization buffer (25 mM Tris pH 7.2, 150 mM NaCl, 1 mM $CaCl_2$; 1 mM $MgCl_2$) that contained 0.5% NP-40 (Thermo Scientific, Waltham, MA, USA) and protease inhibitors (Sigma, St. Louis, MI, USA). The protein concentrations of the lysates were determined by microBCA protein assay (Pierce, Rockford, IL, USA). The samples for SDS-PAGE were prepared at a 1 µg protein/µL concentration using 4X SDS-PAGE buffer (Lifetechnology, San Mateo, CA, USA) and 20 µg of protein was loaded onto each well. Proteins were separated by SDS-PAGE on 4–15% polyacrylamide gels (Lifetechnology, CA, USA) and transferred onto a PVDF membrane (Lifetechnology, CA, USA). After treating with a blocking buffer that contained 0.01% Tween-20, 10% BSA (Lifetechonolgy, CA, USA) for 1 h at room temperature, blots were incubated with primary antibodies diluted in blocking buffer (anti-O_2 1:1000, Millipore, anti-MBP 1:1000, Abcam (Waltham, MA, USA), anti-CNPase 1:1000 and rabbit anti-GAPDH 1:1000, Cell Signaling, CA, USA) overnight at 4 °C, followed by HPR-conjugated secondary antibodies (1:5000, Cell Signaling, CA, USA) for 1 h at room temperature. Detection was carried out using the KODAK Imaging System (Molecular Dynamics, Sunnyvale, CA, USA).

4.10. Determination of the Synaptamide and A8 Level

Synaptamide and A8 were analyzed by reversed phase liquid chromatography coupled to high-resolution tandem mass spectrometry, using a Thermo Scientific Q-Exactive mass spectrometer as described earlier [15]. Briefly, the mice were intravitreally injected with a mixture of synaptamide and A8. At 1 and 24 h after the injection, the mice were perfused with 1× PBS, and the injected eyes were collected and homogenized in a water/methanol (1:1) mixture that contained 2 µM URB597 (a fatty acid amide hydrolase inhibitor) and 50 µg/mL butyl hydroxytoluene (BHT) (Sigma-Aldrich, St. Louis, MO, USA, cat# W218405). The homogenate was brought to BHT-methanol/water (7:3) and centrifuged for 20 min at 4 °C, after the addition of a mixture of deuterated internal standards of d_4-synaptamide and d_6-A8. The supernatants were loaded onto a Strata-X polymeric C18 reverse-phase SPE cartridge (33 µm, 30 mg/mL, Phenomenex, Torrance, CA, USA) that was equilibrated with water. After washing with water, the samples were eluted with 2.5 mL BHT-methanol into glass tubes, dried under N2, and resuspended in a small volume of BHT-methanol and injected onto the LC/MS/MS system. Separation was achieved using an Eclipse C18 HPLC column (1.8 µm, 2.1 mm × 50 mm, Agilent Technologies, Santa Clara, CA, USA) and a tertiary gradient consisting of water (A), methanol (B), and acetonitrile (C), with all solvents containing 0.01% acetic acid (Thermo Scientific). After pre-equilibration of the column with A/B (60%/40%), 5 µL of the extract was injected, and the solvent composition was linearly changed to A/B/C (36.3%/15%/48.7%) in 5 min, followed by a linear gradient to A/B/C (13.5%/68.4%/18.1%) over 22 min. The mass transitions of 372.3 to 62.060, 400.3 to 72.081, 376.3 to 66.085, and 406.4 to 78.118 were used to detect synaptamide, analog 8, d_4-synaptamide, and d_6-A8, respectively. Quantitation of synaptamide and A8 was achieved using d_4-synaptamide and d_6-A8 as the respective internal standards.

4.11. Statistical Analysis

Data were analyzed using GraphPad Prism 7 software (Ver. 7.05). All data are presented as mean ± s.e.m. and are representative of at least two independent experiments. Statistical significance was determined by unpaired Student's *t* test or one-way ANOVA. * $p < 0.05$, ** $p < 0.01$ and *** $p < 0.001$.

Author Contributions: H.-Y.K. conceived the idea and directed the research. H.-S.K. and H.-Y.K. designed the experiments and wrote the manuscript. H.-S.K. performed all the experiments with the help of K.K. for mass spectrometry, M.A.-A. for EM and H.Q. for the analysis of VEP and ERG for the data analysis. S.P. and J.M. designed and synthesized the synaptamide analogue. All authors reviewed and contributed to the manuscript. All authors have read and agreed to the published version of the manuscript.

Funding: The research was supported by the intramural program of NIAAA, NIH.

Institutional Review Board Statement: The study was conducted in accordance with the guiding principles for the care and use of animals approved by the National Institute on Alcohol Abuse and Alcoholism (LMS-HK13).

Informed Consent Statement: Not applicable.

Data Availability Statement: Not applicable.

Acknowledgments: The authors acknowledge the Office of Laboratory Animal Science, NIAAA, for facilitating animal studies.

Conflicts of Interest: The authors declare no competing financial interest.

Abbreviations

CNS, central nervous system; RGC, retinal ganglion cell; GPR110, G-protein coupled receptor 110 (ADGRF1); OEA, N-oleoylethanolamine; ONC, optic nerve crush; CTB, cholera toxin subunit B (CTB); MBP, myelin basic protein; CNPase, 2′, 3′-cyclic-nucleotide 3′-phosphodiesterase; FAAH, fatty acid amide hydrolase; A8, dimethylsynaptamide.

References

1. Fischer, D.; Leibinger, M. Promoting optic nerve regeneration. *Prog. Retin. Eye Res.* **2012**, *31*, 688–701. [CrossRef] [PubMed]
2. He, Z.; Jin, Y. Intrinsic Control of Axon Regeneration. *Neuron* **2016**, *90*, 437–451. [PubMed]
3. Berkelaar, M.; Clarke, D.B.; Wang, Y.C.; Bray, G.M.; Aguayo, A.J. Axotomy results in delayed death and apoptosis of retinal ganglion cells in adult rats. *J. Neurosci.* **1994**, *14*, 4368–4374. [PubMed]
4. Goldberg, J.L.; Barres, B.A. The relationship between neuronal survival and regeneration. *Annu. Rev. Neurosci.* **2000**, *23*, 579–612. [CrossRef]
5. McGee, A.W.; Yang, Y.; Fischer, Q.S.; Daw, N.W.; Strittmatter, S.M. Experience-driven plasticity of visual cortex limited by myelin and Nogo receptor. *Science* **2005**, *309*, 2222–2226. [CrossRef]
6. Park, K.K.; Liu, K.; Hu, Y.; Smith, P.D.; Wang, C.; Cai, B.; Xu, B.; Connolly, L.; Kramvis, I.; Sahin, M.; et al. Promoting axon regeneration in the adult CNS by modulation of the PTEN/mTOR pathway. *Science* **2008**, *322*, 963–966. [CrossRef]
7. Benowitz, L.I.; He, Z.; Goldberg, J.L. Reaching the brain: Advances in optic nerve regeneration. *Exp. Neurol.* **2017**, *287 Pt 3*, 365–373. [CrossRef]
8. Laha, B.S.; Stafford, B.K.; Huberman, A. Regenerating optic pathways from the eye to the brain. *Science* **2017**, *356*, 1031–1034. [CrossRef]
9. Gao, Y.; Deng, K.W.; Hou, J.W.; Bryson, J.B.; Barco, A.; Nikulina, E.; Spencer, T.; Mellado, W.; Kandel, E.R.; Filbin, M.T. Activated CREB is sufficient to overcome inhibitors in myelin and promote spinal axon regeneration in vivo. *Neuron* **2004**, *44*, 609–621. [CrossRef]

10. Hellstrom, M.; Harvey, A.R. Cyclic AMP and the regeneration of retinal ganglion cell axons. *Int. J. Biochem. Cell Biol.* **2014**, *56*, 66–73. [CrossRef]
11. Batty, N.J.; Fenrich, K.K.; Fouad, K. The role of cAMP and its downstream targets in neurite growth in the adult nervous system. *Neurosci. Lett.* **2017**, *652*, 56–63. [CrossRef] [PubMed]
12. Lee, J.W.; Huang, B.X.; Kwon, H.; Rashid, M.A.; Kharebava, G.; Desai, A.; Patnaik, S.; Marugan, J.; Kim, H.Y. Orphan GPR110 (ADGRF1) targeted by N-docosahexaenoylethanolamine in development of neurons and cognitive function. *Nat. Commun.* **2016**, *7*, 13123. [CrossRef] [PubMed]
13. Huang, B.X.; Hu, X.; Kwon, H.S.; Fu, C.; Lee, J.W.; Southall, N.; Marugan, J.; Kim, H.Y. Synaptamide activates the adhesion GPCR GPR110 (ADGRF1) through GAIN domain binding. *Commun. Biol.* **2020**, *3*, 109. [CrossRef] [PubMed]
14. Kwon, H.K.; Kevala, K.; Hu, X.; Patnaik, S.; Marugan, J.; Kim, H.Y. Ligand-Induced GPR110 Activation Facilitates Axon Growth after Injury. *Int. J. Mol. Sci.* **2021**, *22*, 3386. [CrossRef]
15. Chen, H.K.; Kevala, K.; Aflaki, E.; Marugan, J.; Kim, H.Y. GPR110 ligands reduce chronic optic tract gliosis and visual deficit following repetitive mild traumatic brain injury in mice. *J. Neurotrauma* **2021**, *18*, 157.
16. Dorfman, L.J.; Gaynon, M.; Ceranski, J.; Louis, A.A.; Howard, J.E. Visual electrical evoked potentials: Evaluation of ocular injuries. *Neurology* **1987**, *37*, 123–128. [CrossRef]
17. Couto, L.A.; Narciso, M.S.; Hokoc, J.N.; Martinez, A.M.B. Calpain inhibitor 2 prevents axonal degeneration of opossum optic nerve fibers. *J. Neurosci. Res.* **2004**, *77*, 410–419. [CrossRef]
18. Dutta, D.J.; Woo, D.H.; Lee, P.R.; Pajevic, S.; Bukalo, O.; Huffman, W.C.; Wake, H.; Basser, P.J.; SheikhBahaei, S.; Lazarevic, V.; et al. Regulation of myelin structure and conduction velocity by perinodal astrocytes. *Proc. Natl. Acad. Sci. USA* **2018**, *115*, 11832–11837. [CrossRef]
19. Sanchez-Migallon, M.C.; Valiente-Soriano, F.J.; Salinas-Navarro, M.; Nadal-Nicolas, F.M.; Jimenez-Lopez, M.; Vidal-Sanz, M.; Agudo-Barriuso, M. Nerve fibre layer degeneration and retinal ganglion cell loss long term after optic nerve crush or transection in adult mice. *Exp. Eye Res.* **2018**, *170*, 40–50. [CrossRef]
20. de Lima, S.; Koriyama, Y.; Kurimoto, T.; Oliveira, J.T.; Yin, Y.; Li, Y.; Gilbert, H.Y.; Fagiolini, M.; Martinez, A.M.; Benowitz, L. Full-length axon regeneration in the adult mouse optic nerve and partial recovery of simple visual behaviors. *Proc. Natl. Acad. Sci. USA* **2012**, *109*, 9149–9154. [CrossRef]
21. Kim, H.Y.; Spector, A.A. N-Docosahexaenoylethanolamine: A neurotrophic and neuroprotective metabolite of docosahexaenoic acid. *Mol. Asp. Med.* **2018**, *64*, 34–44. [CrossRef] [PubMed]
22. Cai, D.; Shen, Y.; De Bellard, M.; Tang, S.; Filbin, M.T. Prior exposure to neurotrophins blocks inhibition of axonal regeneration by MAG and myelin via a cAMP-dependent mechanism. *Neuron* **1999**, *22*, 89–101. [PubMed]
23. Cai, D.; Qiu, J.; Cao, Z.; McAtee, M.; Bregman, B.S.; Filbin, M.T. Neuronal cyclic AMP controls the developmental loss in ability of axons to regenerate. *J. Neurosci.* **2001**, *21*, 4731–4739.
24. Templeton, J.P.; Geisert, E.E. A practical approach to optic nerve crush in the mouse. *Mol. Vis.* **2012**, *18*, 2147–2152.
25. Rydel, R.E.; Greene, L.A. cAMP analogs promote survival and neurite outgrowth in cultures of rat sympathetic and sensory neurons independently of nerve growth factor. *Proc. Natl. Acad. Sci. USA* **1988**, *85*, 1257–1261. [CrossRef] [PubMed]
26. Bradbury, E.J.; Moon, L.D.; Popat, R.J.; King, V.R.; Bennett, G.S.; Patel, P.N.; Fawcett, J.W.; McMahon, S.B. Chondroitinase ABC promotes functional recovery after spinal cord injury. *Nature* **2002**, *416*, 636–640. [CrossRef]
27. Ruschel, J.; Hellal, F.; Flynn, K.C.; Dupraz, S.; Elliott, D.A.; Tedeschi, A.; Bates, M.; Sliwinski, C.; Brook, G.; Dobrindt, K.; et al. Axonal regeneration. Systemic administration of epothilone B promotes axon regeneration after spinal cord injury. *Science* **2015**, *348*, 347–352. [CrossRef] [PubMed]
28. Park, T.C.H.; Kim, H.Y. GPR110 (ADGRF1) mediates anti-inflammatory effects of N-docosahexaenoylethanolamine. *J. Neuroinflammation* **2019**, *16*, 225. [CrossRef]
29. Desai, A.; Chen, H.; Kim, H. Multiple mild closed head injuries lead to visual dysfunction in a mouse model. *J. Neurotrauma* **2019**, *37*, 286–294.
30. Benchorin, G.; Calton, M.A.; Beaulieu, M.O.; Vollrath, D. Assessment of murine retinal function by electroretinography. *Bio Protoc.* **2017**, *7*, e2218.
31. Abu-Asab, M. *AA Concise Practical Manual of Transmission Electron Microscopy: For Biological & Clinical Specimens*; Kindle Direct Publishing: Seattle, WA, USA, 2021.
32. Friede, R.L.; Beuche, W. Combined scatter diagrams of sheath thickness and fibre calibre in human sural nerves: Changes with age and neuropathy. *J. Neurol. Neurosurg. Psychiatry* **1985**, *48*, 749–756. [CrossRef]

International Journal of
Molecular Sciences

MDPI

Article

Protective Effect of Pioglitazone on Retinal Ganglion Cells in an Experimental Mouse Model of Ischemic Optic Neuropathy

Ming-Hui Sun [1,2,*], Kuan-Jen Chen [1,2], Chi-Chin Sun [2,3] and Rong-Kung Tsai [4,5]

1 Department of Ophthalmology, Linkou Chang Gung Memorial Hospital, Taoyuan 333423, Taiwan
2 College of Medicine, Chang Gung University, Taoyuan 333323, Taiwan
3 Department of Ophthalmology, Keelung Chang Gung Memorial Hospital, Keelung 20401, Taiwan
4 Institute of Medical Sciences, Tzu Chi University, Hualien 970374, Taiwan
5 Institute of Eye Research, Hualien Tzu Chi Hospital, Buddhist Tzu Chi Medical Foundation, Hualien 970473, Taiwan
* Correspondence: minghui0215@gmail.com; Tel.: +886-3-3281200 (ext. 8666); Fax: +886-3-3287798

Abstract: The aim was to assess the protective effect of pioglitazone (PGZ) on retinal ganglion cells (RGCs) after anterior ischemic optic neuropathy (AION) in diabetic and non-diabetic mice. Adult C57BL/6 mice with induced diabetes were divided into three groups: group 1: oral PGZ (20 mg/kg) in 0.1% dimethyl sulfoxide (DMSO) for 4 weeks; group 2: oral PGZ (10 mg/kg) in 0.1% DMSO for 4 weeks; and group 3: oral DMSO only for 4 weeks (control group). Two weeks after treatment, AION was induced through photochemical thrombosis. For non-diabetic mice, adult C57BL/6 mice were divided into four groups after AION was induced: group 1: oral DMSO for 4 weeks; group 2: oral PGZ (20 mg/kg) in 0.1% DMSO for 4 weeks; group 3: oral PGZ (20 mg/kg) in 0.1% DMSO + peritoneal injection of GW9662 (one kind of PPAR-γ inhibitor) (1 mg/kg) for 4 weeks; group 4: peritoneal injection of GW9662 (1 mg/kg) for 4 weeks; One week after the induction of AION in diabetic mice, apoptosis in RGCs was much lower in group 1 (8.0 ± 4.9 cells/field) than in group 2 (24.0 ± 11.5 cells/field) and 3 (25.0 ± 7.7 cells/field). Furthermore, microglial cell infiltration in the retina (group 1: 2.0 ± 2.6 cells/field; group 2: 15.6 ± 3.5 cells/field; and group 3: 14.8 ± 7.5 cells/field) and retinal thinning (group 1: 6.7 ± 5.7 μm; group 2: 12.8 ± 6.1 μm; and group 3: 15.8 ± 5.8 μm) were also lower in group 1 than in the other two groups. In non-diabetic mice, preserved Brn3A$^+$ cells were significantly greater in group 2 (2382 ± 140 Brn3A+ cells/mm^2, $n = 7$) than in group 1 (1920 ± 228 Brn3A+ cells/mm^2; $p = 0.03$, $n = 4$), group 3 (1938 ± 213 Brn3A+ cells/mm^2; $p = 0.002$, $n = 4$), and group 4 (2138 ± 126 Brn3A+ cells/mm^2; $p = 0.03$, $n = 4$), respectively; PGZ confers protection to RGCs from damage caused by ischemic optic neuropathy in diabetic and non-diabetic mice.

Keywords: diabetes; ischemic optic neuropathy; pioglitazone

Citation: Sun, M.-H.; Chen, K.-J.; Sun, C.-C.; Tsai, R.-K. Protective Effect of Pioglitazone on Retinal Ganglion Cells in an Experimental Mouse Model of Ischemic Optic Neuropathy. *Int. J. Mol. Sci.* **2023**, *24*, 411. https://doi.org/10.3390/ijms24010411

Academic Editor: Silvia C. Finnemann

Received: 3 December 2022
Revised: 17 December 2022
Accepted: 20 December 2022
Published: 27 December 2022

1. Introduction

Diabetic retinopathy is the leading cause of adult blindness and is the most common complication of diabetes. It affects >90% of people with diabetes and ultimately leads to retinal edema, neovascularization, and vision loss in some patients [1]. Prolonged hyperglycemia in diabetes is associated with retinal microvasculopathy due to pericyte loss, acellular capillaries [2], capillary cell apoptosis, polyol-pathway-mediated basement membrane thickening [3], the release of vascular endothelial growth factor (VEGF) and proinflammatory cytokines (tumor necrosis factor (TNF)-α, interleukin (IL)-6, and IL-1β) [4], leukostatsis [5], and eventually, vascular hemodynamic changes, which are considered to play a pivotal role in diabetic retinopathy pathogenesis.

Non-arteritic anterior ischemic optic neuropathy (NAION) is the most common acute optic neuropathy in individuals > 50 years old [6,7]. NAION is multifactorial, and its systemic risk factors include arterial hypertension, diabetes, sleep apnea, ischemic heart disease, hyperlipidemia, and atherosclerosis [6]. Although diabetes is one of the most common risk factors for NAION [8,9], the role of diabetes mellitus (DM) in NAION severity is unclear [10–12]. Our previous study in a mice model of anterior ischemic optic neuropathy (AION) showed that diabetes increases the loss of retinal ganglion cells (RGCs), thus increasing the severity of retinal inflammation and damage, which can be reduced with short-term glycemic control [13]. In this study, we investigated the protective effect of long-term hyperglycemia control through treatment with pioglitazone (PGZ), a synthetic ligand of peroxisome proliferator-activated receptor-γ (PPAR-γ), on retinal tissues after AION inducement in mice fed a high-fat diet (HFD) with streptozotocin (STZ)-induced diabetes.

2. Results

2.1. PGZ Normalized Blood Glucose Levels and Did Not Change Body Weight

After rearing mice for 4 weeks on an HFD, their body weight increased ($p = 0.479$) (Figure 1A). Furthermore, 2 weeks after injecting these mice with STZ, their blood glucose increased gradually (Figure 1C), with a slight decrease in body weight (Figure 1B), and they became diabetic. Diabetic mice treated with 20 mg/kg PGZ had lower blood sugar levels (234.0 ± 10.0 mg/dL, $n = 10$) than diabetic mice treated with 10 mg/kg PGZ (271.2 ± 14.1 mg/dL, $n = 10$) and diabetic mice treated with 0 mg/kg PGZ (DMSO only) (368.0 ± 28.3 mg/dL, $n = 10$) ($p = 0.0016$; Figure 1D).

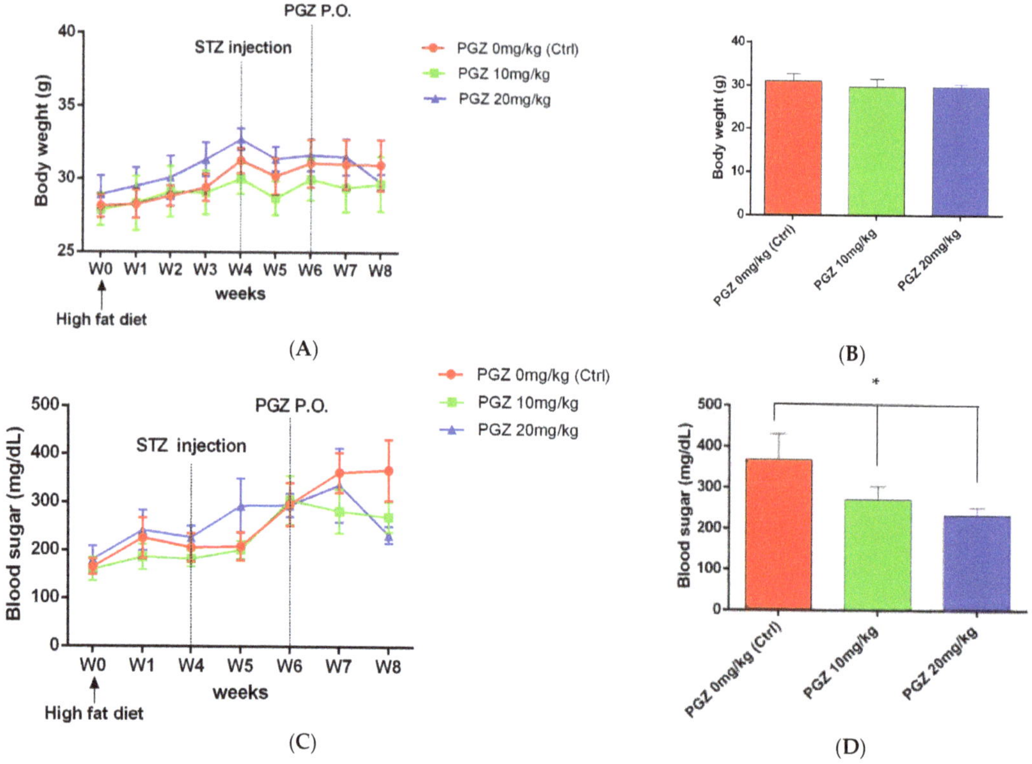

Figure 1. Blood glucose levels and body weights of mice. (**A**) Increase in body weight after high fat diet (HFD) rearing. (**B**) No significant difference in body weight between diabetic mice treated with 20, 10, and 0 mg/kg pioglitazone (PGZ). (**C**) Increase in blood glucose levels after streptozotocin (STZ) injection. (**D**) Diabetic mice treated with 20 mg/kg PGZ for 2 weeks had a lower level of blood sugar than those treated with 10 and 0 mg/kg PGZ (* $p < 0.05$).

2.2. PGZ Preserved Retinal Thickness on OCT Measurement after AION in DM Mice

Since our preliminary study showed that the thinning of peripapillary retinal thickness at the posterior pole scan was more significant than the ganglion cell complex (GCC) thickness at AION W1 and AION W3 in diabetic mice without treatment of PGZ (Figure 2A), we evaluated the protective effect of PGZ on the preservation of peripapillary retinal thickness at AION W1. We found peripapillary retinal thinning was noted 1 week after AION induction in DM mice. Diabetic mice treated with 20 mg/kg PGZ showed lesser thinning compared with that in the other two groups (20 mg/kg PGZ group: 6.7 ± 5.7 μm thinning, N = 15; 10 mg/kg PGZ group: 12.8 ± 6.1 μm thinning, N = 15; and 0 mg/kg PGZ (DMSO only) group: 15.8 ± 5.8 μm thinning, N = 10; $p = 0.041$; Figure 2B,C).

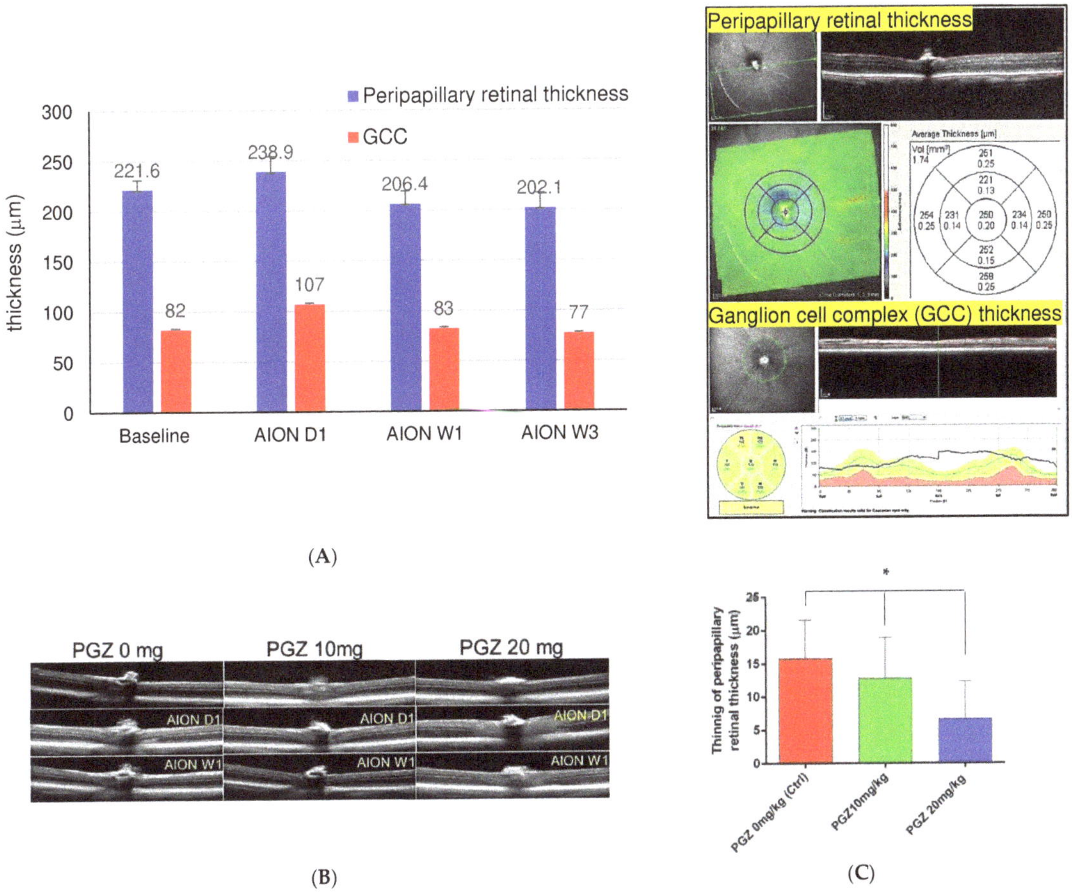

Figure 2. OCT measurement after AION in HFD feeding followed by STZ-induced diabetic mice. (**A**) Peripapillary retinal thickness using posterior pole scan and ganglion cell complex (GCC) thickness were measured through OCT on day 1 (AION D1), week 1 (AION W1), and week 3 (AION W3) in diabetic mice without treatment of PGZ ($n = 17$). The thinning of peripapillary retinal thickness was more significant than (GCC) thickness at AION W1 and W3. The up-right figure showed how the OCT machine measured the peripapillary retinal thickness and GCC thickness. (**B**,**C**) Less retinal thinning of peripapillary retinal thickness at posterior pole scan on AION W1 was noted in DM mice treated with 20 mg/kg PGZ than in the other 2 groups (* $p < 0.05$).

2.3. PGZ Reduced Apoptosis in RGCs 1 Week after AION in DM Mice

One week after ischemic optic neuropathy, RGC apoptosis was much lower in the retina of diabetic mice treated with 20 mg/kg PGZ (8.0 ± 4.9 cells/field, N = 8) than in that of diabetic mice treated with 10 mg/kg PGZ (24.0 ± 11.5 cells/field, N = 8) and diabetic mice treated with 0 mg/kg PGZ (DMSO only) (25.0 ± 7.7 cells/field, N = 6) ($p = 0.013$; Figure 3A,B).

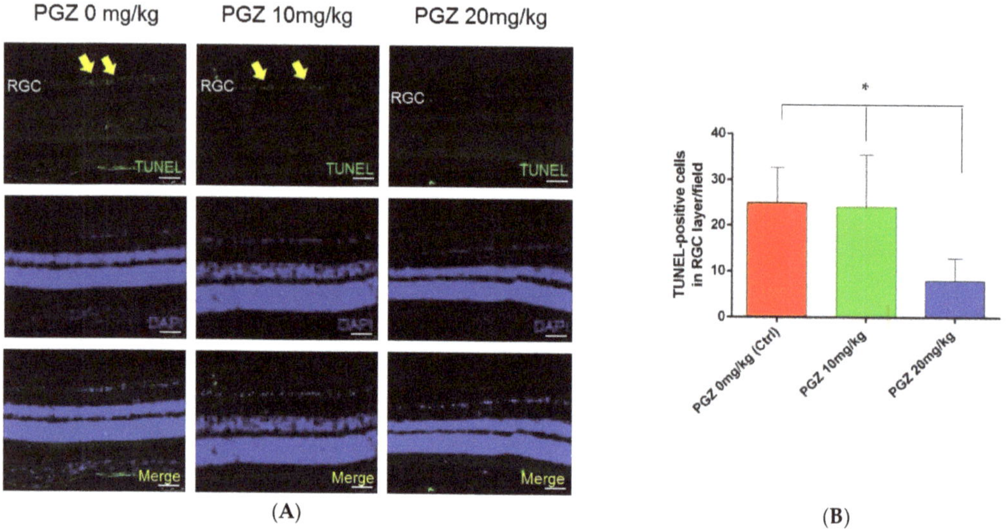

Figure 3. Apoptosis in RGCs 1 week after AION in DM mice. (**A**) Apoptosis in RGCs was evaluated through TUNEL staining. After ischemic optic neuropathy, apoptotic cells (yellow arrows) in RGCs were fewer in diabetic mice treated with 20 mg/kg PGZ than in those treated with 10 and 0 mg/kg PGZ (DMSO only). (**B**) Bar graph shows less apoptotic cells in RGCs in the retina of DM mice treated with 20 mg/kg PGZ compared with that in the other 2 groups (* $p < 0.05$) (scale bar: 75 μm; magnification: 200×).

2.4. PGZ Alleviated Iba1$^+$-Activated Microglia Recruitment to Retina 1 Week after AION

Microglial cells were activated in the retina of diabetic mice 1 week after AION induction (Figure 4A). Activated microglia infiltration in the retina was lesser in diabetic mice treated with 20 mg/kg PGZ compared with that in the other two groups (20 mg/kg PGZ group: 2.0 ± 2.6 cells/field, $n = 8$; 10 mg/kg PGZ group: 15.6 ± 3.5 cells/field, $n = 8$; 0 mg/kg PGZ (DMSO only) group: 14.8 ± 7.5 cells/field, $n = 6$; $p = 0.0016$; Figure 4B).

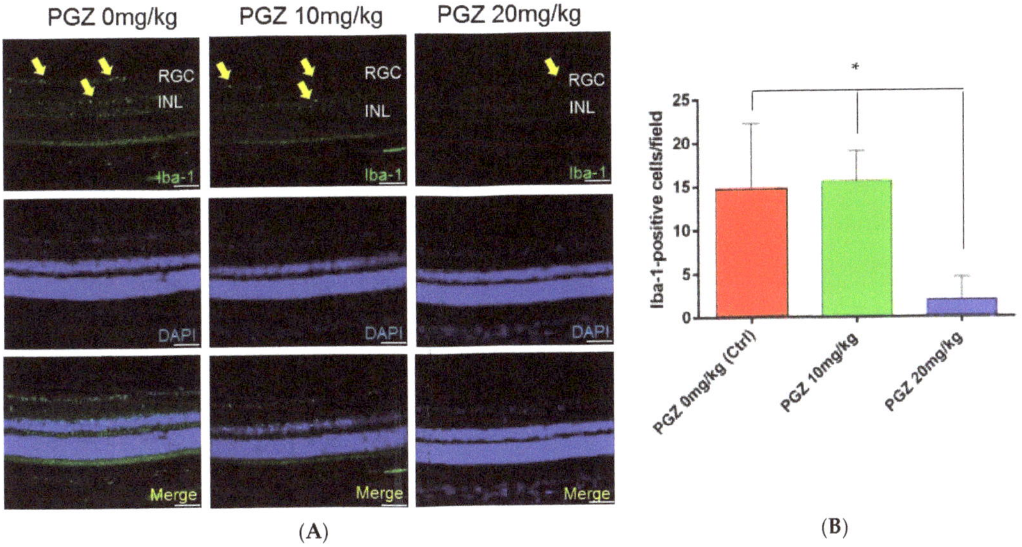

Figure 4. Recruitment of Iba1$^+$-activated microglia to retina 1 week after AION inducement. (**A**) Microglial cells (yellow arrows) were activated in the retina of DM mice 1 week after AION inducement. (**B**) Bar graph shows less microglial cell infiltration in the retina of DM mice treated with 20 mg/kg PGZ compared with that in the other 2 groups (* $p < 0.05$) (scale bar: 75 µm; magnification: 200×).

2.5. PGZ Increased PPAR-γ Expression in Retina

To investigate whether the effects of PGZ are exerted through the PPAR-γ pathway, we performed immunofluorescence staining and found that PPAR-γ expression was barely detected in the retina of diabetic mice without AION and in the retina of AION eyes in diabetic mice without the treatment of PGZ (DMSO only). However, PPAR-γ upregulation after AION inducement was more significant in the retina of diabetic mice treated with 20 mg/kg PGZ than in that of diabetic mice treated with 10 mg/kg PGZ and the retina of normal eyes in diabetic mice treated with 20 mg/kg PGZ. Our results showed that PGZ treatment upregulated PPAR-γ expression in the retina of diabetic mice after AION induction (Figure 5).

2.6. PGZ Preserved RGCs after AION in Diabetic Mice

We counted Brn3A$^+$ RGCs in the retinal whole mount of eyes harvested at 3 weeks after AION induction. The significant loss of Brn3A$^+$ cells was observed after AION induction in diabetic mice treated with 0 mg/kg PGZ (DMSO only) and 20 mg/kg PGZ. However, the loss of Brn3A$^+$ cells was significantly lesser in diabetic mice treated with 20 mg/kg PGZ than in those treated with 0 mg/kg PGZ (DMSO only) (DM-AION eyes treated with 20 mg/kg PGZ orally: 1788 ± 110 Brn3A$^+$ cells/mm^2, DM-control eyes treated with 20 mg/kg PGZ orally: 2441 ± 264 Brn3A$^+$ cells/mm^2, DM-AION eyes without PGZ treatment: 1491 ± 171 Brn3A+ cells/mm^2, DM-control eyes without PGZ treatment: 2131 ± 298 Brn3A+ cells/mm^2; $p = 0.029$; N =10 per group; Figure 6).

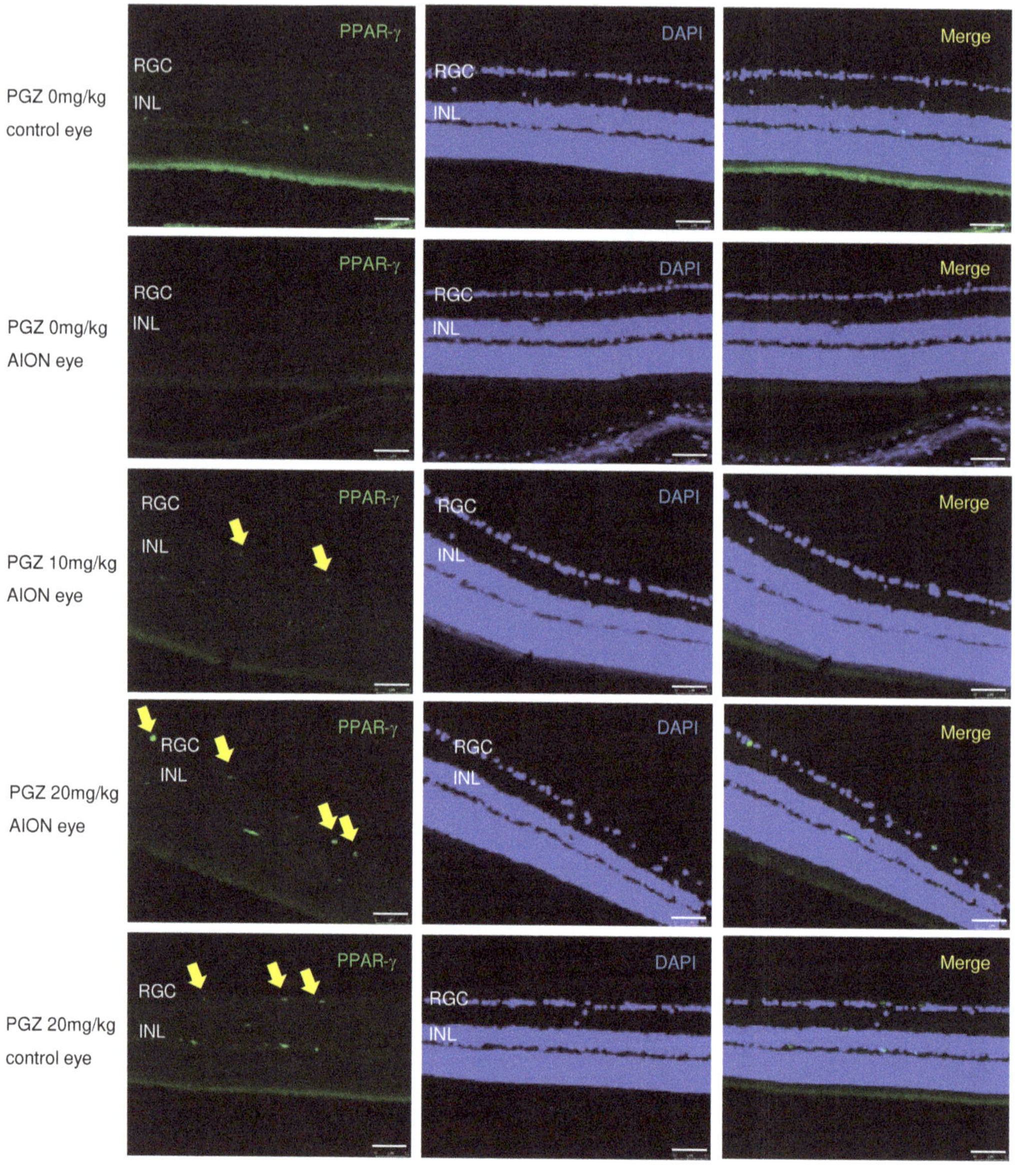

Figure 5. PPAR-γ expression in the retina. The representative figures show that PPAR-γ was barely detected in the retina of diabetic mice without AION and in retina of AION eyes in diabetic mice without treatment of PGZ. PPAR-γ (yellow arrows) expression was more significant in the retina of AION eyes in diabetic mice treated with 20 mg/kg PGZ than in that of diabetic mice treated with 10 mg/kg PGZ and retina of normal eyes in diabetic mice treated with 20 mg/kg PGZ (scale bar: 75 μm; magnification: 200×).

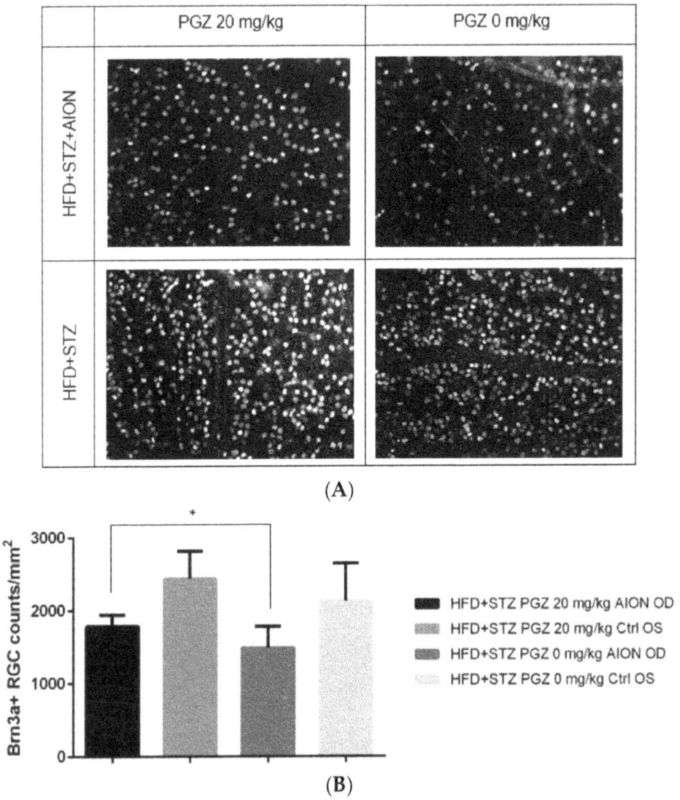

Figure 6. Brn3A$^+$ RGCs in diabetic mice. (**A**) Representative images of immunostaining by using anti-Brn3A antibody in retinal whole-mount preparations of control and AION eyes of diabetic mice treated with 20 and 0 mg/kg PGZ 3 weeks after AION (magnification: 200×). (**B**) Bar graph showing average Brn3A$^+$ cell counts in all 4 conditions 3 weeks after AION (* $p < 0.05$).

2.7. PGZ Preserved RGCs after AION in Non-Diabetic Mice

In order to elucidate whether the mechanism underlying the protective effect of PGZ on diabetic mice is antihyperglycemic-dependent or not, we fed C57BL/6 mice with a regular diet without STZ and counted the Brn3A$^+$ RGCs in the retinal whole mount of non-diabetic eyes harvested at 4 weeks after AION induction. We found the preserved Brn3A$^+$ cells were significantly greater in non-diabetic mice treated with 20 mg/kg PGZ orally every day (2382 ± 140 Brn3A+ cells/mm^2, N = 7) than in those without treatment (1920 ± 228 Brn3A+ cells/mm^2; p = 0.03, N = 4), in those treated with both 20 mg/kg PGZ orally every day and 1 mg/kg GW9662 (one kind of PPAR-γ inhibitor) intraperitoneally injected very other day (1938 ± 213 Brn3A+ cells/mm^2; p = 0.002, N = 4), and in those treated with only 1 mg/kg GW9662 intraperitoneally injected every other day (2138 ± 126 Brn3A+ cells/mm^2; p = 0.03, N = 4), respectively (Figure 7). Our results indicated that PGZ protects RGCs from AION insult through antihyperglycemic-independent effects and through PPAR-γ-dependent effects.

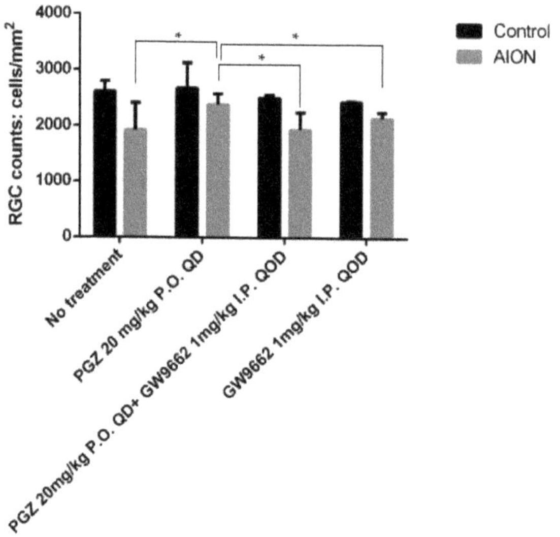

Figure 7. Brn3A$^+$ RGCs in non-diabetic mice. Bar graph showed average Brn3A$^+$ cell counts 4 weeks after AION induction in non-diabetic mice without treatment (oral DMSO only), non-diabetic mice treated with oral (PO) PGZ 20 mg/kg in 0.1% DMSO every day for 4 weeks, oral PGZ 20 mg/kg in 0.1% DMSO every day+ intraperitoneal (IP) injection of GW9662 (PPAR-γ inhibitor) 1 mg/kg every other day for 4 weeks, and intraperitoneal injection of GW9662 (PPAR-γ inhibitor) 1 mg/kg every other day for 4 weeks, respectively (* $p < 0.05$).

3. Discussion

Hyperglycemia could cause endothelial damage through the loss of pericytes and capillary apoptosis in a diabetic mouse model [1]. Moreover, observation under a scanning laser ophthalmoscope showed that in diabetic Ins2Akita mice [5], leukocyte velocity decreased, and the number of rolling leukocytes increased in the retinal arteriole, venule, and vein, and this phenomenon of leukostasis in the endothelial lining suggests inflammation in blood vessels under hyperglycemic status. Furthermore, hyperglycemia could promote vascular perfusion insufficiency from damage to the endothelium through the activation of the polyol pathway, the production of advanced glycation end products, an increase in oxidative stress, the upregulation of the protein kinase C-β pathway [8], and the overproduction of superoxide from the mitochondrial electron transport chain [14]. Producing reactive oxidative species through the overexpression of nuclear factor kappa B contributes to increased inflammatory cytokines, including TNF-α, IL-1β, IL-6, IL-8, vascular cell adhesion molecule-1, and intercellular adhesion molecule-1 [15], which in turn triggers leukocyte infiltration and causes vascular inflammation [16]. Thus, the optic nerve is vulnerable to ischemic insult in patients with diabetes. Some studies have suggested that diabetes increases NAION risk [8,9].

PPAR-γ, a member of the nuclear receptor superfamily, is a ligand-activated transcription factor that plays a crucial role in gene expression associated with various physiological processes including fat cell differentiation, glucose homeostasis, lipid metabolism, aging, and inflammatory and immune responses [17]. In the ocular tissues of mice, PPAR-γ is constitutively expressed in the neuroretina and retinal pigment epithelium [17]. PGZ, a type of thiazolidinedione, improves insulin sensitivity and lipid metabolism through the activation of PPAR-γ [18]; thus, PGZ has been used widely to normalize glucose levels in patients with type 2 diabetes. Moreover, PGZ regulates the lipid metabolism and reduces the levels of inflammatory mediators [19–21]. PGZ has shown protective effects for retinal ischemia/reperfusion injury [22], optic nerve crush injury [23], and normalized insulin signaling in diabetic rat retinas [24]. Our previous study showed that immediate blood sugar control with insulin treatment after AION induction in mice with STZ-induced diabetes reduced damage to the retinal structure [13]. In this study, we further investigated the effect of long-term hyperglycemia control through treatment with PGZ on retinal tissue protection after AION induction in mice with low-dose-STZ-induced diabetes fed an HFD, which mimicked type 2 diabetes through insulin resistance and partial damage to pancreatic β-cells [25]. Two weeks of PGZ (20 mg/kg) treatment could normalize blood glucose levels in HFD-fed mice with STZ-induced diabetes. Moreover, long-term PGZ treatment in HFD-fed mice with STZ-induced diabetes showed reduced apoptosis in RGCs, the decreased recruitment of Iba-1^+-activated microglial cells, preserved retinal thickness on OCT measurement, and less loss of Brn3A^+ RGC counts after AION, and these effects might have occurred through PPAR-γ activation in the retina, as demonstrated via immunofluorescence staining. Furthermore, PPAR-γ expression mainly on the RGC layer was higher in the retina of AION eyes in diabetic mice treated with 20 mg/kg PGZ than in that of diabetic mice without treatment or treated with 10 mg/kg PGZ. In order to elucidate whether the protective effect of PGZ on RGCs from AION insult is antihyperglycemic-dependent or not, we investigated the protective effect of PGZ on RGCs in non-diabetic mice. We found PGZ also preserved more RGCs from AION insult compared with the group without treatment, the group treated with both PGZ and the PPAR-γ inhibitor (GW9662), or the group treated with the PPAR-γ inhibitor alone. Our study suggested that PGZ could also protect RGCs from AION insult through antihyperglycemic-independent and PPAR-γ-dependent effects. To the best of our knowledge, this is the first study reporting the protective effect of PGZ on retinas after AION induction in diabetic mice and non-diabetic mice. Our findings provide insights into the potential therapeutic effect of PGZ on AION.

One limitation in this study is that we did not record the blood glucose levels of the non-diabetic mice treated with PGZ or the PPAR-γ inhibitor; it might be interesting to know if pioglitazone resulted in a decrease in blood glucose (or if the PPAR-γ inhibitor increased it) in non-diabetic mice in a future study.

4. Materials and Methods

4.1. Animals

We used wild-type adult C57BL/6 mice weighing 25–30 g (Charles River, Hollister, CA, USA) housed in a temperature-controlled room with a 12 h light–dark cycle and with free access to food and water. All the animals were treated in accordance with the Statement of the Association for Research in Vision and Ophthalmology for Use of Animals in Ophthalmic and Vision Research. The mice were anesthetized with intraperitoneal injections of 50 to 100 mg/kg ketamine (Hospira Inc., Lake Forest, IL, USA), 2 to 5 mg/kg xylazine (Bedford Laboratories, Bedford, OH, USA), and 0.05 mg/kg buprenorphine (Bedford Laboratories). The pupils of the anesthetized mice were dilated with 1% tropicamide (Alcon Laboratories Inc., Fort Worth, TX, USA) and 2.5% phenylephrine hydrochloride (Akorn Inc., Lake Forest, IL, USA).

4.2. Diabetes Induction

Mice aged 4 to 5 weeks were fed a high-fat diet (HFD) (with 60% energy (Kcal/g) from fat, D12492, TestDiet, St. Louis, MO, USA) for 4 weeks and then intraperitoneally injected with low doses (40 mg/kg) of streptozotocin (STZ) (Sigma, St. Louis, MO, USA) in citrate buffer (pH 4.5) [26] for 3 consecutive days. Two weeks after diabetes induction, we obtained blood from the tail vein to test glucose levels using a basic blood glucose monitoring system (Accu-Check, Aviva Plus, Roche, Indianapolis, IN, USA), and mice with blood glucose levels consistently > 250 mg/dL were considered diabetic. The diabetic mice were divided into 3 groups: (1) mice fed orally with 20 mg/kg PGZ (Sigma) in 0.1% dimethyl sulfoxide (DMSO) with 10 mg/kg cellulose; group; (2) mice fed orally with 10 mg/kg PGZ (Sigma) in 0.1% DMSO with 10 mg/kg cellulose; (3) mice fed orally with DMSO with 10 mg/kg cellulose (control group).

4.3. Experimental AION

Two weeks after treatment, the blood glucose level returned to the normal limit in group 1. We induced AION in all the diabetic mice through photochemical thrombosis [27,28] following an injection of rose bengal (1.25 mM in phosphate-buffered saline; 5 μL/g body weight) into the tail vein by using a trans-pupillary laser in conjunction with a frequency-doubled Nd:YAG laser (Pascal, OptiMedica, Santa Clara, CA, USA) with 400 μm spot diameter, 50 mW power, 1 s duration, and 15 spots.

4.4. Spectral-Domain Optical Coherence Tomography

We performed spectral-domain optical coherence tomography (OCT) scans at baseline and 1 day, 1 week, and 3 weeks after AION induction by using Spectralis HRA + OCT (Heidelberg Engineering, GmbH, Heidelberg, Germany) [27–29]. We performed posterior pole scans (scan angle: 30° × 25°) to measure the peripapillary retinal thickness by using enhanced depth image (EDI) in the high-speed mode (a B scan consisted of 768 A scans, with an average of 9 frames/B scan) as well as 25 line scans (scan angle 25° × 15°) in the high-resolution mode (with an average 16 frames/B scan). The total retinal thickness, defined as the distance from the retinal nerve fiber layer to the Bruch's membrane, was automatically segmented using Spectralis software, and the 1 or 3 mm diameter concentric circle grid with the optic disc in the center was measured. The OCT images of poor quality were excluded.

4.5. Immunohistochemistry and Morphometric Analyses

One week after AION induction, we performed intracardiac perfusion with 4% paraformaldehyde in phosphate-buffered saline, whole-mount retinal dissection, immunohistochemistry, and fluorescence microscopy (Nikon Eclipse TE300 microscope, Nikon Corporation, Tokyo, Japan) by using 4×, 10×, and 20× objectives (Nikon Corporation) and Metamorph software (Molecular Devices, Sunnyvale, CA, USA). To measure activated microglia, we performed morphometric analyses of fluorescence signals after the immunohistochemical analysis of paraffin-embedded retinal sections by using primary rabbit polyclonal anti-Iba1 antibody; these labels activated microglia (1:200 dilution; Wako Chemicals, Richmond, VA, USA). To analyze PPAR-γ expression, we used primary mouse monoclonal anti-PPAR-γ (1:200 dilution; Santa Cruz Biotechnology, Santa Cruz, CA, USA). Immunoreactivity was detected using fluorescein isothiocyanate (FITC)-labeled secondary antibody (Abcam, Cambridge, UK), and cell nuclei were counterstained with 4′-6-diamidino-2-phenylindole (DAPI). To count Brn3A$^+$ RGCs, we performed whole-mount retinal dissection 3 weeks after AION and then stained them with primary mouse monoclonal anti-Brn3A antibody (1:200 dilution; Santa Cruz Biotechnology) and secondary goat antimouse IgG Alexa Fluor 568-labeled antibody (1:200 dilution; Life Technologies). All the retinal whole-mount preparations were mounted with 4′-6-diamidino-2-phenylindole (DAPI)-containing media (Vectashield, Vector Laboratories, Burlingame, CA, USA). To quantify Brn3A$^+$ signals, we obtained 8 images (2 images with 4 quadrants, with each quadrant of 0.14 mm^2) at 200× magnification and used custom-written ImageJ scripts to quantify and calculate the number of Brn3A$^+$ cells/mm^2.

4.6. In Situ TdT-Mediated dUTP Nick-End Labeling

The eyeballs of diabetic mice were harvested 1 week after AION induction and were sectioned along the vertical meridian to include the optic nerve head. For each mouse, two 3 μm thick retinal sections which included the ora serrata and optic nerve were stained by using a TdT-mediated dUTP nick-end labeling (TUNEL)-based kit (TdT FragEL; Oncogene, Darmstadt, Germany). The number of TUNEL-positive cells in each retinal section was obtained through the selection of 6 superior and inferior retinal areas, each 0.425 mm in length. First, we chose 2 segments 0.425 mm superior and inferior to the optic nerve head; second, we chose 2 segments 0.425 mm from the first 2 segments; and third, we chose 2 segments 0.425 mm from the second 2 segments. The total number of TUNEL-positive cells in these 12 retinal areas was averaged as a representative of the number of TUNEL-positive cells per eye sample.

4.7. Statistical Analysis

All data are presented as mean ± SD. We performed statistical analysis by using SPSS 23.0 (SPSS, Inc., Chicago, IL, USA), and statistical significance was defined as $p < 0.05$. We used the Wilcoxon signed-rank test for paired data and the Mann–Whitney U test for unpaired data.

Author Contributions: Conceptualization, M.-H.S.; methodology, M.-H.S.; software, M.-H.S.; validation, M.-H.S., K.-J.C. and C.-C.S.; formal analysis, M.-H.S. and R.-K.T.; investigation, M.-H.S. and R.-K.T.; resources, M.-H.S.; data curation, M.-H.S. and R.-K.T.; writing—original draft preparation, M.-H.S.; writing—review and editing, M.-H.S.; visualization, K.-J.C., C.-C.S. and R.-K.T.; supervision, M.-H.S.; project administration, M.-H.S. and K.-J.C.; funding acquisition, M.-H.S. All authors have read and agreed to the published version of the manuscript.

Funding: This research was funded by a research grant from Chang Gung Memorial Hospital (CMRPG3G1571, and CMRPG3K2271) and the Ministry of Science and Technology of Taiwan (MOST 106-2314-B-182A-046, and MOST 109-2314-B-182A-023).

Institutional Review Board Statement: The animal study protocol was approved by the Institutional Animal Care and Use Committee of Chang Gung Memorial Hospital (Approval number: 2016122020; date of approval: 17 April 2017).

Informed Consent Statement: Not applicable.

Data Availability Statement: Not applicable.

Acknowledgments: We thank Ying-Yi Lin and Yo-Tseng Wen for their kind help in doing animal experiments.

Conflicts of Interest: The authors declare no conflict of interest.

References

1. Feit-Leichman, R.A.; Kinouchi, R.; Takeda, M.; Fan, Z.; Mohr, S.; Kern, T.S.; Chen, D.F. Vascular damage in a mouse model of diabetic retinopathy: Relation to neuronal and glial changes. *Investig. Ophthalmol. Vis. Sci.* **2005**, *46*, 4281–4287. [CrossRef] [PubMed]
2. Weerasekera, L.Y.; Balmer, L.A.; Ram, R.; Morahan, G. Characterization of Retinal Vascular and Neural Damage in a Novel Model of Diabetic Retinopathy. *Investig. Ophthalmol. Vis. Sci.* **2015**, *56*, 3721–3730. [CrossRef] [PubMed]
3. Kern, T.S.; Engerman, R.L. A mouse model of diabetic retinopathy. *Arch. Ophthalmol.* **1996**, *114*, 986–990. [CrossRef] [PubMed]
4. Semeraro, F.; Cancarini, A.; dell'Omo, R.; Rezzola, S.; Romano, M.R.; Costagliola, C. Diabetic Retinopathy: Vascular and Inflammatory Disease. *J. Diabetes Res.* **2015**, *2015*, 582060. [CrossRef]
5. Cahoon, J.M.; Olson, P.R.; Nielson, S.; Miya, T.R.; Bankhead, P.; McGeown, J.G.; Curtis, T.M.; Ambati, B.K. Acridine orange leukocyte fluorography in mice. *Exp. Eye Res.* **2014**, *120*, 15–19. [CrossRef]
6. Hayreh, S.S. Ischemic optic neuropathy. *Prog. Retin. Eye Res.* **2009**, *28*, 34–62. [CrossRef]
7. Biousse, V.; Newman, N.J. Ischemic Optic Neuropathies. *N. Engl. J. Med.* **2015**, *372*, 2428–2436. [CrossRef]
8. Chen, T.; Song, D.; Shan, G.; Wang, K.; Wang, Y.; Ma, J.; Zhong, Y. The association between diabetes mellitus and nonarteritic anterior ischemic optic neuropathy: A systematic review and meta-analysis. *PLoS ONE* **2013**, *8*, e76653. [CrossRef]
9. Lee, M.S.; Grossman, D.; Arnold, A.C.; Sloan, F.A. Incidence of nonarteritic anterior ischemic optic neuropathy: Increased risk among diabetic patients. *Ophthalmology* **2011**, *118*, 959–963. [CrossRef]
10. Hayreh, S.S.; Zimmerman, M.B. Nonarteritic anterior ischemic optic neuropathy: Clinical characteristics in diabetic patients versus nondiabetic patients. *Ophthalmology* **2008**, *115*, 1818–1825. [CrossRef]
11. Odette, J.D.; Okorodudu, D.O.; Johnson, L.N. Early diabetes mellitus or hypertension is not significantly associated with severity of vision loss in nonarteritic anterior ischemic optic neuropathy. *Arch. Ophthalmol.* **2011**, *129*, 1106–1107. [CrossRef] [PubMed]
12. Sharma, S.; Kwan, S.; Fallano, K.A.; Wang, J.; Miller, N.R.; Subramanian, P.S. Comparison of Visual Outcomes of Nonarteritic Anterior Ischemic Optic Neuropathy in Patients with and without Diabetes Mellitus. *Ophthalmology* **2017**, *124*, 450–455. [CrossRef] [PubMed]
13. Sun, M.H.; Shariati, M.A.; Liao, Y.J. Experimental Anterior Ischemic Optic Neuropathy in Diabetic Mice Exhibited Severe Retinal Swelling Associated with VEGF Elevation. *Investig. Ophthalmol. Vis. Sci.* **2017**, *58*, 2296–2305. [CrossRef] [PubMed]
14. Du, X.L.; Edelstein, D.; Rossetti, L.; Fantus, I.G.; Goldberg, H.; Ziyadeh, F.; Wu, J.; Brownlee, M. Hyperglycemia-induced mitochondrial superoxide overproduction activates the hexosamine pathway and induces plasminogen activator inhibitor-1 expression by increasing Sp1 glycosylation. *Proc. Natl. Acad. Sci. USA* **2000**, *97*, 12222–12226. [CrossRef]

15. Grigsby, J.G.; Cardona, S.M.; Pouw, C.E.; Muniz, A.; Mendiola, A.S.; Tsin, A.T.; Allen, D.M.; Cardona, A.E. The role of microglia in diabetic retinopathy. *J. Ophthalmol.* **2014**, *2014*, 705783. [CrossRef]
16. Wang, A.L.; Yu, A.C.; He, Q.H.; Zhu, X.; Tso, M.O. AGEs mediated expression and secretion of TNF alpha in rat retinal microglia. *Exp. Eye Res.* **2007**, *84*, 905–913. [CrossRef]
17. Zhang, S.; Gu, H.; Hu, N. Role of Peroxisome Proliferator-Activated Receptor gamma in Ocular Diseases. *J. Ophthalmol.* **2015**, *2015*, 275435. [CrossRef]
18. Pereira, M.G.; Camara, N.O.; Campaholle, G.; Cenedeze, M.A.; de Paula Antunes Teixeira, V.; dos Reis, M.A.; Pacheco-Silva, A. Pioglitazone limits cyclosporine nephrotoxicity in rats. *Int. Immunopharmacol.* **2006**, *6*, 1943–1951. [CrossRef]
19. Malchiodi-Albedi, F.; Matteucci, A.; Bernardo, A.; Minghetti, L. PPAR-gamma, Microglial Cells, and Ocular Inflammation: New Venues for Potential Therapeutic Approaches. *PPAR Res.* **2008**, *2008*, 295784. [CrossRef]
20. Tawfik, A.; Sanders, T.; Kahook, K.; Akeel, S.; Elmarakby, A.; Al-Shabrawey, M. Suppression of retinal peroxisome proliferator-activated receptor gamma in experimental diabetes and oxygen-induced retinopathy: Role of NADPH oxidase. *Investig. Ophthalmol. Vis. Sci.* **2009**, *50*, 878–884. [CrossRef]
21. Yau, H.; Rivera, K.; Lomonaco, R.; Cusi, K. The future of thiazolidinedione therapy in the management of type 2 diabetes mellitus. *Curr. Diabetes Rep.* **2013**, *13*, 329–341. [CrossRef] [PubMed]
22. Zhang, X.Y.; Xiao, Y.Q.; Zhang, Y.; Ye, W. Protective effect of pioglitazone on retinal ischemia/reperfusion injury in rats. *Investig. Ophthalmol. Vis. Sci.* **2013**, *54*, 3912–3921. [CrossRef] [PubMed]
23. Zhu, J.; Zhang, J.; Ji, M.; Gu, H.; Xu, Y.; Chen, C.; Hu, N. The role of peroxisome proliferator-activated receptor and effects of its agonist, pioglitazone, on a rat model of optic nerve crush: PPARgamma in retinal neuroprotection. *PLoS ONE* **2013**, *8*, e68935. [CrossRef]
24. Jiang, Y.; Thakran, S.; Bheemreddy, R.; Ye, E.A.; He, H.; Walker, R.J.; Steinle, J.J. Pioglitazone normalizes insulin signaling in the diabetic rat retina through reduction in tumor necrosis factor α and suppressor of cytokine signaling 3. *J. Biol. Chem.* **2014**, *289*, 26395–26405. [CrossRef] [PubMed]
25. Gheibi, S.; Kashfi, K.; Ghasemi, A. A practical guide for induction of type-2 diabetes in rat: Incorporating a high-fat diet and streptozotocin. *Biomed. Pharm.* **2017**, *95*, 605–613. [CrossRef]
26. Chaudhry, Z.Z.; Morris, D.L.; Moss, D.R.; Sims, E.K.; Chiong, Y.; Kono, T.; Evans-Molina, C. Streptozotocin is equally diabetogenic whether administered to fed or fasted mice. *Lab. Anim.* **2013**, *47*, 257–265. [CrossRef]
27. Yu, C.; Ho, J.K.; Liao, Y.J. Subretinal fluid is common in experimental non-arteritic anterior ischemic optic neuropathy. *Eye* **2014**, *28*, 1494–1501. [CrossRef]
28. Shariati, M.A.; Park, J.H.; Liao, Y.J. Optical coherence tomography study of retinal changes in normal aging and after ischemia. *Investig. Ophthalmol. Vis. Sci.* **2015**, *56*, 2790–2797. [CrossRef]
29. Ho, J.K.; Stanford, M.P.; Shariati, M.A.; Dalal, R.; Liao, Y.J. Optical coherence tomography study of experimental anterior ischemic optic neuropathy and histologic confirmation. *Investig. Ophthalmol. Vis. Sci.* **2013**, *54*, 5981–5988. [CrossRef]

International Journal of
Molecular Sciences

Article

Transcriptomic Analysis Reveals That Granulocyte Colony-Stimulating Factor Trigger a Novel Signaling Pathway (TAF9-P53-TRIAP1-CASP3) to Protect Retinal Ganglion Cells after Ischemic Optic Neuropathy

Rong-Kung Tsai [1,2,3], Keh-Liang Lin [4], Chin-Te Huang [1,2,5] and Yao-Tseng Wen [1,*]

1 Institute of Eye Research, Hualien Tzu Chi Hospital, Buddhist Tzu Chi Medical Foundation, Hualien 970473, Taiwan; tsai.rk@gmail.com (R.-K.T.); chintehuang@hotmail.com (C.-T.H.)
2 Institute of Medical Sciences, Tzu Chi University, Hualien 970374, Taiwan
3 Doctoral Degree Program in Translational Medicine, Tzu Chi University and Academia Sinica, Hualien 970374, Taiwan
4 Department of Optometry, Mackay Medical College, New Taipei City 252005, Taiwan; eye2020@mmc.edu.tw
5 Department of Ophthalmology, Chung Shan Medical University Hospital, College of Medicine, Chung Shan Medical University, Taichung 402306, Taiwan
* Correspondence: ytw193@gmail.com; Tel.: +886-3-8561825 (ext. 2112)

Abstract: Optic nerve head (ONH) infarct can result in progressive retinal ganglion cell (RGC) death. The granulocyte colony-stimulating factor (GCSF) protects the RGC after ON infarct. However, protective mechanisms of the GCSF after ONH infarct are complex and remain unclear. To investigate the complex mechanisms involved, the transcriptome profiles of the GCSF-treated retinas were examined using microarray technology. The retinal mRNA samples on days 3 and 7 post rat anterior ischemic optic neuropathy (rAION) were analyzed by microarray and bioinformatics analyses. GCSF treatment influenced 3101 genes and 3332 genes on days 3 and 7 post rAION, respectively. ONH infarct led to changes in 702 and 179 genes on days 3 and 7 post rAION, respectively. After cluster analysis, the levels of TATA box-binding protein (TBP)-associated factor were significantly reduced after ONH infarct, but these significantly increased after GCSF treatment. The network analysis revealed that TBP associated factor 9 (TAF9) can bind to P53 to induce TP53-regulated inhibitor of apoptosis 1 (TRIAP1) expression. To evaluate the function of TAF9 in RGC apoptosis, GCSF plus TAF9 siRNA-treated rats were evaluated using retrograde labeling with FluoroGold assay, TUNEL assay, and Western blotting in an rAION model. The RGC densities in the GCSF plus TAF9 siRNA-treated rAION group were 1.95-fold (central retina) and 1.75-fold (midperipheral retina) lower than that in the GCSF-treated rAION group ($p < 0.05$). The number of apoptotic RGC in the GCSF plus TAF9 siRNA-treated group was threefold higher than that in the GCSF-treated group ($p < 0.05$). Treatment with TAF9 siRNA significantly reduced GCSF-induced TP53 and TRIAP1 expression by 2.4-fold and 4.7-fold, respectively, in the rAION model. Overexpression of TAF9 significantly reduced apoptotic RGC and CASP3 levels, and induced TP53 and TRIAP1 expression in the rAION model. Therefore, we have demonstrated that GCSF modulated a new pathway, TAF9-P53-TRIAP1-CASP3, to control RGC death and survival after ON infarct.

Keywords: rat anterior ischemic optic neuropathy model; retinal ganglion cell death; TBP associated factor 9; TP53 regulated inhibitor of apoptosis 1; transcriptome

Citation: Tsai, R.-K.; Lin, K.-L.; Huang, C.-T.; Wen, Y.-T. Transcriptomic Analysis Reveals That Granulocyte Colony-Stimulating Factor Trigger a Novel Signaling Pathway (TAF9-P53-TRIAP1-CASP3) to Protect Retinal Ganglion Cells after Ischemic Optic Neuropathy. *Int. J. Mol. Sci.* **2022**, *23*, 8359. https://doi.org/10.3390/ijms23158359

Academic Editor: Cristoforo Comi

Received: 13 June 2022
Accepted: 26 July 2022
Published: 28 July 2022

1. Introduction

In elderly individuals, the most common type of acute optic neuropathy is non-arteritic anterior ischemic optic neuropathy (NAION), with an estimated annual incidence of 3.72 per 100,000 individuals in Taiwan [1]. NAION is defined clinically as painless visual loss with swelling of the optic disc leading to optic disc atrophy [2]. Currently, there is no effective treatment for NAION. Optic nerve (ON) ischemia induces a series of detrimental events, eventually resulting in retinal ganglion cell (RGC) loss [2]. RGC death and axon degeneration are major complications of ischemic damage and mainly caused by oxidative stress [3–6], pro-inflammatory factors [6,7], aberrant calcium ion homeostasis [8], and macrophage polarization [7,9]. Therefore, a comprehensive investigation on the complex molecular mechanisms of axonal degeneration and RGC death in ON ischemia may bring about new possibilities for treatment.

Several efforts in preventing ON injuries and RGC death have been made using different approaches, such as anti-inflammatory compounds [10,11], neurotropic factors [12,13], oxidative stress regulators [5], calcium channel blockers [14], microglial activation inhibitors [7,15], and blood-borne macrophage infiltration blockers [7,12,16]. These potential treatments provide some possible directions to elucidate how to control the fate of RGCs. In context with our previous study on the neuroprotective effects of granulocyte colony-stimulating factor (GCSF), we found that GCSF exhibited the ability to rescue RGC from apoptosis, which may be involved in modulations of the blood–ON barrier, macrophage infiltration, and inflammatory reactions [7]. Moreover, our previous findings demonstrate that treatment with GCSF can activate the PI3K/AKT pathway to protect RGC from apoptosis [17].

GCSF is a member of the hematopoietic growth factor family. It is widely used in clinical practice for the treatment of neutropenia [18]. Recent findings have suggested that GCSF also has a nonhematopoietic role in memory improvement in Alzheimer's disease and a neuroprotective role in Parkinson's disease [19,20]. It also promotes angiogenesis and inhibits apoptosis and inflammation in rats with ischemic stroke [21–23]. Furthermore, the GCSF receptor (GCSFR) is expressed in various neural and glial cells, such as RGCs, microglia, astrocyte, and oligodendrocyte, which results in the direct activation of GCSFR signaling pathways, including JAK/STAT, PI3K/AKT, and MAPK/ERK pathways [24]. These signaling pathways are involved in cell growth and differentiation. Thus, the mechanisms by which GCSF promotes RGC survival are likely complex.

To deeply investigate and characterize the factors triggered by CGSF treatment, transcriptome analysis of the rat retina is a possible approach that can be used to investigate the transcriptome changes after ON infarct with or without GCSF treatment. The microarray technique is a method of high-throughput analysis to determine the expression levels of large numbers of genes belonging to specific pathways simultaneously. This technique has also been used to evaluate changes after axonal injury in both the retina and isolated RGCs [25,26]. Therefore, we considered that microarray analysis is an adequate tool to explore any possible mechanisms involved in RGC apoptosis and survival.

Different animal models have been used to investigate RGC pathology. Herein, we used a rat anterior ischemic optic neuropathy (rAION) model as it represents similar features and pathology to human and primate AION [27]. The rAION model was achieved by photodynamic therapy, which generates superoxide radicals in the ON capillaries, causing capillary thrombosis, inflammation, and oxidative stress [27]. These pathological changes are important events to induce RGC apoptosis. Thus, this is an appropriate model to use in investigating the mechanisms of RGC apoptosis.

In the present study, a comparative microarray analysis was adopted to explore the dynamic transcriptome changes in the rat retina under ON infarct and GCSF treatment. We identified that the mRNA levels of several TATA-box-binding protein (TBP)-associated factors (TAFs) were significantly reduced after ONH infarct, but significantly increased after GCSF treatment. Among these genes, we targeted one of the most upregulated, transcription initiation factor TFIID subunit 9 (taf9), which encodes for one of the smaller subunits of transcription factor IID (TFIID) that binds to the general transcription factor transcription initiation factor IIB (Gtf2b) and several transcriptional activators, such as p53 and Vp16 [28,29]. Taf9 physically interacts with p53 at its *N*-terminus, where p53 also interacts with its negative regulator, Mdm2, thereby inhibiting Mdm2 degradation of p53 [30]. Functionally, this interaction translates to an increase in p53-induced angiogenesis,

DNA repair, cell arrest, cell survival, or apoptosis [30]. However, it is questionable whether TAF9 drives P53 toward cell survival or apoptosis. Thus, this study aimed to reveal the underlying mechanisms of TAF9 in RGC apoptosis and cell survival.

2. Results

2.1. Identification of Differentially Expressed Genes by Microarray

To investigate RGC death and survival at the transcriptional level, the rAION-inducted rats were treated with phosphate-buffered saline (PBS) or GCSF. The transcriptome profiles were analyzed using oligonucleotide microarrays. Microarray data were analyzed using the Gene Expression Pattern Analysis Suite to identify the differentially expressed genes. From a total of 24,358 analyzed genes, 3101 and 3332 transcripts were regulated by GCSF treatment on days 3 and 7 post rAION, respectively. In addition, 702 and 179 transcripts were regulated by PBS treatment on days 3 and 7 post rAION, respectively (Figure 1A–D). Unsupervised hierarchical clustering analysis of differentially expressed genes from all groups was conducted to investigate the similarity of the whole gene expression between the experimental samples. The result indicated that the profile of gene expression in the GCSF-treated group was similar (Figure 1E). Additionally, the PBS-treated rats on days 3 and 7 post rAION also exhibited similar gene expressions. As stated above, the trend of gene expression is consistent between the PBS- and GCSF-treated groups.

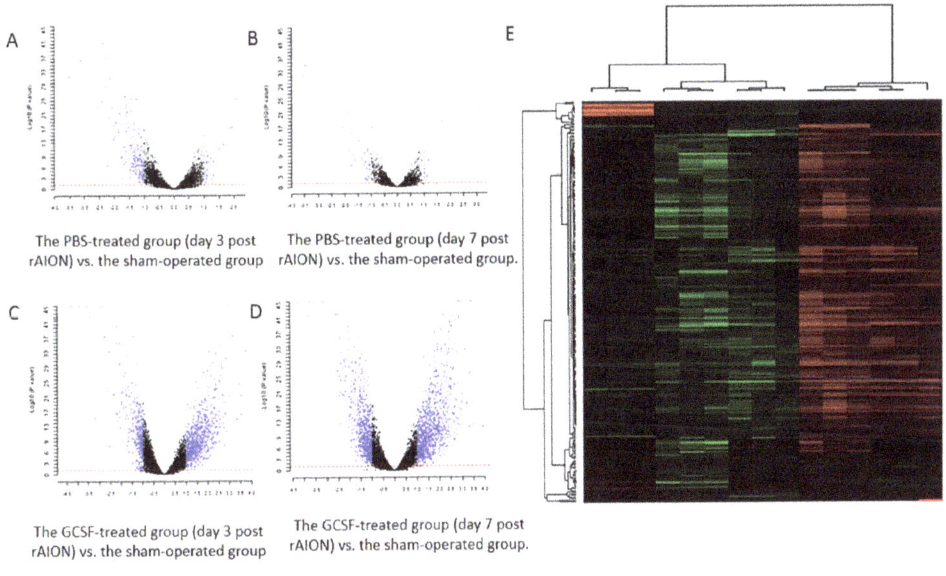

Figure 1. Gene expression profiles of the retina samples. (**A**–**D**) Volcano plot showing the differentially expressed genes in the PBS- and GCSF-treated groups. (**A**) The PBS-treated group (day 3 post rAION) vs. the sham-operated group. (**B**) The PBS-treated group (day 7 post rAION) vs. the sham-operated group. (**C**) The GCSF-treated group (day 3 post rAION) vs. the sham-operated group. (**D**) The GCSF-treated group (day 7 post rAION) vs. the sham-operated group. For each plot, the *X*-axis represents log2 FC, and the Y-axis represents −log10 (*p*-values). The differentially expressed genes are shown as red dots. (**E**) The heatmap of the hierarchical clustering of the differentially expressed genes. Up- and downregulated genes are represented in red and green colors, respectively. The differentially expressed genes were defined as having absolute FC > 1.5 and FDR < 0.1.

2.2. TAFs Involved in Regulation of Cell Death and Proliferation

To classify the biological function of differentially expressed genes, we employed a gene ontology (GO) analysis. After GO analysis, many TBP-associated proteins that were classified into the category of regulation of cell death and proliferation. We found that 18 TAFs, including TAF1, TAF1a, TAF1b, TAF1c, TAF1d, TAF2, TAF5, TAF6l, TAF7, TAF7l, TAF8, TAF9, TAF9b, TAF10, TAF11, TAF12, TAF13, and TAF15, were upregulated by GCSF treatment. Additionally, 17 TAFs, including TAF1, TAF1a, TAF1b, TAF1c, TAF1d, TAF3, TAF5, TAF6, TAF6l, TAF7, TAF7l, TAF8, TAF9, TAF10, TAF11, TAF12, and TAF13, were downregulated by PBS treatment (Figure 2). This indicates that the expression levels of many TAFs were suppressed by ON ischemic injury and induced by GCSF treatment.

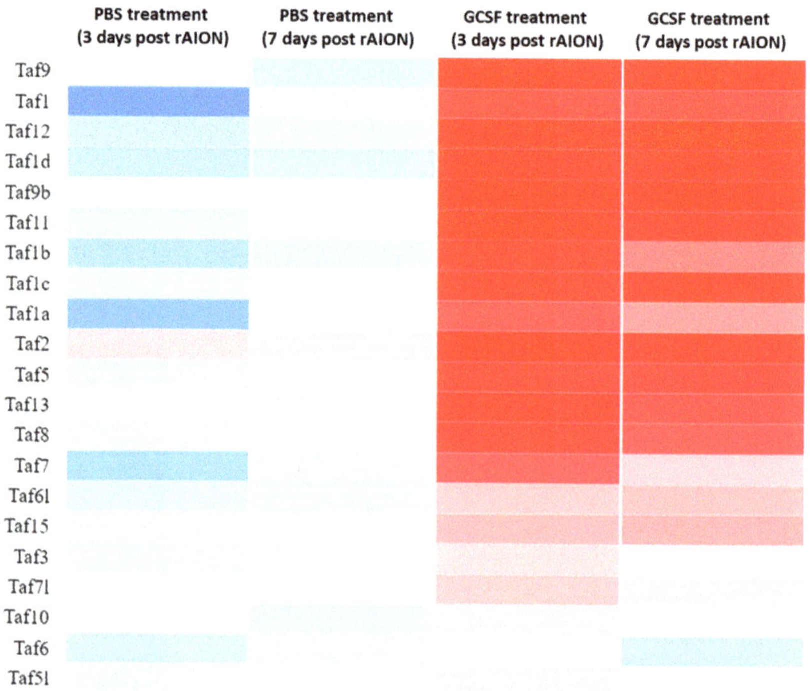

Figure 2. Heatmap of TBP-associated factors expressed in retina samples. After ON infarct, 18 TBP-associated factors were upregulated by GCSF treatment. There were 17 TBP-associated factors that were downregulated by PBS treatment. Genes were clustered into the regulation of cell survival based on gene expression over time. Up- and downregulation are represented in red and blue colors, respectively.

2.3. Network Analysis Revealed That TAFs Directly Interact with TP53 and TBP

The network analysis summarizes the network of predicted associations for a particular group of proteins. In evidence mode, multiple colored lines indicate the different types of interaction evidence. STRING network analysis exhibited that many TAFs interact directly with TP53, including TAF1, TAF1L, TAF2, TAF3, TAF4, TAF5, TAF6, TAF7, TAF7L, TAF9, TAF9b, TAF10, TAF11, TAF12, and TAF13 (Figure 3). Additionally, TAFs have direct interactions with TBP, including TAF1, TAF1a, TAF1b, TAF1c, TAF1d, TAF1L, TAF2, TAF3, TAF4, TAF5, TAF6, TAF7, TAF7L, TAF9, TAF9b, TAF10, TAF11, TAF12, and TAF13. Among these TAFs, TAF9 was predicted to bind with TP53, and the expression level of TAF9 was dramatically elevated by GCSF treatment and suppressed by PBS treatment. The biological function of TAF9 is involved in gene regulation associated with apoptosis [31]. Thus, we selected TAF9 as a candidate gene to evaluate its function in RGC apoptosis and survival after ON ischemia.

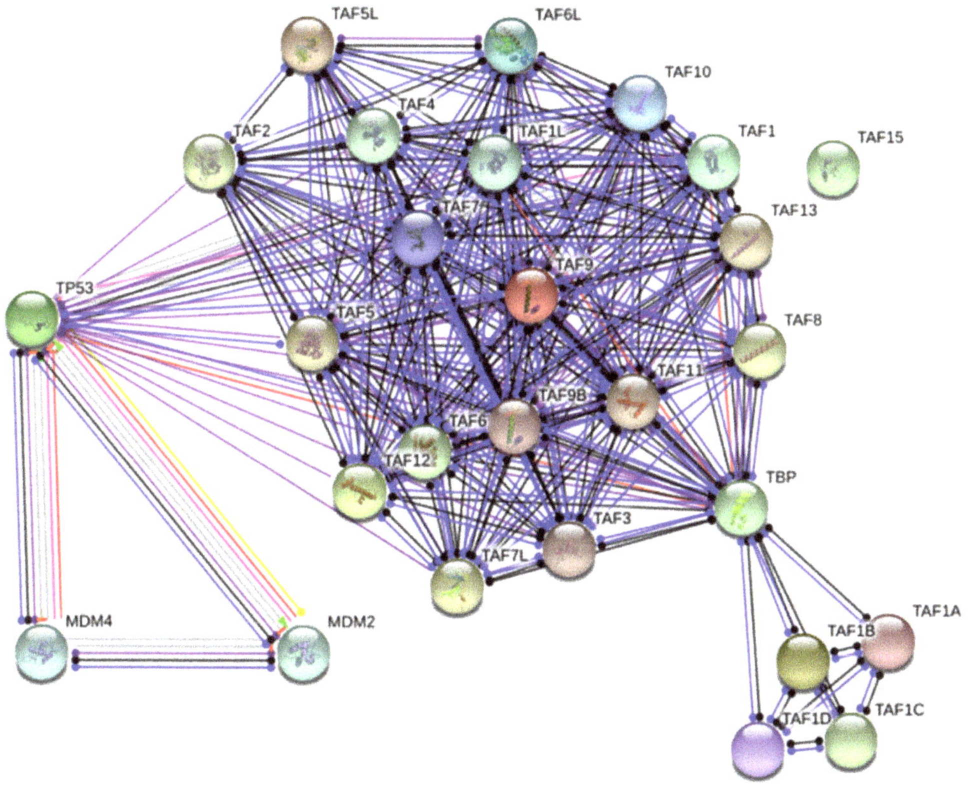

Figure 3. Network analysis of TBP-associated factors. STRING analysis shows that the TBP-associated factors are involved in the known and predicted protein–protein interactions. Network analysis exhibited that many TBP-associated factors directly interact with TP53. The network nodes are proteins. The edges represent the predicted functional associations with 7 differently colored lines representing the existence of the seven types of evidence used in predicting the associations. Red line: the presence of fusion evidence; green line: neighborhood evidence; blue line: cooccurrence evidence; purple line: experimental evidence; yellow line: textmining evidence; light blue line: database evidence; black line: co-expression evidence.

2.4. *Taf9 Knockdown Impaired the Protective Effect of GCSF on the Visual Function*

To evaluate the role of TAF9 in the protection of visual function in rAION, flash visually evoked potentials (FVEPs) were measured at day 28 post infarct (Figure 4A). On TAF9 knockdown, we found no improvement in visual function despite GCSF treatment. The P1-N2 amplitudes in the sham-operated and scrambled siRNA-treated group (Sham + scram si), rAION induction and scrambled siRNA-treated group (rAION + scram si), rAION induction and GCSF plus scrambled siRNA-treated group (rAION + GCSF + scram si), and rAION induction and GCSF plus TAF9 siRNA-treated group (rAION + GCSF + TAF9 si) were 65.8 ± 12.7 μV, 23.4 μV ± 4.2 μV, 49.5 ± 6.6 μV, and 28.9 ± 8.4 μV, respectively (Figure 4B). Treatment with GCSF plus TAF9 siRNA in the rAION group reduced the P1-N2 amplitude by 1.71-fold compared to that of treatment with GCSF plus scrambled siRNA (Figure 4B, $p < 0.05$).

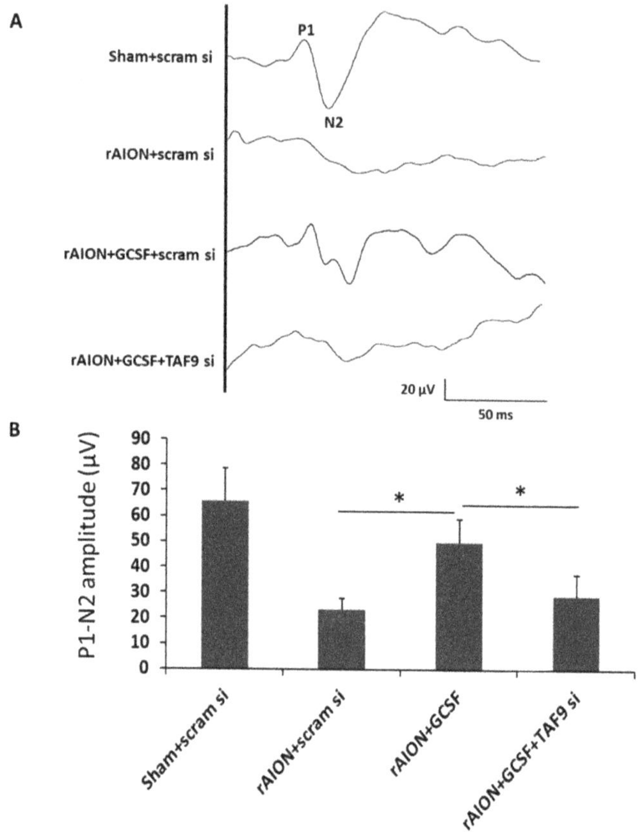

Figure 4. Effect of TAF9 knockdown on FVEP recording in the fourth week after infarct. (**A**) Representative FVEP wavelet in each group. (**B**) GCSF plus TAF9 siRNA treatment reduced the P1-N2 amplitude by 1.71-fold compared to GCSF plus scrambled siRNA treatment in rAION groups (* $p < 0.05$, $n = 12$ per group). Data are expressed as mean ± SD.

2.5. Taf9 Knockdown Impaired the Protective Effect of GCSF on RGC Density

The survived RGCs were labeled with Fluoro-Gold. In the central retina, the RGC densities in the sham-operated and scrambled siRNA-treated group (Sham + scram si), rAION induction and scrambled siRNA-treated group (rAION + scram si), rAION induction and GCSF plus scrambled siRNA-treated group (rAION + GCSF + scram si), and rAION induction and GCSF plus TAF9 siRNA-treated group (rAION + GCSF+ TAF9 si) were 1402.5 ± 99.1, 655.2 ± 199.6, 1265.1 ± 352.5, and 649.7 ± 227.6 cells/mm^2, respectively (Figure 5A). In the midperipheral retina, the RGC densities in the sham-operated and scrambled siRNA-treated group (Sham + scram si), rAION induction and scrambled siRNA-treated group (rAION + scram si), rAION induction and GCSF plus scrambled siRNA-treated group (rAION + GCSF + scram si), and rAION induction and GCSF plus TAF9 siRNA-treated rAION group (rAION + GCSF + TAF9 si) were 1219.4 ± 201.3, 319.2 ± 195.8, 863.3 ± 161.3, and 492.9 ± 250.1 cells/mm^2, respectively (Figure 5). The RGC density in the rAION induction and GCSF plus TAF9 siRNA-treated rAION group was significantly reduced by 1.94- and 1.75-fold in the central and midperipheral retinas, respectively, compared with that in the rAION induction and GCSF plus scrambled siRNA-treated group (Figure 5B, $p < 0.05$).

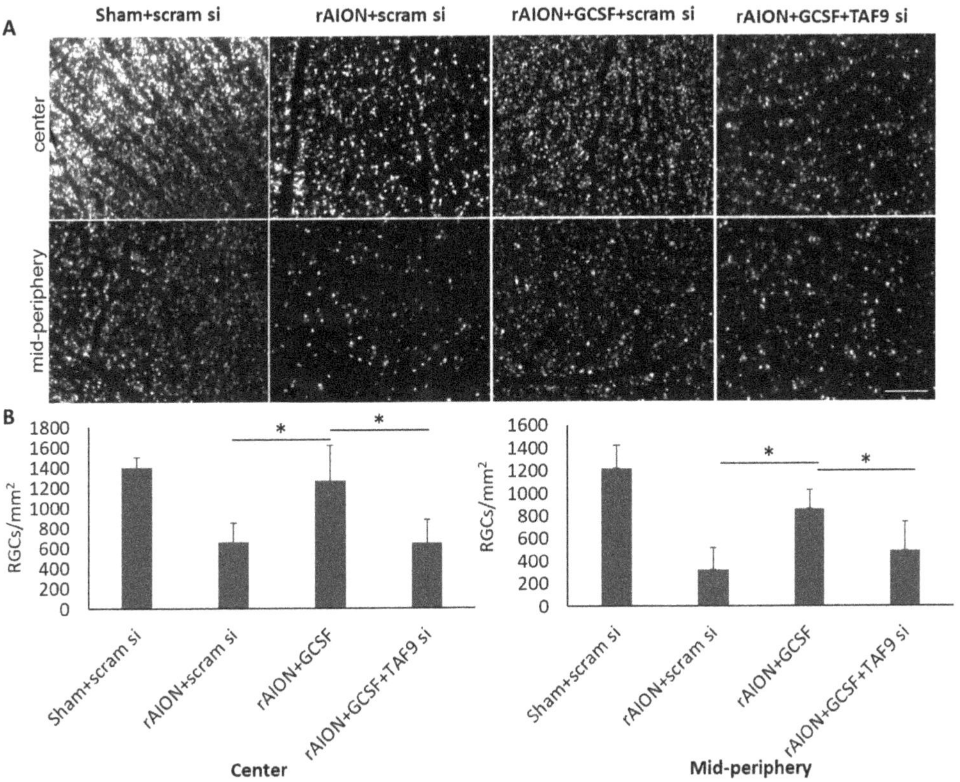

Figure 5. Effect of TAF9 knockdown on RGC density in the fourth week after infarct. (**A**) Representative RGC density of the central and midperipheral retinas in each group. The white spots in the representative figures are the Fluoro-Gold-labeled RGCs in the retina. (**B**) Bar chart showing the RGC density in the rAION induction and GCSF plus TAF9 siRNA-treated rAION group was significantly reduced in the central and midperipheral retinas compared to that in the rAION induction and GCSF plus scrambled siRNA-treated group (* $p < 0.05$, $n = 12$ per group; scale bar = 200 μm).

2.6. TAF9 Knockdown Impaired the Anti-Apoptotic Ability of GCSF

The average numbers of TUNEL-positive cells in each high-powered field (HPF, ×400 magnification) in the sham-operated and scrambled siRNA-treated group (Sham + scram si), rAION induction and scrambled siRNA-treated group (rAION + scram si), rAION induction and GCSF plus scrambled siRNA-treated group (rAION + GCSF + scram si), and rAION induction and GCSF plus TAF9 siRNA-treated group (rAION + GCSF + TAF9 si) were 0.2 ± 0.4/HPF, 7.4 ± 2.7/HPF, 2.1 ± 1.3/HPF, and 6.3 ± 2.2/HPF, respectively. The number of TUNEL-positive celsls in the rAION induction and GCSF plus TAF9 siRNA-treated group significantly increased by three-fold compared to that in the rAION induction and GCSF plus scrambled siRNA-treated group ($p < 0.05$), but there was no significant difference between the scrambled siRNA-treated and GCSF plus TAF9 siRNA-treated rAION groups (Figure 6), further suggesting a survival pathway dependent on TAF9. In addition, the number of TUNEL-positive cells in the rAION induction and scrambled siRNA-treated group was significantly higher than that in the rAION induction and GCSF plus scrambled siRNA-treated group ($p < 0.05$).

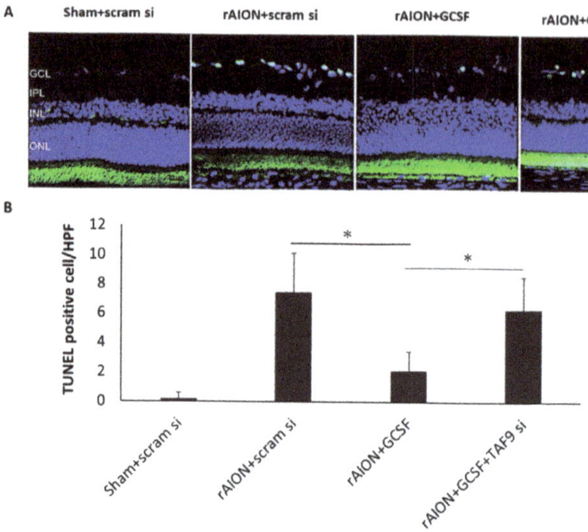

Figure 6. Analysis of RGC apoptosis in the RGC layer through the TUNEL assay in the fourth week after rAION induction. (**A**) Representative images of TUNEL staining. (**B**) Quantification of apoptotic cells per HPF. The number of TUNEL-positive cells in the rAION induction and GCSF plus TAF9 siRNA-treated group significantly increased by threefold compared to that in the rAION induction and GCSF plus scrambled siRNA-treated group (* $p < 0.05$, $n = 6$; scale bar = 50 μm).

2.7. TAF9 Knockdown Suppressed GCSF-Induced TP53 and TRIAP1 Expression

Western blotting confirmed that the rAION induction and GCSF plus scrambled siRNA-treated group exhibited the highest protein level of TAF9 compared with other groups (Figure 7, $p < 0.05$). GCSF plus TAF9 siRNA treatment significantly repressed TAF9 protein expression by 6.9-fold compared to GCSF plus scrambled siRNA treatment ($p < 0.05$). In the rAION induction and GCSF plus TAF9 siRNA-treated group, the TP53 level was reduced by 2.4-fold compared to that in the rAION induction and GCSF plus scrambled siRNA-treated group ($p < 0.05$). One of TP53-regulated genes, the TP53-regulated inhibitor of apoptosis gene 1 (TRIAP1), can inhibit apoptosis through interaction with the APAF1 and heat shock protein 70 (HSP70) complex [32]. Our Western blotting data demonstrate that the TRIAP1 level was reduced by 4.7-fold in the rAION induction and GCSF plus TAF9 siRNA-treated group compared to that in the rAION induction and GCSF plus scrambled siRNA-treated group ($p < 0.05$). In addition, the levels of TAF9, TP53, and TRIAP1 were less in the rAION induction and scrambled siRNA-treated group compared to those in the rAION induction and GCSF plus scrambled siRNA-treated group ($p < 0.05$).

2.8. Overexpression of TAF9 Inhibited RGC Death by Modulating TP53–TRIAP1–CASP3 Axis

To explore the role of TAF9 in the regulation of RGC death and survival, AAV2-rTAF9 was used to overexpress the TAF9 level in the rAION model. Four weeks after rAION, the numbers of TUNEL-positive cells in the PBS-treated and AAV2-r-TAF9-treated groups were 7.4 ± 2.7/HPF and 2.4 ± 1.7/HPF, respectively (Figure 8A). The number of TUNEL-positive cell was 3.1-fold lower in the AAV2-r-TAF9-treated group than that in the PBS-treated group ($p < 0.05$). Western blotting confirmed that the TP53 and TRIAP1 levels in the AAV2-r-TAF9-treated group were significantly increased, by 2.04- and 2.71-fold, respectively, compared to those in the PBS-treated group (Figure 8B, $p < 0.05$). Moreover, the cleaved-caspase 3 (Cl-casp3) level was reduced by 2.33-fold in the AAV2-rTAF9-treated group compared to that in the PBS-treated group (Figure 8B, $p < 0.05$).

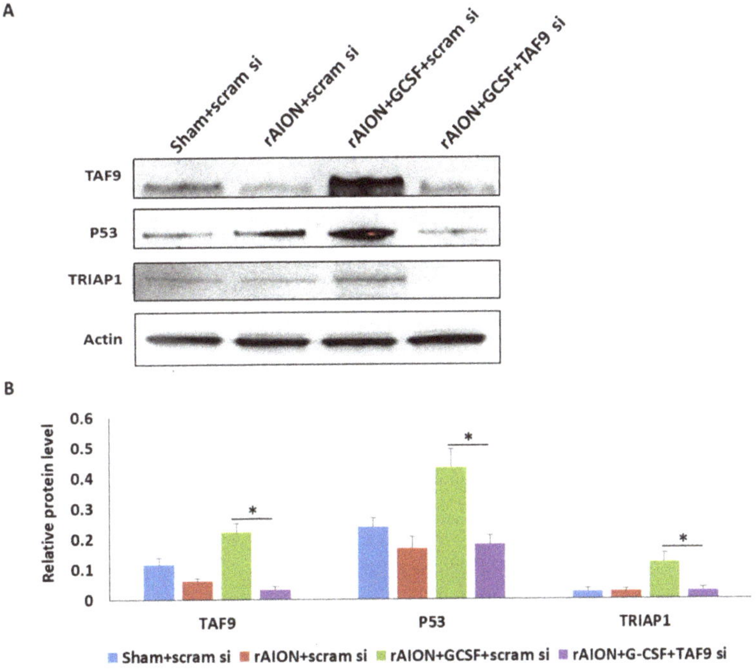

Figure 7. Western blot analysis of TAF9, TP53, and TRIAP1 expression. (**A**) Western blotting image of TAF9, TP53, and TRIAP1. (**B**) Relative protein level of TAF9, TP53, and TRIAP1. Treatment with GCSF plus TAF9 siRNA significantly repressed TAF9, TP53, and TRIAP1 expression by 6.9-, 2.2-, and 4.7-fold compared to treatment with GCSF plus scrambled siRNA in rAION groups (*: $p < 0.05$).

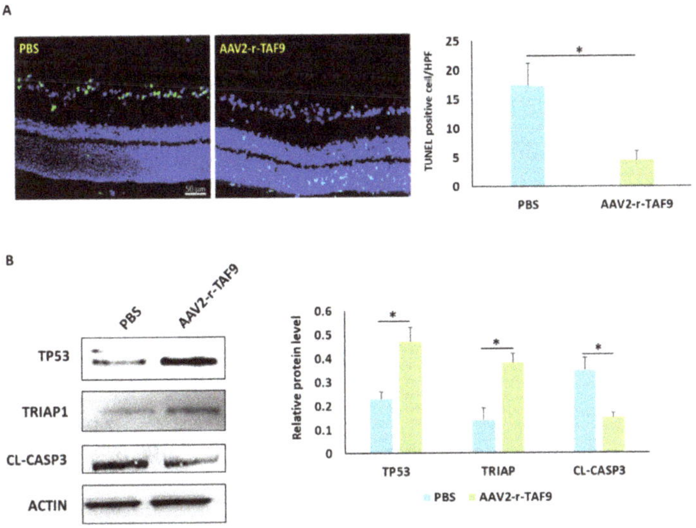

Figure 8. Effects of TAF9 overexpression on RGC apoptosis induced by rAION induction. (**A**) Left: representative images of double-stained apoptotic cells in the ganglion cell layer in each group. The apoptotic cells were stained in green, and the cell nuclei were counterstained with DAPI staining in

blue. Right: Analysis of RGC apoptosis between the PBS- and AAV2-r-TAF9-treated groups. (**B**) Western blot analysis of TP53, TRIAP1, and CASP3 expressions in the PBS- and AAV2-r-TAF9-treated groups. (*: $p < 0.05$).

3. Discussion

In this study, we conducted a microarray analysis of rat retinas to profile the transcriptomic changes in response to ON ischemic injury and GCSF treatments. Dynamic transcriptome profiling revealed many novel differentially expressed genes involved in the regulation of cell death and proliferation. Among the differentially expressed genes, the TAF protein was shown to be the most regulated and intriguing; this is involved in cell death and proliferation. Furthermore, a subsequent in silico pathway analysis revealed significant interactions between TAFs and TP53. One TP53 coactivator, TAF9, was selected to prove its role in the regulation of RGC death and survival because TAF9 is an apoptosis regulator [33]. TAF9 knockdown effectively reduced the neuroprotective effects of GCSF in the rAION model. We found that TAF9 is a key element in modulating the TP53–TRIAP1–CASP3 pathway. The overexpression of TAF9 inhibited RGC apoptosis in the rAION model. This transcriptomic analysis discovered a novel GCSF-regulated pathway, which is involved in RGC death and survival.

The differentially expressed genes found in the study are involved in the regulation of RGC death. Notably, ON ischemia influenced 702 and 179 transcripts on days 3 and 7 post rAION, respectively. We found that the numbers of ON ischemia-influenced genes gradually reduced from days 3 to 7 post rAION. These data indicate that a dramatic change in transcription occurs in the acute stage, but this transcriptional change returns to normal in the subacute stage. A similar observation was found in our previous study, whereby vascular permeability was highly increased in the acute stage and reduced in the subacute stage after ON infarct [7]. Taken together, we consider that ON ischemia may cause severe pathological changes in the acute stage, and the natural course of recovery may be started in the subacute stage. Therefore, the therapeutic window should be focused on the acute stage in ON ischemia. As expected, our previous findings also demonstrated that early treatment with GCSF or methylprednisolone provided good neuroprotective effects in the rAION model [7,34].

Comparing the GCSF-treated groups with the PBS-treated groups, GCSF treatment constantly influenced >3000 transcripts for 7 days, but the PBS-treated rats showed gradually reduced transcriptional changes from the acute to subacute stage. This indicates that immediate treatment with GCSF can influence several genes to trigger the rescue actions after ON ischemia. These remarkable transcriptional changes provide informative messages in discovering the key pathways involved in RGC survival. In this transcriptomic analysis, we found that many TBP-associated proteins were suppressed by ischemic insult, but induced by GCSF treatment. These TAFs were involved in the regulation of RGC death and survival. At the molecular level, gene expression is regulated by many core transcriptional complexes, such as TFIID, along with different cofactors [35]. Previous studies revealed TFIID as an integral component of the core transcriptional machinery for RNA polymerase II in mRNA-encoding genes [35,36], and demonstrated that it is assembled with TBP and multiple TAFs [37]. To date, many TAFs and several tissue-specific variants have been characterized [38]. Some genetic studies have revealed the complex role of TFIID in controlling tissue-specific and context-dependent transcriptional processes, proving the existence of different TFIID complexes and tissue-specific TAFs [39–43]. TFIID subunits regulate many cellular processes in tissue-specific manners, which facilitates research into TAF involvement in moderating biological functions, including proliferation, differentiation, apoptosis, metastasis, and hormone response [44].

After the network analysis, we found that TAF9 was predicted to interact with TBP and TP53. In addition, TAF9 was highly upregulated by GCSF treatment at days 3 and 7 post rAION. This implies that TAF9 plays an important role in modulating RGC death and survival via the P53 signaling pathway. TAF9 was reported to be a crucial P53 coactivator for the stabilization and activation of P53 [28,30]. TAF9 inhibits the MDM2-mediated degradation of p53 by reducing MDM2 binding to p53 [30]. A previous study also demonstrated that one TFIID complex lacking TAF9 in Hela cells causes apoptosis [45]. The interruption of interactions between Hedgehog transcription factors (Gli proteins) and TAF9 reduces Gli/TAF9-dependent transcription, suppresses cancer cell proliferation, and reduces xenograft growth [33]. As mentioned above, we hypothesize that the high TAF9 level activates the P53 pathway to inhibit RGC apoptosis after ON infarct. To verify our hypothesis, the TAF9-knockdown experiment was performed to discover the role of TAF9 in the regulation of RGC death and survival. As expected, TAF9 knockdown effectively reduced the protective effects of GCSF in the rAION model. Therefore, we have demonstrated that TAF9 plays a key role in RGC protection after ON ischemia.

Cell apoptosis is manipulated on multiple levels by the sequence-specific transcription factor TP53, with >100 genes existing TP53 binding sites [46]. Moreover, the function of these genes remains unclear. One of these genes is the TP53-regulated inhibitor of apoptosis gene 1 (TRIAP1), which has a p53 binding site within its coding sequence and is upregulated in many cancer cells [47]. TRIAP1 was reported to protect cancer cells from apoptosis through interaction with HSP70 or the repression of cyclin-dependent kinase inhibitor 1 (p21) [48,49]. Recent findings have demonstrated that TRIAP1 contributes to the resistance of apoptosis in a mitochondria-dependent manner [50,51]. Based on this evidence, we further evaluated the relationship among TAF9, P53, TRIAP1, and CASP3 in the rAION model. Remarkably, immunoblotting data have demonstrated that TAF9 overexpression prevented TP53 degradation and increased TRIAP1 expression in the rAION model. Additionally, we found that TAF9 overexpression reduced apoptotic RGCs and caspase 3 level after ON infarct. Taken together, we can suggest that TAF9 plays a key role in the protection of ischemia-induced RGC apoptosis by modulation of the TP53–TRIAP1–CASPS3 axis.

Therefore, our transcriptomic analysis found a novel signaling pathway to elucidate the anti-apoptotic effects of GCSF on RGCs. In this novel signaling pathway, TAF9 is a key element in the modulation of the TP53–TRIAP1–CASPS3 axis for preventing RGC death (Figure 9). All the evidence suggests that TAF9 is a potential target in developing a new drug for NAION treatment.

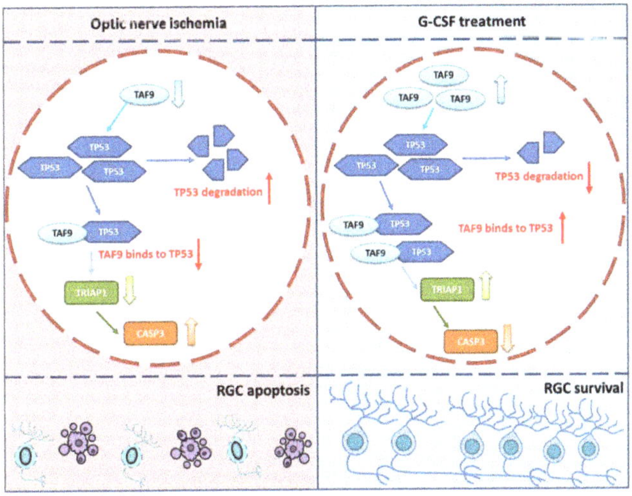

Figure 9. The graphic abstract of the protective mechanism of G-CSF after ON infarct. G-CSF treatment induces the level of TAF9 to prevent TP53 degradation. The binding complex of TP53 and TAF9 induces the level of TRIAP1 to inhibit the level of cleaved CASP3; as a result, the RGC apoptosis is inhibited by treating G-CSF. (↑: increase; ↓: decrease).

4. Materials and Methods

4.1. Study Design

In examining the transcriptome profiles in the retina, the rAION-inducted rats were treated by PBS or GCSF. The GCSF-treated group and the PBS-treated group received a subcutaneous injection of G-CSF (100 μg/kg body weight/day in 0.2 mL of saline; Takasaki Pharmaceutical Plant, Tokyo, Japan) or PBS (0.2 mL) once daily for 3 days, respectively. At day 3 post rAION, the retina samples were collected in the PBS-treated group (n = 3) and GCSF-treated group (n = 3). At day 7 post rAION, the retina samples were again collected in the PBS-treated group (n = 3) and GCSF-treated group (n = 3). The retina samples in the sham-operated group (n = 3) were also collected. All retina samples were used to extract the mRNA. The mRNA samples were analyzed by RNA microarray to profile the transcriptome in each group. The differentially expressed genes were classified by GO analysis. Among the differentially expressed genes, the TBP-associated proteins were classified into the function of cell growth. Therefore, the TBP-associated proteins were selected to predict the protein-to-protein interaction by network analysis (STRING 9.0). The TP53 was predicted to interact with many TBP-associated proteins in the network analysis. One of the TBP-associated proteins, TAF9, was selected to be the target protein to verify the function in the regulation of cell death and survival. TAF9 knockdown and overexpression experiments were performed in the rAION model. The rAION-inducted rats were intravitreally treated with scrambled siRNA (50 pmol; GeneDirex, Keelung, Taiwan), GCSF plus scrambled siRNA (50 pmol; GeneDirex), and GCSF plus TAF9 siRNA (50 pmol; GeneDirex) to evaluate the visual function (n = 12 in each group), RGC density (n = 12 in each group), and apoptotic RGCs (n = 6 in each group). The TAF9, TP53, and TRIAP1 levels were evaluated in each group (n = 6) using Western blot analysis. Moreover, the AAV2-mediated overexpression of TAF9 was intravitreally administered before rAION induction to examine the anti-apoptotic ability of TAF9 in the rAION model. The number of apoptotic RGCs was evaluated in the AAV2-r-TAF9-treated group (n = 6) and PBS-treated group (n = 6). The TP53, TRIAP1, and cleaved-CASP3 levels were determined in the AAV2-r-TAF9-treated group (n = 3) and PBS-treated group (n = 3).

4.2. Animals

Male Wistar rats were used in the study. The rats were aged 6–8 weeks with body weights of 150–180 g. Animal care and experimental procedures were performed in accordance with the Association for Research in Vision and Ophthalmology Statement for the Use of Animals in Ophthalmic and Vision Research, and the Institutional Animal Care and Use Committee (IACUC) at the Tzu Chi Medical Center approved all animal experiments.

4.3. rAION Induction

The procedure of rAION induction was described in our previous study [52]. Before general anesthesia, all rats were administered Mydrin-P (Santan, Osaka, Japan) and Alcaine (Alcon, Fort Worth, TX, USA) eye drops for pupil dilation and topical anesthesia, respectively. Subsequently, the rats were injected intramuscularly with a mixture of ketamine (40 mg/kg body weight, Pfizer, Tadworth, UK) and xylazine (4 mg/kg body weight; Sigma, St. Louis, MO, USA) for general anesthesia. For photosensitization, 2.5 mM Rose Bengal diluted in PBS (1 mL/kg of body weight) was administered intravenously before laser application. After rose bengal injection, the optic disc was immediately exposed to an argon green laser system (MC-500 Multi-color laser, Nidek Co., Ltd., Tokyo, Japan, setting: 532 nm wavelength, 500 μm size and 80 mW power) for 12 1-second pulses. A laser fundus lens (Ocular Instruments, Inc., Bellevue, DC, USA) was used to target the optic disc. At the end of experiment, TobraDex eye ointment (Alcon-Couvreur, Puurs-Sint-Amands, Belgium) was applied to the eyes of all experimented rats.

4.4. RNA Microarray Analysis (Quality Check, Annotation, and Ontology)

The retina samples were collected at day 3 and day 7 post rAION. Total RNA was isolated from retina homogenate using TRIzol reagent (Invitrogen) according to the manufacturer's instructions. Complementary DNAs were synthesized using reverse transcriptase kit. RNA microarray analysis was performed using the Rat OneArray kit according to the manufacturer's protocol. Clustering and principal component analysis were performed to determine the differences among biological sample replicates and their treatment conditions. Raw intensities were normalized with the median scaling normalizing method, and covariance was determined by the error model of the Rosetta Resolver system. Normalized intensity was transformed to the log2 ratio (fold change). Gene annotation was performed with reference to NCBI RefSeq Release 57. EnsEMBL released 70 cDNA sequences and rattus_norvegicus_core_70_5b annotations. Differentially expressed genes that showed both a log2 ratio (fold change) >1 and $p < 0.05$ were considered candidate genes.

4.5. Flash Visual-Evoked Potentials (FVEPs)

FVEP measurements were performed as described in our previous study [52]. After general anesthesia, the sagittal region of the skull was opened in the rats. The 4 mm screw implants were passed through the skull to approximately 1.5 mm and placed at the frontal cortex and primary visual cortex regions of both hemispheres using stereotaxic coordinates. A visual electrodiagnostic system (Diagnosys LLC, Lowell, MA, USA) was used to measure the FVEP. The number of average sweeps was 64 for each rat. A comparison of the average amplitude of the P1-N2 wave in each group was made to evaluate visual function.

4.6. Retrograde Labeling of RGCs and Measurement of RGC Density

RGCs were labeled as described in our previous study [52]. Briefly, retrograde tracer dye fluorogold was injected into the superior colliculus one week before the rats were euthanized. One week after labeling, the rats were euthanized, and retinas were carefully flat-mounted. The central and midperipheral regions in the retina were examined under a 200× fluorescence microscope (Axioplan 2 imaging, Carl Zeiss, New York, NY, USA) with a built-in filter set (excitation filter, 350–400 nm; barrier filter, 515 nm) and connected digital imaging system. Six randomly selected areas in the central and midperipheral regions were used to calculate the number of RGCs in the central and midperipheral regions of each retina. The number of RGCs was calculated using the ImageMaster 2D Platinum Software V 7.0 (GE Healthcare, Chicago, IL, USA).

4.7. Retinal Tissue Preparation and Sections

After euthanizing, the rat eyeballs were fixed in 4% paraformaldehyde overnight. The eyecups and ONs were separated and transferred to 30% sucrose solution; the samples were incubated at 4 °C until they settled at the bottom of the tubes. The retina cross-section and ON longitudinal sections of 10 μm were obtained by using a cryostat-microtome.

4.8. TUNEL Assay

To determine the apoptotic RGCs in the retinal section, the TUNEL assay kit (Click-iT™ Plus TUNEL Assay, Invitrogen, Waltham, MA, USA) was used to stain the apoptotic cells in the ganglion cell layer. Nuclei were stained with 4t,6-diamidino-2-phenylindole (DAPI). The TUNEL-positive cells in the ganglion cell layer of each section were counted in 10 HPF (400×), and an average of six sections per group was used for further statistical analysis.

4.9. Western Blotting Analysis

After euthanizing, the rats' eyes were enucleated. The retinas were homogenized in lysis buffer. The protein sample was separated on 10% bis-acrylamide gel. The proteins were transferred to polyvinylidene difluoride (PVDF) membranes. The membranes were blocked with 5% non-fat dry milk for 1 h. The membranes were incubated with Taf9, TP53, TRIAP1, CASP3 and ACTIN antibody at 4 °C for 12–16 h, followed by incubation with a secondary antibody conjugated to HRP against the appropriate host species for 1 h at room temperature. Then, the membranes were developed using enhanced chemiluminescent (ECL) substrate. Membranes were exposed to a Western blot analyzer, and the relative density was calculated using image master platinum software V 7.0 (GE Healthcare, Chicago, IL, USA).

4.10. Intravitreal Injection of AAV2-rTAF9

The AAV vectors AAV2-CMV-rTAF9 (NovoPro Biotechnology, Shanghai, China) used in this study consisted of the AAV2 capsid, the CMV promoter, and codon-optimized rat TAF9 cDNA. Briefly, rats were anesthetized with ketamine/xylazine and the injected eye was numbed with Alcaine drops. After the general anesthesia, we selected an area on the sclera, devoid of blood vessels, and slowly injected 3 μL of AAV vector preparation into the vitreous cavity for 30 s using a 10 μL Hamilton syringe with a 30 G needle. Tobradex eye ointment was applied after injection to prevent infection in each rat.

4.11. Statistical Analysis

All statistical analyses were performed using IBM SPSS software. The data are presented as mean ± standard deviation. A Mann–Whitney U test was used for comparisons between groups. p-values < 0.05 were considered statistically significant, with * representing $p < 0.05$.

5. Conclusions

In conclusion, we proved that GCSF has an anti-apoptotic effect on RGCs after ON infarct via modulating the TAF9–TP53–TRIAP1–CASPS3 axis. TAF9 is highly induced by GCSF to prevent MDM2-mediated degradation of TP53. The binding complex of TAF9 and TP53 upregulates the level of TRIAP1 to inhibit RGC apoptosis after ON infarct (Figure 9). However, GCSF treatment may result in leukocytosis, fever, muscle pain, and joint pain in patients with NAION. Induction of TAF9 and TRIAP1 in the retinal cells using the transfection system may provide therapeutic effects similar to GCSF, and may preclude the side effects from GCSF treatment. Thus, we believe that TAF9 and TRIAP1 may be the potential targets of gene therapy for NAION patients in the future.

Author Contributions: R.-K.T. and Y.-T.W. conceptualized and designed the research project. Y.-T.W. and R-KT contributed to all the necessary materials, financial support, and laboratory facilities. C.-T.H. and Y.-T.W. executed all the experiments in this study. K.-L.L., Y.-T.W. and C.-T.H. contributed to the discussion and interpretation of the raw data. Y.-T.W. and K.-L.L. contributed to data evaluation and drafting. All authors have read and agreed to the published version of the manuscript.

Funding: This research was funded by the Buddhist Tzu Chi Medical Foundation under the research grant number "TCRD107-69".

Institutional Review Board Statement: The animal study protocol was approved by the Institutional Review Board of Tzu-Chi Hospital (protocol code: 107-26; date of approval: 10 December 2018).

Informed Consent Statement: Not applicable.

Data Availability Statement: Data as reported in this study are available from corresponding author upon reasonable request.

Acknowledgments: The authors acknowledge the Institute of Eye Research, Hualien Tzu Chi Hospital for experiment assistance.

Conflicts of Interest: The authors declare no conflict of interest.

References

1. Lee, Y.C.; Wang, J.H.; Huang, T.L.; Tsai, R.K. Increased Risk of Stroke in Patients With Nonarteritic Anterior Ischemic Optic Neuropathy: A Nationwide Retrospective Cohort Study. *Am. J. Ophthalmol.* **2016**, *170*, 183–189. [CrossRef] [PubMed]
2. Bernstein, S.L.; Johnson, M.A.; Miller, N.R. Nonarteritic anterior ischemic optic neuropathy (NAION) and its experimental models. *Prog. Retin. Eye Res.* **2011**, *30*, 167–187. [CrossRef]

3. Yang, Y.; Xu, C.; Chen, Y.; Liang, J.J.; Xu, Y.; Chen, S.L.; Huang, S.; Yang, Q.; Cen, L.P.; Pang, C.P.; et al. Green Tea Extract Ameliorates Ischemia-Induced Retinal Ganglion Cell Degeneration in Rats. *Oxidative Med. Cell. Longev.* **2019**, *2019*, 8407206. [CrossRef] [PubMed]
4. Park, J.W.; Sung, M.S.; Ha, J.Y.; Guo, Y.; Piao, H.; Heo, H.; Park, S.W. Neuroprotective Effect of Brazilian Green Propolis on Retinal Ganglion Cells in Ischemic Mouse Retina. *Curr. Eye Res.* **2020**, *45*, 955–964. [CrossRef] [PubMed]
5. Lin, W.N.; Kapupara, K.; Wen, Y.T.; Chen, Y.H.; Pan, I.H.; Tsai, R.K. Haematococcus pluvialis-Derived Astaxanthin Is a Potential Neuroprotective Agent against Optic Nerve Ischemia. *Mar. Drugs* **2020**, *18*, 85. [CrossRef] [PubMed]
6. Guan, L.; Li, C.; Zhang, Y.; Gong, J.; Wang, G.; Tian, P.; Shen, N. Puerarin ameliorates retinal ganglion cell damage induced by retinal ischemia/reperfusion through inhibiting the activation of TLR4/NLRP3 inflammasome. *Life Sci.* **2020**, *256*, 117935. [CrossRef]
7. Wen, Y.T.; Huang, T.L.; Huang, S.P.; Chang, C.H.; Tsai, R.K. Early applications of granulocyte colony-stimulating factor (G-CSF) can stabilize the blood-optic-nerve barrier and ameliorate inflammation in a rat model of anterior ischemic optic neuropathy (rAION). *Dis. Model Mech.* **2016**, *9*, 1193–1202. [CrossRef]
8. Melamed, S. Neuroprotective properties of a synthetic docosanoid, unoprostone isopropyl: Clinical benefits in the treatment of glaucoma. *Drugs Under Exp. Clin. Res.* **2002**, *28*, 63–73.
9. Georgiou, T.; Wen, Y.T.; Chang, C.H.; Kolovos, P.; Kalogerou, M.; Prokopiou, E.; Neokleous, A.; Huang, C.T.; Tsai, R.K. Neuroprotective Effects of Omega-3 Polyunsaturated Fatty Acids in a Rat Model of Anterior Ischemic Optic Neuropathy. *Invest. Ophthalmol. Vis. Sci.* **2017**, *58*, 1603–1611. [CrossRef]
10. Nguyen Ngo Le, M.A.; Wen, Y.T.; Ho, Y.C.; Kapupara, K.; Tsai, R.K. Therapeutic Effects of Puerarin Against Anterior Ischemic Optic Neuropathy Through Antiapoptotic and Anti-Inflammatory Actions. *Invest. Ophthalmol. Vis. Sci.* **2019**, *60*, 3481–3491. [CrossRef] [PubMed]
11. Huang, T.L.; Wen, Y.T.; Chang, C.H.; Chang, S.W.; Lin, K.H.; Tsai, R.K. Early Methylprednisolone Treatment Can Stabilize the Blood-Optic Nerve Barrier in a Rat Model of Anterior Ischemic Optic Neuropathy (rAION). *Invest. Ophthalmol. Vis. Sci.* **2017**, *58*, 1628–1636. [CrossRef]
12. Kapupara, K.; Wen, Y.T.; Tsai, R.K.; Huang, S.P. Soluble P-selectin promotes retinal ganglion cell survival through activation of Nrf2 signaling after ischemia injury. *Cell Death Dis.* **2017**, *8*, e3172. [CrossRef] [PubMed]
13. Goldenberg-Cohen, N.; Avraham-Lubin, B.C.; Sadikov, T.; Askenasy, N. Effect of coadministration of neuronal growth factors on neuroglial differentiation of bone marrow-derived stem cells in the ischemic retina. *Invest. Ophthalmol. Vis. Sci.* **2014**, *55*, 502–512. [CrossRef] [PubMed]
14. Ribas, V.T.; Koch, J.C.; Michel, U.; Bähr, M.; Lingor, P. Attenuation of Axonal Degeneration by Calcium Channel Inhibitors Improves Retinal Ganglion Cell Survival and Regeneration After Optic Nerve Crush. *Mol. Neurobiol.* **2017**, *54*, 72–86. [CrossRef]
15. Mehrabian, Z.; Guo, Y.; Weinreich, D.; Bernstein, S.L. Oligodendrocyte death, neuroinflammation, and the effects of minocycline in a rodent model of nonarteritic anterior ischemic optic neuropathy (rNAION). *Mol. Vis.* **2017**, *23*, 963–976. [PubMed]
16. Huang, T.L.; Wen, Y.T.; Chang, C.H.; Chang, S.W.; Lin, K.H.; Tsai, R.K. Efficacy of Intravitreal Injections of Triamcinolone Acetonide in a Rodent Model of Nonarteritic Anterior Ischemic Optic Neuropathy. *Invest. Ophthalmol. Vis. Sci.* **2016**, *57*, 1878–1884. [CrossRef]
17. Tsai, R.K.; Chang, C.H.; Sheu, M.M.; Huang, Z.L. Anti-apoptotic effects of human granulocyte colony-stimulating factor (G-CSF) on retinal ganglion cells after optic nerve crush are PI3K/AKT-dependent. *Exp. Eye Res.* **2010**, *90*, 537–545. [CrossRef]
18. Ghalaut, P.S.; Sen, R.; Dixit, G. Role of granulocyte colony stimulating factor (G-CSF) in chemotherapy induced neutropenia. *J. Assoc. Physicians India* **2008**, *56*, 942–944.
19. Ghahari, L.; Safari, M.; Rahimi Jaberi, K.; Jafari, B.; Safari, K.; Madadian, M. Mesenchymal Stem Cells with Granulocyte Colony-Stimulating Factor Reduce Stress Oxidative Factors in Parkinson's Disease. *Iran. Biomed. J.* **2020**, *24*, 89–98. [CrossRef]
20. Wu, C.C.; Wang, I.F.; Chiang, P.M.; Wang, L.C.; Shen, C.J.; Tsai, K.J. G-CSF-mobilized Bone Marrow Mesenchymal Stem Cells Replenish Neural Lineages in Alzheimer's Disease Mice via CXCR4/SDF-1 Chemotaxis. *Mol. Neurobiol.* **2017**, *54*, 6198–6212. [CrossRef] [PubMed]
21. Lee, S.T.; Chu, K.; Jung, K.H.; Ko, S.Y.; Kim, E.H.; Sinn, D.I.; Lee, Y.S.; Lo, E.H.; Kim, M.; Roh, J.K. Granulocyte colony-stimulating factor enhances angiogenesis after focal cerebral ischemia. *Brain Res.* **2005**, *1058*, 120–128. [CrossRef] [PubMed]
22. Bu, P.; Basith, B.; Stubbs, E.B., Jr.; Perlman, J.I. Granulocyte colony-stimulating factor facilitates recovery of retinal function following retinal ischemic injury. *Exp. Eye Res.* **2010**, *91*, 104–106. [CrossRef]
23. Popa-Wagner, A.; Stocker, K.; Balseanu, A.T.; Rogalewski, A.; Diederich, K.; Minnerup, J.; Margaritescu, C.; Schabitz, W.R. Effects of granulocyte-colony stimulating factor after stroke in aged rats. *Stroke A J. Cereb. Circ.* **2010**, *41*, 1027–1031. [CrossRef] [PubMed]
24. Dwivedi, P.; Greis, K.D. Granulocyte colony-stimulating factor receptor signaling in severe congenital neutropenia, chronic neutrophilic leukemia, and related malignancies. *Exp. Hematol.* **2017**, *46*, 9–20. [CrossRef] [PubMed]
25. Laboissonniere, L.A.; Goetz, J.J.; Martin, G.M.; Bi, R.; Lund, T.J.S.; Ellson, L.; Lynch, M.R.; Mooney, B.; Wickham, H.; Liu, P.; et al. Molecular signatures of retinal ganglion cells revealed through single cell profiling. *Sci. Rep.* **2019**, *9*, 15778. [CrossRef] [PubMed]
26. Ueno, S.; Yoneshige, A.; Koriyama, Y.; Hagiyama, M.; Shimomura, Y.; Ito, A. Early Gene Expression Profile in Retinal Ganglion Cell Layer After Optic Nerve Crush in Mice. *Invest. Ophthalmol. Vis. Sci.* **2018**, *59*, 370–380. [CrossRef]
27. Bernstein, S.L.; Guo, Y.; Kelman, S.E.; Flower, R.W.; Johnson, M.A. Functional and cellular responses in a novel rodent model of anterior ischemic optic neuropathy. *Invest. Ophthalmol. Vis. Sci.* **2003**, *44*, 4153–4162. [CrossRef]

28. Buschmann, T.; Lin, Y.; Aithmitti, N.; Fuchs, S.Y.; Lu, H.; Resnick-Silverman, L.; Manfredi, J.J.; Ronai, Z.; Wu, X. Stabilization and activation of p53 by the coactivator protein TAFII31. *J. Biol. Chem.* **2001**, *276*, 13852–13857. [CrossRef]
29. Uesugi, M.; Nyanguile, O.; Lu, H.; Levine, A.J.; Verdine, G.L. Induced alpha helix in the VP16 activation domain upon binding to a human TAF. *Science* **1997**, *277*, 1310–1313. [CrossRef]
30. Jabbur, J.R.; Tabor, A.D.; Cheng, X.; Wang, H.; Uesugi, M.; Lozano, G.; Zhang, W. Mdm-2 binding and TAF(II)31 recruitment is regulated by hydrogen bond disruption between the p53 residues Thr18 and Asp21. *Oncogene* **2002**, *21*, 7100–7113. [CrossRef] [PubMed]
31. Frontini, M.; Soutoglou, E.; Argentini, M.; Bole-Feysot, C.; Jost, B.; Scheer, E.; Tora, L. TAF9b (formerly TAF9L) is a bona fide TAF that has unique and overlapping roles with TAF9. *Mol. Cell. Biol.* **2005**, *25*, 4638–4649. [CrossRef] [PubMed]
32. Fook-Alves, V.L.; de Oliveira, M.B.; Zanatta, D.B.; Strauss, B.E.; Colleoni, G.W. TP53 Regulated Inhibitor of Apoptosis 1 (TRIAP1) stable silencing increases late apoptosis by upregulation of caspase 9 and APAF1 in RPMI8226 multiple myeloma cell line. *Biochim. Biophys. Acta* **2016**, *1862*, 1105–1110. [CrossRef] [PubMed]
33. Bosco-Clément, G.; Zhang, F.; Chen, Z.; Zhou, H.M.; Li, H.; Mikami, I.; Hirata, T.; Yagui-Beltran, A.; Lui, N.; Do, H.T.; et al. Targeting Gli transcription activation by small molecule suppresses tumor growth. *Oncogene* **2014**, *33*, 2087–2097. [CrossRef] [PubMed]
34. Huang, T.L.; Huang, S.P.; Chang, C.H.; Lin, K.H.; Chang, S.W.; Tsai, R.K. Protective effects of systemic treatment with methylprednisolone in a rodent model of non-arteritic anterior ischemic optic neuropathy (rAION). *Exp. Eye Res.* **2015**, *131*, 69–76. [CrossRef]
35. Hampsey, M. Molecular genetics of the RNA polymerase II general transcriptional machinery. *Microbiol. Mol. Biol. Rev. MMBR* **1998**, *62*, 465–503. [CrossRef]
36. Huh, J.R.; Park, J.M.; Kim, M.; Carlson, B.A.; Hatfield, D.L.; Lee, B.J. Recruitment of TBP or TFIIB to a promoter proximal position leads to stimulation of RNA polymerase II transcription without activator proteins both in vivo and in vitro. *Biochem. Biophys. Res. Commun.* **1999**, *256*, 45–51. [CrossRef]
37. Wu, S.Y.; Chiang, C.M. TATA-binding protein-associated factors enhance the recruitment of RNA polymerase II by transcriptional activators. *J. Biol. Chem.* **2001**, *276*, 34235–34243. [CrossRef]
38. Klaus, E.S.; Gonzalez, N.H.; Bergmann, M.; Bartkuhn, M.; Weidner, W.; Kliesch, S.; Rathke, C. Murine and Human Spermatids Are Characterized by Numerous, Newly Synthesized and Differentially Expressed Transcription Factors and Bromodomain-Containing Proteins. *Biol. Reprod.* **2016**, *95*, 4. [CrossRef] [PubMed]
39. Deato, M.D.; Marr, M.T.; Sottero, T.; Inouye, C.; Hu, P.; Tjian, R. MyoD targets TAF3/TRF3 to activate myogenin transcription. *Mol. Cell* **2008**, *32*, 96–105. [CrossRef]
40. Deato, M.D.; Tjian, R. Switching of the core transcription machinery during myogenesis. *Genes Dev.* **2007**, *21*, 2137–2149. [CrossRef]
41. Deato, M.D.; Tjian, R. An unexpected role of TAFs and TRFs in skeletal muscle differentiation: Switching core promoter complexes. *Cold Spring Harb. Symp. Quant. Biol.* **2008**, *73*, 217–225. [CrossRef] [PubMed]
42. Dikstein, R.; Zhou, S.; Tjian, R. Human TAFII 105 is a cell type-specific TFIID subunit related to hTAFII130. *Cell* **1996**, *87*, 137–146. [CrossRef]
43. Martianov, I.; Brancorsini, S.; Gansmuller, A.; Parvinen, M.; Davidson, I.; Sassone-Corsi, P. Distinct functions of TBP and TLF/TRF2 during spermatogenesis: Requirement of TLF for heterochromatic chromocenter formation in haploid round spermatids. *Development* **2002**, *129*, 945–955. [CrossRef]
44. Ribeiro, J.R.; Lovasco, L.A.; Vanderhyden, B.C.; Freiman, R.N. Targeting TBP-Associated Factors in Ovarian Cancer. *Front. Oncol.* **2014**, *4*, 45. [CrossRef] [PubMed]
45. Bell, B.; Scheer, E.; Tora, L. Identification of hTAF(II)80 delta links apoptotic signaling pathways to transcription factor TFIID function. *Mol. Cell* **2001**, *8*, 591–600. [CrossRef]
46. Resnick, M.A.; Tomso, D.; Inga, A.; Menendez, D.; Bell, D. Functional diversity in the gene network controlled by the master regulator p53 in humans. *Cell Cycle* **2005**, *4*, 1026–1029. [CrossRef]
47. Adams, C.; Cazzanelli, G.; Rasul, S.; Hitchinson, B.; Hu, Y.; Coombes, R.C.; Raguz, S.; Yagüe, E. Apoptosis inhibitor TRIAP1 is a novel effector of drug resistance. *Oncol. Rep.* **2015**, *34*, 415–422. [CrossRef]
48. Staib, F.; Robles, A.I.; Varticovski, L.; Wang, X.W.; Zeeberg, B.R.; Sirotin, M.; Zhurkin, V.B.; Hofseth, L.J.; Hussain, S.P.; Weinstein, J.N.; et al. The p53 tumor suppressor network is a key responder to microenvironmental components of chronic inflammatory stress. *Cancer Res.* **2005**, *65*, 10255–10264. [CrossRef]
49. Andrysik, Z.; Kim, J.; Tan, A.C.; Espinosa, J.M. A genetic screen identifies TCF3/E2A and TRIAP1 as pathway-specific regulators of the cellular response to p53 activation. *Cell Rep.* **2013**, *3*, 1346–1354. [CrossRef]
50. Potting, C.; Tatsuta, T.; König, T.; Haag, M.; Wai, T.; Aaltonen, M.J.; Langer, T. TRIAP1/PRELI complexes prevent apoptosis by mediating intramitochondrial transport of phosphatidic acid. *Cell Metab.* **2013**, *18*, 287–295. [CrossRef] [PubMed]
51. Miliara, X.; Garnett, J.A.; Tatsuta, T.; Abid Ali, F.; Baldie, H.; Pérez-Dorado, I.; Simpson, P.; Yague, E.; Langer, T.; Matthews, S. Structural insight into the TRIAP1/PRELI-like domain family of mitochondrial phospholipid transfer complexes. *EMBO Rep.* **2015**, *16*, 824–835. [CrossRef] [PubMed]
52. Liu, P.K.; Wen, Y.T.; Lin, W.; Kapupara, K.; Tai, M.; Tsai, R.K. Neuroprotective effects of low-dose G-CSF plus meloxicam in a rat model of anterior ischemic optic neuropathy. *Sci. Rep.* **2020**, *10*, 10351. [CrossRef] [PubMed]

International Journal of
Molecular Sciences

MDPI

Perspective

Using Noninvasive Electrophysiology to Determine Time Windows of Neuroprotection in Optic Neuropathies

Vittorio Porciatti * and Tsung-Han Chou

Bascom Palmer Eye Institute, University of Miami, Miami, FL 33136, USA; tchou@med.miami.edu
* Correspondence: vporciatti@med.miami.edu

Abstract: The goal of neuroprotection in optic neuropathies is to prevent loss of retinal ganglion cells (RGCs) and spare their function. The ideal time window for initiating neuroprotective treatments should be the preclinical period at which RGCs start losing their functional integrity before dying. Noninvasive electrophysiological tests such as the Pattern Electroretinogram (PERG) can assess the ability of RGCs to generate electrical signals under a protracted degenerative process in both clinical conditions and experimental models, which may have both diagnostic and prognostic values and provide the rationale for early treatment. The PERG can be used to longitudinally monitor the acute and chronic effects of neuroprotective treatments. User-friendly versions of the PERG technology are now commercially available for both clinical and experimental use.

Keywords: neuroprotection; retinal ganglion cells; optic neuropathy; glaucoma; pattern electroretinogram

Citation: Porciatti, V.; Chou, T.-H. Using Noninvasive Electrophysiology to Determine Time Windows of Neuroprotection in Optic Neuropathies. *Int. J. Mol. Sci.* **2022**, *23*, 5751. https://doi.org/10.3390/ijms23105751

Academic Editors: Rong-Kung Tsai and Neil R. Miller

Received: 26 April 2022
Accepted: 13 May 2022
Published: 20 May 2022

1. Introduction

The death of retinal ganglion cells (RGCs) and their axons is the final common pathway of optic neuropathies resulting in loss of vision [1,2]. Neuroprotective strategies aimed at preventing loss of RGCs and sparing their function have been an area of intense investigation in animal models [3–5]. The great majority of experimental studies on neuroprotective strategies have been performed in glaucoma models using a large variety of neuroprotectants targeting multiple molecular pathways, often with impressive positive effects [2,6]. While neuroprotection studies in experimental models provide powerful proofs of principle, translation of neuroprotective strategies to the clinical application remains elusive [7–9]. One caveat of experimental models is that they are a gross approximation of the corresponding clinical condition [10,11], resulting in limited concordance of treatment effects between preclinical models and clinical trials. Another limitation is that results obtained in animal models most often reflect neuroprotective protocols started in temporal proximity of the induction of the pathological condition, while in the clinical condition therapeutical options are generally initiated after diagnosis that may occur relatively late over the course of the disease. A further limitation is that the sophisticated methods to assess RGC structure and function in experimental models are not generally applicable in the clinical setting. Here, we offer a perspective on the optimal time window for neuroprotective treatments to rescue RGC from death and preserve their function based on noninvasive methods to assess RGC functional integrity that can be used both in experimental models and clinical trials.

2. The Tipping Point

In progressive optic neuropathies, the tipping point represents the idealized transition from a physiological state to a pathological state. During the period preceding the tipping point (critical period) [12–14] accumulating adverse factors eventually overwhelm homeostatic mechanisms and cause irreversible and progressive cell death. The duration of the critical period of transition can be of the order of years, as in glaucoma, [15] or months, as in Leber's Hereditary Optic Neuropathy (LHON) [16], and its identification would provide a red flag of impending disease and an opportunity to consider neuroprotective treatment in a time window where altered conditions may be still capable of reversal. While the tipping point is a well-established intuitive concept (Figure 1), its identification is challenging as phenotypic expression and molecular changes occurring during the critical period overlap with those of the normal condition, and homeostatic neuroplasticity mechanisms to maintain normal vision offset pathological alteration [17]. Later stages are dominated by cell survival and associated maladaptive processes including rewiring of the neural tissue and disruption of function that define the manifest disease state [18]. As sketched in Figure 1, there are several potential therapeutical time windows for neuroprotection, each of them probably resulting in a different outcome. Prophylactic neuroprotection (Rx_t0 in Figure 1) based on risk factors only is not currently considered in the clinical setting [19]. Typically, neuroprotective actions are considered by the time the disease is manifest (Rx_t3, Rx_t4 in Figure 1) [20,21] with the goal of slowing further damage. If a goal of neuroprotective therapy is to preserve RGC integrity and have a long-term efficacy, then it should be initiated as early as possible, ideally at pre-clinical stages (Rx_t1, Rx_t2, in Figure 1) where adaptive neural mechanisms may be still reversible. At preclinical stages, noninvasive structural RGC and RNFL assessments are unlikely to provide meaningful clinical indications [22,23]. In contrast, adaptive changes occurring during the critical period may impair the electrophysiological response of RGCs to visual stimuli, which can be used as biomarker of impending disease, to monitor its progression, and to provide a rationale for initiating neuroprotective treatment.

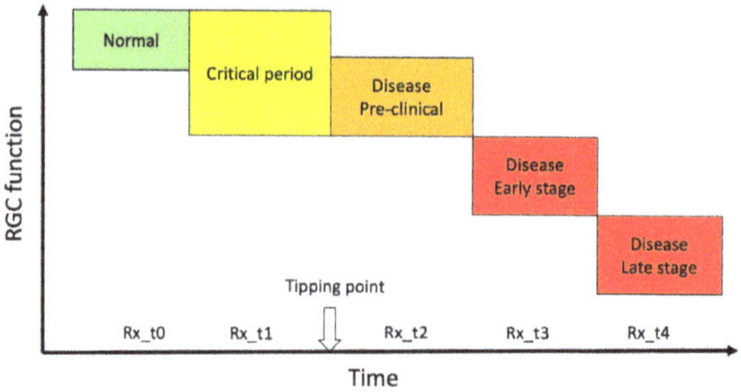

Figure 1. Hypothetical transitional stages of retinal ganglion cell function over the course of a progressive optic neuropathy. The vertical arrow on the time axis represents the idealized transition from a physiological state to a pathological state (tipping point). Abbreviations on the time axis (Rx_t0-t4) represent the idealized time windows of neuroprotective treatment over the course of the disease. Rx_t0 represents prophylaxis. In the time window immediately preceding the tipping point (critical period), early pathological processes may induce RGC dysfunction that is identifiable using sensitive electrophysiological tests such as PERG. Neuroprotective treatment during the critical period (Rx_t1) may interrupt the pathological process and even reverse RGC dysfunction. Neuroprotective treatments at increasing time after the tipping point (Rx_t2, Rx_t3, Rx_t4) may slow progression of RGC dysfunction.

3. Electrophysiological Testing of Retinal Ganglion Cell Function

The electrophysiological activity of RGCs and their axons can be tested with specific variants of the electroretinogram (ERG) [24]. The best-understood and most sensitive technique is the ERG in response to contrast-reversing patterns (Pattern Electroretinogram, PERG). While the precise cellular sources of the PERG signal are not known, the PERG depends on the presence of functional RGCs, as it is rapidly abolished after the optic nerve crush that results in RGC degeneration, while the standard ERG remains unaffected. Both spiking and nonspiking electrical activity contribute to the PERG. Compared to the standard ERG, the PERG has a much smaller amplitude. However, using state-of-the-art equipment with robust averaging and processing to improve the signal-to-noise ratio, the PERG can now be easily recorded from surface adhesive electrodes in human and subdermal electrodes in mice (Figure 2) [25,26].

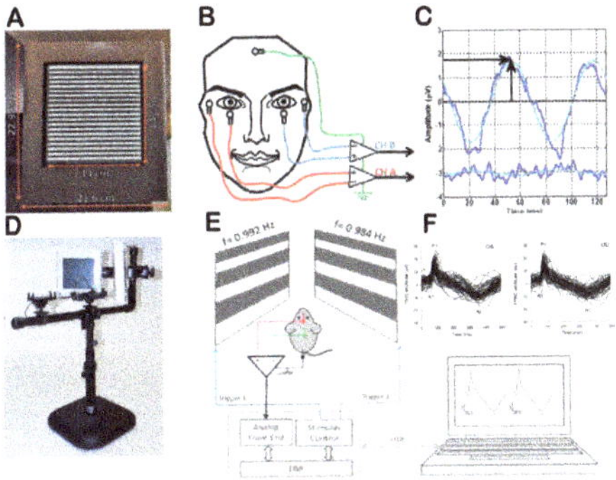

Figure 2. Outline of PERG setup for clinical (**A–C**) and experimental (**D–F**) use. (**A**) Pattern stimulus. (**B**) Taped skin electrode placement. (**C**) Example of steady-state PERG and noise waveforms (continuous lines) in response to one stimulus cycle (two pattern reversals). The dashed sinusoidal waveforms superimposed to the SS-PERG waveforms represent the frequency-domain component that is measured in amplitude (vertical arrow) and latency (horizontal arrow). (**D**) Tiltable pattern displays to change body posture. (**E**) Binocular pattern stimuli reverse at slightly different frequency to retrieve uniocular PERG using a common subcutaneous needle in the snout. (**F**) Examples of PERG waveforms recorded simultaneously for both eyes consisting of a major positive component (P1) at 80–100 ms and a negative component (N2) at about 350 ms. Amplitude is measured from P1 to N2, and latency is measured as time-to-peak of P1. From Monsalve et al., 2017 and Chou et al., 2014.

The PERG may be altered before histological loss of RGCs in glaucoma and optic neuropathies in both human and animal models [27–29]. The PERG can also inform about the response dynamics over a range of visual stimuli of different strength [30] as well as the ability to autoregulate under physiologically stressful conditions such as body inversion [31,32] or flicker-induced increase in metabolic demand [33]. Both response dynamics and autoregulation may provide useful biomarkers to establish altered RGC function not associated with cell death [30,34]. Typically, neuroprotection studies in experimental models of optic neuropathies quantify the effect of treatment by comparing the RGC/axon number of an independent control group with that of the study group at a given endpoint. Noninvasive electrophysiology such as PERG provides longitudinal information on overall RGC function from baseline to endpoint, and additionally it provides unique information on the acute effect of treatment and the time course of the effect, which includes the potential neuroenhancement effect as well as the potential toxic effect and is useful for screening purposes.

4. Comparing RGC Function with RGC Number

A strong proof of concept for the use of PERG as a biomarker of premanifest disease is offered by the DBA/2J mouse strain, which spontaneously develops a pigment-liberating iris disease, resulting in age-related IOP elevation and glaucoma [35,36]. Figure 3A compares the time course of IOP, PERG amplitude, and optic nerve axon number as a function of age of DBA/2J mice [29]. The IOP increases moderately between 2 and 7 months, and more sharply thereafter, when the optic nerve starts losing axons. By the time axon loss is noticeable at about 8 months of age, the PERG signal has already lost over 50% of baseline amplitude at 2 months of age. This indicates that RGCs become dysfunctional before they die. Multiple regression analysis of data shown in Figure 3A reveals that age (Log p = 28.5) plays a larger role than IOP (Log p = 3.8) in progressive loss of PERG signal. The horizontal distance between the decay curves of function and structure provides an estimate of the lifespan of sick RGCs, which represents the time window of opportunity for treatment to prevent RGC death. The vertical distance between the decay curves of function and structure provides an estimate of RGC dysfunction that is not accounted for by cell death, which is potentially reversible [37].

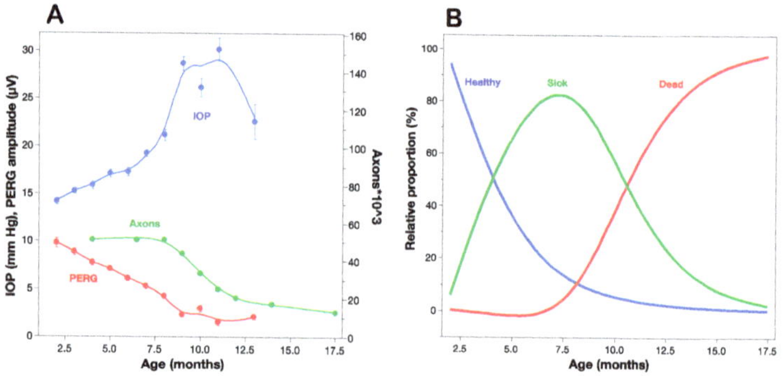

Figure 3. Structure–function relationships in DBA/2J mice. (**A**) IOP, PERG amplitude, and optic nerve axon counts as a function of age of mice. (**B**) Estimated proportion of healthy, sick, and dead retinal ganglion cells at different ages based on a mathematical model that accounts for the structural/functional differences shown in panel (**A**). (**A**) replotted from Saleh et al., IOVS 2007; (**B**) replotted from Porciatti and Chou, Cells 2021.

The comparison between the time courses of PERG amplitude and axon number (Figure 3A) offers an opportunity to investigate the relationship between RGC dysfunction and death [13]. The working hypothesis assumes that at any given time point the residual PERG amplitude reflects the summed contribution of still normal RGCs, the reduced contribution of sick RGCs, and the null contribution of dead/lost RGCs, each in relative proportions. The residual axon count reflects the remaining number of RGCs. The hypothesis also assumes that at each successive timepoint a constant proportion of RGCs becomes sick (decay rate **b**), functions at reduced capacity (dysfunction coefficient **d**) and survives for a limited amount of time (time lag τ between sick and dead RGCs). These events will be reflected in progressive loss of PERG amplitude and axon number, with the former expected to anticipate loss compared to the latter. These parameters can be included in a simple mathematical model [13] that best fits the structural (axon number) and functional (PERG amplitude) time courses. In the example of Figure 3A the parameters that best fit the curves are decay rate **b** = 0.3/month, dysfunction coefficient **d** = 0.5 of normal, and sick-to-dead time τ = 6.5 months. Using these parameters, it is possible to estimate at each timepoint the proportion of healthy, sick, and dead RGCs (Figure 3B). Although the simple model shown in Figure 3B has obvious limitations, it is useful to show that by the time RGCs start dying at about 7.5 months of age, most RGCs are sick and there are fewer healthy RGCs left. By 10 months of age there are no heathy RGGs left, while there are fewer sick RGCs to repair together with a growing population of dead RGCs. This has implications for choosing the appropriate time window for preventing RGC dysfunction (Rx_t1 in Figure 1), preventing RGC dysfunction and repairing ongoing RGC dysfunction (Rx_t2 in Figure 1), or limiting the rate of RGC death (Rx_t3, Rx_t4 in Figure 1). Neuroprotective strategies in different time windows do not necessarily use similar pharmacological approaches and may result in distinctive outcomes for residual RGC function and RGC number. Analogue models to that shown in Figure 3 may be hypothesized for a variety of conditions impacting the susceptibly and lifespan of RGCs together with their ability to generate electrical signals under a protracted degenerative process. Longitudinal clinical data in early glaucoma patients [27] also show progressive loss of PERG signal, anticipating comparable loss of retinal nerve fiber thickness by several years. The rate of progressive PERG loss in glaucoma suspects may be reduced with IOP-lowering treatment [38]. In human LHON, sudden and severe visual loss often begins with one eye first, usually followed by similar loss in the fellow eye few months later [16]. In unilateral LHON cases, the PERG signal is much altered not only in the symptomatic eye, but also in the asymptomatic eye [39]. This suggests that in the asymptomatic eye there is manifest RGC dysfunction preceding RGC death that may be potentially prevented with a timely neuroprotective intervention, including gene therapy [40,41]. It is conceivable that PERG testing in LHON carriers may anticipate conversion from asymptomatic to symptomatic stage and thus inform timing of neuroprotective therapy.

5. Saving RGC Function vs. Saving RGC Bodies

Neuroprotection refers to the relative preservation of neuronal structure and/or function independently of the primary cause of neuronal insult [9]. Ideally, neuroprotection should extend the lifespan of functional RGCs, but this may not always be the case. In principle, neuroprotective strategies that target downstream molecular pathways of cell death such as caspases [42] may keep RGCs on life support for a long time, but these RGCs are not expected to be fully functional. In contrast, strategies that enhance RGC function in the short term do not necessarily alter the rate of progression and may even accelerate RGC death [43]. Noninvasive electrophysiology such as PERG provides the necessary functional outcome to assess the ability of RGCs to generate electrical signals under a protracted degenerative process with or without the presence of neuroprotective treatments. Notably, the PERG can provide a unique contribution to document altered dynamics of RGC function before the tipping point (critical period in Figure 1), which would also represent a rationale for early treatment.

5.1. RGC Excitability

The PERG signal depends not only on the presence of functional RGCs, but also on the molecular environment that controls neuronal excitability, such as neurotrophic factors [44]. For example, BDNF/TrkB interaction controls RGC intrinsic excitability by shifting polarization of the membrane potential [45,46]. In healthy mice, a retrobulbar injection of lidocaine (axon transport blocker) does not induce RGC death but rapidly and reversibly reduces the PERG signal [47] (Figure 4). These effects are believed to be induced by deficiency of retrograde signaling in the optic nerve, in particular shortage of neurotrophic factors derived from brain targets via retrograde axonal transport [48]. Axon transport defects are known to play a critical role in the early stage in neurodegenerative disease [49] including glaucoma and LHON [50,51]. Early PERG impairment in glaucoma and optic neuropathies may be at least in part due to altered axonal transport that reduces RGC excitability.

Changes in RGC excitability are reflected in the dynamics of the PERG response [30]. In the normal mouse, the PERG amplitude increases with increasing contrast approximately in a linear manner (i.e., the PERG amplitude at 20% contrast is about 20% of the amplitude at 100% contrast). Although there are measurable differences in PERG contrast dependence in different mouse strains [52] a strong departure from linearity occurs when availability of neurotrophic factors is altered [30]. Figure 5 shows that in naive C57BL/6J mice, the PERG amplitude at 20% contrast is much lower than that at 100% contrast. In C57BL/6J mice receiving an intravitreal injection of BDNF or in C57BL/6J mice who had a chronic lesion of the superior colliculus—resulting in a compensatory upregulation of endogenous BDNF in the retina [53]—the PERG amplitude at low contrast is higher than that of control C57BL/6J mice. Although the mechanisms underlying altered PERG contrast dependence (neurotrophic support/expression, synaptic transmission, plasticity) are only conjectural, changes of PERG dynamics can be used to detect and monitor early changes in RGC excitability.

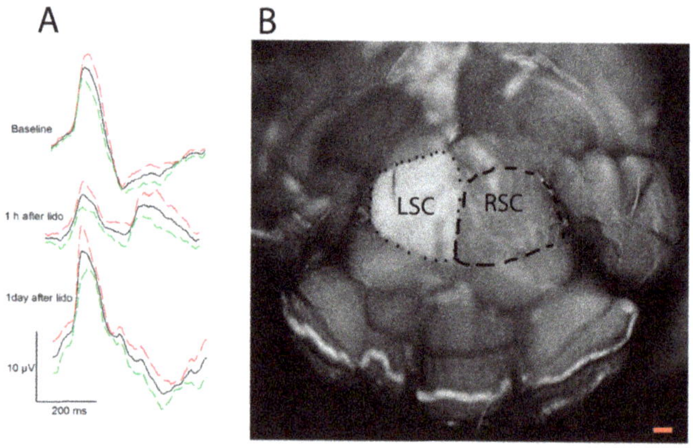

Figure 4. Retrobulbar lidocaine blocks axon transport and reversibly reduces PERG amplitude. The axon transport marker Alexa Fluor 488 Cholera Toxin B was intravitreally injected in both eyes of young DBA/2J mice, and lidocaine was immediately injected in the retrobulbar space of the left eye. (**A**) The PERG signal (average of 5 mice ± SE) was much reduced 1 h after retrobulbar lidocaine compared to baseline and fully recovered one day after. (**B**) After PERG recording, the entire brain was fixed, and both superior colliculi (SC) exposed by aspirating the overlying cortex. The dorsal view shows the surface of both left SC (LSC) and right SC (RSC), roughly outlined with a dotted line and a dashed line, respectively. Confocal scanning laser ophthalmoscopy was performed to identify Alexa Fluor 488 Cholera Toxin B fluorescence. Note the bright fluorescence of the LSC and the absent fluorescence of the RSC, indicating blockage of axon transport along the retinocollicular pathway of the lidocaine-treated eye; scale bar, 200 µm. Replotted from Chou et al., Int. J. Mol. Sci. 2018.

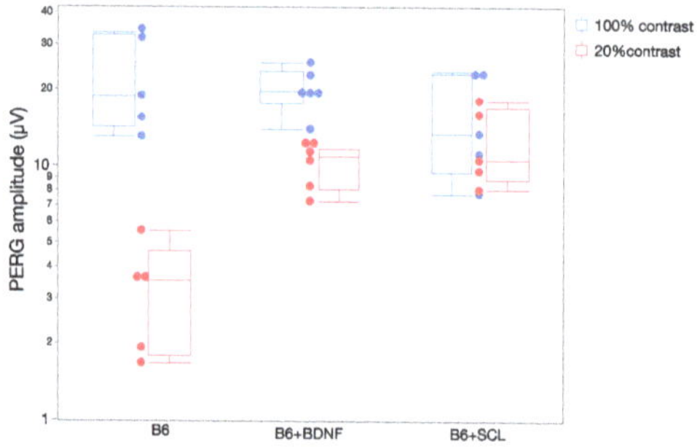

Figure 5. Contrast dependence of PERG amplitude in control C57BL/6J (B6) mice and in B6 mice in which neurotrophic support has been altered ((B6 + BDNF): intravitreal injection of BDNF; (B6 + SCL): chronic lesion of the contralateral superior colliculus). Replotted from Chou et al., Exp. Eye Res. 2016.

5.2. RGC Adaptation

Rapid dilation of retinal vessels in response to flickering light or fast-reversing patterns (functional hyperemia) is a well-known autoregulatory response driven by increased neural activity in the inner retina [54]. Sustained metabolic stress may in turn influence RGC function, and this is reflected in a progressive decline of the PERG signal to a plateau (adaptation) over 2–4 min [55] (Figure 6). PERG adaptation occurs in mice [33] as well as in humans [56], and represents an index of normal neurovascular autoregulation triggered by a metabolic challenge. PERG adaptation may be reduced or absent when RGCs are dysfunctional as in glaucoma [57] or in optic neuritis [58]. For hypothesis-testing purposes, several models can explain the PERG adaptation dynamics. The model sketched in Figure 6C is based on an energy budget model in a neurovascular-glial network that can be reduced to a simple electrical circuit and mathematical equation [14].

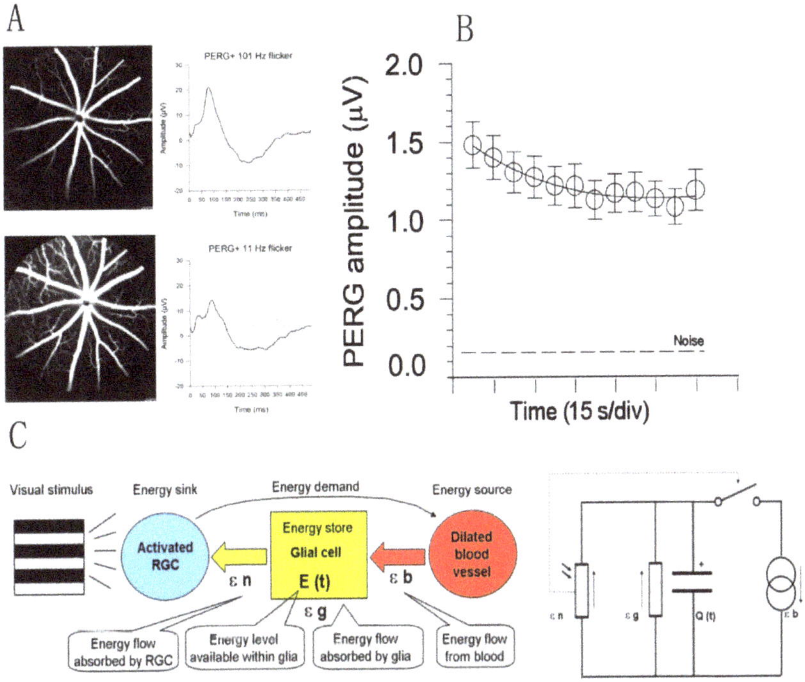

Figure 6. Flicker-induced PERG adaptation. (**A**) Flickering light at 11 Hz superimposed to a pattern stimulus induces vasodilation in C57BL/6J mouse, as shown by fluorescein angiography, and reduces the PERG amplitude compared to the same pattern stimulus with superimposed flicker at 101 Hz (invisible to photoreceptors). (**B**) In human subjects, the PERG signal in response to sustained pattern reversal at 16 rps becomes progressively reduced to a plateau over 2 min. (**C**) Energy budget model that accounts for the temporal dynamics of PERG adaptation in mice and human subjects. At any given time, the energy available to activated neurons (ε n, photoresistor) depends on the energy flow provided by glial stores (ε g capacitor) and vascular supply (ε b, current generator) minus the energy absorbed in the process (ε g, resistor). The switch connecting activated neurons to vascular supply represents the neurovascular coupling. The direction of arrows indicates the energy flow. (**A**) Replotted from Chou et al., Sci. Rep. 2019; (**B**) replotted from Porciatti et al., IOVS 2005; (**C**) replotted from Porciatti and Ventura, Vis. Res. 2009.

Independently of the underlying mechanisms, PERG adaptation dynamics can be used to detect and monitor altered autoregulation of RGCs together with the neurovascular-glial network impinging on them. As shown in Figure 3, in DBA/2J glaucoma the PERG amplitude progressively decreases with increasing age followed by loss of RGCs [28,29]. In DBA/2J mice, retinal levels of nicotinamide adenine dinucleotide (NAD+, a key molecule in energy and redox metabolism) decrease with age and render aging neurons vulnerable to disease-related insults [6]. Oral administration of the NAD+ precursor nicotinamide (vitamin B3) spares RGCs and their function at older ages [6]. The magnitude of PERG adaptation also decreases with increasing age (Figure 7) [59]. However, prophylaxis with a diet rich in vitamin B3, in addition to saving functional RGCs, also spares the PERG autoregulatory dynamic range in response to flicker [59].

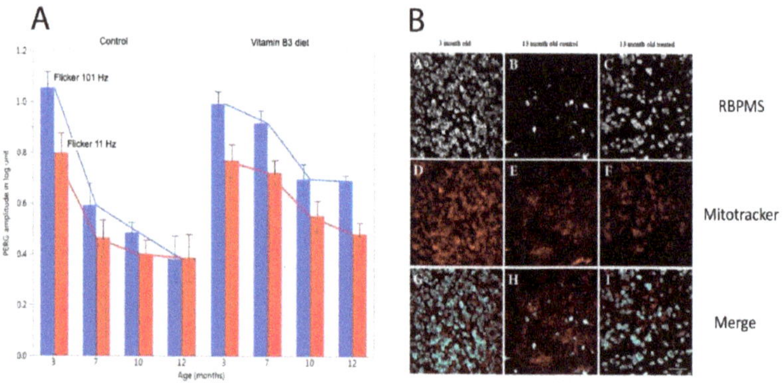

Figure 7. Flicker-PERG amplitude adaptation and RGC survival in control DBA/2J mice fed with standard diet and in DBA/2J mice fed with vitamin B3-enriched diet. (**A**) Amplitude of PERG recorded with superimposed flickering light at either 101 Hz (baseline, blue bars) or 11 Hz (test, red bars) in mice of different ages. The difference between baseline and test represents the magnitude of flicker-PERG adaptation. Note in control mice that flicker-PERG adaptation progressively decreases with increasing age, whereas in vitamin B3-treated mice PERG adaptation is preserved together with a slower decline of PERG amplitude with age. Error bars represent the SEM (n = 10 for each group). (**B**) Representative examples of RBPMS (RNA-binding protein with multiple splicing)-immunostained RGCs and Mitotracker-immunostained mitochondria in flat mounted retinas of DBA/2J mice 3 months old and 13 months old fed with either standard diet or vitamin B3-enriched diet. Note the rescue effect of vitamin B3-enriched diet on RGCs and mitochondria in mice 13 months old. Replotted from Chou et al., Nutrients 2020.

5.3. RGC Susceptibility to Stress

Stress tests such as physical exercise are widely employed to investigate altered heart dynamics and are also used in eye diseases. Recovery of vision and VEP amplitude after exposure to a bright light (photostress) may be prolonged in macular diseases [60] and in optic neuritis [61]. Temporary IOP elevation can be induced with head-down (HD) body posture. In DBA/2J mice of different ages, head-down (HD) tilt of 60 degrees causes an IOP elevation of about 5 mm Hg [31]. The PERG of young mice is unaffected by HD, but it becomes substantially depressed in older mice even before the onset of RGC death, suggesting susceptibility to HD stress [31]. In human subjects, HD tilt of 10 degrees induces IOP elevation of about 3 mm Hg on average [32]. While the PERG of normal subjects is not altered by HD tilt, it becomes substantially depressed in a subpopulation of glaucoma suspects [32]. Longitudinal observation of HD-susceptible glaucoma suspects has shown that most of them developed RNFL thinning over 5 years [34].

6. Conclusions

Noninvasive, longitudinal assessment of RGC function appears to be a needed diagnostic tool in optic neuropathies. A substantial body of evidence supports the use of PERG to assess the ability of RGCs to generate electrical signals under a protracted degenerative process with or without the presence of neuroprotective treatments, which may have both diagnostic and prognostic values. Further, the PERG can provide a unique contribution to document altered dynamics of RGC function in response to stimuli of different intensity and under different physiological stressors, which may occur before the tipping point and provide the rationale for early treatment. Indeed, a goal of neuroprotective approaches should be preserving and restoring RGC integrity. The PERG can also be useful to screen acute neuroenhancement and toxic effects of neuroprotective drugs. User-friendly versions of the PERG technology are now commercially available for both clinical and experimental use.

Author Contributions: Conceptualization, analysis, and draft preparation, V.P.; review and editing, T.-H.C.; funding acquisition, V.P. All authors have read and agreed to the published version of the manuscript.

Funding: NIH-NEI RO1EY019077; NIH-NEI RO1EY014957, NIH-NEI R24EY028785; NIH-NEI P30EY014801; unrestricted grant to Bascom Palmer Eye Institute from Research to Prevent Blindness, Inc.

Conflicts of Interest: The authors declare no conflict of interest.

References

1. Levin, L.A. Axonal loss and neuroprotection in optic neuropathies. *Can. J. Ophthalmol.* **2007**, *42*, 403–408. [CrossRef] [PubMed]
2. Levin, L.A. Neuroprotection in Optic Neuropathy. *Asia Pac. J. Ophthalmol.* **2018**, *7*, 246–250.
3. Osborne, N.N.; Chidlow, G.; Layton, C.J.; Wood, J.P.; Casson, R.J.; Melena, J. Optic nerve and neuroprotection strategies. *Eye* **2004**, *18*, 1075–1084. [CrossRef] [PubMed]
4. Ghaffarieh, A.; Levin, L.A. Optic nerve disease and axon pathophysiology. *Int. Rev. Neurobiol.* **2012**, *105*, 1–17. [PubMed]
5. Khatib, T.Z.; Martin, K.R. Neuroprotection in Glaucoma: Towards Clinical Trials and Precision Medicine. *Curr. Eye Res.* **2020**, *45*, 327–338. [CrossRef] [PubMed]
6. Williams, P.A.; Harder, J.M.; Foxworth, N.E.; Cochran, K.E.; Philip, V.M.; Porciatti, V.; Smithies, O.; Jpohn, S.W.M. Vitamin B3 modulates mitochondrial vulnerability and prevents glaucoma in aged mice. *Science* **2017**, *355*, 756–760. [CrossRef] [PubMed]
7. Almasieh, M.; Levin, L.A. Neuroprotection in Glaucoma: Animal Models and Clinical Trials. *Annu. Rev. Vis. Sci.* **2017**, *3*, 91–120. [CrossRef]
8. Haefliger, I.O.; Fleischhauer, J.C.; Flammer, J. In glaucoma, should enthusiasm about neuroprotection be tempered by the experience obtained in other neurodegenerative disorders? *Eye* **2000**, *14 Pt 3B*, 464–472. [CrossRef]
9. Casson, R.J.; Chidlow, G.; Ebneter, A.; Wood, J.P.; Crowston, J.; Goldberg, I. Translational neuroprotection research in glaucoma: A review of definitions and principles. *Clin. Exp. Ophthalmol.* **2012**, *40*, 350–357. [CrossRef]
10. Perlman, R.L. Mouse models of human disease: An evolutionary perspective. *Evol. Med. Public Health* **2016**, *2016*, 170–176. [CrossRef]
11. Ioannidis, J.P. Extrapolating from animals to humans. *Sci. Transl. Med.* **2012**, *4*, 151ps15. [CrossRef] [PubMed]
12. Liu, X.; Chang, X.; Leng, S.; Tang, H.; Aihara, K.; Chen, L. Detection for disease tipping points by landscape dynamic network biomarkers. *Natl. Sci. Rev.* **2019**, *6*, 775–785. [CrossRef] [PubMed]
13. Porciatti, V.; Chou, T.H. Modeling Retinal Ganglion Cell Dysfunction in Optic Neuropathies. *Cells* **2021**, *10*, 1398. [CrossRef] [PubMed]
14. Porciatti, V.; Ventura, L.M. Adaptive changes of inner retina function in response to sustained pattern stimulation. *Vis. Res.* **2009**, *49*, 505–513. [CrossRef] [PubMed]
15. Heijl, A.; Bengtsson, B.; Hyman, L.; Leske, M.C.; Early Manifest Glaucoma Trial Group. Natural history of open-angle glaucoma. *Ophthalmology* **2009**, *116*, 2271–2276. [CrossRef]
16. Yu-Wai-Man, P.; Newman, N.J.; Carelli, V.; La Morgia, C.; Biousse, V.; Bandello, F.M.; Clermont, C.V.; Castillo Campillo, L.; Leruez, S.; Moster, M.L.; et al. Natural history of patients with Leber hereditary optic neuropathy-results from the REALITY study. *Eye* **2022**, *36*, 818–826. [CrossRef]
17. Turrigiano, G. Homeostatic synaptic plasticity: Local and global mechanisms for stabilizing neuronal function. *Cold Spring Harb. Perspect. Biol.* **2012**, *4*, a005736. [CrossRef]
18. Li, X.Y.; Wan, Y.; Tang, S.J.; Guan, Y.; Wei, F.; Ma, D. Maladaptive Plasticity and Neuropathic Pain. *Neural Plast.* **2016**, *2016*, 4842159. [CrossRef]
19. Newman, N.J.; Biousse, V.; David, R.; Bhatti, M.T.; Hamilton, S.R.; Farris, B.K.; Lesser, R.L.; Newman, S.A.; Turbin, R.E.; Chen, K.; et al. Prophylaxis for second eye involvement in leber hereditary optic neuropathy: An open-labeled, nonrandomized multicenter trial of topical brimonidine purite. *Am. J. Ophthalmol.* **2005**, *140*, 407–415. [CrossRef]
20. Mallah, K.; Couch, C.; Borucki, D.M.; Toutonji, A.; Alshareef, M.; Tomlinson, S. Anti-inflammatory and Neuroprotective Agents in Clinical Trials for CNS Disease and Injury: Where Do We Go from Here? *Front. Immunol.* **2020**, *11*, 2021. [CrossRef]
21. Yang, J.P.; Liu, H.J.; Yang, H.; Feng, P.Y. Therapeutic time window for the neuroprotective effects of NGF when administered after focal cerebral ischemia. *Neurol. Sci.* **2011**, *32*, 433–441. [CrossRef] [PubMed]
22. Cordeiro, M.F.; Hill, D.; Patel, R.; Corazza, P.; Maddison, J.; Younis, S. Detecting retinal cell stress and apoptosis with DARC: Progression from lab to clinic. *Prog. Retin. Eye Res.* **2022**, *86*, 100976. [CrossRef] [PubMed]
23. Guo, L.; Cordeiro, M.F. Assessment of neuroprotection in the retina with DARC. *Prog. Brain Res.* **2008**, *173*, 437–450. [PubMed]
24. Porciatti, V. Electrophysiological assessment of retinal ganglion cell function. *Exp. Eye Res.* **2015**, *141*, 164–170. [CrossRef] [PubMed]
25. Chou, T.H.; Bohorquez, J.; Toft-Nielsen, J.; Ozdamar, O.; Porciatti, V. Robust mouse pattern electroretinograms derived simultaneously from each eye using a common snout electrode. *Investig. Ophthalmol. Vis. Sci.* **2014**, *55*, 2469–2475. [CrossRef]

26. Monsalve, P.; Triolo, G.; Toft-Nielsen, J.; Bohorquez, J.; Henderson, A.D.; Delgado, R.; Miskiel, E.; Ozdamar, O.; Feuer, W.J.; Porciatti, V. Next Generation PERG Method: Expanding the Response Dynamic Range and Capturing Response Adaptation. *Transl. Vis. Sci. Technol.* **2017**, *6*, 5. [CrossRef]
27. Banitt, M.R.; Ventura, L.M.; Feuer, W.J.; Savatovsky, E.; Luna, G.; Shif, O.; Bosse, B.; Porciatti, V. Progressive loss of retinal ganglion cell function precedes structural loss by several years in glaucoma suspects. *Investig. Ophthalmol. Vis. Sci.* **2013**, *54*, 2346–2352. [CrossRef]
28. Howell, G.R.; Libby, R.T.; Jakobs, T.C.; Smith, R.S.; Phalan, F.C.; Barter, J.W.; Barbay, J.M.; Marchant, J.K.; Mahesh, N.; Porciatti, V.; et al. Axons of retinal ganglion cells are insulted in the optic nerve early in DBA/2J glaucoma. *J. Cell Biol.* **2007**, *179*, 1523–1537. [CrossRef]
29. Saleh, M.; Nagaraju, M.; Porciatti, V. Longitudinal evaluation of retinal ganglion cell function and IOP in the DBA/2J mouse model of glaucoma. *Investig. Ophthalmol. Vis. Sci.* **2007**, *48*, 4564–4572. [CrossRef]
30. Chou, T.H.; Feuer, W.J.; Schwartz, O.; Rojas, M.J.; Roebber, J.K.; Porciatti, V. Integrative properties of retinal ganglion cell electrical responsiveness depend on neurotrophic support and genotype in the mouse. *Exp. Eye Res.* **2016**, *145*, 68–74. [CrossRef]
31. Nagaraju, M.; Saleh, M.; Porciatti, V. IOP-dependent retinal ganglion cell dysfunction in glaucomatous DBA/2J mice. *Investig. Ophthalmol. Vis. Sci.* **2007**, *48*, 4573–4579. [CrossRef] [PubMed]
32. Ventura, L.M.; Golubev, I.; Lee, W.; Nose, I.; Parel, J.M.; Feuer, W.J.; Porciatti, V. Head-down posture induces PERG alterations in early glaucoma. *J. Glaucoma* **2013**, *22*, 255–264. [CrossRef] [PubMed]
33. Chou, T.H.; Toft-Nielsen, J.; Porciatti, V. Adaptation of retinal ganglion cell function during flickering light in the mouse. *Sci. Rep.* **2019**, *9*, 18396. [CrossRef] [PubMed]
34. Porciatti, V.; Feuer, W.J.; Monsalve, P.; Triolo, G.; Vazquez, L.; McSoley, J.; Ventura, L.M. Head-down Posture in Glaucoma Suspects Induces Changes in IOP, Systemic Pressure, and PERG That Predict Future Loss of Optic Nerve Tissue. *J. Glaucoma* **2017**, *26*, 459–465. [CrossRef]
35. Libby, R.T.; Anderson, M.G.; Pang, I.H.; Robinson, Z.H.; Savinova, O.V.; Cosma, I.M.; Snow, A.; Wilson, L.A.; Smith, R.S.; Clark, R.F.; et al. Inherited glaucoma in DBA/2J mice: Pertinent disease features for studying the neurodegeneration. *Vis. Neurosci.* **2005**, *22*, 637–648. [CrossRef]
36. Howell, G.R.; Libby, R.T.; Marchant, J.K.; Wilson, L.A.; Cosma, I.M.; Smith, R.S.; Anderson, M.G.; John, S.W.M. Absence of glaucoma in DBA/2J mice homozygous for wild-type versions of Gpnmb and Tyrp1. *BMC Genet.* **2007**, *8*, 45. [CrossRef]
37. Porciatti, V.; Ventura, L.M. Retinal ganglion cell functional plasticity and optic neuropathy: A comprehensive model. *J. Neuroophthalmol.* **2012**, *32*, 354–358. [CrossRef]
38. Ventura, L.M.; Feuer, W.J.; Porciatti, V. Progressive loss of retinal ganglion cell function is hindered with IOP-lowering treatment in early glaucoma. *Investig. Ophthalmol. Vis. Sci.* **2012**, *53*, 659–663. [CrossRef]
39. Porciatti, V.; Alba, D.E.; Feuer, W.J.; Davis, J.; Guy, J.; Lam, B.L. The Relationship Between Stage of Leber's Hereditary Optic Neuropathy and Pattern Electroretinogram Latency. *Transl. Vis. Sci. Technol.* **2022**, *11*, 31. [CrossRef]
40. Newman, N.J.; Yu-Wai-Man, P.; Carelli, V.; Biousse, V.; Moster, M.L.; Vignal-Clermont, C.; Sergott, R.C.; Kloptstock, T.; Sadun, A.A.; Girmens, J.-F.; et al. Intravitreal Gene Therapy vs. Natural History in Patients with Leber Hereditary Optic Neuropathy Carrying the m.11778G>A ND4 Mutation: Systematic Review and Indirect Comparison. *Front. Neurol.* **2021**, *12*, 662838. [CrossRef]
41. Lam, B.L.; Feuer, W.J.; Davis, J.L.; Porciatti, V.; Yu, H.; Levy, R.B.; Vanner, E.; Guy, J. Leber Hereditary Optic Neuropathy Gene Therapy: Adverse Events and Visual Acuity Results of all Patient Groups. *Am. J. Ophthalmol.* **2022**. [CrossRef] [PubMed]
42. Hotchkiss, R.S.; Strasser, A.; McDunn, J.E.; Swanson, P.E. Cell death. *N. Engl. J. Med.* **2009**, *361*, 1570–1583. [CrossRef] [PubMed]
43. Zádori, D.; Klivényi, P.; Szalárdy, L.; Fülöp, F.; Toldi, J.; Vécsei, L. Mitochondrial disturbances, excitotoxicity, neuroinflammation and kynurenines: Novel therapeutic strategies for neurodegenerative disorders. *J. Neurol. Sci.* **2012**, *322*, 187–191. [CrossRef] [PubMed]
44. Fiedler, D.; Sasi, M.; Blum, R.; Klinke, C.M.; Andreatta, M.; Pape, H.C.; Lange, M.D. Brain-Derived Neurotrophic Factor/Tropomyosin Receptor Kinase B Signaling Controls Excitability and Long-Term Depression in Oval Nucleus of the BNST. *J. Neurosci.* **2021**, *41*, 435–445. [CrossRef]
45. Van Welie, I.; van Hooft, J.A.; Wadman, W.J. Homeostatic scaling of neuronal excitability by synaptic modulation of somatic hyperpolarization-activated Ih channels. *Proc. Natl. Acad. Sci. USA* **2004**, *101*, 5123–5128. [CrossRef]
46. Demb, J.B. Functional circuitry of visual adaptation in the retina. *J. Physiol.* **2008**, *586*, 4377–4384. [CrossRef]
47. Chou, T.H.; Park, K.K.; Luo, X.; Porciatti, V. Retrograde signaling in the optic nerve is necessary for electrical responsiveness of retinal ganglion cells. *Investig. Ophthalmol. Vis. Sci.* **2013**, *54*, 1236–1243. [CrossRef]
48. Morgan, J.E. Circulation and axonal transport in the optic nerve. *Eye* **2004**, *18*, 1089–1095. [CrossRef]
49. Morfini, G.A.; Burns, M.; Binder, L.I.; Kanaan, N.M.; LaPointe, N.; Bosco, D.A.; Brown, J.H., Jr.; Brown, H.; Tiwari, A.; Hayward, L.; et al. Axonal Transport Defects in Neurodegenerative Diseases. *J. Neurosci.* **2009**, *29*, 12776–12786. [CrossRef]
50. Quigley, H.A.; McKinnon, S.J.; Zack, D.J.; Pease, M.E.; Kerrigan–Baumrind, L.A.; Kerrigan, D.F.; Mitchell, R.S. Retrograde axonal transport of BDNF in retinal ganglion cells is blocked by acute IOP elevation in rats. *Investig. Ophthalmol. Vis. Sci.* **2000**, *41*, 3460–3466.
51. Bahr, T.; Welburn, K.; Donnelly, J.; Bai, Y. Emerging model systems and treatment approaches for Leber's hereditary optic neuropathy: Challenges and opportunities. *Biochim. Biophys. Acta—Mol. Basis Dis.* **2020**, *1866*, 165743. [CrossRef] [PubMed]

52. Porciatti, V.; Chou, T.H.; Feuer, W.J. C57BL/6J, DBA/2J, and DBA/2J.Gpnmb mice have different visual signal processing in the inner retina. *Mol. Vis.* **2010**, *16*, 2939–2947. [PubMed]
53. Yang, X.; Chou, T.H.; Ruggeri, M.; Porciatti, V. A new mouse model of inducible, chronic retinal ganglion cell dysfunction not associated with cell death. *Investig. Ophthalmol. Vis. Sci.* **2013**, *54*, 1898–1904. [CrossRef] [PubMed]
54. Riva, C.E.; Logean, E.; Falsini, B. Visually evoked hemodynamical response and assessment of neurovascular coupling in the optic nerve and retina. *Prog. Retin. Eye Res.* **2005**, *24*, 183–215. [CrossRef]
55. Chou, T.H.; Porciatti, V. Adaptable retinal ganglion cell function: Assessing autoregulation of inner retina pathways. *Neural Regen. Res.* **2020**, *15*, 2237–2238.
56. Porciatti, V.; Sorokac, N.; Buchser, W. Habituation of retinal ganglion cell activity in response to steady state pattern visual stimuli in normal subjects. *Investig. Ophthalmol. Vis. Sci.* **2005**, *46*, 1296–1302. [CrossRef]
57. Porciatti, V.; Bosse, B.; Parekh, P.K.; Shif, O.A.; Feuer, W.J.; Ventura, L.M. Adaptation of the steady-state PERG in early glaucoma. *J. Glaucoma* **2014**, *23*, 494–500. [CrossRef]
58. Fadda, A.; Di Renzo, A.; Martelli, F.; Marangoni, D.; Batocchi, A.P.; Giannini, D.; Parisi, V.; Falsini, B. Reduced habituation of the retinal ganglion cell response to sustained pattern stimulation in multiple sclerosis patients. *Clin. Neurophysiol.* **2013**, *124*, 1652–1658. [CrossRef]
59. Chou, T.H.; Romano, G.L.; Amato, R.; Porciatti, V. Nicotinamide-Rich Diet in DBA/2J Mice Preserves Retinal Ganglion Cell Metabolic Function as Assessed by PERG Adaptation to Flicker. *Nutrients* **2020**, *12*, 1910. [CrossRef]
60. Parisi, V.; Falsini, B. Electrophysiological evaluation of the macular cone system: Focal electroretinography and visual evoked potentials after photostress. *Semin. Ophthalmol.* **1998**, *13*, 178–188. [CrossRef]
61. Parisi, V.; Pierelli, F.; Restuccia, R.; Spadaro, M.; Parisi, L.; Colacino, G.; Bucci, M.G. Impaired VEP after photostress response in multiple sclerosis patients previously affected by optic neuritis. *Electroencephalogr. Clin. Neurophysiol.* **1998**, *108*, 73–79. [CrossRef]

MDPI
St. Alban-Anlage 66
4052 Basel
Switzerland
Tel. +41 61 683 77 34
Fax +41 61 302 89 18
www.mdpi.com

International Journal of Molecular Sciences Editorial Office
E-mail: ijms@mdpi.com
www.mdpi.com/journal/ijms

www.ingramcontent.com/pod-product-compliance
Lightning Source LLC
LaVergne TN
LVHW070210100526
838202LV00015B/2028